M000288381

Medical Response to

Adult Sexual Assault

A Resource for Clinicians and Related Professionals

STM **Learning,** Inc.

Leading Publisher of Scientific, Technical, and Medical Educational Resources

Saint Louis

www.stmlearning.com

Our Mission

To become the world leader in publishing and information services on child abuse, maltreatment, diseases, and domestic violence. We seek to heighten awareness of these issues, and provide relevant information to professionals and consumers.

A portion of our profits is contributed to nonprofit organizations dedicated to the prevention of child abuse and the care of victims of abuse and other children and family charities.

We dedicate the book to the Internal Association of Forensic Nursing, which has provided a valuable professional forum in which we, as well as many of our contributors, have been able to enhance our understanding of how the various forms of sexual victimization manifest and from which we continue to advocate for appropriate policies and resources to serve victims, ultimately seeking to prevent the problem entirely.

Linda E. Ledray, RN, SANE-A, PhD, FAAN
Ann Wolbert Burgess, DNSc, APRN, BC, FAAN
Angelo P. Giardino, MD, PhD, MPH, FAAP

Medical Response to

Adult Sexual Assault

A Resource for Clinicians and Related Professionals

Linda E. Ledray, RN, SANE-A, PhD, FAAN
Director
SANE-SART Resource Service
Minneapolis Medical Research Foundation
Minneapolis, Minnesota

Ann Wolbert Burgess, DNSc, APRN, BC, FAAN
Professor of Psychiatric Nursing
William F. Connell School of Nursing
Boston College
Chestnut Hill, Massachusetts

Angelo P. Giardino, MD, PhD, MPH, FAAP
Medical Director
Texas Children's Health Plan
Clinical Professor of Pediatrics
Baylor College of Medicine
Attending Physician
Children's Assessment Center
Texas Children's Hospital
Houston, Texas

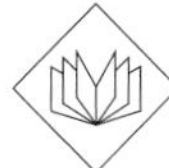

STM **Learning,** Inc.

Leading Publisher of Scientific, Technical, and Medical Educational Resources

Saint Louis

www.stmlearning.com

Publishers: Glenn E. Whaley and Marianne V. Whaley
Art Design Director: Glenn E. Whaley
Associate Editor: Mallory C. Skinner
Book Design/Page Layout: G.W. Graphics
Heather N. Green
Print/Production Coordinator: Heather N. Green
Cover Design: G.W. Graphics
Color Prepress Specialist: Kevin Tucker
Acquisition Editor: Glenn E. Whaley
Developmental Editor: Elaine Steinborn
Shawn Greene
Copy Editor: Julie Dill
Proofreader: Katie Sharp
Indexer: Donna M. Drialo

Printed in China.

Publisher:
STM Learning, Inc.
8045 Big Bend Blvd., Suite 202, Saint Louis, Missouri 63119-2714 USA
Phone: (314)993-2728 Fax: (314)993-2281 Toll Free: (800)600-0330
http://www.stmlearning.com

Library of Congress Cataloging-in-Publication Data

Medical response to adult sexual assault : a resource for clinicians and related professionals / [edited by] Linda E. Ledray, Ann Wolbert Burgess, and Angelo P. Giardino.
p. ; cm.
Includes bibliographical references and index.
ISBN 978-1-878060-11-2 (alk. paper)
1. Rape victims--Medical care--United States. 2. Rape--United States. 3. Sex crimes--United States. I. Ledray, Linda E. II. Burgess, Ann Wolbert. III. Giardino, Angelo P.
[DNLM: 1. Rape. 2. Crime Victims. 3. Forensic Medicine. 4. Forensic Nursing. W 795]
HV6250.3.U5M43 2011
614'.1--dc23

2011018159

Contributors

Donna M. Barry, RN, MSN, APN-C, FN-CSA
Director
University Health Center
Coadministrator
Sexual Assault Response Team
Montclair State University
Montclair, New Jersey

Kathleen M. Brown, RN, MSN, CRNP, PhD, FAAN
Assistant Professor
School of Nursing
University of Pennsylvania
Philadelphia, Pennsylvania

Imelda Buncab, BA
Social Change Agent and Consultant
Sherman Oaks, California

Rebecca Campbell, PhD
Professor
Department of Psychology
Michigan State University
East Lansing, Michigan

Susan Chasson, JD, MSN, SANE-A
Lecturer
College of Nursing
Brigham Young University
Provo, Utah

Diana Faugno, MSN, RN, CPN, SANE-A, SANE-P, FAAFS, DF-IAFN
Forensic Registered Nurse Consultant
Founding Board Director
EVAW International
Escondido, California

Patricia A. Frazier, PhD
Distinguished McKnight University Professor
Department of Psychology
University of Minnesota
Minneapolis, Minnesota

Donna A. Gaffney, DNSc, PMHCNS-BC, FAAN
Faculty
International Trauma Studies Program
Advisor for Education and Research
Project Rebirth
New York, New York

Annie Heirendt, LCSW
Los Angeles, California

Jill Kapur, MSN, RN
Hanover, Massachussetts

Robert D. Laurino, JD
Short Hills, New Jersey

Marc A. LeBeau, PhD
Unit Chief
Federal Bureau of Investigation Laboratory
Quantico, Virginia

Jenifer Markowitz, ND, RN, WHNP-BC, SANE-A, DF-IAFN
Medical Advisor
AEquitas, The Prosecutor's Resource on Violence Against Women
Washington DC

CDR Barbara Mullen, (FNP), NC, USN
Family Nurse Practitioner
United States Naval Academy
Annapolis, Maryland

Katherine Nash Scafide, PhD(c), RN, FNE-A, FNE-P, SANE-A, SANE-P
Forensic Clinical Nurse Specialist
Johns Hopkins University School of Nursing
Baltimore, Maryland

Colleen O'Brien, RN, MS, SANE-A, SANE-P
Forensic Nurse Consultant
Ridgeway, Wisconsin

Tawnne O'Connor, RN, BSN
Sexual Assault Nurse Examiner
Patient Care Coordinator
Naval Medical Center San Diego
San Diego, California

Debra Patterson, PhD, LMSW, MA
Assistant Professor
Wayne State University
Detroit, Michigan

Susan B. Patton, DNSc, PNP-BC, SANE-A, SANE-P
DNP Forensic Nursing Option Coordinator
Associate Professor
College of Nursing
University of Tennessee Health Science Center
Memphis, Tennessee

Mark E. Safarik, MS, VSM (FBI Ret.)
Executive Director
Forensic Behavioral Services International
Fredericksburg, Virginia

Daniel J. Sheridan, PhD, RN, FNE-A, SANE-A, FAAN
Assistant Professor
Forensic Clinical Nurse Specialist
School of Nursing
John Hopkins University
Baltimore, Maryland

Margaret L. Simpson, MD
Medical Director
Hennepin County Sexually Transmitted Infections
Clinic
Physician
Department of Internal Medicine
Hennepin County Medical Center
Minneapolis, Minnesota

Patricia M. Speck, DNSc, APN, FNP-BC, DF-IAFN, FAAFS, FAAN
Associate Professor
Public Health Nursing Option Coordinator
College of Nursing
University of Tennessee Health Science Center
Memphis, Tennessee

Anjali R. Swienton, MFS, JD
President and CEO
SciLawForensics, Ltd.
Germantown, Maryland

Supplemental Photo Contributions

Rick Castro
Jill Crum, BSN, RN, SANE-A
Merle Endo, RN, SANE-A, SANE-P
Diana Faugno, MSN, RN, CPN, SANE-A, SANE-P, FAAFS, DF-IAFN
Reena Isaac, MD
Mary Reina, RN, MSN

Foreword

Medical Response to Adult Sexual Assault is a testament to the maturity of our understanding of the unfortunate reality of adult sexual assault. In many ways, it is the reference bible for adult sexual assault, reflecting the collective science and wisdom of an increasingly professional response to the needs of sexual assault victims. This tome does a superb job of reflecting the history of society's response to sexual assault. Whether the reader is looking to fully understand legislative responses, addressing the medical needs of victims, the significance of and how to collect forensic evidence, the mental health impact of sexual assault, or the critical importance of treatment, each and every aspect of these topics is fully covered.

The most important first steps following disclosure of sexual assault are critically important to substantiation, protection, and, ultimately, securing the treatment services that victims need and deserve. Whether the reader is a new graduate of a SANE/SART program or a seasoned clinician, a law enforcement investigator or prosecutor, a mental health clinician, or a community agency professional, this reference text provides the most up-to-date information to understand and respond to the needs of victims.

It is not enough to simply be able to know one's own discipline and be competent in that discipline. Successful outcomes depend on interdisciplinary collaboration. This reference is organized in a manner that provides not only an understanding of what each discipline must do to address the needs of victims, but how to work with other disciplines in a manner that ultimately provides a collective insight and best serves the needs of victims.

The unique needs of special populations, such as college students, drug-facilitated assault victims, elder sexual assault victims, or victims whose assault occurs while on duty, are addressed.

For the health care professional, it is not enough to just identify the physical evidence of assault, collect evidence, and treat the patient. Clinicians must understand the legal implications of everything they do and the importance of how they document their observations and the histories they obtain that speak to the truth of an assault victim's experience. They must maintain a balanced, objective demeanor and formulate defensible diagnostic assessments. The knowledge to accomplish the tasks just outlined is in this text from the most basic to the most nuanced information.

These 20 chapters, written by recognized authorities, are well constructed, simple to read, and richly illustrated, making this text the reference of choice for emergency rooms and professionals who serve the needs of sexual assault victims.

Martin A. Finkel, DO, FAAP
Professor of Pediatrics
Medical Director
Child Abuse Research and Service Institute
School of Osteopathic Medicine
University of Medicine and Dentistry of New Jersey
Stratford, New Jersey

Foreword

If there has been a downside to the development and institution of sexual assault nurse or forensic examiner (SANE/SAFE) programs, it has been that medical communities with these programs have become complacent about the needs of this and other closely linked forensic patient populations. It has become easy for emergency department (ED) personnel to transfer the care of the sexual assault patient to the SANE without feeling an obligation to understand the medical and forensic needs of the patient, and equally easy to avoid education around these patient populations. This perception has predisposed the ED staff to miss other closely linked forensic patients, such as the patient who is experiencing intimate partner violence, human trafficking, drug-facilitated sexual assault, or elder abuse.

More than 2 decades have passed since former surgeon general of the United States, Dr. C. Everett Koop, informed us that violence was a major public health issue. *Medical Response to Adult Sexual Assault* allows us to see where we began, how far we have come, and the path to where we want to go in service to our patients. It offers directive for both the trained and untrained examiner, as each provides effective, comprehensive care to the sexual assault patient population.

Medical professionals, whether registered nurses or advanced practice providers, have an obligation to provide comprehensive medical and forensic care to all sexually assaulted patients; however, our abilities extend beyond simply the provision of care. We have the duty to comprehend and improve both the short- and long-term health consequences associated with having been sexually victimized. In the words of Dr. Koop, "medicine does have a contribution to make and we should be bound, in all good conscience, to make it."

Medical Response to Adult Sexual Assault is a must for all emergency departments regardless of size, as it will guide personnel through the details of the sexual assault examination as well as the special circumstances that very often arise. Additionally, the text will identify the coordinated, collaborative community response to sexual assault that occurs with the existence of sexual assault response teams; the importance of the sexual assault response team concept; and the individual roles and responsibilities of the professionals involved.

Jennifer Pierce-Weeks, RN, SANE-A, SANE-P
Forensic Nurse Examiner Program
Memorial Health System
Colorado Springs, Colorado

FOREWORD

I am a relative newcomer to the field of sexual assault forensic health care compared to some of the pioneers in this field. Unlike many of my colleagues who had watched well-intentioned, but poorly prepared, clinicians fumbling through sexual assault evidentiary exams, I participated in a sexual assault nurse examiner (SANE) course after realizing that victimization and health were at polar ends of the wellness spectrum. As a women's health nurse practitioner, I needed to learn how to move my patients away from one end of the spectrum and closer to the other. I had never seen a sexual assault evidence collection kit; had never stood beside a patient watching in frustration as a physician read the directions on the box; and had never been confronted by angry or distraught patients waiting hours for care. I only knew that, in my practice, violence seemed like the thread in an unraveling sweater—pull at it a bit and discover there is more of it in your hands.

I completed the SANE course in the mid-1990s, only to wait several years before I found a community where SANE programming was not only feasible, but also thriving. In the 16 years since I was educated as a forensic nurse examiner, a great deal has changed. SANEs (or the more profession-neutral SAFEs [sexual assault forensic examiners]) are not a curiosity, but a standard of care in many communities across North America. Where once there were only a handful of SANEs, now we number in the thousands. We are in all 50 states, throughout the Canadian provinces, and abroad. Large urban trauma centers, suburban community hospitals, rural and tribal health clinics, freestanding rape crisis programs, and police departments—SANE/SAFE programs thrive in all of these settings.

Higher quality responses to victims of sexual violence are a result of multidisciplinary collaboration. In the past, law enforcement, victim advocacy, prosecutors, and clinicians remained in silos with little to no contact with each other; now we have sexual assault response/resource teams (SARTs) and an expectation of communication and shared education across disciplines. The forthcoming SART Toolkit, a project of the National Sexual Violence Resource Center, was created "to provide resources that will help communities customize their outreach and expand services to underserved communities." To borrow from the environmental movement, we are now discussing sexual assault response globally while encouraging communities to adapt (and act) locally.

The clinical approach to sexual assault patients has also made great strides during these past 15 years, again within the framework of multidisciplinary (as well as *inter*disciplinary) collaboration. The President's DNA Initiative brought about such pivotal documents as the *National Protocol for Sexual Assault Medical Forensic Examinations*, and its companion, the *National Training Standards for Sexual Assault Forensic Examiners*. The International Association of Forensic Nurses' *Sexual Assault: Forensic and Clinical Management* virtual practicum provides an opportunity for clinicians to obtain hands-on experience with all aspects of medicolegal care. Health care is even sitting at the sexual violence prevention table, thanks in part to the vision and encouragement of the Centers for Disease Control and Prevention and the World Health Organization, who recognize sexual violence as a public health issue. Never has the prospect of working myself out of a job been so enticing.

It is only fitting then that in this era of greater standardization and burgeoning evidence-based practice we have a new text that examines the complexities and nuances of sexual assault medical-forensic care. While there have been others before it, *Medical Response to Adult Sexual Assault* is notable in that it examines the issue holistically and avoids the pitfalls of analysis in a vacuum. The authors, all of who have storied careers that can be measured in decades and not years, have had the foresight to offer context, as well as presentation. When paging through this book, you will find information that looks at the dynamics and clinical issues of adult victimization, and the text also covers the unique challenges of elderly, male, and incarcerated patients. It examines sexual violence as it co-occurs with intimate partner violence, human trafficking, and homicide. There is also considerable discussion about the unique issues accompanying sexual assault in the military, on college campuses, and within jails and prisons. Most notably, however, is a chapter devoted to evaluating the SANE's work. For years, SANEs have theorized that a targeted, multidisciplinary approach to sexual violence makes a difference. Anecdotal evidence, patient feedback, and stakeholder testimonials support that theory. It is only within the past 10 years that data has been collected that confirms what our instincts have told us: SANE/SAFE practice matters.

The evolution of sexual assault medical-forensic care has, in part, shined a bright light on the gaps that still exist in the field. As a clinician who has worked closely with struggling SANE programs around the country, I am keenly aware of the need for current and applicable health care resources. A text like *Medical Response to Adult Sexual Assault* expands our clinical knowledge of the topic and builds our capacity to better respond to the health care and forensic needs of our patients. Its publication is well-timed, complemented by several federally funded projects, including the SANE Sustainability Technical Assistance Project (National Sexual Violence Resource Center), the SAFE Technical Assistance Project (International Association of Forensic Nurses), and the Violence Against Women Act Forensic Compliance Project (End Violence Against Women, International), that give SANEs/SAFEs the programmatic tools they need to provide quality care for victims of sexual violence.

Following more than a decade of rich and varied developments, it is hard to imagine what the next decade will bring: greater emphasis on program infrastructure; widespread expansion of clinical services; or engagement in the policy arena. The possibilities are infinite when the foundation is a solid one.

Jenifer Markowitz, ND, RN, WHNP-BC, SANE-A, DF-IAFN
Medical Advisor
AEquitas, The Prosecutor's Resource on Violence Against Women
Washington DC

PREFACE

When Ann Burgess wrote her seminal article, "Rape Trauma Syndrome," in 1974 and Linda Ledray started the first sexual assault nurse examiner (SANE) program in Minneapolis in 1977, neither dreamed that over 30 years later there would be SANE and sexual assault forensic examiner (SAFE) programs across the United States, Canada, and many other countries. While the initial drive to improve services clearly came from the advocate movement, the medical community—led by nurses—was quick to respond. We hope the time has come when it is no longer acceptable to just read the directions in the sexual assault evidence collection kit while providing care to the victim. We would certainly think this behavior unacceptable within any other patient population.

Another milestone for the forensic nursing movement came in 1992 when 72 nurses from 26 programs throughout the United States came together in Minneapolis, excited about the new role that was developing. Since two members of our group were from Canada, we decided to call this new organization the International Association of Forensic Nurses (IAFN). Once we combined the enthusiasm and expertise of the many nurses across the country, the model began to flourish. This new role officially became known as the SANE role 5 years later in 1997 at an IAFN meeting in Kansas City. Around the same time, the Office for Victims of Crime took the opportunity to further support program development through grants, many of which have gone to the IAFN and to member programs. To a great extent, it was the support for the SANE model from the staff and members of IAFN that took it from only a few programs to every state in the United States as well as to many countries throughout the world. The US military also strives to have this high quality of care available for all soldiers who may be victimized, regardless of where they are stationed.

Medical Response to Adult Sexual Assault is intended to summarize these 30 years of experience and research and provide the reader with up-to-date information based upon this research. It is intended to provide the reader with an easily accessible guide to providing all men, women, and adolescents who have been sexually assaulted with the best care possible, anticipating and meeting all of their needs. It is also intended to walk the reader through the court process and address their role, should the case go to trial. Knowing what can be expected in a court of law is the best preparation for our work and documentation of that work in the medical setting. The better job we do with the initial exam and documentation, the more likely an offender will be identified, and the more likely the case will settle out of court (and the less likely we will be called to testify). When we provide good patient care and evidence collection, there is less secondary trauma for our patients, and more offenders are identified and apprehended, resulting in fewer future sexual assaults. This is clearly an opportunity to impact not only the way our patients are treated, but—by assisting the criminal justice system to identify the offenders—also assist them with preventing future victimization.

Those of us who were a part of that initial meeting in Minneapolis are especially grateful to the continued efforts of IAFN staff and members to further the SANE model. That is why we have chosen to dedicate this book to IAFN and its members. Our hope is that it will help further our mutual goal of improving the medical, legal, forensic, and supportive response to victims of sexual assault.

Linda E. Ledray, RN, SANE-A, PhD, FAAN
Ann Wolbert Burgess, DNSc, APRN, BC, FAAN
Angelo P. Giardino, MD, PhD, MPH, FAAP

REVIEWS

In Medical Response to Adult Sexual Assault, *Dr. Ledray leads the way for medical and allied health professionals to improve their medical care giving to this population. According to the Rape, Abuse, and Incest National Network, in 2007 there were 243 300 victims of adult sexual assault in the United States. This population has specific unmet needs, some of which can be met with the emergence into practice of the content knowledge from Dr. Ledray's book. This text is comprehensive in scope, covering the history of specialization care, categorizations of victims of adult sexual assault with common threads for identification and treatment, and includes a chapter on evidence collection, preservation, and identification that will strongly support the legal machinations that must occur. This text should become a necessary and well-worn resource to medical professionals working with adult sexual assault victims.*

Karyn E. Holt, CNM, PhD
Associate Clinical Professor
Drexel University
Philadelphia, Pennsylvania

Medical Response to Adult Sexual Assault *offers a comprehensive, holistic, and collaborative approach to adult sexual assault, and is an invaluable resource to any professional who may provide care to this population. This book provides the content and framework to expand and improve the quality of an interdisciplinary assessment and treatment of adult sexual assault. This resource also provides a broader scope of the specific dynamics of the adult sexual assault response in settings such as the military and college campuses, and informs the reader with greater understanding of the male sexual assault victim, elder sexual abuse, and human trafficking. Having all the relevant content in one textbook like this is an effective and informative tool for professionals in health care as well as other important disciplines serving these victims.*

Philip V. Scribano, DO, MSCE
Associate Professor of Pediatrics
College of Medicine
Ohio State University
Columbus, Ohio

Medical Response to Adult Sexual Assault *is an outstanding text that mimics an encyclopedia as it covers a wide range of pertinent issues that include historical, medical, SANE, and legal perspectives. The book provides hard-to-find information about topics such as conducting a sexual assault examination, providing courtroom testimony, and identifying the complexities associated with crimes against vulnerable individuals, such as the elderly and incarcerated. The seasoned contributors bring the content alive with their experience, anecdotes, and superb writing. This text is most worthy of some precious space on your bookshelf.*

Carol Anne Marchetti, PhD, RNCS, SANE
Southeast Regional Coordinator
MA Sexual Assault Nurse Examiner Program
Boston, Massachusetts

The authors of Medical Response to Adult Sexual Assault *provide an invaluable resource for the professionals who collaborate to provide services to victims of sexual assault. The range of chapters and the comprehensiveness with which each chapter is written demonstrates a complete and detailed understanding of the issues associated with sexual assault cases. The reader will find that reference and the use of this resource to be most rewarding. This superbly edited text by three of the most well-respected clinicians in the area of sexual assault will undoubtedly become a standard in educational settings across a diverse professional spectrum.*

L. Kathleen Sekula, PhD, APRN-BC
Associate Professor
Director, Forensic Graduate Programs
School of Nursing
Duquesne University
Pittsburgh, Pennsylvania

This text is a must read for all health care professionals who work in hospital emergency departments and other professionals who come in contact with sexual assault victims. Topics covered include the history and importance of SARTs; physiological and psychological consequences of sexual assault; conducting the examination; collecting evidence; and qualifications of SART members. Registered nurses interested in becoming SANEs will find this text particularly informative. This text clearly articulates the highest standards of care and is both a valuable reference book and an excellent instructional source for educating professionals in the care of sexual assault victims.

Ana Maria Catanzaro, RN, PhD
Associate Professor
Chair, Master of Science in Nursing Programs
Holy Family University
Philadelphia, Pennsylvania

Contents in Brief

Contents in Detail

Medical Response to

Adult Sexual Assault

A Resource for Clinicians and Related Professionals

STM **Learning,** Inc.

Leading Publisher of Scientific, Technical, and Medical Educational Resources

Saint Louis

www.stmlearning.com

Chapter 1

Sexual Assault Nurse Examiner and Sexual Assault Response Team Overview and History

Linda E. Ledray, RN, SANE-A, PhD, FAAN
Ann Wolbert Burgess, DNSc, APRN, BC, FAAN

A New Standard of Care

With the implementation of sexual assault nurse examiner (SANE) programs across the United States, a new standard of care has been implemented for sexual assault patients. It is no longer acceptable to have untrained medical personnel reading the directions of the exam while they are treating sexual assault victims and collecting evidence. As such practices would never be considered reasonable for a physician or nurse to perform in the emergency department (ED) with other patient populations, they should not be acceptable with victims of rape.

In many medical institutions, rape victims still encounter long waits and inadequate, substandard care. Some may wait up to 12 hours for a rape exam in even several of the best medical facilities.[1] On a national level, only 20% of rape victims who receive medical care after a rape are given emergency contraception (EC), and only 58% are screened or given medication to prevent sexually transmitted infections (STIs).[2] In medical facilities with SANE programs, care is far superior. Although more program evaluation and outcomes research is needed, the evidence indicates that SANE programs offer EC 97% of the time and medication to prevent STIs 99% of the time.[3]

In 1989, the California State Court of Appeals ruled that a woman who was not given the right to choose EC could sue the hospital that provided the inadequate care.[4] This kind of lawsuit takes place in a very public forum—one that a rape victim may not be willing or able to endure. Smugar et al recognize that while it can be therapeutic for some, these lawsuits will further prolong the trauma for others.[5] It should not be necessary for rape victims to sue in order to access the care they need and deserve. To prevent this from being necessary, many states have passed laws requiring sexual assault victims be provided information about EC or given these medications by health care providers. As health care providers, we are responsible to know the best practices and to have a system in place that meets the needs of this often vulnerable population.

Over the past several decades, our awareness of the magnitude and the trauma of crime victimization has increased considerably. The costs incurred by society include medical and psychological services to aid victim recovery, the apprehension and disposition of offenders, and the invisible climate of fear that makes safety a paramount consideration in scheduling normal daily activities. In addition to the monetary costs associated with sexual victimization, the impact of such abuse on the victim has been well documented.[6,7]

This chapter reviews the social and political forces in place in the 1970s when the antirape movement began; the impact of rape victimization, which includes the history of rape trauma syndrome and posttraumatic stress disorder; and the development and implementation of victim services, specifically SANE programs and sexual assault response teams (SARTs).

The Antirape Movement: The Beginning

The women's rights movement in the 19th century was focused on the legal recognition of women to secure their rights to vote, to own and control property, and to participate in public affairs. In the 20th century, the movement focused on confronting restrictions on women's personal lives. Analysis of these restrictions began in ***consciousness-raising groups*** (CR), a new organizing tool of the women's movement whereby women discussed their experiences and the problems of being female in a modern society. Often described by men as hot beds of radical feminism, the reality was that simply attending such a discussion group was the most assertive act many of these women were capable of taking. Within the supportive environment of the CR groups, women found the courage to share private experiences never before shared, such as incest and rape.[8]

These anecdotal disclosures of former victims had a profound effect on their listeners. The revelations represented an unprecedented breakthrough of the silence that surrounded the topic of rape for centuries. The act of rape has been an inherent part of women's lives throughout recorded history—a theme commonly found in literature, poetry, theater, art, and war.

Police departments and rape crisis centers first began to address the crime of rape in the early 1970s when little was known about rape victims or sex offenders. The issue of rape was just beginning to be raised by feminist groups. The 1971 New York Speak-Out on Rape was held. Susan Brownmiller wrote the history of rape and urged people to deny its future.[9] The general public, however, was not particularly concerned about rape victims. Few academic publications or special services existed, funding agencies did not see the topic as important, and health policy was almost nonexistent.

The antirape movement began to attract women from all walks of life and political persuasions. Various strategies began to emerge, one of which was the self-help program now widely known as the "rape crisis center." One of the first such centers was founded in Berkeley in early 1972, known as Bay Area Women Against Rape (BAWAR). Within months of the opening of the Berkeley center, similar centers were established in Ann Arbor, Michigan; Washington, DC; and Philadelphia, Pennsylvania. Hospital-based rape counseling services began in Boston and Minneapolis.[10] Centers were soon replicated, and services flourished. Although volunteer ranks tended to include a large number of university students and instructors, they also included homemakers and working women. The volunteer makeup usually reflected every age, race, socioeconomic class, sexual preference, and level of political consciousness. Volunteers were, however, exclusively women. The most common denominators were commitments to aiding victims and bringing about social change.[8,10] As Susan Brownmiller noted, the amazing aspect of the proliferation of the grassroots women's groups was that such an approach to the problem of rape had never been suggested by men—that women should organize to combat rape was a result of the women's movement.[9]

In retrospect, the history of the rape crisis centers in the United States has been one of enormous struggle. The struggle was to overcome indifferences, apathy, changing social trends, and the lack of stable resources, yet the struggle was willingly undertaken from the belief in the rightness of the cause—a cause that, despite the struggles, had its share of successes. Feminists identified a social need and a way of responding to it. Rape crisis centers began to adapt their services to assist other crime victims, specifically battered women and their children. Although they never reached the goal of eradicating rape through social change, they were the instigators of social change essential to the rights of women.[8,10]

Rape Law Reform

Laws greatly shape public opinion and attitudes. Legislation in the form of law reform can be both instrumental and symbolic. Such was the case with rape law reform, especially in conveying the concept of rape as a physically and emotionally damaging act. Changes in rape laws helped to influence attitudes within both the criminal justice and the general communities, although some would argue that jurors/citizens are still inclined to view rape in moral rather than criminal terms.

United States' criminal rape laws were derived from British common law. Three elements needed to be proved in cases of rape: (1) sexual contact, (2) force/coercion or lack of consent, and (3) the identity of the assailant. In addition, most state laws today consider the sexual assault a more serious crime, because it carries more severe penalties when penetration (however slight) occurred, the victim was injured, a weapon was used, or the victim was under the age of consent. It varies by state. Two influential legal theorists were 17th-century jurist, Lord Chief Justice Matthew Hale, and the Edwardian-era scholar, John Henry Wigmore. Hale's belief that rape was "...an accusation easily made, and hard to be proved, and harder to be defended by the party accused, though ever so innocent" was reflected in both American jury instructions and standards of proof.[11] Similarly, Wigmore's concern about sexually precocious minors and unchaste women who fantasize about rape gave rise to the corroboration doctrine and influenced such practices as the routine polygraph examination of victims.[12] Though neither man's assertions were supported by empirical data, they received widespread endorsement by legal bodies. As a result, US law reflected a concept of rape as a sexual rather than a violent offense and imposed a vast array of safeguards against false accusations by the turn of the 20th century.[13]

The need for rape law reform was clearly noted by women's rights movement participants who encouraged former victims to speak publicly about insensitive and indifferent treatment they experienced in the criminal justice system. These disclosures fostered recognition for systematic change that women activists felt must begin with the law itself. Movement activists organized to develop a rape law reform agenda, solicit public support for reform, and present their case to state legislators. The political climate was favorable to these citizen-initiated efforts, but it was a growing presence of women and sympathetic men within the legal and lawmaking professions that reduced most of the resistance to change. As evidenced by the radical shift in the concept of unacceptable behavior, a review of rape law reform by Largen suggested, among other things, that in most states, social concepts of sexual assault were changing more rapidly than legal concepts.[13] Politicians also recognized the need for more research on the impact of rape on the victim and the development of programs to meet apparent needs.

Congressional Support

Financial help came from Congress. In response to a rising crime rate and growing community concern over the problem of rape, Senator Charles Mathias of Maryland introduced a bill in September 1973 to establish the National Center for the Prevention and Control of Rape. The purpose of the bill was to provide a focal point within the National Institute of Mental Health from which a comprehensive national effort would be undertaken to conduct research, develop programs, and provide information leading to aid for victims and their families. Also, efforts could be made to address rehabilitation of offenders and the ultimate curtailment of rape crimes. The bill was passed overwhelmingly in the 93rd Congress, vetoed by President Ford, and successfully reintroduced. The National Center was established through Public law 94-63 in July 1975. The chair of the first advisory committee to the new center was a nurse, Ann Wolbert Burgess.

By the late 1970s, the battered women's movement became an extension of the antirape movement and focused on male violence against domestic partners. Violence emerged as a public health issue with Surgeon General C. Everett Koop's convening of a workshop on violence and public health in 1985. The closing of the National Center for the Prevention and Control of Rape, however, in the late 1980s left a void for funding until 1994. Again, organized efforts were needed to keep rape crisis centers operating and lobbying for government funding. Congress once again recognized violence against women as a national problem in its 1994 passage of the Violence Against Women Act (VAWA) as part of the Violent Crime Control and Law Enforcement Act and by President Clinton's establishment of an Office on Violence Against Women in the US Department of Justice. The National Research Council established a Panel on Research on Violence Against Women in 1995 to fulfill a congressional request to develop a research agenda to increase understanding and control of violence against women. This report highlights the major literature on the scope of violence against women in the United States, the causes and consequences of that violence, the interventions needed for both women victims of violence and male perpetrators, and funding needed to meet research goals.[7]

History and Need for SANE-SART Programs

The impetus to develop SANE programs in the United States began about the same time as the first rape crisis centers were opened—the early 1970s—with nurses, other medical professionals, counselors, and advocates working with rape victims who came for medical care in traditional settings such as hospital EDs. It was obvious to these individuals that the services to sexual assault victims were inadequate, as they failed to meet the standard of care required for other medical patients.[14,15] Rape victims often had to wait 4 to 12 hours in a busy, public area, competing unsuccessfully with the critically ill for medical staff time.[14,16,17] They were often not allowed to eat, drink, or urinate while they waited for fear of destroying evidence.[18]

Emergency department services were inconsistent and problematic. The typical rape survivor faced a time-consuming, cumbersome succession of examiners, some with only a few hours of orientation and little experience. Many doctors and nurses were not sufficiently trained to do the medicolegal exam and were unwilling or unable to provide expert witness testimony if the case went to court.[19] When they had the training to complete the evidentiary exam, staff often did not complete a sufficient number of exams to maintain their level of proficiency.[20-22] Even when the victim's medical needs were met, their emotional needs were often overlooked and they, too, were often blamed by police and others when they made a report.[23]

Often, only male physicians were available to do the vaginal exam.[20] While approximately half of the rape victims in one study were unconcerned with the gender of the examiner, the other half found this extremely problematic. Even male victims indicated they preferred to be examined by a woman, as they were most often raped by a man and experienced the same generalized fear and anger toward men that female victims experienced.[24] More research is needed, however, to explore gender issues. With the proper skills and awareness, either gender should be able to provide the highest standard of care to victims of violent crimes. The issue likely has more to do with demeanor, sensitivity, and understanding than gender.

Many anecdotal and published reports depict physicians as reluctant to do the rape exam. Key factors that have led to this reluctance include a lack of experience and training in forensic evidence collection[17,19,25]; the time-consuming nature of the evidentiary exam in a busy ED with many other medically urgent patients waiting to be seen[26,27]; and the potential that if they complete the exam they may be subpoenaed and taken away from their work in the ED to testify in court and be questioned by a sometimes hostile defense attorney.[17,18,27] Documentation of evidence was rushed, inadequate, or incomplete because of these factors.[27] Staff physicians in teaching hospitals often assigned residents to do the forensic examinations when they were available; physicians have refused to do the exam.[26] In one case, a rape victim was reportedly sent home without having an evidentiary exam completed because no physician could be found to do it.[28]

As information has become more readily available on the complex medical-forensic needs of rape victims, nurses and other professionals have realized the importance of providing the best ED care possible.[20] For 75% of victims in a study evaluating care received in the ED, the initial ED visit was the only known contact they had with medical or professional support staff.[29] Nurses became aware that while they were often only credited with "assisting the physician with the exam," in reality they were typically doing all of the medical-forensic examination except the pelvic speculum exam.[26,29] It was clear to these nurses that it was time to reevaluate the system and consider a new approach.

Pioneer Sexual Assault Nurse Examiner Programs

To better meet the needs of the sexually assaulted population, SANE programs were established in Memphis, Tennessee, in 1976,[17] Minneapolis, Minnesota, in 1977,[30,31] and Amarillo, Texas, in 1979.[32] Unfortunately, these nurses worked in isolation, unaware of other very similar programs' existence until the late 1980s. In 1992, 72 individuals from 31 SANE programs across the United States and Canada came together for the first time at a meeting hosted by the Sexual Assault Resource Service and the University of Minnesota School of Nursing in Minneapolis. At this meeting the International Association of Forensic Nurses (IAFN) was formed.[24]

Development of SANE programs today is progressing rapidly, especially with the high program visibility afforded by the publication of the US Department of Justice, Office for Victims of Crime (OVC) document, *The SANE Development and Operation Guide*.[33] While only 86 SANE programs were identified and included in the October 1996 listing of SANE programs published in the *Journal of Emergency Nursing*,[24] there are currently nearly 600 SANE programs registered on the OVC grant-funded Web site www.sane-sart.com.[34] The Joint Military Task Force on Sexual Assault (2004) also recognized the need for improved services for members of the Armed Forces and has begun the process of implementing SART teams for every military unit.

The American Nurses' Association (ANA) officially recognized forensic nursing as a new specialty in 1995.[35] SANEs make up the largest subspecialty of forensic nursing internationally. At the 1996 IAFN meeting in Kansas City, Geri Marullo, executive director of ANA, predicted that the Joint Commission on Accreditation of Health Care Organizations (JCAHO) would eventually require every hospital to have a forensic nurse available.[36] Smugar et al also recommend that the JCAHO or legislation require health care providers to meet a higher standard of care.[5] SANE-SART programs have raised the standard of care for victims of sexual assault, but this standard is typically not being met in facilities that do not have SANE nurses.[37]

The Role of the SANE and SAFE

Since forensic nurse examiner programs began and functioned independently until the founding of IAFN in Minneapolis in 1992, different terminology has been used across the country to define this new role. At the October 1996 IAFN annual meeting held in Kansas City, the SANE Council voted on the terminology it wanted to use. The overwhelming decision was to use the title "SANE"—Sexual Assault Nurse Examiner. A SANE is a registered nurse (RN) who has advanced education in the forensic examination of sexual assault victims. In programs where physicians are also used, the more inclusive term of Sexual Assault Forensic Examiners (SAFE), or Forensic Examiners (FE) is typically used. Advanced education in sexual assault forensic evidence collection is vital.

The primary mission of a SANE/SAFE program is to meet the needs of all male and female victims of sexual assault or abuse by providing immediate, compassionate, culturally sensitive, and comprehensive forensic evaluation and treatment by trained, professional nurse experts within the parameters of the individual's state Nurse Practice Act, the SANE standards of the IAFN, and the individual agency policies. With proper training, SANE programs may provide services to child, adolescent, and adult victims. Nearly half of SANE programs in 2007 provide services for all age groups.

In addition to documentation and collection of forensic evidence, prophylactic treatment of STIs and EC are provided by the SANE. The SANE also conducts a medicolegal examination, not a routine physical examination, to identify trauma.

While SANEs are not advocates, they do provide the rape survivor with information to assist her in anticipating what may happen next, to aid her in making choices about reporting and deciding whom to tell, and to ensure that she is safe and gets the support needed after she leaves the SANE facility. This usually includes a discussion between the victim and the SANE about reporting to law enforcement.

If the victim has made a choice not to report, the SANE will need to discuss and determine why she may be hesitant to report. While the decision to report is always ultimately the victim's, in most cases the SANE will encourage the survivor to report the crime and make referrals to advocacy agencies that can provide the support necessary to help her through the criminal justice process and to aid in a successful recovery from the rape. The SANE will also provide emotional support and crisis intervention, working with advocacy support groups such as rape crisis counselors when available.

Typical SANE-SART Program Operation

To be optimally effective and provide the best service possible to victims of sexual assault, the SANE/FE must function as a part of a team of individuals from community organizations, usually referred to as a sexual assault response team (SART). At a minimum, the SART will include the SANE/FE, advocate, law enforcement officer, and prosecutor. It is important to understand that SARTs can function in a variety of ways, both formally and informally. To be a functioning SART, it is not necessary for all team members to respond to the survivor at the same time. In fact, most SARTs do not function this way. Research that evaluates these models of response is necessary.

There are 2 primary methods of SART operation: the *multiple-initial interview model* and the *single-initial interview model.* In the more common multiple-initial interview model the SANE is available on call, off premises, 24 hours a day, 7 days a week. The on-call SANE is paged immediately whenever a sexual assault or abuse survivor enters the community's response system. If a rape advocate is available, the staff or SANE will also page the advocate on call. During the time it takes for the SANE to respond (usually no more than one hour), the ED or clinic staff will evaluate and treat any urgent or life-threatening injuries. If treatment is medically necessary, the ED staff will treat the patient, always considering and documenting the forensic consequences of the life-saving and stabilizing medical procedures. Once the SANE arrives, consent for the forensic medical examination is obtained, and the SANE conducts the forensic evidentiary examination. The law enforcement officer either conducts the initial interview before or after the SANE exam is completed.

In the single-initial interview model the SANE/FE, advocate, and law enforcement officer respond together and conduct one joint interview of the victim. Chapter 12 and Chapter 13 address options for effective SART operation in detail and describe the impact SANE-SART programs have had on both treatment of sexual assault victims and prosecution of cases.

The SANE Evidentiary Exam

With the development of the SANE role, a trained medical professional was available to provide complete care to the survivor of sexual assault. In facilities with SANEs on call, it was no longer necessary for the survivor to wait until someone, often with minimal to no special training, could be freed up to provide care that was often incomplete.

The SANE's forensic medical exams include the following:

— Collection of evidence using a sexual assault evidence collection kit

— Further assessment and documentation for drug-facilitated sexual assault (DFSA)

— Assessment and documentation of injuries

— Risk evaluation and prophylactic care of STIs

— Evaluation of pregnancy risk and EC

— Crisis intervention

— Referrals for medical and psychological follow-ups.

In most agencies, a complete evidentiary exam is conducted for up to 72 hours from the time of the sexual assault, as recommended by the American College of Emergency Physicians,[38] the SANE Development and Operation Guide,[33] and the *National Protocol for Sexual Assault Medical Forensic Exams: Adults/Adolescents.*[39] As DNA recovery techniques improve, some programs have extended this time frame and now collect evidence up to 96 or even 120 hours after the assault. Research is still needed to better evaluate the value of this decision. The publication of *A National Protocol for Sexual Assault Medical Forensic Exams: Adults and Adolescents* was a major step toward encouraging consistent treatment for victims of sexual assault throughout the US.[39] Chapter 4 discusses the SANE/FE exam in detail.

The Psychological Impact of Sexual Assault

The fact that rape occurs and is an act of conquest is documented in the Bible as well as in war annals. It is endemic to humankind and was undoubtedly practiced by cavemen. But in 1972, when Burgess and Holmstrom launched their research, there were very few clinically based articles that dealt with the incidence of rape or the impact of rape on the victim or family. There was also little information on the offender. While the violent acts and the suffering they caused had been noted since the origins of humanity, few considered these events from a health standpoint.

In the early 1970s, there were 2 common stereotypes of the rapist that, in turn, greatly influenced how the rape victim was viewed. At one extreme, he was regarded as a perfectly healthy, "red-blooded," sexually aggressive, macho male whose offense was simply an extreme product of his cultural conditioning elicited by a provocative and seductive but punitive woman. At the other extreme, he was thought of as a bizarre, demented, oversexed "fiend" filled with lust and perverted desire who stalked his prey at night when the moon was full. In the former situation, the offender was seen as a totally normal individual who was essentially a victim of circumstance; in the latter, he was an inhuman creature whose predatory assaults were his only source of gratification. Both stereotypes reflected the erroneous but popular belief that rape was motivated primarily by sexual desire—the normal desires of a healthy male or the warped impulses of a sex fiend. This mistaken notion was an insidious assumption, for it followed from such a premise that if the offender was sexually aroused, then it must have been the victim who aroused him as it was toward her that these impulses were directed. From that point on, responsibility and accountability for the offense, to a large extent, shifted from the offender to the victim, and she became the accused by police, family, friends, and even herself. In court, it became the central aim of the defense attorney to impeach the victim's credibility by showing that by her dress, conduct, conversation, or behavior she invited the assault and, either deliberately or unintentionally, that she aroused the sexual urges of her assailant. He was seen as the victim of her provocative behavior. Some high-profile cases have continued to foster this notion.

Rape, until the 1970s, thrived on prudery, misunderstanding, and silence. It was not until the 1980s that academic and scientific publications on the subject multiplied. A review of articles on the psychological effects of rape and interventions for rape victims in the posttraumatic period located 78 references between 1965 and 1976, with 36 on the effects of rape and 42 on intervention.

History of Rape Trauma Syndrome

Rape trauma syndrome was one of 3 typologies identified by Burgess and Holmstrom in 1974 and published in the *American Journal of Psychiatry*.[40] The typologies were the result of personal interviews of 146 people who ranged in age from 3 to 73 years at the time of admission to the Boston City Hospital Emergency Department. The individuals were all admitted with the complaint, "I've been raped." Three types of sexual trauma were conceptualized from the sample of 146 and based on consent (or not) to have sex: rape trauma (no consent), pressured sex (coerced sex), and sex stress (initial consent but then denial of consent). Of the 146 individuals, 92 women age 18 to 73 years were classified as rape trauma victims, and their responses to the assaultive experience formed the basis for the rape trauma syndrome. These women were interviewed at the emergency ward of the hospital and followed 4 to 6 years later in regard to the problems they experienced as a result of being forced into nonconsensual sex.[41]

One of the conclusions reached by Burgess and Holmstrom as a result of studying 92 adult rape victims was that victims suffer a significant degree of physical and emotional trauma during a rape. This trauma can be noted immediately following the assault and over a considerable time period afterward. Victims consistently described certain symptoms that included flashbacks; intrusive thoughts of the rape, fear, anxiety, nightmares, and daymares; and development of phobias. A cluster of symptoms that most victims experienced was described as the rape trauma syndrome. This syndrome has 2 phases: the immediate or acute phase, in which the victim's lifestyle is completely disrupted by the rape crisis, and the long-term process, in which the victim must reorganize this disrupted lifestyle. The syndrome includes physical, emotional, and behavioral stress reactions that result from the person being faced with a dire threat to life or integrity.

Victims expressed other feelings in conjunction with fear, ranging from humiliation, degradation, guilt, shame, and embarrassment to self-blame, anger, and revenge. Victims reported feeling distress over reminders (or cues) of the assault. Victims become cautious and distrustful with all people; they expect the assailant to be everywhere.

The prevailing stereotype of rape in the 1970s was that women should feel ashamed and guilty after being raped, but that was not the primary reaction in most victims. Instead, most expressed a fear of physical injury, death, or retaliation.

The Burgess and Holmstrom study was twofold, with a clinical focus on victim response and an institutional focus. The study made clear that rape does not end with the assailant's departure; rather, the profound suffering of the victim can be diminished or heightened by the response of those who staff the police stations, hospitals, and courthouses. Ironically, the institutions that society has designated to help victims may in fact cause further damage.[42] The clinical findings from the Burgess and Holmstrom study were published and used by rape crisis staff as well as mental health staff.

Rape trauma syndrome was accepted as a nursing diagnosis into the North American Nursing Diagnosis Association official nomenclature in 1979. Also included were 2 variations of rape trauma syndrome: silent response to rape and compounded reaction to rape. The silent response to rape was observed in persons who had never told anyone of a rape experience but later (months or years) the assault was revealed. In the Burgess and Holmstrom study, women talked freely of these early experiences in the context of the new assault experience. In the compounded rape trauma, the individual has a primary presenting medical or psychological disorder through which the rape trauma symptoms are filtered. Examples include elders with dementia, persons with a psychiatric disorder or physical disorder, persons with a mental retardation, and persons with somatic complaints, multiple ED visits, substance abuse, eating disorders, and depressive disorders.

History of Psychological Trauma

Rape trauma syndrome preceded the term *posttraumatic stress disorder* (PTSD) by 6 years. When the American Psychiatric Association's Work Group on Anxiety Disorders was considering how to classify a number of traumatic events (eg, combat stress, natural disasters, rape trauma), it decided to make PTSD an umbrella term under which the various life-threatening events could fall.[43]

The term PTSD came into the official nosology of the American Psychiatric Association in 1980 with the publication of the third edition of the *Diagnostic and Statistical Manual of Mental Disorders* (DSM).[43] The history of the development of this term is believed to date back to an account of Merlin of King Arthur's court. He was said to be have been a wild man who went away to live alone in the woods for some years because he was affected by the sounds and sights of terrible battle. He avoided people and lived as a hermit for several years, only to return refreshed and with his special powers. In 1666, Samuel Pepys described his intense emotional reaction to having observed the London fire.

The theme of traumatic memories haunting people after experiencing overwhelming terror has been used in literature from Homer to Shakespeare's *Macbeth*. By the late 1850s, Briquet suggested a link between the symptoms of hysteria and childhood histories of trauma. During this time, a small Anglo-Saxon literature emerged documenting responses to accidents (eg, "railway spine" after train accidents) and war trauma ("soldier's heart"). The relationship between trauma and psychiatric illness, however, only began to be explored in the last two decades of the 19th century when neurologist Charcot lectured on the functional effects of trauma on behavior.[44]

Charcot's student Pierre Janet undertook one of the first systematic studies of the relationship between trauma and psychiatric symptoms and delivered a major paper at the Harvard Medical School in 1906. Janet realized that different temperaments predisposed people to deal with trauma with different coping styles. He coined the term "subconscious" to describe the collection of memories that form the mental schemes that include the person's interaction with the environment. He suggested it was the interplay of memory systems and temperament that made each person unique and complex.[44]

Although one of Freud's earliest published works was *Studies on Hysteria,* he later shifted from a PTSD paradigm of neurosis to a paradigm that centered on intrapsychic fantasy. In a later work, *Beyond the Pleasure Principle,* he once again addressed the issue of traumatic neurosis and looked at trauma as disequilibrium. The history of the development of PTSD was intensified around war and combat stress. Despite such recognition, though, systematic inquiry into the phenomenon of posttraumatic stress was remarkably late in coming. It was not until 1980 that the condition was determined to be a separate and distinct diagnostic category by the American Psychiatric Association.

There are 4 main criteria of PTSD symptoms. A diagnosis of PTSD requires the presence of all categories of symptomatic responses:

1. ***Reexperiencing the trauma:*** flashbacks, nightmares, intrusive memories, and exaggerated emotional and physical reactions to triggers that remind the person of the trauma.

2. ***Emotional numbing:*** feeling detached, lack of emotions (especially positive ones), loss of interest in activities.

3. ***Avoidance:*** avoiding activities, people, or places that remind the person of the trauma.

4. ***Increased arousal:*** difficulty sleeping and concentrating, irritability, hypervigilance (being on guard), and exaggerated startle response.

There have been several revisions to the PTSD diagnosis.[43,45] The last major revision was the fourth edition ("DSM-IV"), published in 1994, although a text revision was produced in 2000. The fifth edition ("DSM-V") is currently in consultation, planning, and preparation, and is due for publication in May 2012.[43,45]

Terminology

Rape or Sexual Assault?

While legal definitions of rape and sexual assault vary greatly from state to state, in this book the terms will be used interchangeably. They will refer to any unwanted contact of the sexual organs of one person, whether male or female, by another person, regardless of gender, with penetration, however slight, or without penetration, and with or without resulting physical injury.

He or She?

While it is acknowledged that men are also victims of sexual assault, female pronouns will primarily be used for the purpose of this book because women are more often victims. When different needs of male and female victims are addressed, the appropriate pronouns will be used.

Victim or Survivor?

As this book, for the most part, focuses on the period directly after the rape, we have chosen to use the term *victim of rape*. ***Victims*** are those who present acutely after experiencing an assault; ***survivors*** are those who are not in the acute stages and have survived the assault; and ***thrivers*** are those who in the aftermath of an assault are thriving and functioning well despite the trauma of sexual violence. We do, however, recognize that an important goal of recovery is to help the victim move from feeling like a victim of the rape to becoming a survivor and then, ultimately, a thriver. This process may happen very quickly for some individuals and very slowly for others. It may take days, weeks, months, or even years, but it rarely occurs during the first few hours.

SANE or SAFE?

Because today the majority of medical practitioners with advanced training in sexual assault management and evidence collection are nurses, we will primarily use the term SANE. When we refer to the SAFE, we are also referring to a non-nurse, usually a physician or physician assistant, who has also had advanced training in sexual assault management and evidence collection.

Sexual Assault Response Team

When we refer to SART, we are referring to formal as well as informal collaborative "teams." They may respond as a unit, or they may work independently, but they work cooperatively in meeting the needs of victims of rape. It is important to remember that there are many options for SART operation. These are discussed in detail in Chapters 12 and 13.

Role of Nursing

Nursing is and will continue to be a major player in the trauma field. The antirape movement helped catapult nursing to the status of a major provider of health care services to victims of abuse. The Joint Commission on Accreditation of Health Care Organizations has suggested that, in the future, forensic nurses be staffed in EDs. The requirement to educate nurses in the fundamentals of forensic science was firmly established in 1997 when the JCAHO published its revised standards for patient assessment. The guidelines required that all staff members be educated to identify victims of abuse, violence, and neglect, and be able to collect and safeguard physical evidence associated with a known or potential criminal act.[46] It opened doors for nurses to develop interdependent relationships with other health care providers, initiate courses and programs of research in victimology and traumatology, influence legislation and health care policy, provide expert testimony in criminal and civil legal cases, and define the new specialty of forensic nursing. However, sexual violence still affects hundreds of thousands of women's and children's lives each year, and health care professionals could be even more influential in case finding and treatment of trauma as well as in designing research and outcome protocols for the interventions aimed at preventing abuse and decreasing the number of victims. Such interventions must target the perpetrators or potential perpetrators of sexual assault. The foothold of skilled investigator nurses in EDs and their preparation for collecting and presenting evidence as well as testifying in judicial proceedings is a major contribution. The advance of the nurse to become a certified SANE-A or SANE-P has firmly established a forensic nursing role.

Rape trauma is now on the radar screen for all disciplines. The pioneers have provided the foundation for the next generation, and they need to keep motivating young clinicians and scholars to forge ahead.

References

1. Katz M. Rape victims often denied proper care. *Courier-Post*. August 27, 2006:B1A.

2. von Hertzen H, Piaggio G, Peregoudov A, et al. For the WHO research group on post-ovulatory methods of fertility regulation. *Lancet*. 2003;360(9348):1803-1810.

3. Cianone A, Wilson C, Collette R, et al. Sexual assault nurse examiner programs in the United States. *Ann Emerg Med*. 2000;35:353-357.

4. California State Court of Appeals, BO32109, 1989.

5. Smugar SS, Spina BJ, Merz JF. Respond. *Am J Public Health*. 2001;91(8):1169-1170.

6. Prentky RA, Burgess AW. *Forensic Management of Sexual Offenders*. New York, NY: Kluwer Academic/Plenum Publishers; 2000.

7. Crowell N, Burgess AW, eds. *Understanding Violence Against Women*. Washington, DC: National Academy of Science Press; 1996.

8. Largen MA. The anti-rape movement: past and present. In: Burgess AW, ed. *Rape and Sexual Assault*. New York, NY: Garland Press; 1985:1-13.

9. Brownmiller S. *Against Our Will: Men, Women, and Rape*. New York, NY: Simon & Schuster; 1975.

10. Burgess AW, Fredericks A. Sexual violence and trauma: Nursing's Contribution. *Nurs Health Policy*. 2002;1(1):17-36.

11. Hale M. The history of the pleas of the crow. In: *Encyclopædia Britannica*. Encyclopædia Britannica Online. Published 2007. http://www.britannica.com/eb/article-2978. Accessed August 25, 2009.

12. Wigmore JN. *A treatise on the Anglo-American system of evidence in trials at common law: including the statutes and judicial decisions of all jurisdictions of the United States and Canada*. Boston, MA: Little, Brown; 1923.

13. Largen MA. Rape-law reform: an analysis. In: Burgess AW, ed. *Rape and Sexual Assault II*. New York, NY: Garland Press;1988:271-292.

14. Holloway M, Swan A. A & E management of sexual assault. *Nurs Stand*. 1993; 7(45):31-35.

15. O'Brien C. Improved forensic documentation of genital injuries with colposcopy. *J Emerg Nurs*. 1997;23(5):460-462.

16. Sandrick K. Tightening the chain of evidence. *Hosp Health Netw*. 1996;6:646.

17. Speck PM, Aiken MM. 20 years of community nursing service. *Tenn Nurs*. 1995:15-18.

18. Thomas M, Zachritz H. Tulsa sexual assault nurse examiners (SANE) program. *J Okla State Med Assoc*. 1993;86:284-286.

19. Lynch V. Forensic nursing: diversity in education and practice. *J Psychosoc Nurs.* 1993;31(11):7-14.

20. Lenehan GP. Sexual assault nurse examiners. *J Emerg Nurs.* 1991;17:1-2.

21. Yorker B. Nurses in Georgia care for survivors of sexual assault. *Ga Nurs.* 1996; 56(1):5-6.

22. Tobias G. Rape examinations by GPs. *Practitioner.* 1990;234:874-877.

23. Rennison CM. *Rape and sexual assault: Reporting to police and medical attention, 1992-2000.* Washington, DC: Bureau of Justice Statistics; 2002.

24. Ledray L. The sexual assault resource service: a new model of care. *Minn Med.* 1996;79(3):43-45.

25. Bell K. Tulsa sexual assault nurse examiners program. *Okla Nurs.* 1995;40(3):16.

26. DiNitto D, Martin PY, Norton DB, et al. After rape: who should examine rape survivors? *Am Journal Nurs.* 1986;86(5):538-540.

27. Frank C. The new way to catch rapists. *Redbook.* 1996:104-105,118,120.

28. Kettleson D. Nurses trained to take evidence. *Unit News/District News.* 1995:1.

29. Ledray LE. The sexual assault nurse clinician: a fifteen-year experience in Minneapolis. *J Emerg Nurs.* 1992;18:217-222.

30. Ledray L, Chaignot MJ. Services to sexual assault victims in Hennepin County. *Eval Change.* 1980;Special Issue:131-134.

31. Ledray L. Evidence collection: an update. *J Child Sex Assault.*1993;2(1):113-115.

32. Antognoli-Toland P. Comprehensive program for examination of sexual assault victims by nurses: a hospital-based project in Texas. *J Emerg Nurs.* 1985;11(3):132-136.

33. Ledray L. *Sexual Assault Nurse Examiner (SANE) Development and Operation Guide.* US Department of Justice, Office of Victims of Crime: 1999.

34. Sexual Assault Resource Service. Sexual Assault Nurse Examiners, Sexual Assault Response Team. http://www.sane.sart.com. Accessed September 16, 2009.

35. Lynch VA. President's report: goals of the IAFN. Presented at: 4th Annual Scientific Assembly of Forensic Nurses; November 1996; Kansas City, MO.

36. Marullo G. The future and the forensic nurse: new dimensions for the twenty-first century. Paper presented at: 4th Annual Scientific Assembly of Forensic Nurses; November 1996; Kansas City, MO.

37. Goldenring JM, Allred G. Post-rape care in hospital emergency rooms. *Am J Public Health.* 2001;91(8):1169.

38. American College Emergency Physicians. *Evaluation and Management of the Sexually Assaulted or Sexually Abused Patient.* Irving, TX: American College Emergency Physicians; 1999.

39. USDOJ, Office on Violence Against Women. *A National Protocol for Sexual Assault Medical Forensic Examinations: Adults/Adolescents.* September 2004; NCJ

206554.

40. Burgess AW, Holmstrom LL. Rape trauma syndrome. *Am J Psychiatry*. 1974; 131:981-986.

41. Burgess AW, Holmstrom LL. *Violence through a Forensic Lens*. King of Prussia, PA: Nursing Spectrum; 2000.

42. Holmstrom LL, Burgess AW. *The Victim of Rape: Institutional Reactions*. New York, NY: Wiley; 1979.

43. American Psychiatric Association. *Diagnostic and Statistical Manual*. 3rd ed. Washington, DC: American Psychiatric Association; 1980.

44. Van der Kolk, Bessel A. The neurobiology of childhood trauma and abuse. *Child Adolesc Psychiatr Clin N Am*. 2003;12(2):293-317.

45. American Psychiatric Association. Summary of Practice-Relevant Changes to the DSM-IV-TR. http://www.psych.org/mainmenu/research/dsmiv/dsmivtr.aspx. Accessed August 27, 2009.

46. Joint Commission on Accreditation of Healthcare Organizations. *Comprehensive Accreditation Manual for Hospitals: The Official Handbook*. Oakbrook Terrace, IL: Joint Commission on Accreditation of Healthcare Organizations; 1997.

Chapter 2

Basic Anogenital and Oral Anatomy

Diana Faugno, MSN, RN, CPN, SANE-A, SANE-P, FAAFS, DF-IAFN
Patricia M. Speck, DNSc, APN, FNP-BC, DF-IAFN, FAAFS, FAAN

Recognition and understanding of the genital, anal, and oral anatomy is essential when evaluating patients for sexual assault. The examiner must be familiar with the appearance of normal anatomy in order to recognize injury and/or medical conditions that can influence the physical appearance of the tissue and mimic sexual assault injury. This chapter will identify the genital, anal, and oral anatomy of adolescents and adults as well as review the terminology of injury.

Female Genital Anatomy

The Genitalia

Female external genitalia vary in size, shape, and color (**Figure 2-1**).[1] For the purposes of this text, the term *external genitalia* will not be used as it is confusing to those outside the health care professions and the term *external genitalia* has been used in court to argue that external genitalia are actually outside structures. In reality, the introitus contains structures only visible with separation of the labia majora. These anatomical structures are covered with nonkeratinized epithelium making them *internal* structures. The exposed skin structures, including the mons and the external surfaces of the labia majora, are covered with keratinized cellular structures, hair, and glands, and they are external to the nonkeratinized introitus and vulva structures. The introitus extends from the mons to the perianal areas and has 3 vulvar openings that are visible.

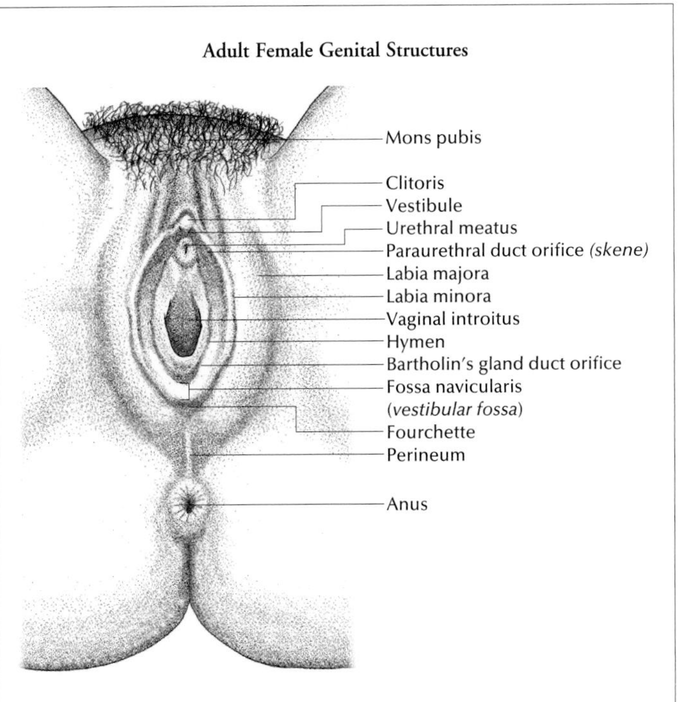

Figure 2-1. *The genital structures of the adult female.*

The *mons pubis* is the rounded fleshy prominence created by underlying adipose tissue that lies over the pubic symphysis bone (**Figure 2-2**). The area is covered in keratinized skin and, at puberty, with hair that persists throughout life. Evidence demonstrates that this anatomical area is typically not injured during sexual assault or rape because the mons pubis is exterior to and located superior to the vestibular area. The bone of the mons pubis also protects the internal sexual and reproductive organs.

The *vulva* is a general term for an area that includes the mons pubis, clitoris and prepuce, labia minora and majora, vestibule (or introitus) and its contents, posterior fourchette, and fossa navicularis. Postmenopausal women lacking estrogen can develop a condition called *lichen sclerosus* (**Figure 2-3**). This chronic skin disorder has a predilection for the vulva. The typical lesions of lichen sclerosus are white plaques, often with areas of bruising and ulceration. The vulvar architecture may be disfigured or destroyed with scarring that results in adhesion of the clitoral prepuce tissue, reabsorption of the labia minora, and narrowing of the lumen of the vagina. Symptoms of lichen sclerosus include chronic itching, burning, and soreness of the vulvar area. There often is splitting of the vulvar skin, causing stinging, pain, inflammation, swelling, and risk for common skin infections. The skin becomes fragile and pale white in appearance. These skin changes often cause difficulties with sexual intercourse. Lichen sclerosus must be followed closely, as 3% to 6% of women with the disorder develop vulvar cancer.

The *vestibule* is an area without hair. Although the area is labeled "external genitalia" in many texts, the vestibule is actually internal to the visible structures of the lateral surfaces of the labia major (eg, skin). The internal structures of the vestibule are covered with mucous membrane, and the area contains the openings of the vagina, urethra, and Skene's and Bartholin's glands. The vestibule border is the margin of the mucous membrane and skin and includes the lateral surfaces of the clitoral hood, the inner surfaces of the labia major, and posterior fourchette (also called posterior commissure or Hart's Line).

The *clitoral hood* or prepuce is a structure in the vestibule that is a fold of skin covering the clitoris. It is homologous with the foreskin in the male. The hood/prepuce that covers the clitoris varies in size and must be retracted to observe clearly. This is best accomplished with a modified labial separation technique. The technique requires the examiner to use the dorsal surface of the index and middle finger of the dominant hand to spread the labia minora and with an upward motion, exposing the urethra and the surface of the glans clitoris by retracting the prepuce. The examiner should never touch the glans exposed with this technique. Note any injury and collect any trace evidence left under the clitoral hood. This area is subject to erythema and edema from contact with irritants, poor hygiene, or trauma.

The *clitoris* is a small, cylindrical, bulbous structure capable of erection at the anterior portion of the vulva, covered by the clitoral hood or prepuce (**Figure 2-4**). It is normally 3 to 6 cm in size and is the most sensitive part of the female genital anatomy.[2] The clitoris consists of stratified squamous cell epithelium with a rich supply of nerve endings.[3] With stimulation, the clitoris enlarges and may protrude from under the prepuce.

Additional considerations for the forensic examiner include the cultural practice of infibulation or piercing. Since ancient times, infibulation is a procedure performed primarily on males worldwide, but the practice fell by the wayside when circumcision became the norm after the 19th century[4]; however, some third-world cultures continue to perform infibulation-type procedures on young females in a process where the clitoris is cut, modified, or mutilated, either in part or wholly. Infibulation remains illegal in the United States and in other parts of the world. When the effect of infibulation is seen in health care settings, the genital modification may have been performed for religious or cultural purposes. Health care providers should recognize the appearance of and rationale for the modified anatomical presentations along with the implications for health.[5]

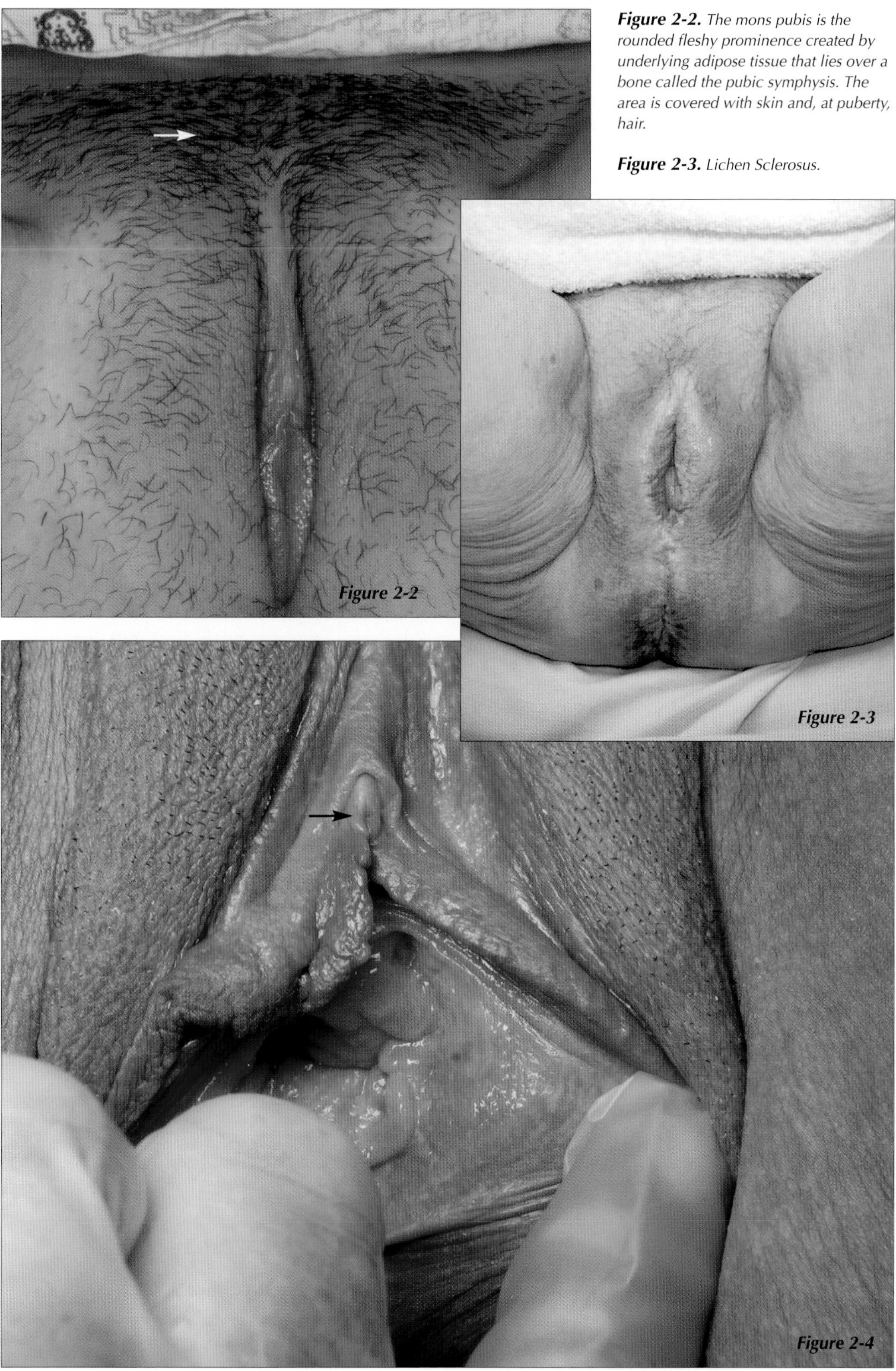

Figure 2-2. *The mons pubis is the rounded fleshy prominence created by underlying adipose tissue that lies over a bone called the pubic symphysis. The area is covered with skin and, at puberty, hair.*

Figure 2-3. *Lichen Sclerosus.*

Figure 2-4. *The clitoris is smooth, pink, and partially covered by the prepuce.*

Piercing of the clitoris is becoming increasingly popular, and early evidence reports increased desire by women who pierce (**Figures 2-5**).[6] Clitoral piercing may not be anatomically advisable as the clitoral structure must be substantial enough to support the jewelry because downward pull on the clitoral hood can constrict erect tissue and result in injury to the nerves. Most women are not suitable candidates for this piercing for this reason.[7] Another common type of piercing that the health care provider may encounter is the navel piercing (**Figures 2-6**).

Competent nursing care is more than simply noting the presence or absence of body piercings or modifications. It should include accurate assessment, cultural sensitivity, and related patient education for treatment challenges during trauma or postassault care.

Vestibular bands (also called urethral ligaments) are structures that support the urethra and are often confused with adhesive scarring. When unrecognized, some examiners have labeled the finding as scars from sexual abuse. These bands can be difficult to see if there is significant estrogen effect, injury, or infectious discharge present. When seen, these bands are usually symmetrical, found in pairs, and attached to the pubic symphysis area.[8,9] The vestibular bands not only support the urethra, they also support the pelvic floor.[10]

Urethral meatus is a location on the urethra that encircles the lumen of the external opening of the urethral tube (**Figure 2-7**). The urethra connects the urinary bladder to the urethral meatus for the purpose of releasing urine. This opening in the female is located in the anterior vestibule, which is external to the hymen, and can be difficult to locate. Females with varying degrees of hypospadius can also present challenges to the examiner. Hypospadius is the result of congenital and/or genetic conditions when the urethral opening is located adjacent to or in the vagina

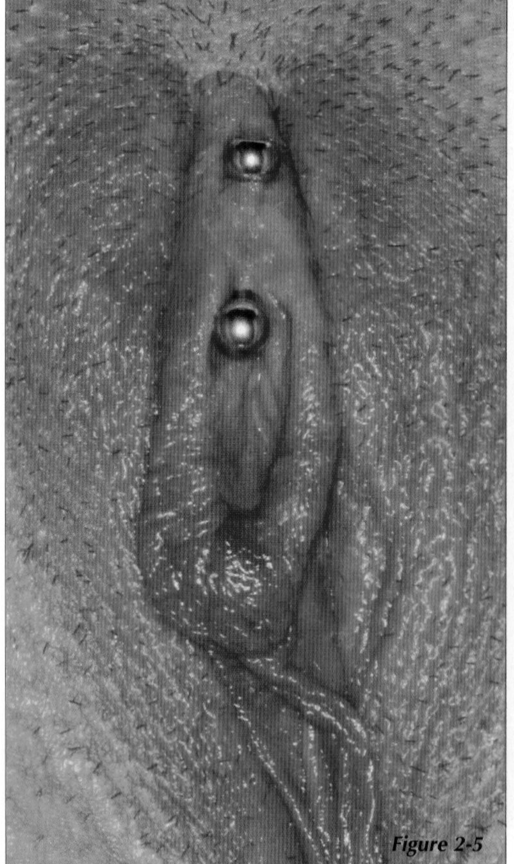

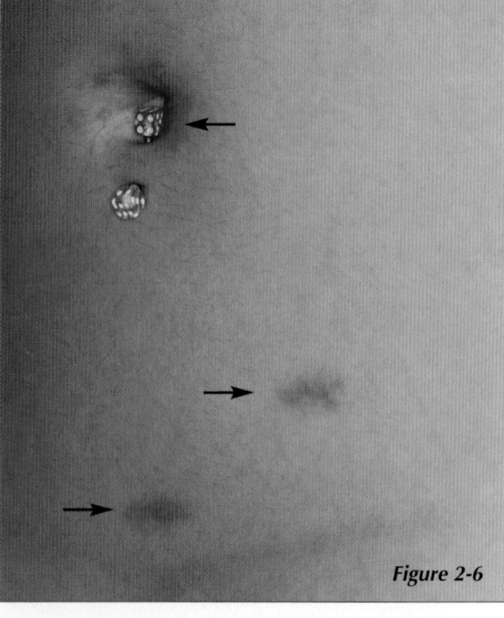

Figure 2-5. *Shaved genital area with prepuce hood piercing.*

Figure 2-6. *This is a navel piercing. The lower abdomen shows 2 old scars from laparoscopic surgery.*

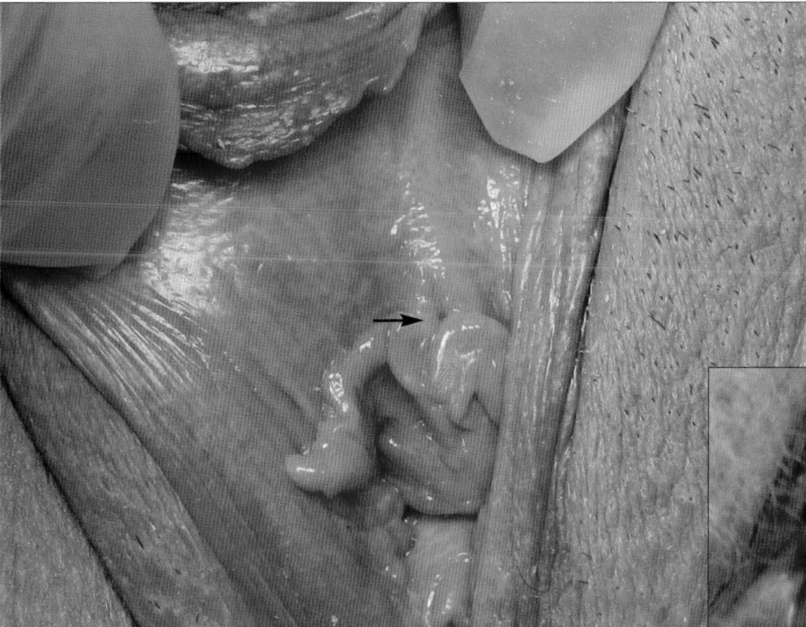

Figure 2-7. *The urethral meatus is superior to the hymen and vaginal orifice. In this photograph, the examiner has lifted the tissue to expose the opening.*

Figure 2-8. *This is a herniation of the urethra, creating a urethrocele. The urethrocele is a direct result of weakening pelvic ligaments and stretching of the urethral body, readily seen in older females or females with multiple births.*

inferior to the hymen, and not the vestibule. Lateral retraction of the labia majora frequently will dilate the urethral meatus allowing for better visualization and catheterization of this structure. The periurethral area is located around and adjacent to the urethra. Urethrocele is a direct result of stretching and weakening pelvic ligaments that support the urethral body (**Figure 2-8**). When the urethra is not supported by the muscles and tissues around it, it can curve, widen, or become herniated. This is called a urethrocele. It is common for a bladder herniation (cystocele) to develop along with a urethrocele. This is because the pubo-cervical fascia is damaged or torn during childbirth or there is a genetic weakening of the fascia. Both types of urinary herniations can press against the wall of the vagina, creating a balloon-like appearance (**Figure 2-9-a** and **b**). When the superior vaginal membrane is bulging, inexperienced examiners may mistake this finding as a sign of trauma, including early hematoma (without discoloration). Finally, cystocele and urethrocele are different from urethral prolapse. Urethral prolapse is a condition with unknown causes seen frequently in 4-year-old African American girls and less often in other ages and races. The urethral lining protrudes from the urethral meatus resulting in a "donut-shaped" circle of tissue around the meatus. In some cases, the urethral tissue is traumatized as a result of exposure to external factors and will appear beefy red to necrotic; however, when protected from the external environment, the condition may go undetected until seen by the examiner. Both injured and uninjured urethral prolapse are easily treated, when indicated, with external application of estrogen.

Paraurethral ductal openings (Skene's glands) are located inferior and slightly posterior to the urethra in the female. Their rudimentary glands are located near the neck of the bladder. They are derived embryologically from the same tissues that differentiate to become the prostate gland in males.[11]

Normal Female Pelvic Anatomy

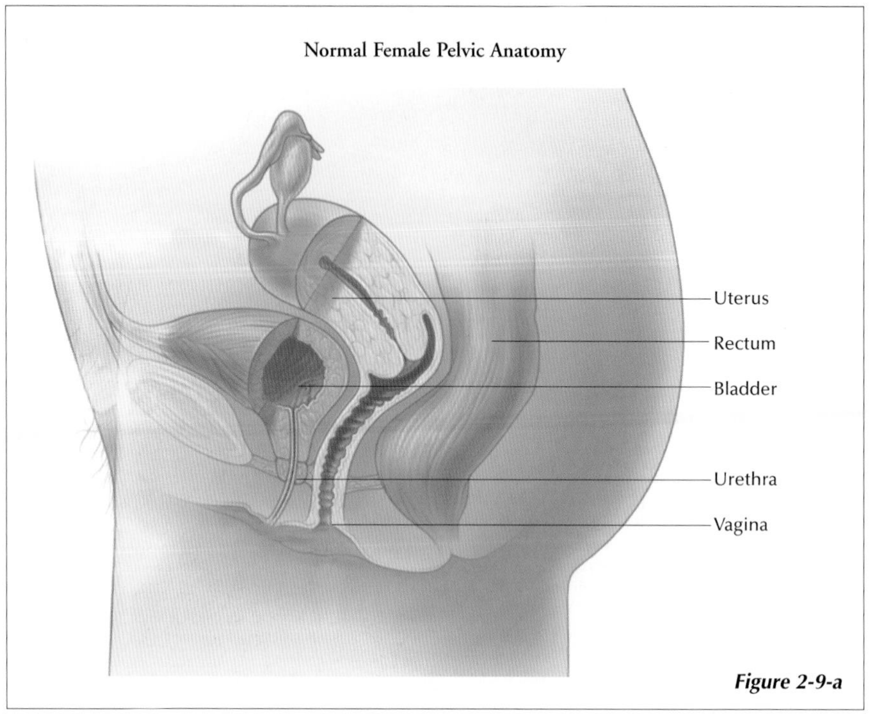

Figure 2-9-a

Urethrocele with Moderate Cystocele

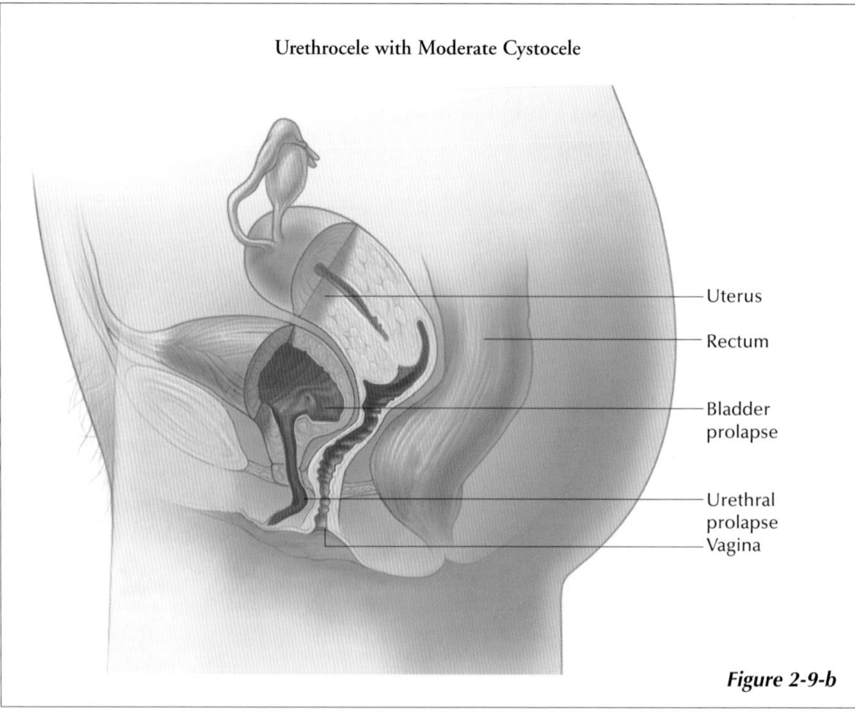

Figure 2-9-b

Figure 2-9-a *and* ***b.*** *The urethra is the tube that carries urine from the bladder to the outside of the body. When the urethra is not well supported by the muscles and tissues around it, it can curve and widen. This is called a urethral prolapse. It is common for a bladder prolapse to develop along with a urethral prolapse. Both kinds of prolapse can press against the wall of the vagina. Reprinted with permission from Proprietory Rights Notice. Copyright 2007 Healthwise, Incorporated, PO Box 1989, Boise, Idaho 83701. Copying of any portion of this material is not permitted without express written permission of HEALTHWISE, Incorporated.*

The *labia majora* (**Figure 2-10**) are the two folds of skin on either side of the labia minora. This area is usually covered with hair that appears during puberty. In some females of African and Mediterranean descent, pubic hair also appears along the medial labia majora and central labial fold, and over the mons as much as a year before puberty; some females have sparse but thickened hair over the entire surface of the mons and labia throughout their lives. While many of these presentations will be normal, the precocious appearance of hair outside the parameters of expected appearance deserve a referral to an endocrinologist to eliminate pathology associated with early appearance of pubic hair. Today many adolescents and adults cut hair designs or shave bald this part of their genital area. The labia majora is covered with squamous epithelium and is less sensitive than the labia minora.[3]

The skin of the labia majora forms the lateral boundaries of the vulva and vestibule and includes all surfaces covered by mucous membrane, including the inner aspects of the labia majora. The labia majora meet at the midline, providing a mechanical barrier that protects the internal structures of the genitalia, including the medial aspects of the labia majora, the vestibule, vulva, labia minora, clitoris, clitoral prepuce, frenulum structures, urethra and periurethral areas, Skene's glands, vagina, hymen, fossa navicularis, anterior, lateral and posterior commissure, and the posterior fourchette. It is important to point out that the term *external genitalia* is a misnomer that includes all the distal internal structures of the genitalia (noted above) and that the only true external portion of the genitalia is the lateral aspects of the labia majora that are not covered by mucous membrane and are visible without separation of the labia majora. Forensic examiners should be aware of the language discrepancy and the local laws that define rape. Explanations about what is external and internal should be addressed in education programs for health care providers and interprofessional forensic personnel.

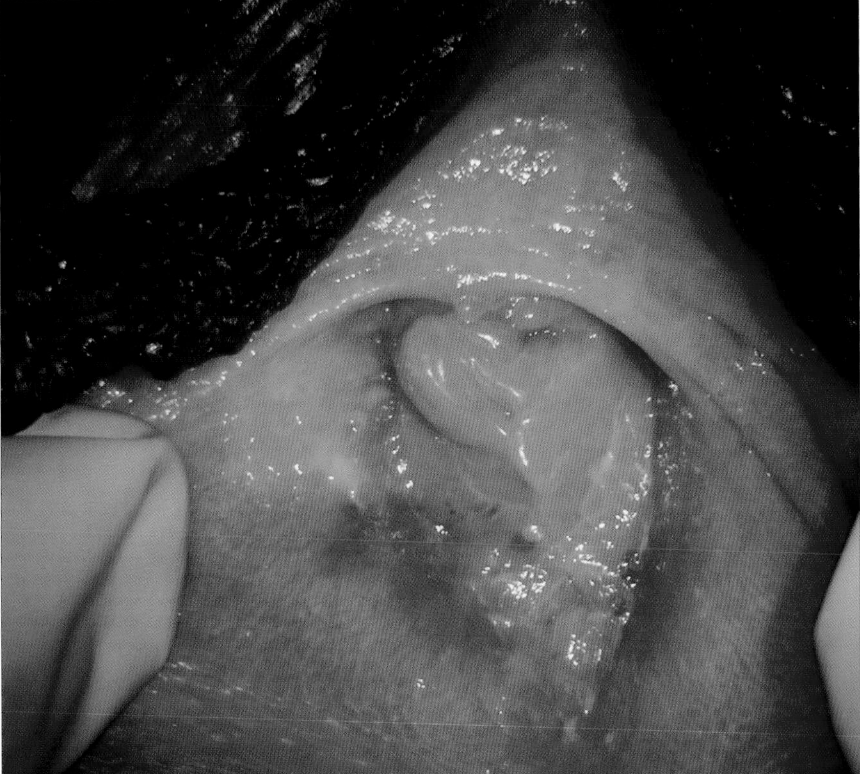

Figure 2-10. *Labial majora separation with an estrogenized pale closed hymen, and scattered focal redness is noted from 3 to 9 o'clock on the fossa navicularis hymen sulcus area. A follow-up examination can confirm if the finding is bruising.*

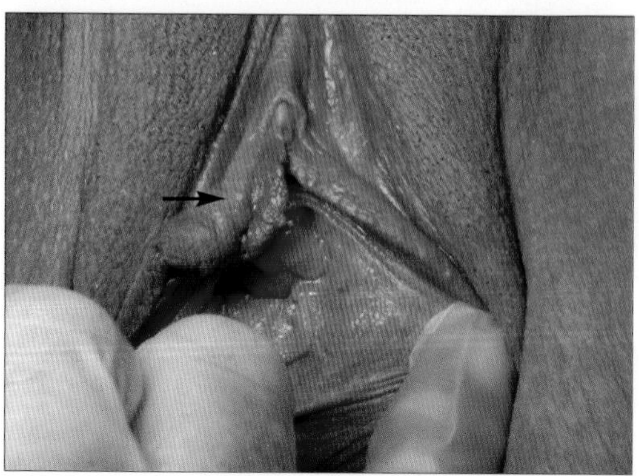

Figure 2-11. *The right labia minora represents the hyperplastic response to hormonal influence during the reproductive phase of life; it is normal to have variations in size and appearance of the labia minora. However, when injury is suspected, the examiner should determine with a follow-up evaluation if it is hyperplastic response or swelling.*

The *labia minora* are the longitudinal, thin folds of nonkeratinized skin medial to the labia majora. The labia minora are hairless but have many sensory nerve endings. The labia minora are located in the vestibule and meet midline in the adult female. In children and infants, the labia minora often terminate at the 3 o'clock and 9 o'clock positions of the vestibule, only to enlarge during puberty, meeting at the midline of the posterior fourchette. Labia minora regress again in the menopausal female. This outer area is covered with keratinized epithelium.[12]

The function of the labia minora is twofold. First, the location and position during normal activity protect the inner structures of the vestibule, including the urethra, hymen, and vaginal outlet. Second, the tissue becomes erect with stimulation. During the human sexual response, the labia minora become engorged (thickened) and elevated, opening the lumen of the vagina in preparation for penetration of the vaginal vault.[11,13] The incidence of injury to this structure following a complaint of rape is second only to the posterior fourchette,[14] but the reasons why are largely unknown.

During puberty and throughout reproductive age, the labia minora may enlarge asymmetrically (**Figure 2-11**). This is due to a hypertrophic and hyperplastic response of the tissue to estrogen. It is important that the examiner not confuse this normal presentation for some sign of past or recent trauma.[15,16] In obvious hyperplastic response to estrogen, the examiner should lift and gently stretch the flap of tissue to examine all surfaces of this structure for trauma.

Bartholin's glands are small and located adjacent to the vaginal opening within the labia minora at the 5 o'clock and 7 o'clock positions. They can produce several drops of lubrication when stimulated. They also contribute to the moisture for the vulva. The gland is frequently the site of swelling when infected.

The Hymen

The *hymen* is named after Hymenaeus, the Greek god of marriage and weddings. Girardin et al describes the hymen as a collar or semicollar of tissue surrounding the vaginal orifice.[10] Crowley describes hymenal tissue as comprising of fibrous bands covered by epithelium composed of squamous cells.[15] The hymen structure is the least understood of the genital structures. Evidence reveals that the hymen is not an indicator of virginity nor can an examiner tell if an individual is a virgin. It is not unusual for the inexperienced health care provider to refer a patient to the forensic nurse in sexual assault care to evaluate the hymen because it is thought to be "gone" or "not intact." Myths about the hymen abound, and it is not an uncommon, albeit mistaken, belief that once a female has been penetrated by a penis during intercourse, the hymen no longer exists.

Some cultures view the female as property whose value is diminished when the hymen is injured and may consider that a female is not marriageable if she does not have an intact hymen. The terms *intact* and *intact hymen* in medical journals are defined as an absence of injury in the hymen. But *intact* implies property value that is attached to the female's body part rather than the female person (eg, intact is good, not intact or ruptured is bad and not valued; even "dirty" or "unclean"). In addition, the language about the hymen is burdened with significant and differing cultural meanings throughout the world. For these reasons, the words *intact, intact hymen, virgin,* or *virginal* should not be used by forensic nurses and physicians to describe the hymen in any medical or medicolegal documentation.[17] The terms *intact, virginal,* or *marital hymen* are inexact and confusing terms. The examiner should not use this terminology for identification of the type of hymen. The examiner should document a description of the hymen and surrounding structures in order to create a visual picture of the area. Early evaluators of patients complaining of sexual assault recognized this, and the evidence demonstrates a trend away from the use of these words in documentation by forensic nurses and physicians in sexual assault care.[18]

The hymen membrane separates the vulva from the distal vaginal vault. The physical appearance changes with (1) age, (2) positioning during evaluation, and (3) the degree of relaxation of the patient.[1] When exposed, the tissue responds to estrogen with hypertrophic (eg, larger cells) and hyperplastic (eg, more cells) growth, producing a structure that may be larger than the vulva space available. A folding results in redundancy of appearance, making evaluation of the margins difficult.

The hymen's appearance also changes throughout the life span. The effects of estrogen on the tissue are predictable, caused by activation of the hormonal cycles that provide a response in the physical receptors in the hymen and surrounding tissue (**Figure 2-12** and **Table 2-1**). The maximum visible effect of estrogen is most evident on a female at

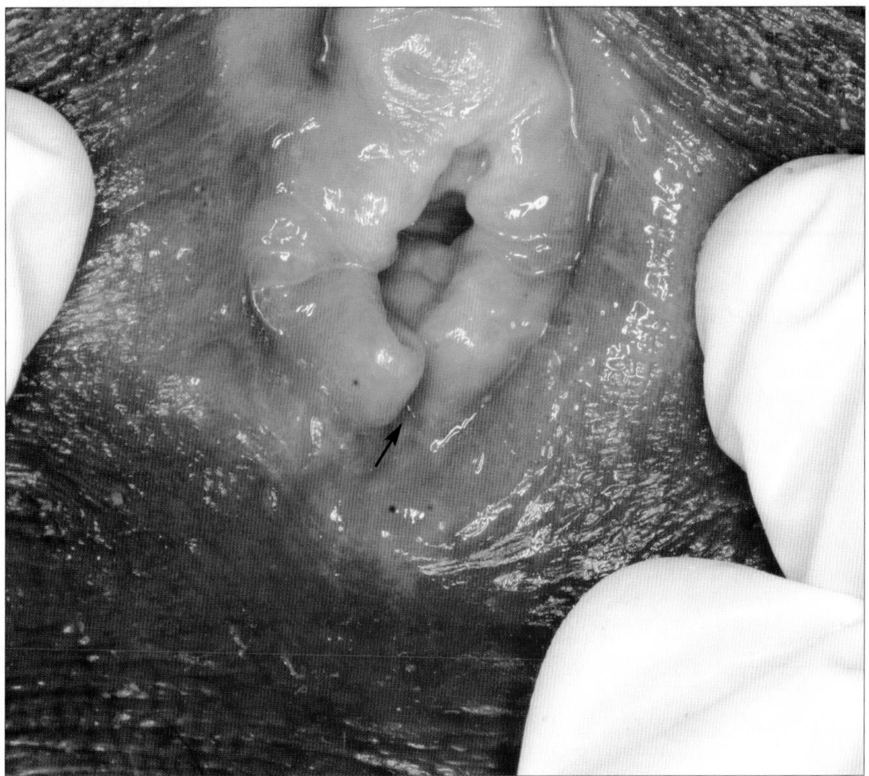

Figure 2-12. *Hymen tissue appearance is different both in shape and size, and the appearance changes throughout the life cycle. This hymen is fully estrogenized with irregularities visible at 3, 6, and 9 o'clock. The irregular appearance could represent a redundancy in a fold at 3 and 9 o'clock or a tear at 6 o'clock. Further evaluation of each of these areas would be necessary to determine if there is healed injury.*

birth and during the reproductive years, particularly with pregnancy.[19,20] The appearance may also be influenced, even changed, by minor and major penetrating injury to the tissue.[20,21] For instance, without the influence of estrogen, the hymen is generally thin tissue that may tear easily or slough after injury and lack of capillary structures. The injury creates a void where hymen tissue previously existed. Evidence demonstrates that the tissue will *anastomose* when approximated, either surgically or accidentally during healing, creating a unique appearance for the individual. With estrogen stimulation, tissue that appears to be gone in a prepubertal state will "magically" reappear with estrogen stimulation. This phenomenon is due to the hypertrophic and hyperplastic response of the tissue to hormonal influence.[22] In these types of cases, if routine screening by the primary health care provider determines the hymen type and estrogenic phase, then a critical determination of penetrating injury can be made after assault. Many providers who work with victims of sexual assault believe that this type of routine screening of the hymen in the pediatric patient is as important as immunizations, height, and weight.[23] However, in the medical literature, there is no consistent description for hymen membrane at all stages of development.

The Hymen Estrogen Response Scale (HERS) is a useful tool in evaluating changes to the hymen and surrounding structures related to developmental and cyclic changes throughout the life span.[20,24] While not previously available, literature has described elements supporting the assumptions listed in **Table 2-1**, and the assumptions support the need for development of an easy to use descriptive tool that results in consistency among providers in the documentation of a description of the hymen and surrounding tissue.

Table 2-1. Hymen Tissue Response to Estrogen

Response
— *Estrogen effect* is clinically absent at certain developmental ages.
— Maternal estrogen effect is present at birth until age 2-3 in hymenal, vaginal, and uterine tissue.
— A reduction in estrogen results in thinning of the hymenal tissue circumferentially and narrowing of the hymen laterally.
— Estrogen creates a response in the tissue resulting in hypertrophy and hyperplasia of the hymen, vagina, and vestibular tissues.
— Estrogen reduces sensitivity to palpation of the vestibular structures, hymen, and vagina.
— Physiological discharge (leukorrhea) is present with estrogenized tissue.
— Estrogen levels decrease after birth and increase during puberty throughout the child bearing years only to diminish with aging.
— Exogenous estrogens have been used medically to enhance the healing process.
— Vagina pH becomes more acidic with estrogen and more basic in the absence of estrogen.
— The acid base of the vestibule and vagina change from acidic at birth to basic in early childhood, to acidic in puberty and throughout reproductive years, and finally to basic in menopause.
— Bacterial and glycogen counts increase with estrogen and decrease in the absence of estrogen.

Using the Huffman Scale as a model from birth to puberty, the HERS was developed as a descriptive tool for use with females throughout the cycles and at any stage of development, including menopause.[20] The ordinal HERS for estrogen effect on the hymen was developed in 1998 and validated in 2001 at a large mid-south SANE program, and assessments from HERS have been used to explain injury patterns in females. The ordinal HERS described the appearance in color and thickness of the tissue, motion and pain, and discharge of the female hymen and surrounding tissue. Using the ordinal HERS Levels, 100 photographs of female vulva and hymen were randomly chosen from the patient files in 2001. The patients ranged in age from 2 weeks to 87 years. Three expert SANE nurse practitioners (eg, 1 FNP, 1 ANP, 1 PNP) with over 50 years combined clinical experience as advanced practice nurses were blinded to score the photographs using the ordinal HERS Levels. There was 97% inter-rater reliability in scoring when using the descriptive classifications among the raters. Once validated, the tool was implemented in the large mid-south agency; however, use of the tool among providers at the same agency with less experience or education resulted in increased variance among providers using the HERS. While variance is expected between raters, it was soon discovered that there was lack of understanding about the tool by some nonadvanced practice-prepared SANEs that resulted in several menopausal octogenarian females classified as fully estrogenized. While not impossible, being fully estrogenized at 80 years of age is unlikely. The variation in use and understanding among SANEs was the impetus for development of a new method for staging the hymen and vestibular structures. In 2006, a numerical HERS was developed and validated with 10 content expert nurse practitioners and SANEs with greater than 1000 medical and sexual assault and abuse evaluations of females of all ages.[24] Feedback was incorporated into the current HERS, and it was introduced to forensic nurses at an international meeting for use in their programs.[25] Again, the need for conversion to a numerical tool was based on the belief that, like other numerical tools (eg, Apgar, Glascow), the HERS would be easy to learn and use, the inter-rater variability would be minimized, and reliability could be established.[24] Pre- and posttests demonstrated ease of use of the tool in one session. Validation studies are currently underway.

The HERS scores are 0, 1, or 2 and describe 5 variables including color, thickness, lubrication, distensibility, and sensitivity. The score of 0 reflects the assignment of characteristics expected when estrogen is in low amounts or absent. Scores between 0 and 10 are assigned when there is variability in characteristics when varying levels of estrogen are present and other unknown variables, such as genital changes throughout the life span, cyclic variability, medications, and activities that impact the appearance of the hymen and surrounding tissues. A score of 10 implies the presence of characteristics expected in the presence of high levels of estrogen (eg, pregnancy). The entire scale is demonstrated in **Table 2-2**.

The HERS scored items are added up to create a total score. The score determines the level of estrogen effect as noted in the table. To date, when intentional and unintentional injury is not circumferential, the HERS has been used to evaluate pain (currently mandated by the Joint Commission), explain pain and bleeding in vulvar disease, and explain bleeding following consensual intercourse.[26] It has been anecdotally reported that forensic nurses in sexual assault care are using it to evaluate and treat pain in patients before catheterization in emergency rooms.

Once the female enters reproductive age, the hymen will stretch, but the amount of stretch varies individually. For the purpose of quality assurance and peer review, the visible effects of estrogen in a photograph may give a clue as to the distensibility of the

Table 2-2. Hymen Estrogen Response Scale and Scoring

VARIABLE	0	1	2	SCORE
Color	Red	Pink	White	
Thickness	Translucent	Partial translucency	No translucency	
Lubrication	None/Scant clear	Scant white caked	Clear to white mucous	
Distensibility	None – flat	Some folds/scallops	Redundancy/layers	
Sensitivity	Painful to touch	Sensitive to touch	No pain to touch	
			HERS Score TOTAL	

SCORE	HERS INTERPRETATION
0-1	No estrogen effect (NEE)
2-4	Early transition (ET)
5-7	Late transition (LT)
8-10	Full estrogen effect (FEE)

hymen.[20] When using photographs for evaluation of estrogen effects, be sure to evaluate the photograph for clarity, naturalness, color, and usefulness.[27] Certain hormones (Depo-Provera), medications (Tamoxifen), and activities (exercise) can diminish the protective effects of estrogen.[28] Therefore, a hymen membrane that is exposed and responds to estrogen during the reproductive years is not expected to have injury when stretched during penetration with tampons or fingers, nor significant injury—if any at all—when stretched by a penis or other items (**Figure 2-13**). Conversely, the elder postmenopausal female may have pain and injury following penetration even in consensual intercourse that includes the vulva, hymen, and vagina, made worse when there is an absence of endogenous/exogenous estrogens. The hymen's capacity for distensibility and stretch before tearing is demonstrated in populations of reproductive

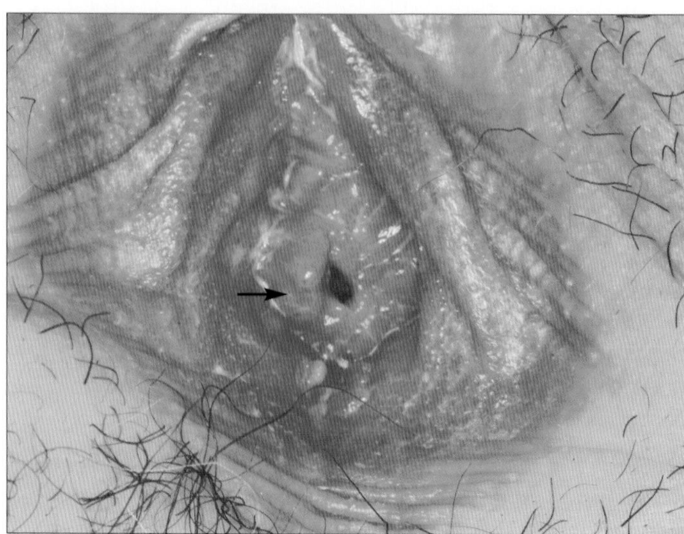

Figure 2-13. *Annular hymen fully estrogenized in a 21-year-old female. Tampon, finger, and penis were inserted into the vagina 12 hours ago. This has resulted in an increase in redness. The diminishing of redness can be evaluated in a follow-up evaluation to determine if it is related to the complaint.*

females; however, the capacity for stretch is unique to the individual and cannot be predicted for the court in an individual or single case without knowledge of the pre-existing presentation. When slight force is used, injury may be explained if there is an absence of estrogen, as in the menopausal woman or child. When there is significant evidence of the effect of estrogen, force may be the only explanation for minor injury to the hymen and surrounding structures. Hence, evidence demonstrates that the hymen is not the most common site of injury in sexual assault.[14] Consensual intercourse may also produce evidence of injury[26,29-31]; therefore, the forensic nurse in sexual assault care must not only consider the maturation of the hymen in response to estrogen, but also consider the patient's history when forming nursing diagnoses and treatment because the risks for disease and pregnancy, upheaval in the core family structure, and mental health sequelae are considerable.

Hymenal Types

The hymen has multiple appearances reflecting differing shapes and configurations. The forensic nurse in sexual assault care must be aware of all possible presentations (**Figures 2-14-a** through **e**).

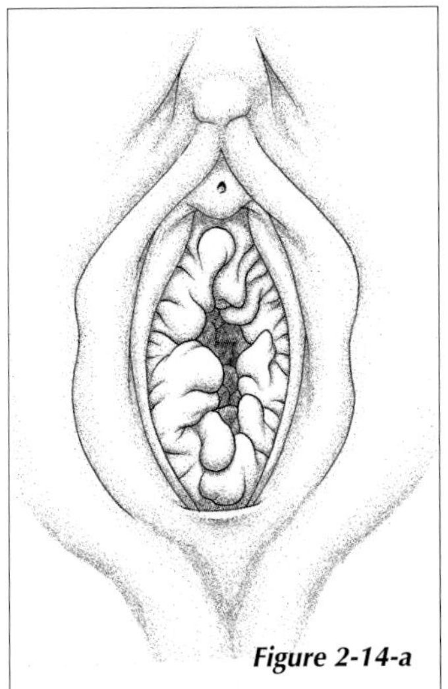

Figure 2-14-a

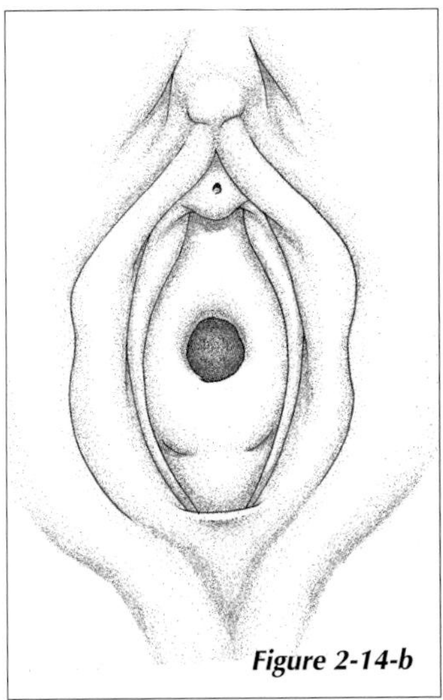

Figure 2-14-b

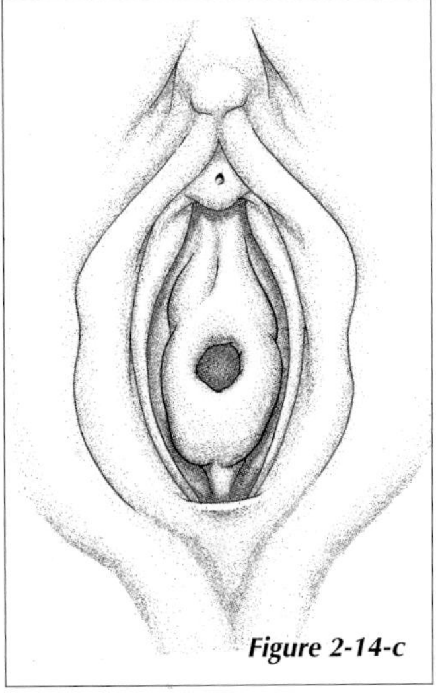

Figure 2-14-c

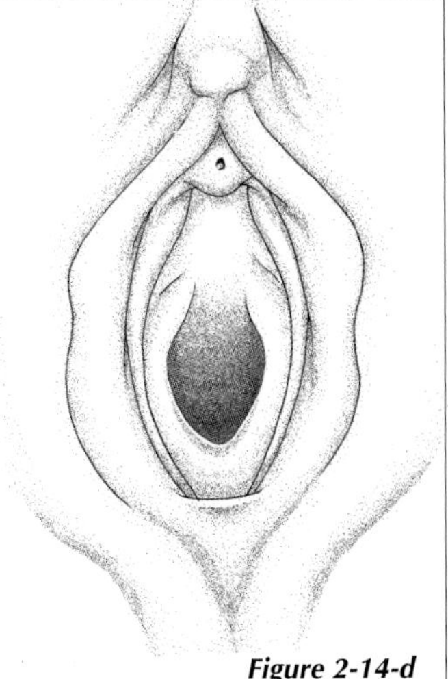

Figure 2-14-d

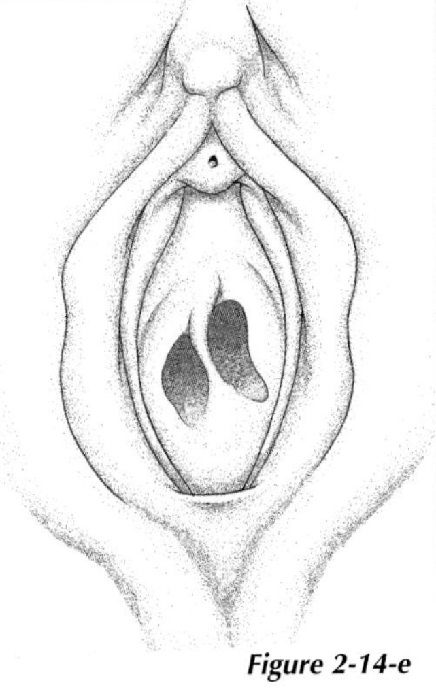

Figure 2-14-e

Figures 2-14-a. *A fimbriated or denticular hymen orifice diagram.*

Figures 2-14-b. *The annular hymen orifice diagram.*

Figures 2-14-c. *The redundant or sleeve-like hymen orifice diagram.*

Figures 2-14-d. *The crescentic hymen orifice diagram.*

Figures 2-14-e. *The septate hymen orifice diagram.*

The most common type of hymen is annular. An *annular hymen* has tissue that encircles the entire vaginal opening that may or may not connect at the 12 o'clock position.[32] The *cresentric hymen* is the second most common type of hymen. The tissue does not attach in the suburethral area in this type of hymen. Another description might be an open collar where the hymen is present from the 1 o'clock to 11 o'clock position and absent from the 11 o'clock to 1 o'clock position. Emans et al looked at 200 sexually inactive adolescents and found that 62% had annular hymens, and 38% had cresentric hymens; of the latter, 70% were redundant.[32] The absence in redundancy for those evaluated by Emans et al may be related to the amount of estrogen effect noted.[20,32] In addition to *redundancy*, the fully estrogenized hymen can also be labeled as *fimbriated*, with multiple layers and finger-like projections creating an edge or multiple layers. The irregular margins are not due to tearing but rather the estrogen effect on the hymen primarily seen in some adolescents and adults during their reproductive years (**Figure 2-15**). The effect of estrogen changes the hymen appearance and mobility, including its distensibility, thickness, color, lubrication, and sensitivity.[20] Fully estrogenized tissue becomes marginally pale (even bleached in appearance), thickened at the base of the tissue, and redundant. This additional tissue allows for distensibility and stretch without injury. Tissue that is without visible estrogen effect is taut, and flat and may be translucent, reddened with visible capillaries, dry, and sensitive to touch.[20] Transitions throughout hymenal maturation may result in combinations of visibly thick and thin tissue.

For a difficult-to-explain injury, hymens in transition to full estrogenization may injure with minor manipulation (eg, digital penetration) in ways that destroy the thin areas and preserve the thickened areas. This will result in an irregular appearance, possibly with thinning of the tissue from its original thickness from the base. Human subject protections prohibit the study of this particular hypothesis; however, routine evaluations of the hymen in primary care practices could result in the data necessary to evaluate these characteristics. Seminal work to refute the notion of congenital absence of hymen has largely been completed through studies that have evaluated the presence or absence of the hymen in newborns, where the congenital absence of a hymen has never been reported.[19,33]

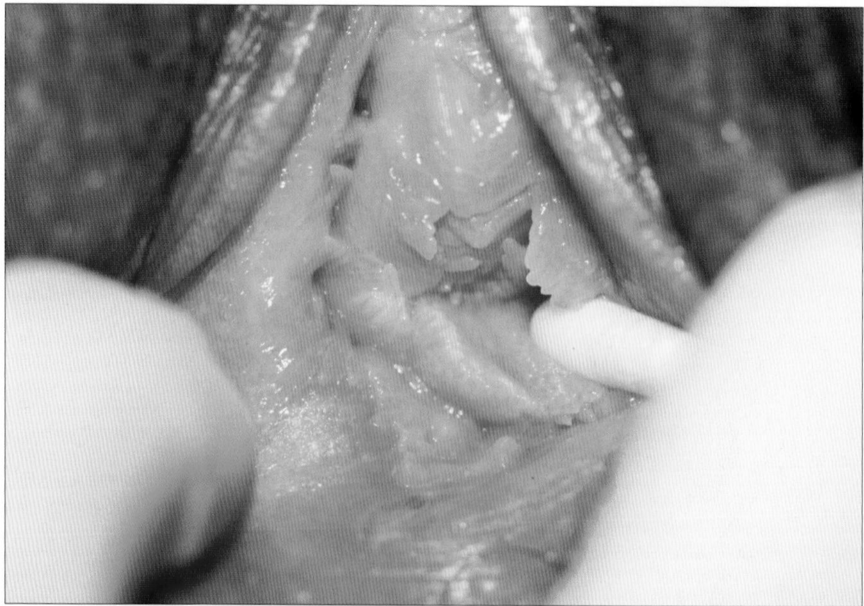

Figure 2-15. *This fully estrogenized hymen can also be labeled as frimbriated with multiple layers and finger-like projections creating an edge. The irregular margins are not due to tearing but are due to the estrogen effect on the hymen primarily seen in some adolescent and adults in their reproductive years.*

The imperforate hymen has been described as a "sealed door" or a piece of tissue that "completely covers" the entrance to the vagina.[10] This is a rare presentation of a medical condition.[34] Rarely, the imperforate hymen is identified at birth or soon thereafter. Most are identified much later when the female begins menstruation.[35] The imperforate hymen has no opening for escape of menstrual blood or vaginal discharge. Typically, patients with this condition are diagnosed with imperforate hymen in the emergency department or in the primary care office of their health care provider after complaints of abdominal pain during adolescence. Treatment may include a lance or puncture of the hymen centrally to allow the discharge to exit the vaginal vault.

Septate hymens have fibrous bands that create two lumen openings; they are seen in children and adolescents and occasionally in the sexually active adult female (**Figure 2-14-e**). A septate hymen is a band of tissue that divides the hymenal lumen and is connected anteriorly to the posterior hymen; the appearance reflects 2 openings into the vaginal vault. This tissue may also be thick and join a vaginal septum. The hymen septum may be torn away after tampon insertion, first-time penile/vaginal intercourse, or some other type of trauma. When discovered, it is always important to refer the patient to a primary physician (eg, family practice or pediatrician), pediatric urologist, or OB/GYN for further evaluation to identify any other anatomical malformations in the genitourinary system. A hymenal tag is a protrusion of hymenal tissue, and the etiology is unknown. Tags are seen in newborns and estrogenized adults. Those tags located at 6 o'clock on the hymen may have been an incomplete septum. Other tags may be a result of incomplete tears or estrogenic hyperplasia. See **Figures 2-16-a** and **b** for examples of hymenal tags.

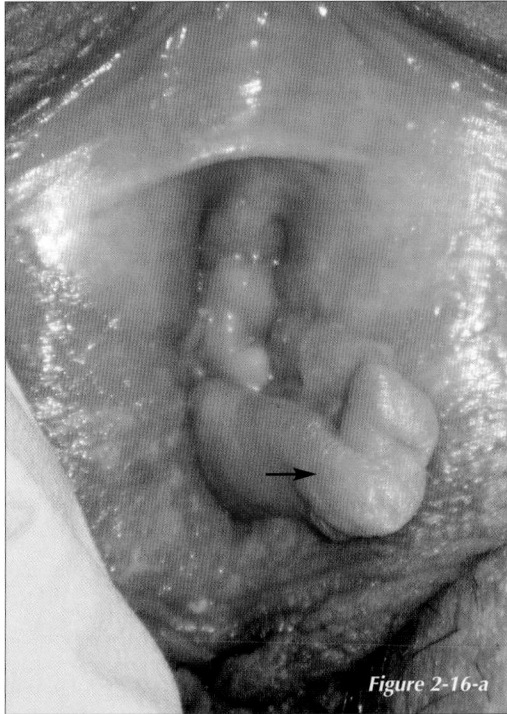

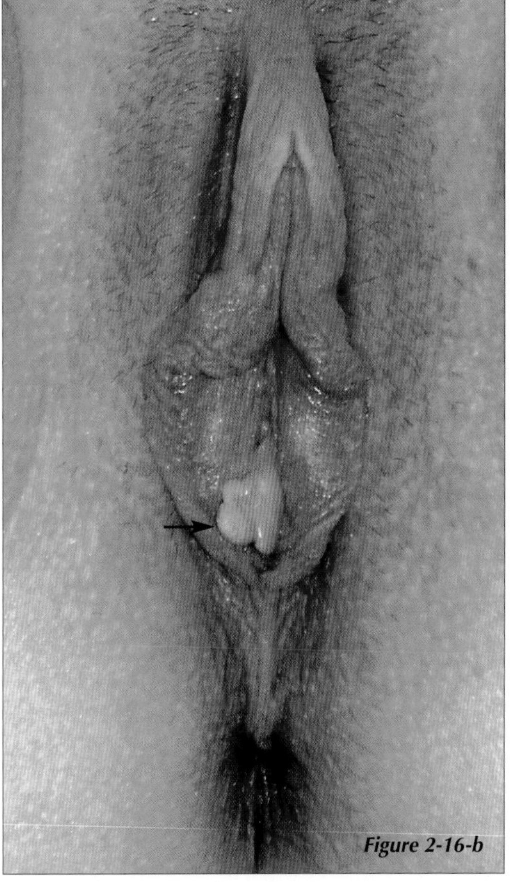

Figure 2-16-a. *In this case of hymenal tag, the patient reported no problems with consensual intercourse or vaginal delivery.*

Figure 2-16-b. *Normal female genitalia with hymenal tag visible externally.*

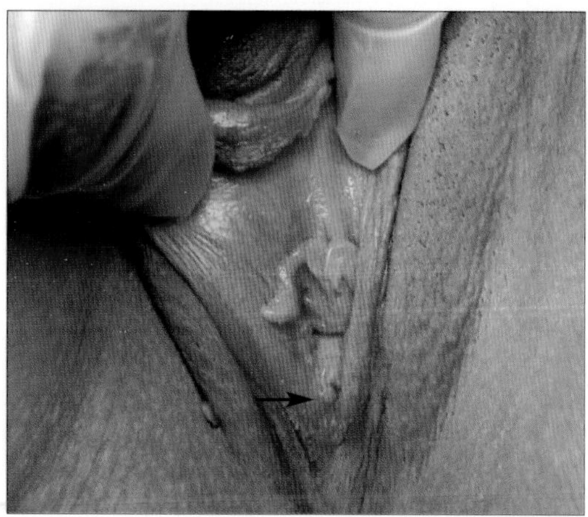

Figure 2-17. *The absence of hymen remnants from 6 to 9 o'clock implies a deeper injury to the hymen membrane during penetration (may be consensual) or vaginal delivery. The periurethral area at 12 o'clock is estrogenized tissue in finger-like projections and implies hymenal tissue, but the tissue could represent estrogenized periurethral tissue. With all these projections, some providers use the term "fimbriation" to describe finger-like projections of the hymen membrane.*

Postinjury Hymen

Injury to the hymen and surrounding structures occurs when the tissue exceeds its capacity to stretch and it tears.[20] Variables, such as amount of force, estrogen effect, and object, will determine the severity and location of the injury in the genital structures. On healing, the hymen is not generally identified in the documentation or even recognized by health care providers. When it is identified, the hymen remnants are called *caruncululae myrtiformis* (**Figure 2-17**). These remnants may be small elevations in the menopausal female or larger rounded or triangular mounds of hymen tissue encircling the vaginal orifice in the reproductive female. Birthing scars create an absence of hymen remnants from the 5 o'clock to 7 o'clock position, but in reality, the absence of hymen in these areas reflects a failure of the perineum to rejoin—usually because the perineum was not stitched after an uncomplicated birth. Hymen tears and subsequent remnants are created from tearing of the tissue and are typically seen in women who have complained of bleeding with their first penile/vaginal intercourse or had one or more vaginal deliveries with tears through the base of the hymen or episiotomy cuts that are not stitched. These areas are easily palpated for scar formation or absence of connective tissue and musculature following significant injury. It is important to remember that hymen tissue that approximates after injury may bond and create a normal appearance to the hymen. McCann et al support this assertion in children and adolescents who were studied to determine healing of the hymen in acute injuries when they were due to penetration following complaints of sexual assault or accident.[36] In this body of work, if there was a complete tear through the hymen, the remnants did not grow back together, and in follow-up exams, the resulting appearance was a transection or defect.

Inspection of the Hymen

The hymen can sometimes be visualized using labial separation (**Figures 2-18** and **2-19**). Labial separation is best used to initially evaluate the flat and minimally folded structures of the introitus (eg, labia minora, urethra, periurethra, pairs of urethral bandings, clitoral hood, and clitoris). Modifying the labial separation technique for examination of the clitoris and under the clitoral hood can result in full visualization of the structures (**Figure 2-20**). The labial separation modification instructs the forensic nurse to use the back of the dominant hand's index and middle finger to lift the internal labia minora and retract the prepuce. It is recommended that the back of the hand be used whenever possible to avoid a "personal touch" during the evaluation.

Labial traction (or labial tunneling) allows the examiner to visualize the area containing the structures of the introitus (**Figure 2-21**). Care should be taken to avoid significant pulling until a full assessment is complete, as iatrogenic injury to the posterior fourchette is a possibility in all females and is difficult to explain in court. The structures visible with labial traction may include the structures visible in labial separation; however, the type of hymen and the presence or absence of an acute or chronic injury, in particular to the fossa navicularis, is best seen using this technique (**Figure 2-22**).[37] In addition, the

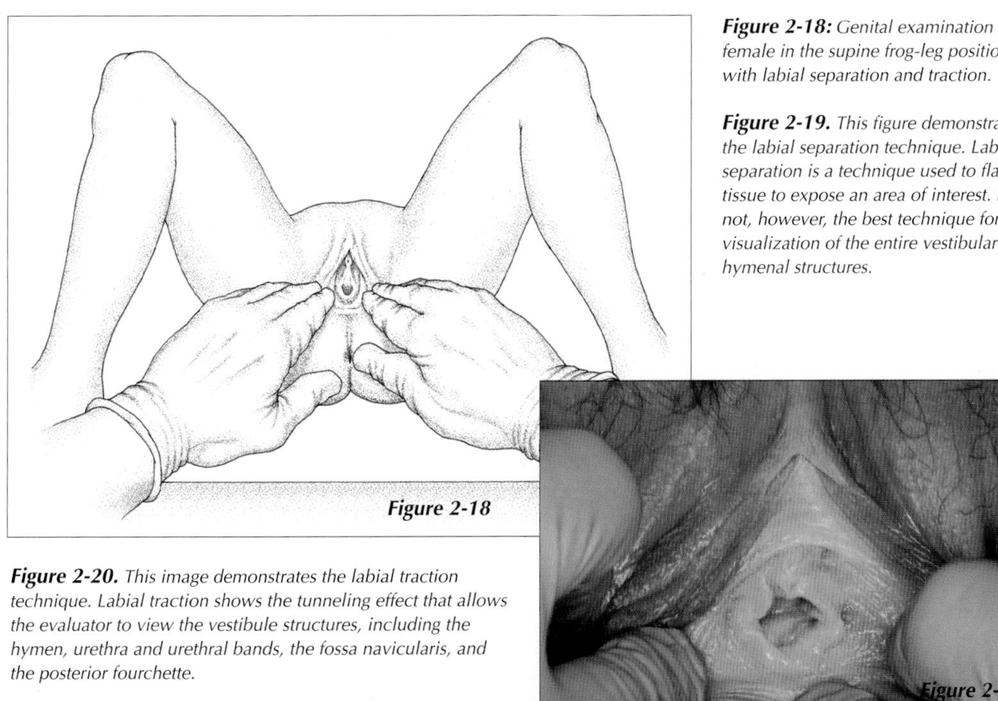

Figure 2-18

Figure 2-18: *Genital examination of the female in the supine frog-leg position with labial separation and traction.*

Figure 2-19. *This figure demonstrates the labial separation technique. Labial separation is a technique used to flatten tissue to expose an area of interest. It is not, however, the best technique for visualization of the entire vestibular and hymenal structures.*

Figure 2-19

Figure 2-20. *This image demonstrates the labial traction technique. Labial traction shows the tunneling effect that allows the evaluator to view the vestibule structures, including the hymen, urethra and urethral bands, the fossa navicularis, and the posterior fourchette.*

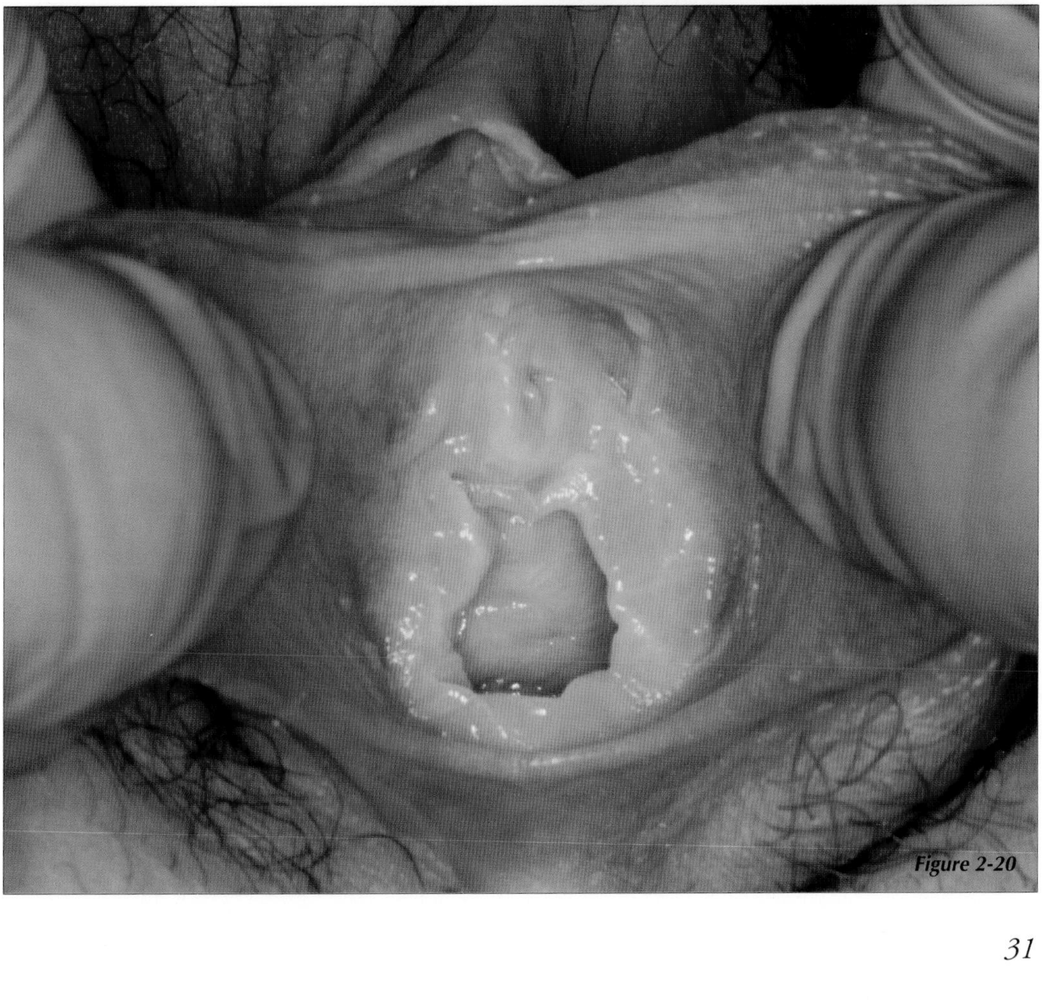

Figure 2-20

labial traction technique flattens the posterior fourchette, fossa navicularis, perineum, and other introital vestibular areas when the patient is in supine lithotomy position and legs in stirrups. In patients who are comfortable with traction, the external urethra will dilate and the pelvic floor will relax exposing the vaginal tissue. In morbidly obese women, labial traction is minimally valuable due to the obstructing adipose tissue, and the labial separation method may need to be used and documented for all aspects of the evaluation. The prone or supine knee-chest, lateral Sims, or lateral decubitus positions are also helpful, but use of the vestibular tunneling technique is difficult in all except the prone knee-chest position. The position chosen should offer the best visualization of the genital area given the patient's physical, emotional, or psychological limitations; and the choice of methods should always be directed toward patient-centered care and comfort. During documentation, the genital structures are described and the position is stated using a fixed imaginary clock for locations of injury, noninjury, or structures. While nurses may vary in the positioning of the clock, a full description will clearly tell those reading or reviewing the report where the injury is located (for example, one may describe the hymen as missing from the 5 o'clock to 7 o'clock position in the supine position using the lateral traction method) (**Figure 2-23**).

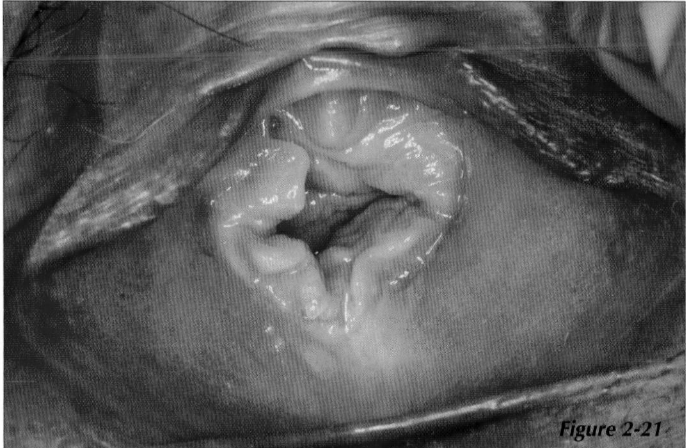

Figure 2-21. *Labial traction exposes an estrogenized, pale, and thick annular hymen and surrounding tissue.*

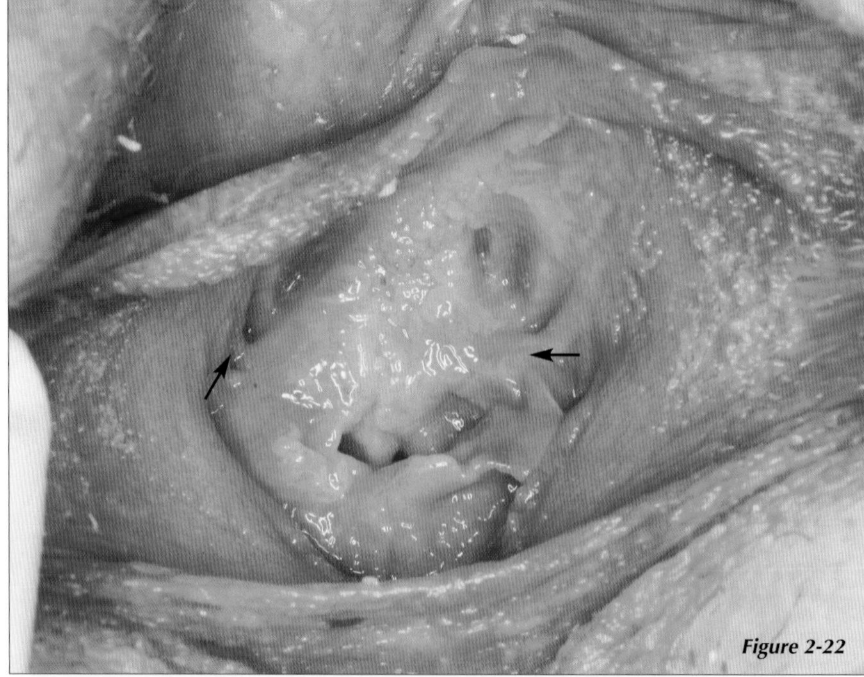

Figure 2-22. *Using labial traction, periurethal vestibular bands are present on both sides of the hymen from 9 to 3 o'clock. These bands support and connect to the vestibular wall.*

The hymen type should be identified, described, and documented in each evaluation of the genitalia in primary care settings (**Figures 2-24-a, b,** and **c**).[38] When the hymen is injured, the type of hymen may not be discoverable because pain or injury prevents full visualization of the tissue using labial traction. In these cases, the patient should return for a follow-up visit not only to document hymen type, but also to assess the healing process.[36,39]

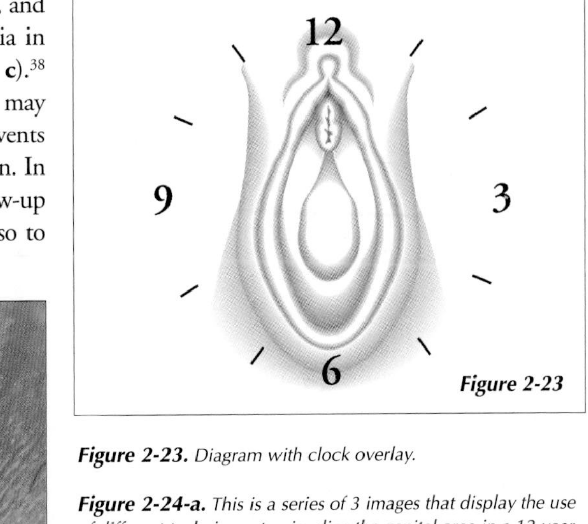

Figure 2-23. Diagram with clock overlay.

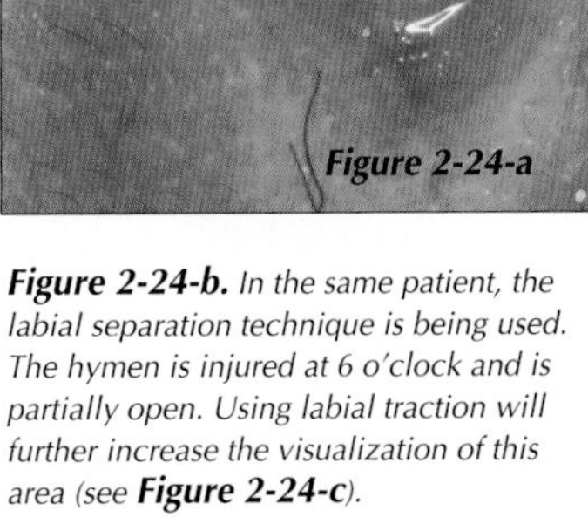

Figure 2-24-a. *This is a series of 3 images that display the use of different techniques to visualize the genital area in a 12-year-old patient who had consensual sex with three 17-year-old males. This image shows the examiner pulling upwards without labial traction or labial separation. The periurethral area is visible, however the hymen is not fully exposed. There is hymen injury seen at 4 o'clock. Further examination techniques will be needed to expose and explore potential injury and to visualize the entire area on this patient.*

Figure 2-24-b. *In the same patient, the labial separation technique is being used. The hymen is injured at 6 o'clock and is partially open. Using labial traction will further increase the visualization of this area (see **Figure 2-24-c**).*

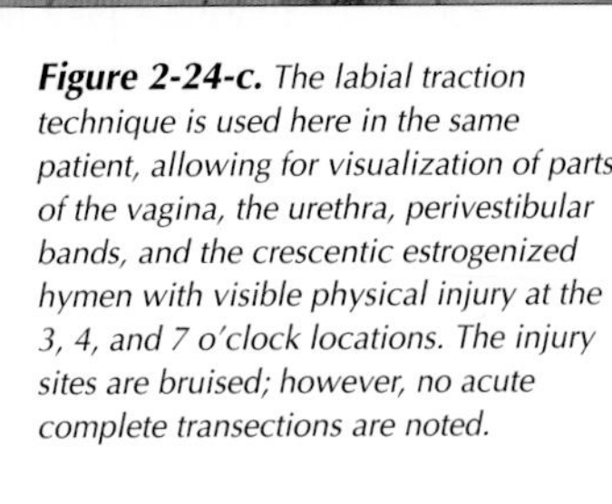

Figure 2-24-c. *The labial traction technique is used here in the same patient, allowing for visualization of parts of the vagina, the urethra, perivestibular bands, and the crescentic estrogenized hymen with visible physical injury at the 3, 4, and 7 o'clock locations. The injury sites are bruised; however, no acute complete transections are noted.*

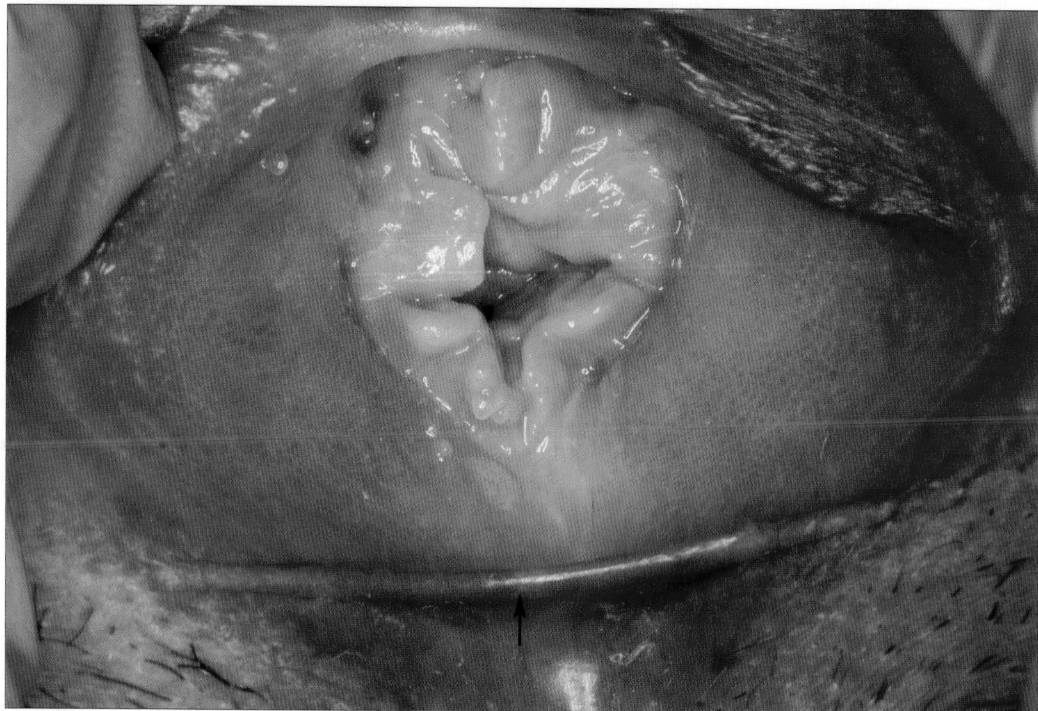

Figure 2-25. *This image highlights the posterior fourchette (also called the posterior commissure or Hart's line).*

Posterior Fourchette

The *posterior fourchette* (also called Hart's line and the posterior commissure) is an area that represents the union of the 2 labia posteriorly (**Figure 2-25**). It is the most frequently injured site in females reporting rape.[14] This location is also often injured in straddle injury in children or consensual sexual penetration in adults.[40] This area typically is the point of first contact with the penis or foreign object when the female is on her back. Tears with consenting or nonconsenting sex are common.[26,41]

The *fossa navicularis* is an area where there is a concavity of the lower part of the vestibule and is posterior and inferior to the hymen corona (**Figure 2-10**). It covers the surface of the introitus area that extends from the base of the hymen to the posterior fourchette between the 5 o'clock and 7 o'clock positions in the supine position. When visualizing this area, the examiner may see that a fully estrogenized, redundant hymen usually obstructs the view. It may be necessary to move the hymen to visualize the complete fossa navicularis in fully estrogenized tissue and determine if there is injury, lack of injury, or evidence to collect.

Female Reproductive Parts

The reproductive organs in the female include the vagina, the cervix, the uterus, the fallopian tubes, and the ovaries. The *vagina* is a muscular, hollow tube that extends from the vaginal opening to the cervix. It is lined by nonkeratinizing, stratified, squamous epithelium that undergoes hormone-related cyclical changes.[42] The vagina does not contain secretion glands, but it is rich with capillaries and veins.[3,43] The vagina is about 8 to 12 cm (3 to 5 inches) long in an adult female. The vagina has muscular walls that allow it to expand and contract. This ability to become wider or narrower is multi-factored across the life span and allows the vagina to accommodate something as slim as a tampon and as large as a baby's head. The *vaginal introitus* is an anatomical area where the pubo-vanalis muscle forms the entrance to the vagina bounded by the internal border of the mons to the perianal areas and has 3 openings that are visible.

Vaginal rugae develop as a result of estrogen receptor stimulation and are a result of hypertrophy and hyperplasia resulting in a redundancy of normal folds of the epithelium. After menopause the vaginal walls will thin significantly and flatten again unless estrogen is replaced.[44] These folds run circumferentially around the vaginal columns that keep it protected and moist. Vaginal columns support the vaginal canal and may be visible. In the adolescent and adult, the pH of vaginal secretions is acidic and normally between 4 and 5. In those without estrogen effect, the vaginal pH is basic, between 7.0 and 8.0. The acidic vaginal pH is thought to be protective against infection and will influence the growth of normal flora.[45-48] This basic vaginal pH is demonstrated by tissue that is pink and may be flat or adherent if scarred. The vagina functions as a receptacle for sexual intercourse, the birth canal, and the route for the menstrual blood and vaginal secretions to be discharged from the body. The outer third of the vagina, especially the area near the vaginal introitus, contains nearly 90% of the vaginal nerve endings and, therefore, is much more sensitive to touch than the inner two-thirds of the vaginal vault.[3] However, if the sensation of pressure is felt and the underlying structure is inflamed, a complaint of pain is likely during palpation or speculum insertion.

The *posterior fornix* is a location adjacent to where the cervix attaches inferiorly to the vagina. This area allows for pooling of discharge and is where the cervix rests in seminal products after intercourse.[11]

The *uterus* is a hollow, thick-walled, pear-shaped, muscular organ between the bladder and rectum. The uterus is held loosely in place by 6 ligaments, and its position varies. The uterus changes size throughout the life span. It is the site of implantation of the fertilized ovum (egg), where the fetus develops during pregnancy, and the structure that sheds its lining monthly during menstruation.

The *cervix* is located at the neck of the uterus, between the isthmus and the vagina. It should be pink, smooth, and evenly colored (**Figures 2-26-a** and **b**). The cervix

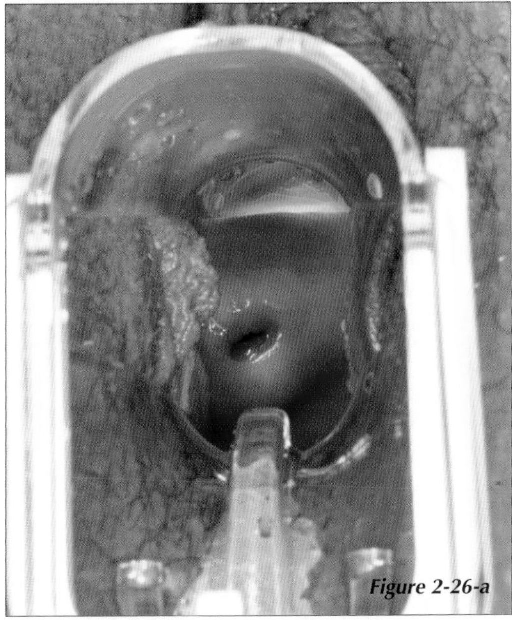

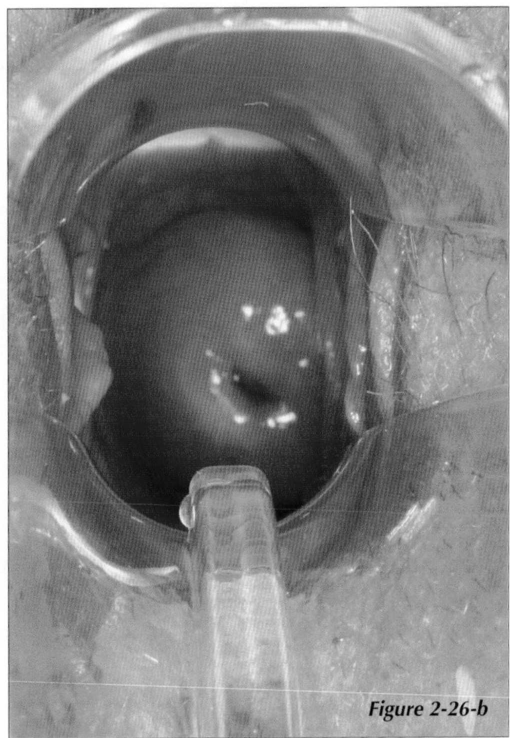

Figure 2-26-a. *Small speculum in place in the vaginal vault exposing the pink cervix and cervical os.*

Figure 2-26-b. *This image displays a normal pink cervix.*

protrudes 1 to 3 cm into the vagina and has no nerve endings (**Figures 2-27-a** through **2-28-b**). The ectocervix, or the part that protrudes into the vagina, is lined with squamous epithelium. The endocervical canal, also known as the cervical os, is the opening of the cervix. This area consists of unstratified, columnar epithelium cells.[10] There may be a circumscribed area around the cervical os of exposed columnar epithelium from the cervical os. This is called *extropion* or *eversion* and is prominent in young adolescents who present with an immature physical appearance. Cervical eversion is common in women of all ages, depending on the stage or day in their menstrual cycle. An inexperienced examiner may confuse cervical eversion with injury (**Figures 2-29-a** through **g**). Photographic peer review is helpful for the forensic nurse examiner in sexual assault care to maintain proficiency in this area where descriptions of cervical findings may create experiential conflict among providers.[27]

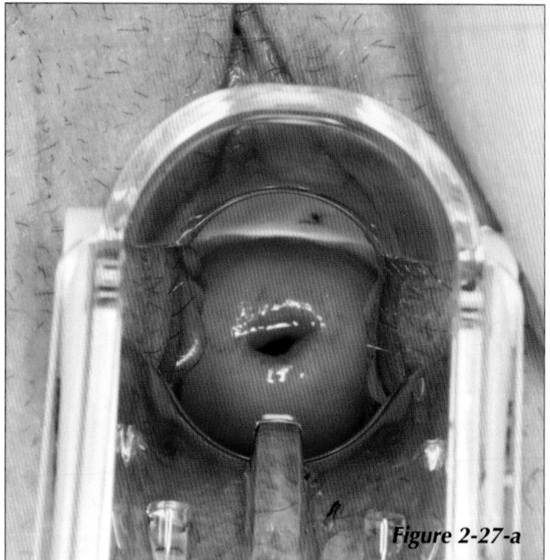
Figure 2-27-a

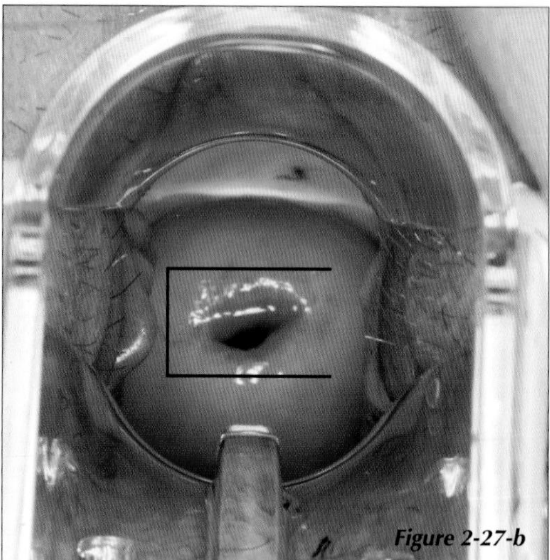
Figure 2-27-b

Figure 2-27-a. *This is a shaved female genital area with a clear speculum that is inserted into the vaginal tube exposing a nullaparous cervix.*

Figure 2-27-b. *The superior cervical neck is stretched to expose the squamocolumnar junction, primarily seen from 9 to 3 o'clock but visible circumferentially. The increased redness of the junction is normal and should not be confused with injury.*

Figure 2-27-c. *The petechiae lesions (arrow) on the surface of the cervical body could be due to consensual intercourse, infection (eg, Trichomonas), or other mechanisms, such as opening the speculum on the cervix rather than in the vaginal vault. Further evaluation of these potential causes of injury would be necessary to determine if it is injury or infection.*

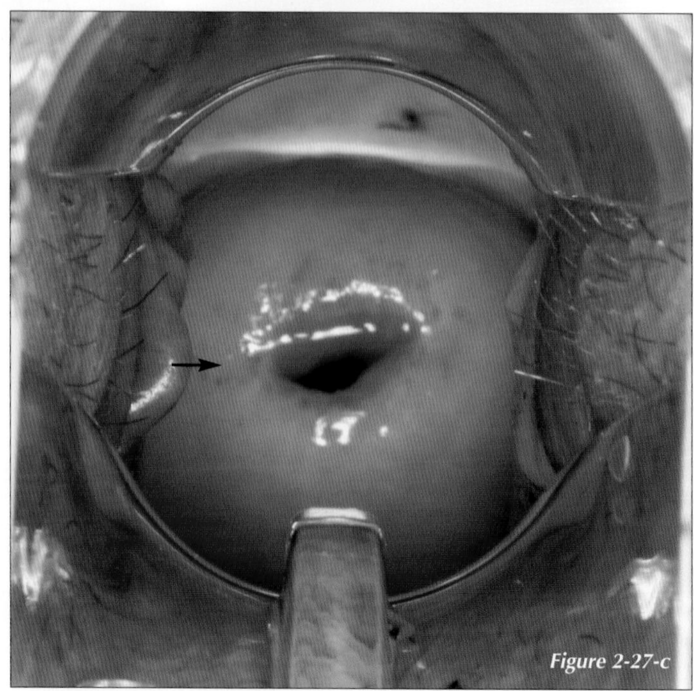
Figure 2-27-c

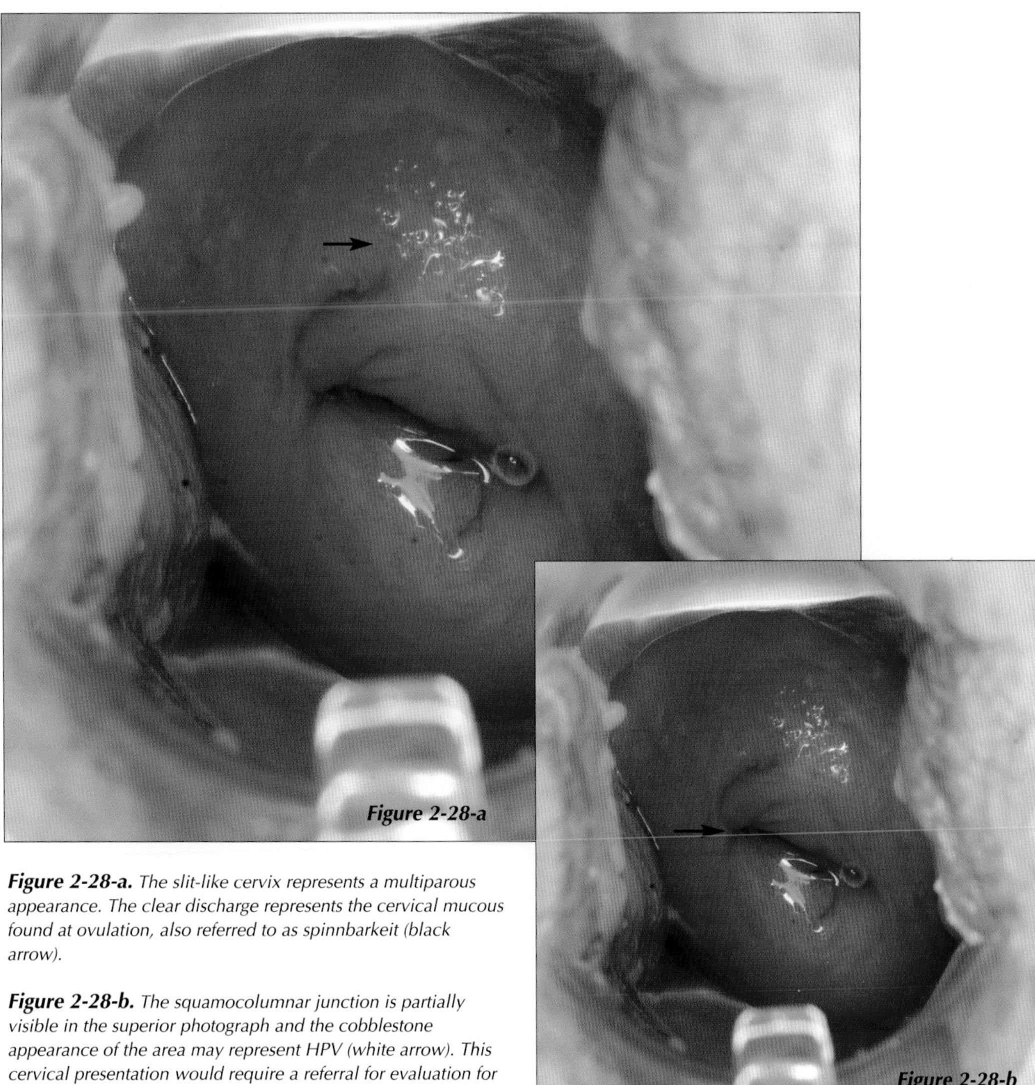

Figure 2-28-a. *The slit-like cervix represents a multiparous appearance. The clear discharge represents the cervical mucous found at ovulation, also referred to as spinnbarkeit (black arrow).*

Figure 2-28-b. *The squamocolumnar junction is partially visible in the superior photograph and the cobblestone appearance of the area may represent HPV (white arrow). This cervical presentation would require a referral for evaluation for medical reasons.*

The *squamous-columnar junction* is the line of demarcation between the squamous epithelium of the vaginal part of the cervix and the columnar epithelium of the endocervical canal (**Figure 2-29-a**).[15] Cervical secretions vary throughout the monthly cycle from thin and watery to thick mucus.[11] When there are high levels of estrogen, cervical mucus can be stretched 15 to 20 cm before breaking when placed between two glass slides that are then pulled apart. This property of cervical mucus is termed *spinnbarkeit* (**Figure 2-29-b**).[2] In addition, when dried on a slide, the mucus can produce the "ferning" effect seen during ovulation.[2] Both methods are used to predict ovulation when using natural family planning methods.[11]

The *fallopian tubes* (the oviducts) are a pair of tubes that extend about 10 cm (4 inches) from the upper uterus out toward the ovaries (but not touching them), through which ova (eggs) travel from the ovaries toward the uterus where fertilization of the ovum takes place.[11] The fallopian tubes have internal cilia that direct ova produced and released by the nearby ovary into the tube where the tube serves as the meeting ground for ova and sperm.

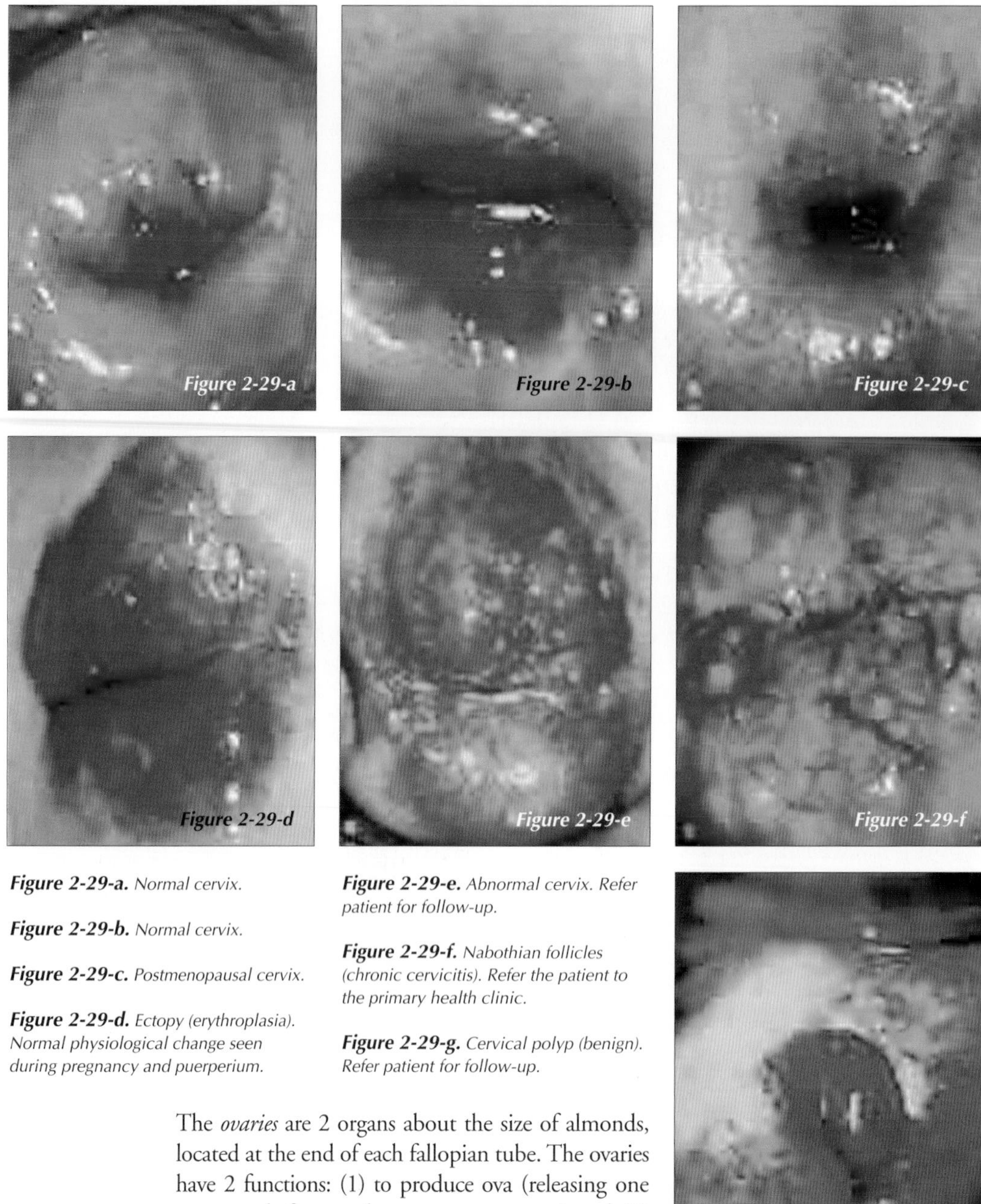

Figure 2-29-a. *Normal cervix.*

Figure 2-29-b. *Normal cervix.*

Figure 2-29-c. *Postmenopausal cervix.*

Figure 2-29-d. *Ectopy (erythroplasia). Normal physiological change seen during pregnancy and puerperium.*

Figure 2-29-e. *Abnormal cervix. Refer patient for follow-up.*

Figure 2-29-f. *Nabothian follicles (chronic cervicitis). Refer the patient to the primary health clinic.*

Figure 2-29-g. *Cervical polyp (benign). Refer patient for follow-up.*

The *ovaries* are 2 organs about the size of almonds, located at the end of each fallopian tube. The ovaries have 2 functions: (1) to produce ova (releasing one per month from puberty to menopause) and (2) to produce estrogen and progesterone. These hormones are responsible for the development of sex characteristics.

The *perineum* is the external surface or base of the perineal body, lying between the vulva and the anus (**Figures 2-30** and **2-31**). This network of muscles is located between and surrounding the vagina and the anus, and it supports the pelvic cavity and maintains the structure of the pelvic floor by keeping the organs in place. The perineal body consists of the central tendon of the perineum that separates the lower end of the vagina from the rectum in the female and the anus and scrotum in the male. This area has an injury rate of 11% in sexual assault.[14]

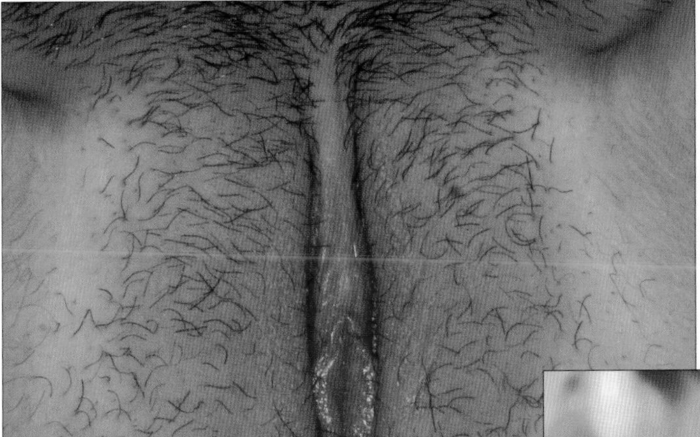

Figure 2-30

Figure 2-30. *Normal female genital anatomy. The mons pubis, clitoris and prepuce, labia minora and majora, vestibule and its contents, posterior fourchette, and fossa navicularis are contained in the vulva. The perineum lies between the vulva and the anus.*

Figure 2-31. *The perineum is further exposed when traction is applied to the external genital area. In this case, the multiparous female has multiple areas of hypopigmentation, implying multiple vaginal deliveries.*

Figure 2-31

Male Genital Anatomy

External Genitals

The visible male genitals consist of the penis and the scrotum, both of which are covered with skin (**Figure 2-32**). Puberty is the sequence of events in which children develop secondary sex characteristics and changes to the genitalia. Male puberty begins between ages 9 and 13.5 years. The mean age for spermarche is between 13.5 and 14 years.[1] The *penis* is the male sex organ composed of 3 chambers of elastic erectile tissue through which the urethra passes (**Figure 2-33**). It is a cylindrical structure with the capacity to be flaccid or erect. The penis is homologous with the clitoris of the female, as they are derived embryologically from the same tissue.[11] The average length of a nonerect penis is 8.5 to 10.5 cm. The length of an erect penis averages 16 to 19 cm with an average diameter of 3.5 cm.[49] Masters and Johnson evaluated the size of the penis, nonerect and erect, in the initial sample of participants in the 1960s and concluded that there was more varied size in the nonerect penis than in the erect penis.[11] An erection occurs when the 3 chambers of elastic tissue expand as blood flows into them. Two chambers are called corpora cavernosa, which absorb most of the blood. The third chamber, the corpus spongiosum, covers the urethra. The rise in blood pressure is caused by the veins at the base of the penis constricting so that blood flow out of the penis is less than blood flow in. The result is an erection.[50]

The *glans* is the principal source of induction and maintenance of sexual responses and it is innervated by the dorsal nerve.[51] The *glans penis* (balanus) is the cap-shaped expansion of corpus spongiosum at the head of the penis, which is covered by loose skin (foreskin or prepuce), that enables it to expand freely during an erection.

Figure 2-32. *Frontal view of the external male genitalia.*

Figure 2-33. *Tanner V flaccid circumcised penis. The urethra is midline, and there is no erythema or discharge present.*

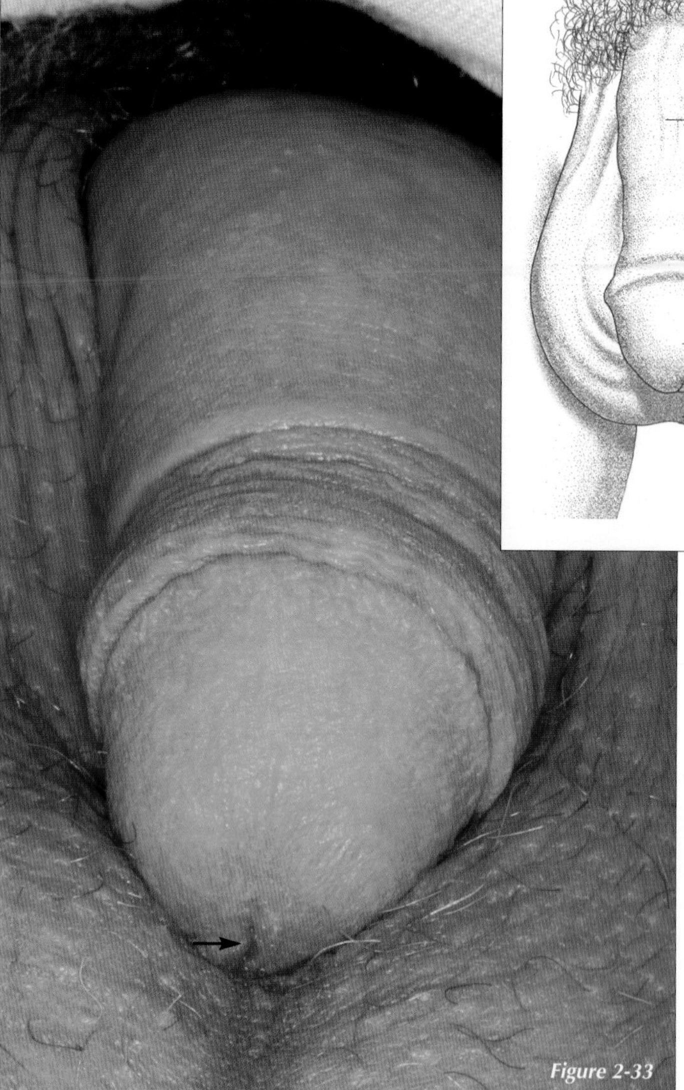

Figure 2-33

External Adult Male Genitalia

Shaft
Dorsal vein
Corona
Scrotum
Glans
Urethral meatus
Median raphe

Figure 2-32

The *corona of the glans* is the rounded and prominent border of the glans on the distal portion of the penile shaft. It is the most sensitive part of the glans.[51] The frenulum is a small fold of membrane attaching prepuce to the central ventral surface of corona.

The *urethral meatus* is a slit-like opening primarily located at the tip of the glans. This is where the urine and seminal products (including spermatozoa) will exit the body. Sometimes the urethral meatus is located on the distal third of the ventral surface of the glans or on the shaft instead of on the upper two-thirds of the glans.[52,53] This is a congenital birth finding known as hypospadius. The word *hypospadias* comes from Greek: *hypo* means below and *spadon* means opening. In 1993, 39.7% per 10 000 births of both sexes had this condition.[54] Recent evidence has suggested that the location of the urethral meatus on the glans is variable and represents a normal presentation among the populations, where surgical repair for functional outcomes remains the intervention of choice.[55] The *foreskin,* also called the prepuce, is analogous to the prepuce in the female that covers the clitoris.[56,57] All males are born with foreskin that completely covers the glans. Parents often do not realize that the foreskin of a baby boy is not designed to retract. The foreskin adheres to the glans until a boy is between age 5 to 15 years, and any attempt to force it back before it separates naturally can result in painful tearing and scar tissue formation.[50] Circumcisions date back to 4000 BC among tribal cultures. Some cultures will circumcise the foreskin so that the glans is exposed for religious reasons. In the United States in the early 1990s, circumcisions were done more for health and hygiene.[11] Many parents today opt to leave the foreskin in place as this surgical procedure has become elective, and most insurance companies will no longer pay for it.[58] The examiner must remember to retract the foreskin in uncircumcised males for complete assessment in this area. By the end of the first year, the foreskin can be retracted in most uncircumcised infants. By 4 years, the foreskin is easily retractable in 80% of uncircumcised boys.[2] Recent research has linked the length of the foreskin and exposure to venereal disease, particularly human papilloma virus (HPV), to penile cancer. Others argue that the foreskin is important to sensation and should not be removed, so the practice of circumcision remains controversial.[59-62]

Male patients or suspects will need to be assessed for potential injury and evidence by retracting the foreskin. Care must be taken to avoid stripping any adhesions that may have formed as a result of lack of hygiene or infection. Possible DNA evidence may be trapped and retained between the coronal glans and the foreskin or in the folds of the skin of the frenulum. The examiner must also ensure that the foreskin is replaced over the glans when the inspection or collection of evidence during the forensic nursing assessment is complete.

The *scrotum* is the pouch that contains the testicles and their accessory organs. It is located inferiorly to the penis and is covered with hair in the reproductive-aged male (**Figures 2-34** and **2-35**). The right side of the scrotum usually hangs lower because of the longer length of the left spermatic cord.[15,17] The scrotum protects the testes and maintains the temperature needed for the production of viable sperm. Typically this is 2° to 3°C lower than the body temperature. The lower body temperature is necessary for the production of viable spermatazoa. This area should be swabbed in the suspect or victim exam because discharge will have drained here.[63]

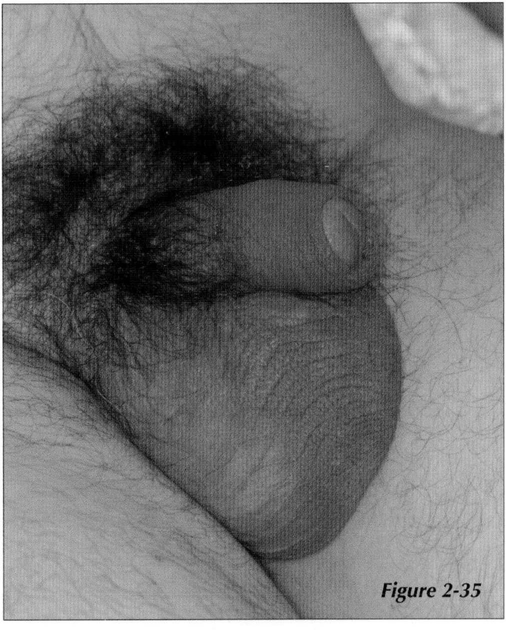

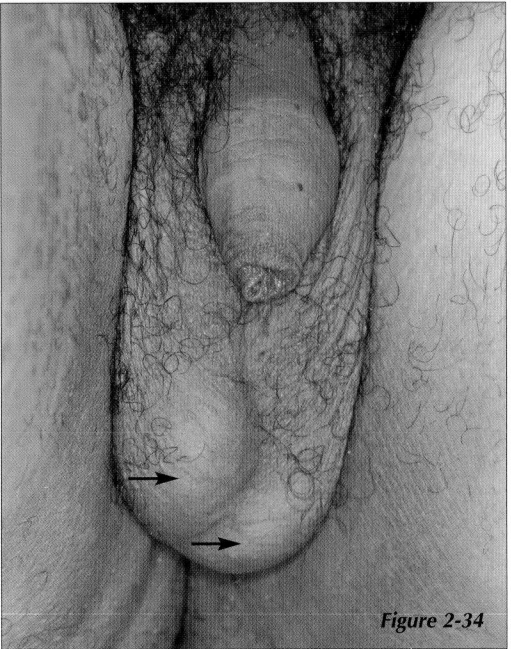

Figure 2-34. *Tanner V uncircumcised flaccid penis and scrotum. The testes are visible bilateral in the scrotal sac (arrows).*

Figure 2-35. *This image displays the area on the scrotum to swab in evidentiary evaluations. This area should be swabbed in addition to the penis and its structures (eg, corona, frenulum, and base).*

Male Reproductive Parts

The male reproductive parts are the testes, epididymides, vasa deferentia, seminal vesicles, prostate gland, and Cowper's glands.

The *testes* are paired, oval-shaped organs that produce sperm and male sex hormones; they are located in the scrotum (**Figure 2-34**). They are highly innervated and sensitive to touch and pressure. Each testicle is an oval structure about 5 cm long and 2.5 to 3 cm in diameter.[64] The testes produce *testosterone,* which is responsible for the development of male sexual characteristics and sex drive (libido). Testosterone starts dropping in the early 30s, with a long, gradual decline over decades. Low testosterone increases the risk of heart disease, prostate cancer, and Alzheimer's disease.[65]

At age 1 year, about 1% of boys have undescended testes (cryptorchidism). Most experts recommend that orchiopexy be performed before age 2 years because some research has suggested a link between testicular cancer and older aged males with undescended testicles at surgery.[66]

The *epididymides* are the 2 highly coiled tubes against the posterior side of the testes where sperm mature and are stored until they are released during ejaculation. The *vasa deferentia* (singular, vas deferens) are the paired tubes that carry the mature sperm from the epididymides to the urethra.

The *seminal vesicles* are a pair of glandular sacs that secrete about 60% to 70% of the fluid that makes up the semen in which sperm are transported. Seminal fluid provides nourishment for sperm. Seminal fluid ranges in color from whitish to tones of yellow or gray and has a creamy, sticky texture. The seminal fluid initially forms a gel that can be mistaken for spinnbarkeit. The gel liquefies within a short period of time and drains from the vagina. The drainage is called "backflow." Semen consists of water, mucus, and a large number of chemical substances that include sugar bases and prostaglandins that change the semen to gel and also cause contraction in the uterus and fallopian tubes.[11] Through the process of spermatogenesis, sperm are produced within the seminiferous tubules. The mature sperm cell has a head, midpiece, and a tail. The tail propels the sperm with a lashing movement. After a vasectomy, sperm is no longer present in the ejaculate, but the quantity of seminal fluid remains the same.[49] The head of the sperm contains the 23 chromosomes (DNA). The entire process, beginning with a primary spermocyte, takes about 74 days due to different phases of production.[64] Sperm production begins at puberty and continues throughout the life of the adult male, whereas the number of eggs is fixed at birth in the female.[49] Spermatozoa are mature male sperm cells. A sperm is only 1/1500 inch long and is only visible by using a microscope. Semen is discharged during rhythmic contractions called climax. A single discharge of about 2.5 to 5 mL of semen contains 50 to 150 million mL. When the number of spermatozoa falls below 20 million mL, the male is likely to be infertile. Semen has a slightly alkaline pH of 7.20 to 7.60. Semen provides spermatozoa with a transportation medium and nutrients, and it neutralizes the acid environment of the male urethra and the female vagina.

The *prostate gland* is a walnut-sized glandular structure that secretes about 30% of the fluid that makes up semen.[49] The alkaline quality of the fluid neutralizes the acidic environment of the male and female reproductive tracts. A muscle at the bottom of the prostate gland keeps the sperm out of the urethra until ejaculation begins. The prostate gland is very sensitive to stimulation and can be a source of sexual pleasure for some men.[11]

Cowper's glands are two pea-sized glands at the base of the penis under the prostate that secrete a clear alkaline fluid into the urethra during sexual arousal and before orgasm and ejaculation. These glands produce mucoid, preejaculatory fluid in the urethra that acts as a lubricant for the sperm and coats the urethra as semen flows out of the penis. These glands were first identified by Cowper in 1698.[67] *Median raphe* is raised midline connective tissue extending from the scrotum to the anus (**Figure 2-36**).

Ejaculation

Ejaculation occurs when the prostate gland contracts and semen with sperm is thrust into the urethra. Rhythmic contractions during ejaculation insure the bolus is deposited outside the body. There are 3 other principal forms of ejaculation: premature, retarded, and retrograde. Retrograde ejaculation happens when the opening from the bladder does not close during erection and semen spurts backward into the bladder. You can test for this by obtaining urine after ejaculation for sperm count. Retrograde ejaculation frequently follows a prostatectomy and other injuries or diseases. The female typically cannot be fertilized if the male has this condition.[67] Premature or retarded ejaculation is likely due to environmental and psychological factors.

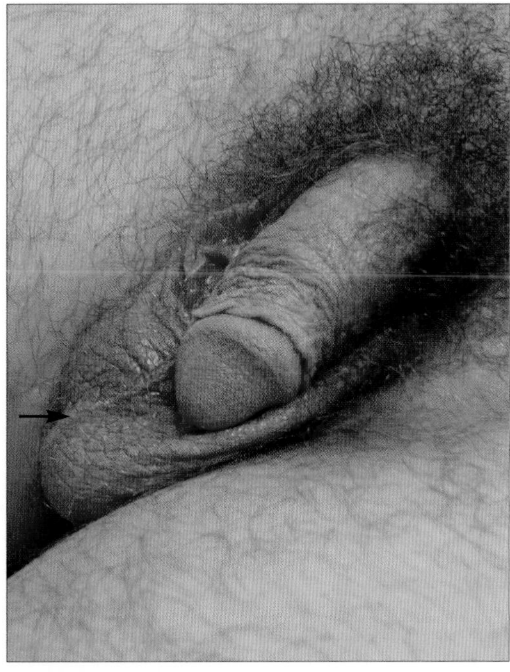

Figure 2-36. *This is a Tanner V circumcised flaccid penis and a scrotum. The glans, corona, foreskin, and penile shaft along with the media raphe and rugae of the scrotal sac are visible.*

Female and Male Anal Anatomy

The *anus orifice* is at the lower opening of the digestive tract that lies in the fold between the buttocks. Functionally the anus dilates routinely to allow the passage of feces and could readily admit an object the size of a penis with minimal or no residual findings.[68] *Perianal skin folds* are wrinkles of perianal skin created by the contraction of the anal sphincter (**Figure 2-37**). These skin folds are also called *rugae* and are symmetrical, circumferentially radiating folds formed by relaxation of corrugator cutis ani muscle. This structure is the first thing the examiner sees on separation of the buttocks. This area has more pigmentation and is more sensitive to pain. The area can be swabbed, but the examiner must realize that if the patient is a female, because of backflow of semen, the swabbed area around the perianal folds may be contaminated with vaginal, seminal, or condom discharge. Through understanding the anatomy and proper labeling of swabs, the examiner will provide accurate and comprehensive testimony in court at a later date. Anal tags are extra skin that develops on the anus after trauma, including fissures or lacerations (**Figure 2-38**).[49]

The *anus* is viewed as a linear slit-like outlet opening visible with retraction of the buttocks; however, the anus is a 3-4 cm tubular canal in the adult.[10] The anal opening is surrounded by and kept closed with 2 sphincter muscles (**Figure 2-39**). The internal sphincter is located at the internal end of the anal canal. The external anal sphincter surrounds the anus posterior to the perineum.[15] These internal and external anal sphincters are located around the anal canal and will relax or contract depending on the fecal mass. There is no lubricating glans around the anus. The anal tone is relaxed and will readily dilate after gentle traction on the buttocks if feces are present.[15] This is a normal physiological finding that should not be confused with recent or past injury. The anal canal is distensible and lined with pain-insensitive mucous membrane that is pink to salmon in color.[49]

Figure 2-37. *Anal folds are generally visible with limited traction. In a pre-injury state, they are symmetrical and form a slit-like opening. With relaxation of the external anal sphincter, the anus opens to form a cylindrical tube that allows visibility of the rectum.*

Figure 2-38. *This image displays an anal tag. Some anal tags form as a result of injury and healing cycles (eg, hemorrhoids, fissures), while others may be congenital.*

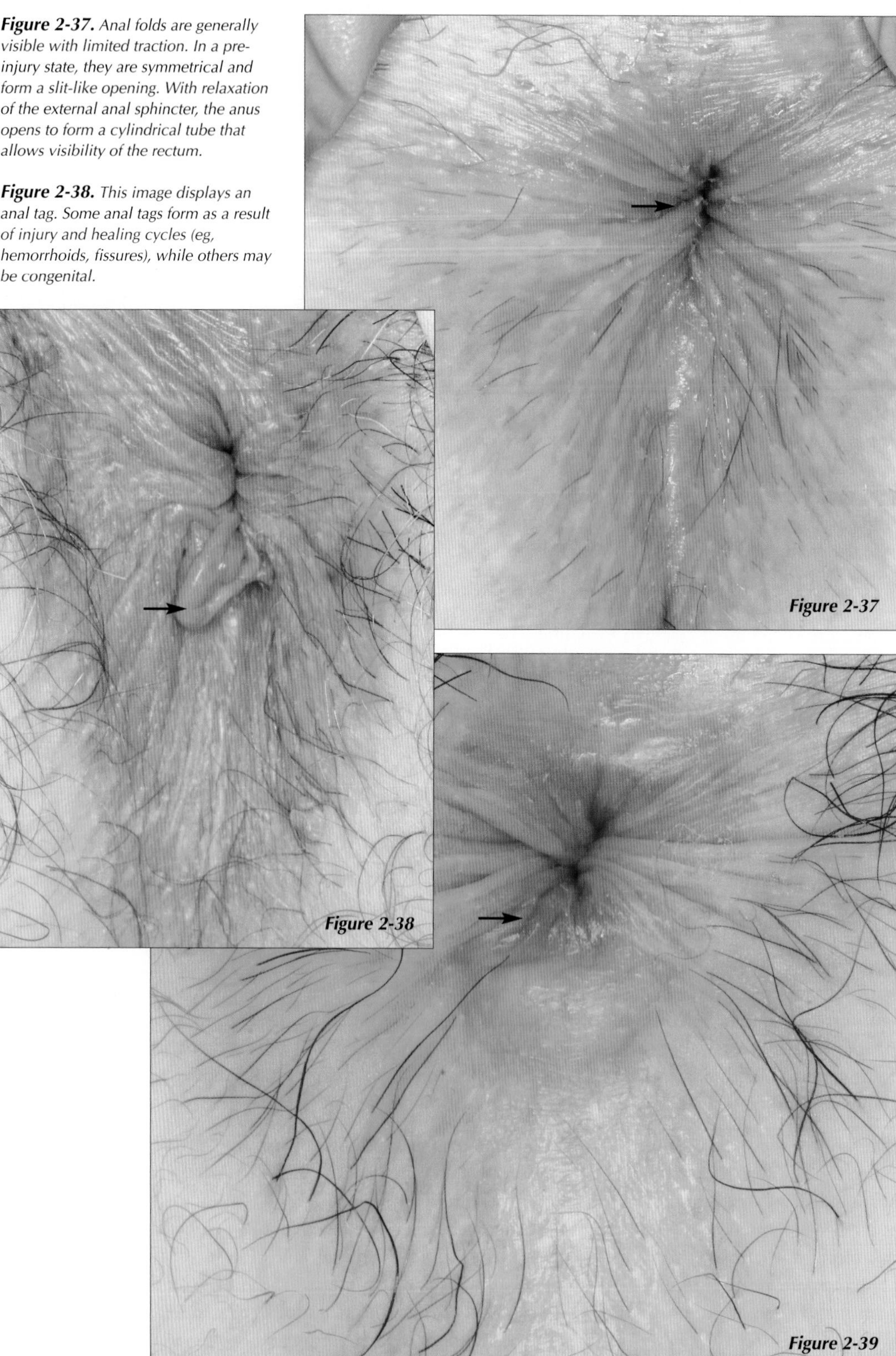

Figure 2-39. *With abdominal pressure, the anal veins (ie, hemorrhoidal plexus) will engorge. A change in position will change the appearance of the anal vein.*

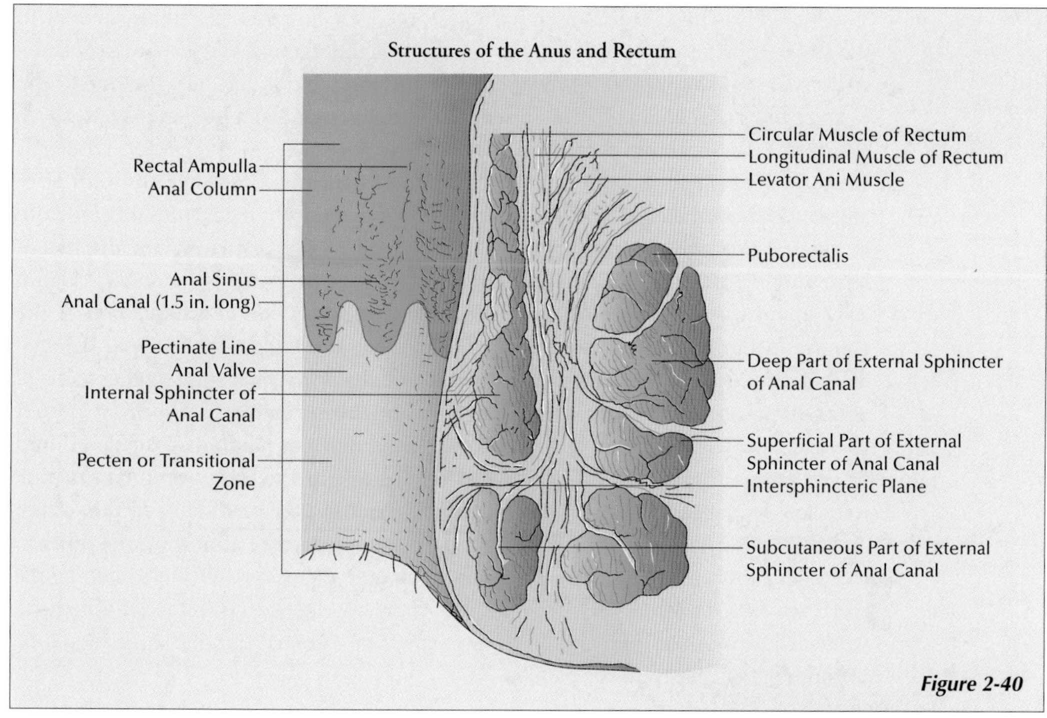

Figure 2-40

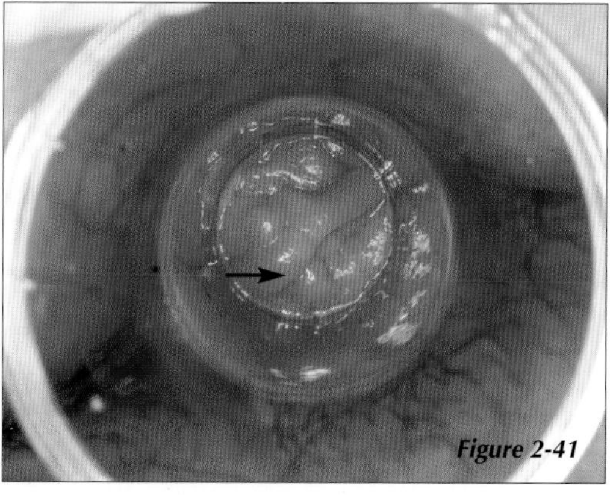

Figure 2-41

The *anal verge* overlies the subcutaneous tissue of the external anal sphincter at distal end of the anal canal and extends exteriorly to the margin of anal skin.[69] This is a transitional area between the mucous membrane of the anal canal and the perianal skin.[70] The external sphincter extends the entire length of the anal canal (**Figure 2-40**). This sphincter muscle is usually contracted. It will voluntarily relax for defecation. If a finger is inserted into the anus during an exam, the external sphincter tightens to resist the insertion. Asking the patient to push relaxes the muscle. The anterior portion of the sphincter ring is more vulnerable to trauma. The external hemorrhoidal plexus of perianal space is within the loose connective tissue surrounding the proximal anal orifice.[68] This vein frequently becomes engorged when the patient is in supine or prone position and may be mistaken for a bruise. The examiner can differentiate a contusion from an engorged vein by changing the position of the patient or with claudication through active pressure.[68]

The *pectinate* (dentate) line is the saw-toothed line of demarcation between the lower portion of the anal valves and the pectin, a smooth zone of stratified squamous epithelium extending to the anal verge.[69] Simply stated, it separates the anus from the rectum and reveals the sinuses and columns. This area has no hair, sweat glands, or sebaceous glands, so penetration may cause superficial trauma.[68] The pectin-smooth zone of simple stratified epithelium extends to the anal verge. Typically, an examiner is not able to visualize this area on general inspection. Knee-chest positioning with relaxation may result in dilation exposing the pectinate. A clear plastic anoscope allows the examiner to see this area (**Figure 2-41**).

Figure 2-40. *Cross section of anus, normal.*

Figure 2-41. *An anal scope has been inserted through the anus into the rectum. The mucosal tissue is normally pink or salmon color. Swab the rectum for both trace and biological evidence.*

The *rectum* is defined as the distal portion of the large intestine, beginning anterior to the third sacral vertebra. It is the continuation of the sigmoid and is bordered at the anal canal and the terminal (lower) end of intestine (colon). It lies superior to the dentate line. It is about 13 cm in length. The walls are glandular mucosa with an autonomic nerve supply that is pain insensitive. A rectal prolapse (rectocele) occurs when the tissues and muscles that hold the end of the large intestine (rectum) in place are stretched or weakened. In females, rectal prolapse results in the rectum moving from its natural position to press against the back wall of the vagina. When the tissues separating the two are weak, the rectum bulges into the back wall of the vagina (**Figure 2-42-a** and **b**). The associated causes include fecal impaction and herniation of the rectum. In this case, the rectocele may be transient and visible only when a bolus of feces is present in the rectum. For many older adults or patients with varying levels of paralysis (eg, spina bifida), the appearance of the rectocele is chronic. Another associated cause is a vaginal wall tear following childbirth or rape where the distal third of the vagina is unrepaired (eg, delayed reporting). In this case, the inflammation following injury and pain with defecation will result in pooling of feces in the rectum and a separation of the healing vaginal tear. Depending on the size of the bolus of feces, the healing process will result in adhesions that fix the vagina to the rectum, altering the space between, known as the cul de sac. The visual appearance is a rectocele. Whether a weakened pelvic floor from childbirth or paralysis or a vaginal tear, the cause should be historically available from the patient.

The perianal area of the anus and rectum are frequently involved in consenting and nonconsenting sex. One study looked at college-age women who practiced consenting anal sex. About 33% stated they have anal sex on a consistent basis.[71] Anal sex is also

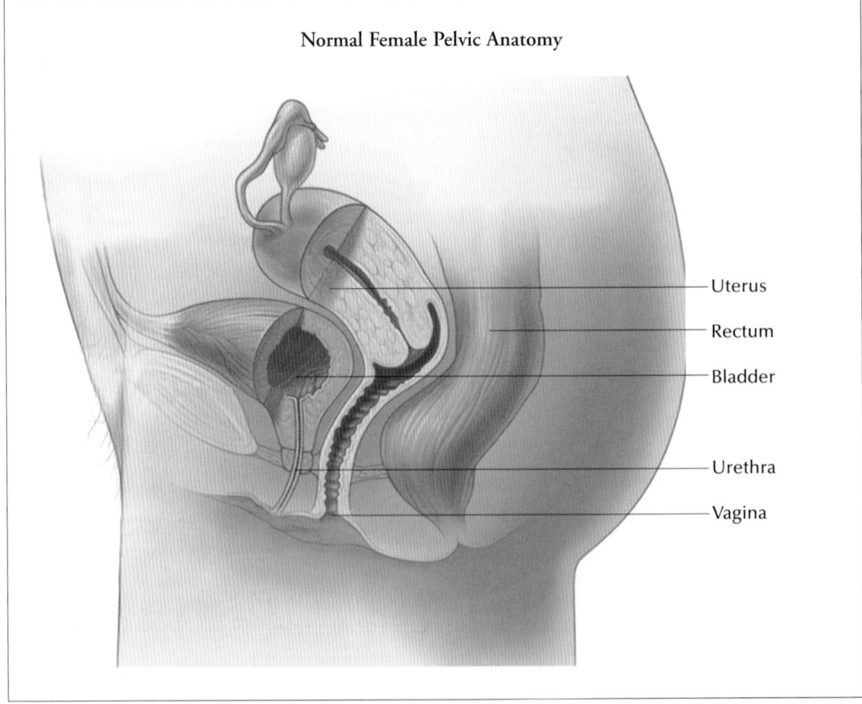

Figure 2-42-a. *Normal female pelvic anatomy. Reprinted with permission from Proprietory Rights Notice. Copyright 2007 Healthwise, Incorporated, PO Box 1989, Boise, Idaho 83701. Copying of any portion of this material is not permitted without express written permission of HEALTHWISE, Incorporated.*

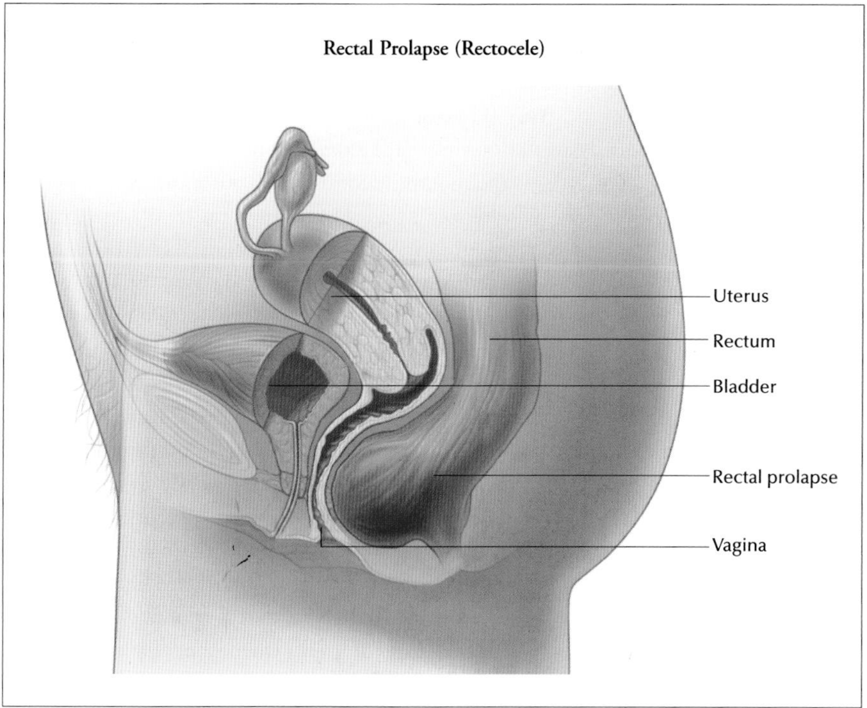

Figure 2-42-b. *A rectal prolapse (rectocele) occurs when the tissues and muscles that hold the end of the large intestine (rectum) in place are stretched or weakened. This results in the rectum moving from its natural position to press against the posterior wall of the vagina. Sometimes the tissues separating the two are so weak that the rectum bulges into the back wall of the vagina. Reprinted with permission from Proprietory Rights Notice. Copyright 2007 Healthwise, Incorporated, PO Box 1989, Boise, Idaho 83701. Copying of any portion of this material is not permitted without express written permission of HEALTHWISE, Incorporated.*

practiced at a higher rate in some of the developing countries because this is a form of birth control. Some cultures also believe that unless sexual activity involves vaginal-penile penetration, it is not sex; therefore, anal sex becomes one way to preserve the virginity of the female. The examiner should be culturally sensitive and communicate with full acceptance in order to obtain the correct history. Assumptions and bias create barriers to effective care by the health care provider and may also prevent statements from the patient about penetration of the anus or other activities considered risky by mainstream health care systems.

Oral Anatomy

The anatomy of the oral cavity begins at the lips and extends to the pharynx (**Figure 2-43**). Many things can be inserted in the oral cavity. The mouth is an integral part of the digestive, speech, and respiratory systems of all human beings. The oral cavity is the upper opening of the digestive tract and begins with the facial lips and contains the teeth, gums, tongue, and tonsils. The cheeks are muscular structures that form the lateral walls of the oral cavity. The most common sites of injury following a sexual penetration, in order, are the soft and hard palate, the lips, frenulum, uvula, and the arch. The lips are 2 fleshy folds that surround the orifice of the mouth and are covered with mucous membrane on the inside and skin on the outside. The transition zone where the 2 kinds of covering tissue meet is called the vermillion. This portion of the lips is nonkeratinized. The color of the blood in the underlying blood vessels is visible through the transparent surface layer of the vermillion.[64]

The *frenulum* is a membrane (a thin layer of tissue) that connects the tongue to the sublingual area of the floor of the throat. In fact, the whole base of the tongue is firmly anchored to the floor of the mouth. This is an area that can be injured and torn if there are forceful penetrations of the cavity (**Figures 2-44** through **2-46**). The dorsal surface of the tongue is covered with a layer of bumps called *papillae*. The *palate* forms the roof of the mouth; it consists of 2 portions: the hard palate and soft palate. The palate is the hard and soft tissue forming the roof of the mouth. The hard palate is the bony front portion of the roof of the mouth. The hard palate is the anterior portion of the roof of the mouth and is formed by the maxillae and palatine bones and covered by mucous membrane. This palate forms a bony partition between the oral and nasal cavities. The soft palate forms the posterior portion of the roof of the mouth (**Figure 2-47**). It is an arch-shaped muscular partition between the oropharynx and the nasopharynx and is lined by mucous membrane.[64] The uvula is an area on the soft palate that is centrally located and may be a site of injury when objects are forced into the mouth.[72]

Illustration of Oral Anatomy

Upper lip
Gingiva
Hard palate
Soft palate
Pharynx
Uvula
Tonsil
Tongue
Gingiva
Frenulum
Lower lip

Figure 2-43

Figure 2-43. *Illustration of oral anatomy.*

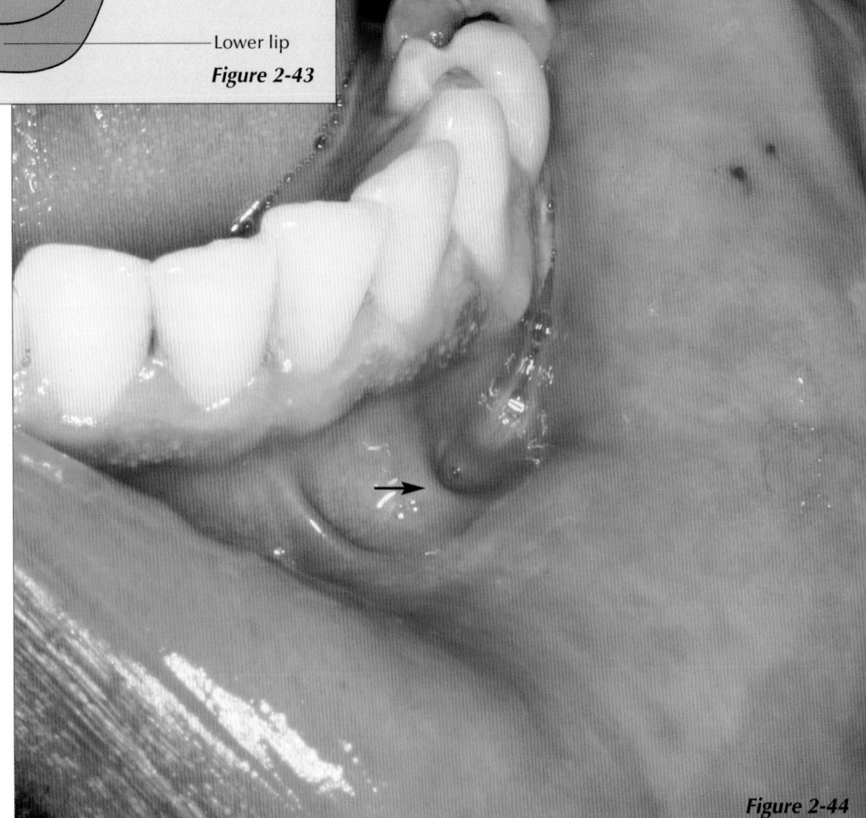

Figure 2-44. *The frenulum is visible when the lower lip is retracted. The frenulum is midline and attaches the lower and upper lip to the gingival tissue surrounding the teeth. This is a frequent area of injury in forced penetration of the oral cavity.*

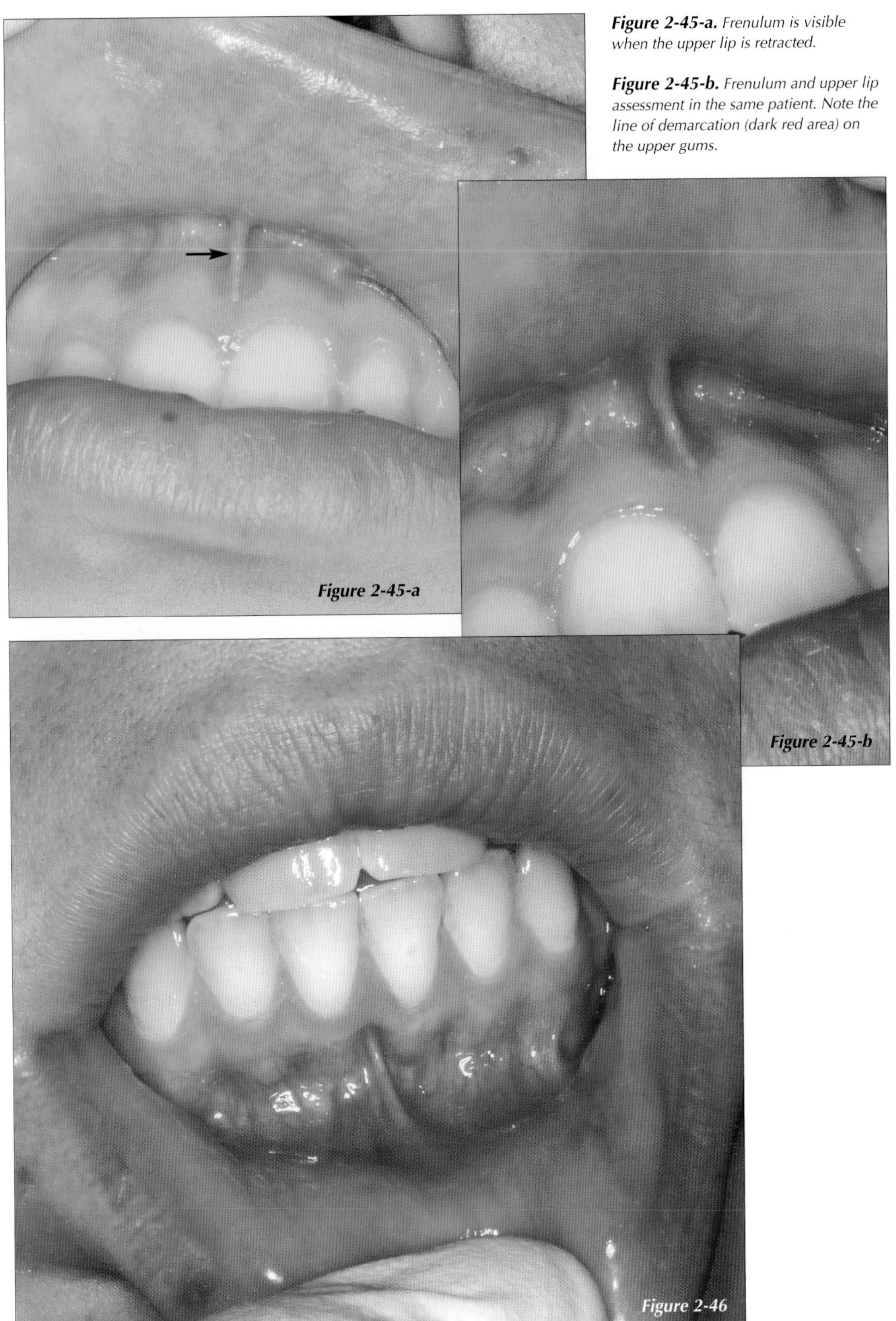

Figure 2-45-a. *Frenulum is visible when the upper lip is retracted.*

Figure 2-45-b. *Frenulum and upper lip assessment in the same patient. Note the line of demarcation (dark red area) on the upper gums.*

Figure 2-46. *Frenulum and lower lip assessment. Note the line of demarcation (dark red area) on the lower gums.*

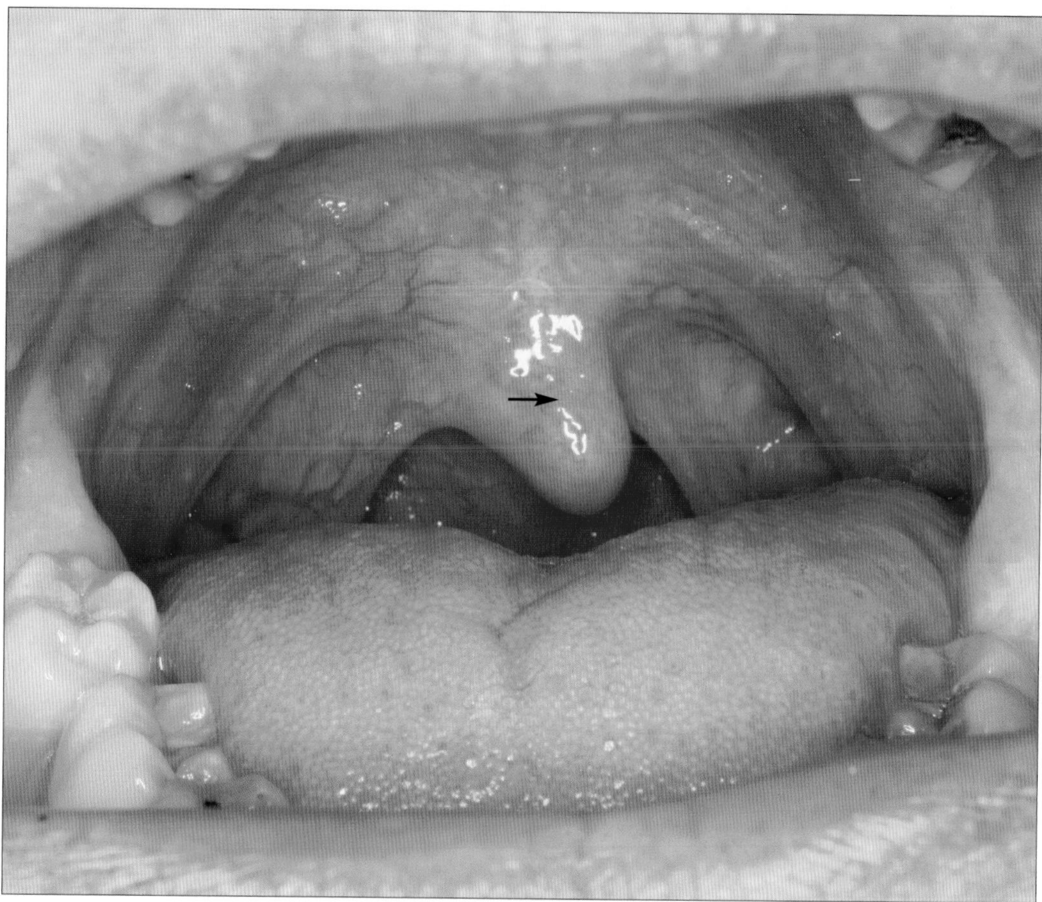

Figure 2-47. *Hypervascularization is visible in the soft palate. Further, the palatoglossal and palatropharyngeal arches also have hypervascularization, although minimal. If vascularization is related to injury, a follow-up visit can capture the healing process and injury can be observed in any of these areas in consensual or nonconsensual copulation.*

Petechial hemorrhages may be found on the soft palate or pharynx after oral copulation (**Figures 2-48**).[73] The tongue and associated muscles form the floor of the oral cavity.[64] The muscles move the tongue back and forth and from side to side. The lingual frenulum, a fold of mucous membrane in the midline of the undersurface of the tongue, aids in limiting the movement of the tongue posteriorly. Breath over the vocal cords, along with the tongue and teeth work together to form words. If the frenulum is too short or limits the movement of the tongue, speech is faulty, and the person is said to be "tongue-tied."[64] The upper portion of the tongue is covered with papillae and epithelium, and the sensations associated with the tongue during mastication is governed by cranial nerves I (smell), V (chewing), VII (anterior tongue taste, saliva glands), IX (sensation of pharynx, taste from posterior tongue), X (pharynx sensation, swallowing), and XII (movements of tongue). Evidence collection from this area may reveal tongue piercing and studs that are considered sources of potential evidence to collect (**Figure 2-49**). The examiner should swab the stud, around the stud and tongue, and into the hole of the piercing.

The teeth are the hardest bone in the body. Deciduous teeth are commonly called baby teeth or primary teeth; the first set usually consists of 20 teeth. Children begin losing their primary and baby teeth around age 6 years. The last baby tooth is lost around age 12 years. There are a total of 32 permanent or adult teeth. The *cusp* is the pointed

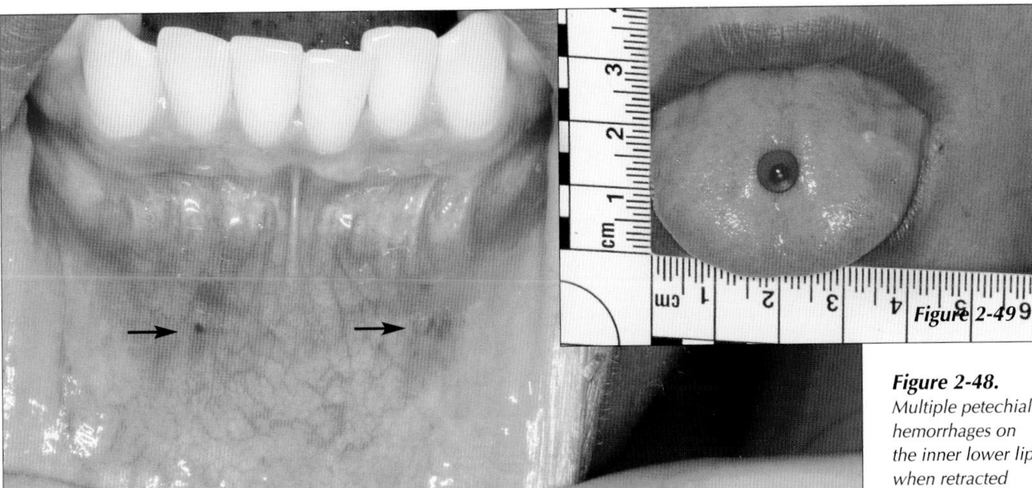

Figure 2-48. *Multiple petechial hemorrhages on the inner lower lip when retracted downward as well as the back palate.*

Figure 2-49. *Tongue piercing. Evidence collection should be considered around and in the hole of the piercing as trapped body fluids could be collected here.*

portion of the tooth. The surfaces of the teeth are named with relation to fixed oral landmarks. *Mesial* means toward the midline of the mouth; *distal* means the opposite. *Lingual* (also called palatal) connotes the surface of the tooth adjacent to the tongue; labial, buccal, and facial all signify the opposite. *Bicuspids* are the fourth and fifth teeth from the center of the mouth to the back of the mouth. These are the back teeth that are used for chewing; they only have 2 points (cusps). Adults have 8 bicuspids (also called premolars), 2 in front of each group of molars. *Cuspids,* also known as canines, are the third tooth from the center of the mouth to the back of the mouth. These are the front teeth that have one rounded or pointed edge used for biting. *Incisors* are the 4 upper and 4 lower front teeth, excluding the cuspids (canine teeth). These teeth are used primarily for biting and cutting. *Molars* are the 3 back teeth in each dental quadrant used for grinding food. *Pulp* is the connective tissue that contains blood vessels and nerve tissue, essentially the living part of the tooth, located inside the dentin. It supplies the nutrients to the tooth. The *gingiva* is the soft tissue overlying the crowns of unerupted teeth and encircling the necks of those that have erupted. *Wisdom teeth* are the third (last) molars that usually erupt at age 18 to 25 years. The teeth in an adolescent frequently are encased in braces. This area must also be considered for potential evidence collection and photography when oral copulation has been reported.

Saliva is the clear lubricating fluid in the mouth and contains water, enzymes, bacteria, mucus, viruses, blood cells, and undigested food particles. *Salivary glands* produce fluid and are located under the tongue and in the buccal areas of the cheeks.[74] Most saliva is secreted by the salivary glands. The amounts of saliva secreted daily vary considerably but range from 1000 to 1500 mL.[64] Saliva in the mouth is slightly acidic, with a pH of 6.35 to 6.85.[64] There are other glands that also secrete salivary fluid. Evidence collection for forced oral copulation should include swabbing and photography. Teeth are often used as weapons when one person attacks another or when a victim tries to ward off an assailant. Traces of saliva deposited during biting can be recovered to acquire DNA evidence.[75]

Some medical oral conditions can also mimic injury. A *hemangioma* is a blood vessel lesion that is caused by an abnormality during development. It usually occurs on the lip or tongue. It is a bluish-colored swelling that may increase/decrease in size or remain unchanged. The examiner must be aware of these potential visible findings that are not due to forceful injury. This may require a follow up visit to observe change in the pattern of injury or continued evidence of hemangiomas.

Frequently, bite marks may be involved in some patients who state they have been sexually assaulted. Forensic odontology has an important consultant role on the sexual assault team. Recent studies are seeing a pattern of bite marks in different patient groups that show how the pattern can relate to the age of the patient.[76] The forensic odontologist can determine and compare teeth markings when no DNA is available. Swabbing the area and photographing the injury meet the standards of practice for forensic nurses and local protocols for evidence collection. Potential injury to the gingiva from flossing may expose the victim to remaining (and potentially infective) body fluids left by the assailant; therefore, flossing for evidence is discouraged. While there may be anecdotal evidence of occasional DNA recovery with flossing post–oral coitus, the potential for injuring the intact gingiva resulting in disease transmission outweighs the need to floss for evidence. In lieu of flossing, it is recommended that a cotton-tipped applicator be used by the examiner to gently touch areas for potential evidence.

Many adolescents today do not consider oral sex to be sex.[77] An adolescent's primary source of information regarding sexuality is his or her peer group, all of whom are experiencing and reinforcing the same behaviors.[78] The forensic examiner must be aware of this adolescent attitude when providing and preparing information about the prevention of sexually transmitted diseases.[79]

This chapter was written for the purpose of standardizing the language for anatomical structures and locations of anogenital and oral structures among SANEs and SAFEs. Health care personnel should understand the genesis of anatomical structures and use a common language not only for legal reasons but also for quality health care. Networks of experienced advanced nursing and physician practitioners assist in quality review of cases where proper anatomical terms for anatomy are used. Language for anatomical structures and locations that are common and understandable to the expert providers facilitates the reconstruction of visual images from words when the actual photograph is unavailable, making it possible for an understanding of the injury and conditions discovered during a SANE/SAFE evaluation. Anatomical language may also describe injury that mimics abuse so the diagnostic criteria for conditions and disease should be considered when creating a diagnostic opinion for injury, whether intentional or unintentional.

References

1. Heger A, Emans S, Muram D, eds. *Evaluation of the Sexually Abused Child.* 2nd ed. New York, NY: Oxford University Press; 2000.

2. Swartz M. *Textbook of Physical Diagnosis: History and Examination.* 5th ed. Philadelphia, PA: Saunders/Elsevier; 2006.

3. Gaffney D. Genital injury and sexual assault. In: Giardino A, Datner E, Asher J, Girardin BW, Faugno D, Spencer M, eds. *Sexual Assault: Victimization Across the Life Span.* St. Louis, MO: GW Medical; 2003:223-239.

4. Schultheiss D, Mattelaer JJ, Hodges FM. Preputial infibulation: from ancient medicine to modern genital piercing. *BJU Int.* 2003;92(7):758-763.

5. Crane P. Female genital mutilation. In: Lynch VA, Duval J, eds. *Forensic Nursing.* St. Louis, MO: Mosby; 2006:43-51.

6. Milner VS, Eichold BH II, Sharpe TH, Lynn SC Jr. First glimpse of the functional benefits of clitoral hood piercings. *Am J Obstet Gynecol.* 2005;193(3):675-676.

7. Hudson K. Female Genital Piercings: Clitoris. About.com. http://tattoo.about.com/cs/beginners/a/blclitoris.htm. Accessed July 23, 2007.

8. de la Taille A, Delmas V, Lassau JP, Boccon-Gibod L. Anatomic study of the pubic-urethral ligaments in women: role of urethral suspension. *Progres en Urologie.* 1997;7(4):604-610.

9. Wilson PD, Dixon JS, Brown AD, Gosling JA. Posterior pubo-urethral ligaments in normal and genuine stress incontinent women. *J Urology.* 1983;130(4):802-805.

10. Girardin B, Faugno D, Seneski P, Slaughter L, Whelan M. *The Color Atlas of Sexual Assault.* St Louis, MO: Mosby; 1997.

11. Masters W, Johnson V, Kolodny R. Sexual Physiology. *Human Sexuality.* 5th ed. New York, NY: Harper Collins Publishers; 1995.

12. Sanders M. Normal Vulva. Path Web. http://pathweb.uchc.edu/frame.php?whatorgan=Vulva. Accessed January 14, 2010.

13. Kolodny RC, Johnson VE, Masters WH. *Human Sexuality.* Boston, MA: Allyn & Bacon; 1995.

14. Slaughter L, Brown C, Shackeford S, et al. Patterns of genital injury in victims of sexual assault. *Am J Obstet Gynecol.* 1997;176:609-619.

15. Crowley SR. *Sexual Assault: The Medical Legal Examination.* Ontario, Canada: Appleton & Lange; 1999.

16. Giardino A, Datner E, Asher J, Girardin BW, Faugno D, Spencer M. *Sexual Assault: Victimization Across the Lifespan.* St Louis, MO: GW Medical Publishing; 2003.

17. Finkel M. Physical examination. In: Finkel M, Giardino A, eds. *Medical Evaluation of Child Sexual Abuse.* 3rd ed. Elk Grove, IL: American Academy of Pediatrics; 2009:63.

18. Linden J, Lewis-O'Connor A, Jackson M. Forensic examination of adult victims and perpetrators of sexual assault. In: Olshaker J, Jackson M, Smock W, eds. *Forensic Emergency Medicine.* 2nd ed. Philadelphia, PA: Lippincott, Williams and Wilkins; 2006:85-125.

19. Berenson AB, Heger AH, Hayes JM, Bailey RK, Emans SJ. Appearance of the hymen in prepubertal girls. *Pediatrics.* 1992;89:387-394.

20. Speck PM. Recognition of child assault in the emergency care setting. Presented at: 3rd Annual Tennessee Emergency Nurses Association Conference; October 1998; Nashville, TN.

21. Speck PM. From the president. *On the Edge.* 2003;9(1-4):2.

22. Myher AK, Berntzen K, Bratlid D. Genital anatomy in non-abused preschool girls. *Acta Pediatr.* 2003;92:1353-1462.

23. Muram D, Speck PM, Cassinello B. *Teaching Forensic Evaluation of Sexual Abuse Victims to Medical Residents.* Memphis, TN: Tennessee Department of Human Services; 1989.

24. Speck PM. Hymen morphology: Estrogen effect across the life span. Baptist Regional SANE/SAFE Education. Pensacola, FL: Baptist Regional Health Center; 2007.

25. Speck PM, Patton SB. Hymen morphology updated: classifying estrogen effect across the life span. Presented at: 15th Annual Scientific Assembly; 2007; Salt Lake City, UT.

26. Faugno DK, Speck PM, Rossman L. Elder abuse. Presented at: 16th Annual Scientific Assembly of the International Association of Forensic Nurses; 2008; Dallas, TX.

27. Ernst E. *Evaluation of Image Quality of Digital Photo Documentation of Female Genital Injuries After Sexual Assault* [unpublished dissertation]. Cleveland, OH: Case Western Reserve University; 2009.

28. Rauh MJ, Macera CA, Trone DW, Shaffer RA, Brodine SK. Epidemiology of stress fracture and lower-extremity overuse injury in female recruits. *Med Sci Sports Exerc.* 2006;38(9):1571-1577.

29. Anderson S, McClain N, Riviello R. Genital findings of women after consensual and nonconsensual intercourse. *J Int Forensic Nurs.* 2006;2(3):59-64.

30. Jones JS, Rossman L, Harman M, Alexander CC. Anogenital injuries in adolescents after consensual sexual intercourse. *Acad Emerg Med.* 2003;10(12):1378-1383.

31. White C, McLean I. Adolescent complaints of sexual assault: injury patterns in virgin and non-virgin group. *J Clin Forensic Med.* 2006;12(4):172-180.

32. Emans SJ, et al. Hymenal findings in adolescent women: impact of tampon use and consensual sexual activity. *J Pediatr.* 1994;124:153.

33. Jenny C. *Medical Evaluation of Physical and Sexually Abused Children.* Thousand Oaks, CA: Sage Publications; 1996.

34. Dane C et al. Imperforate hymen—a rare cause of abdominal pain: two cases and review of the literature. *J Pediatr Adolesc Gynecol.* 2007;20(4):245-247.

35. Goto K, Yoshinari H, Tajima K, Kotsuji F. Microperforate hymen in a primigravida in active labor: a case report. *J Reprod Med.* 2006;51(7):584-586.

36. McCann J, Sheridan M, Boyle C, Rogers K. Healing of hymenal injuries in prepubertal and adolescent girls: a descriptive study. *Pediatrics.* 2007;119(5):989.

37. Muram D. Treatment of prepubertal girls with labial adhesions. *J Pediatr Adolesc Gynecol.* 1999;12:67-70.

38. Heger AH, Ticson L, Guerra L, Lister J, Zaragoza T, McConnell G, Morahan M. Appearance of the genitalia in girls selected for nonabuse: review of hymenal morphology and nonspecific findings. *J Pediatr Adolesc Gynecol.* 2002;15(1):27-35.

39. Edwards L, Dunphy J. Wound healing. Injury and normal repair. *N Engl J Med.* 1958;259:275-285.

40. Biggs M, Stermac LE, Divinsky M. Genital injuries following sexual assault of women with and without prior sexual intercourse experience. *Can Med Assoc J.* 1998;159(1):33-37.

41. Anderson S, Annan S, McClain N, Parker B, Bourguignon C, Byverud S. A comparison of injury patients in women after consensual intercourse. *J Emerg Nursing.* 2005;30:206.

42. Berman L, Adhikari S, Goldstein I. Anatomy and physiology of sexual functions and dysfunction: classification, evaluation and treatment options. *Eur Urol.* 2000;38:20-26.

43. Slaughter L. Binocular microscopy in sexual assault examinations. In: Lynch VA, Duval J, eds. *Forensic Nursing.* St. Louis, MO: Mosby; 2006:160.

44. Cardozo L, Bachmann G, McClish D, Fonda D, Birgerson L. Meta-analysis of estrogen therapy in the management of urogenital atrophy in post menopausal women: second report of the Hormones and Urogenital Therapy Committee. *Obstet Gynecol.* 1998;92:722-727.

45. Das S, Allan S. Higher vaginal pH is associated with Neisseria gonorrhoeae and Chlamydia trachomatis infection in a predominantly white population. *Sex Transm Dis.* 2006;33(8):527-528.

46. Mahmoud EA, Svensson LO, Olsson SE, Mardh PA. Antichlamydial activity of vaginal secretion. *Am J Obstet Gynecol.* 1995;172(4):1268-1272.

47. Pavletic AJ, Hawes SE, Geske JA, Bringe K, Polack SH. Experience with routine vaginal pH testing in a family practice setting. *Infect Dis Obstet Gynecol.* 2004; 12(2):63-68.

48. Sheffield JS, Andrews WW, Klebanoff MA, et al. Spontaneous resolution of asymptomatic chlamydia trachomatis in pregnancy. *Obstet Gynecol.* 2005;105(3): 567-562.

49. Olshaker J, Jackson M, Smock W. *Forensic Emergency Medicine.* 2nd ed. Philadelphia, PA: Lippincott, Williams and Wilkins; 2006:119.

50. "Penis Structure." Available at: www.penis-size-info.com. Accessed Aug. 25, 2007.

51. Yang CC, Bradley WE. Innervation of the human glans penis. *J Urology.* 1999; 161(1):97-102.

52. Uygur MC, Ersoy E, Erol D. Analysis of meatal location in 1244 healthy men: definition of the normal site justifies the need for meatal advancement in pediatric anterior hypospadias cases. *Pediatr Surg Int.* 1999;15:119-120.

53. Fichtner J, Filipas D, Mottrie AM, Voges GE, Hohenfellner R. Analysis of meatal location in 500 men: wide variation questions need for meatal advancement in all pediatric anterior hypospadias cases. *J Urology.* 1995;154:833-884.

54. Bukowski T, Zeman P. Hypospadias: of concern but correctable. *Contemp Pediatr.* 2001;2:89-99.

55. Hutton KAR, Babu R. Normal anatomy of the external urethral meatus in boys: implications for hypospadias repair. *BJU Int.* 2007;100(1):161-163.

56. Cold CJ, Taylor JR. The prepuce. *Br J Urol Int.* 1999;83:33-34.

57. Velazquez EF, Bock A, Soskin A, Codas R, Arbo M, Cubilla AL. Preputial variability and preferential association of long phimotic foreskins with penile cancer: an anatomic comparative study of types of foreskin in a general population and cancer patients. *Am J Surg Pathol.* 2003;27(7):994-998.

58. Rockney R. Newborn circumcision. *Am Fam Physician.* 1988;38(4):151-155.

59. Fetus and Newborn Committee, Canadian Paediatric Society. Neonatal circumcision revisited. *Can Med Assoc J.* 1996;154:769-780.

60. Baskin LS. Circumcision. In: Baskin LS, Kogan BA, Dukett JW, eds. *Handbook of Pediatric Urology.* Philadelphia, PA: Lippincott-Raven; 1997:1-9.

61. Hodges FM. The ideal prepuce in ancient Greece and Rome: male genital aesthetics and their relation to lipodermos, circumcision, foreskin restoration, and the kynodesme. *Bull Hist Med.* 2001;75:375-405.

62. Schoen EJ. The status of circumcision of newborns. *N Engl J Med.* 1990;322: 1308-1312.

63. Traughber M, Spear T. Hidden treasure on the family jewels. *Tieline.* 2000;23:11.

64. Tortora G, Anagnostakos N. *Principles of Anatomy and Physiology.* 6th ed. Harper Collins; 1990:736-738.

65. Weede T. When testosterone falls: a hormone deficiency zaps energy and libido. Is supplementing the solution? *Nat Health.* 2005;36(1):104-106.

66. Pettersson A, Richiardi L, Nordenskjold A, Kaijser M, Akre O. Age at surgery for undescended testis and risk of testicular cancer. *N Engl J Med.* 2007;356:1835-1841.

67. Gilbaugh J. *Men's Private Parts: An Owner's Manual.* New York, NY: Crown Publishers; 1993.

68. Giardino A, Alexander, R, eds. *Child Abuse: Quick Reference for Healthcare, Social Service, and Law Enforcement Professionals.* 2nd ed. St. Louis, MO: GW Medical Publishing; 2006.

69. American Professional Society on the Abuse of Children. *Descriptive Terminology in Child Sexual Abuse Medical Examinations.* Chicago, IL: APSAC; 1995.

70. Stedman TL. *American Heritage Stedman's Medical Dictionary.* 2nd ed. Boston, MA: Houghton Mifflin Company; 2004.

71. Flannery D, Lyndall E, Karen S, Votaw B, Schaefer E. Anal intercourse and sexual risk factors among college women, 1993-2000. *Am J Health Behav.* 2003;27(3): 228-234.

72. Gray H. *Anatomy of the Human Body.* Philadelphia, PA: Lea & Febiger; 1918. Available at: www.bartleby.com/107/. Accessed January 20, 2010.

73. Maguire SA, Hunter B, Hunter LM, Sibert J, Mann MK, Kemp AM. Diagnosing abuse: a systematic review of torn frenum and intra-oral injuries. *Arch Dis Child.* 2007;92:1113-1117.

74. Mathis CEG. WebMD Medical Reference provided in collaboration with The Cleveland Clinic. Revised May 1, 2005. Accessed July 20, 2007.

75. Sweet D, Pretty IA. A look at forensic dentistry—Part 2: teeth as weapons of violence—identification of bitemark perpetrators. *Br Dent J.* 2001;190(8):415-418.

76. Freeman AJ, Senn DF, Arendt DM. Seven hundred seventy eight bite marks: analysis by anatomic location, victim and biter demographics, types of crime and legal disposition. *J Forensic Sci.* 2005;20(6):1436-1441.

77. Halpern-Feisher B, Cornell J, Kropp R, Tschann J. Oral versus vaginal sex among adolescents: perceptions, attitudes, and behavior. *Pediatrics.* 2005;115(4):845-851.

78. Grant L, Demetriou E. Adolescent sexuality. *Pediatr Clin North Am.* 1988;35(6): 1271-1289.

79. Bersamin MM, Fisher DA, Walker S, Hill DL, Grube JW. Defining virginity and abstinence: adolescents' interpretations of sexual behaviors. *J Adolesc Health.* 2007;41(2):182-188.

Chapter 3

Body Injury and Dynamics of Sexual Assault

Kathleen M. Brown, RN, MSN, CRNP, PhD, FAAN
Ann Wolbert Burgess, DNSc, APRN, BC, FAAN
Donna A. Gaffney, DNSc, PMHCNS-BC, FAAN

Recognition of injury requires knowledge of anatomy and physiology, the refined skills of observation and examination, and an understanding of the dynamics of victimization that may contribute to injuries. The clinician must be aware that genital injury can occur in consensual sex, especially between partners who have never been sexually active. Conversely, in nonconsensual penetration, there may be no indication of genital injury. Therefore, the clinician must remember that each case must be viewed on its own merits, including factors such as the relationship between the parties involved and their interaction. Because of this complex relationship, it is nearly impossible to predict if genital injury will be found under a particular set of circumstances. It is also impossible to use the evidence of, or absence of, injury to determine whether or not sexual contact was consensual.

Statistics

Of all victims of assault seen in emergency rooms in the United States, 4.2% were sexual assault victims.[1] Data on injury related to sexual assault originates from the sexual assault victims seen in the emergency departments; however, the National Violence Against Women survey estimates that only about one-third of women received medical care after their most recent rape.[2] An emergency department sample of sexual assault victims is, therefore, not representative of all victims of sexual violence.

In a study of 819 victims of sexual assault, Eckert et al[3] reports 52% had injury to the body, 20% had genital trauma, and 41% were without injury. General body trauma in this study was associated with being hit, kicked, strangled, penetrated orally or anally, and stranger assault. Genital trauma was related to age (victims younger than 20 and older than 49), virginity, and time of exam. In another recent study, two-thirds of 1038 victims who reported sexual assault in Baltimore had physical injury or genital injury and almost one-third (30%) had injury to both the body and the genitalia.[4]

Dynamics of Victimization

Two basic defenses are used by defendants in a criminal (or civil) suit. The first is mistaken identity. This defense is used less with the careful evidence collection by examiners and the scientific advances in DNA fingerprinting. The second defense is consent, which is used more often as social boundaries and rules of dating have loosened and substance use has expanded. From a clinical view, rape and sexual assault are not mistakes or miscommunication; they are nonconsensual sex with an unwilling partner. The forensic examiner's role in the assessment, treatment, and care of sexual assault patients is critical.

Sexual assault rarely occurs in a public place. It is highly unusual for this crime to be witnessed. The victim interview is an important step in understanding the dynamics of victimization and provides direction on how to examine the victim. These dynamics include the relationship between the victim and offender, the method of approach, the control tactics used by the offender, and the reaction of the victim.

Relationship Between Victim and Offender

The relationship, from the victim's standpoint, can be described as known or unknown. If known, the role could be as casual as an acquaintance or a date, or as intimate as a family member. If unknown, the relationship could range from never having seen the assailant to not being able to see the assailant because of the method of approach.

Method of Approach

When an individual decides on a behavioral act (as in rape), it is human nature to choose a method with which he or she feels most comfortable. This is the logical course used by an assailant in choosing a method of approaching and subduing the intended victim. Because each aspect of a sexual assault can provide information about the perpetrator, it is necessary to categorize the style of approach used, with the broad categories being the *con*, *blitz*, and *surprise*.

Con

With the con approach, the offender approaches his victim openly using a ruse, trick, or confidence line. He may offer assistance or request directions. He is initially pleasant and friendly. Verbal strategies can be used to convince the target to accompany the offender to a second, more private location. The offender may be able to convince the victim to allow him to drive to her or his home or to give him a ride home. The victim may willingly accompany the offender. Often the victim goes with the offender because he has convinced her that he is interested in a date. The victim is unaware that a sexual assault or rape is planned.

This rapist's goal is to gain the victim's confidence, reach a position to overcome her resistance, and capture her. Often, and for different reasons, he exhibits a sudden change in attitude once she is under his control. In some instances, the rapist alters his behavior to convince the victim he is serious. In other instances, the change merely reflects inner hostility toward the victim or women in general. This style of approach suggests an individual who has confidence in his ability to interact with women and is not intimidated by them.

Blitz

A person using a blitz approach immediately employs injurious force in subduing his victim. He allows her no opportunity to react physically or negotiate verbally and frequently gags, blindfolds, or binds his victim. His attack may occur from either the front or the rear. Usually he uses his fists or other blunt force, but he also may use chemicals, strangulation, or suffocation techniques. This approach suggests hostility toward women.

Surprise

In the surprise approach, the rapist may either approach the victim while she is sleeping or lie in wait for the victim (eg, back seat of a car, behind a wall, in the woods). Taking control of a sleeping victim also allows the offender to gain control. In these cases, an offender awakens the victim by mounting him or her. Typically, this individual uses verbal threats and/or the presence of a weapon to subdue the victim. There are 2 possibilities for using this style: the victim may have been targeted or preselected for assault or the offender does not feel sufficiently confident to use a con approach and does not want to use violence to capture her via the blitz approach.

Control of the Victim

To commit a sexual assault, the offender must maintain control of his victim. How the offender maintains control primarily depends on the motivation for committing the sexual assault. When the offender has the victim controlled in a private location, the assault occurs. The offender may continue to use a weapon, to offer drugs and alcohol until the victim loses consciousness, or apply physical force to complete the rape. Five control methods are commonly observed: mere presence, verbal threats, display of a weapon, use of physical force, and substance use.

Mere Presence

Depending on the fear and passivity of the victim, the offender's mere presence can be sufficient to control the victim. This control strategy is commonly seen in victims with learning disabilities, mental illness or retardation, cognitive compromise, and the elderly.

Threats

Many victims are understandably intimidated by threats of violence. Clues to the motivation for the assault often lie in these verbal threats. Clinicians should elicit (verbatim if possible) the context of the threats and document whether or not the threat was carried out.

Weapon

Many rapists display a weapon, which tends to ensure that the victim will do as the offender commands. It is important to ascertain if the rapist had a weapon, and at what point he displayed or indicated he had one. The clinician can document if it was a weapon of choice and brought to the scene (eg, gun, switchblade) or of opportunity (eg, kitchen knife, screwdriver); if the offender relinquished control of it (ie, gave it to the victim or put it down); and whether he inflicted any physical injury with the weapon. See **Figures 3-1** through **3-3**.

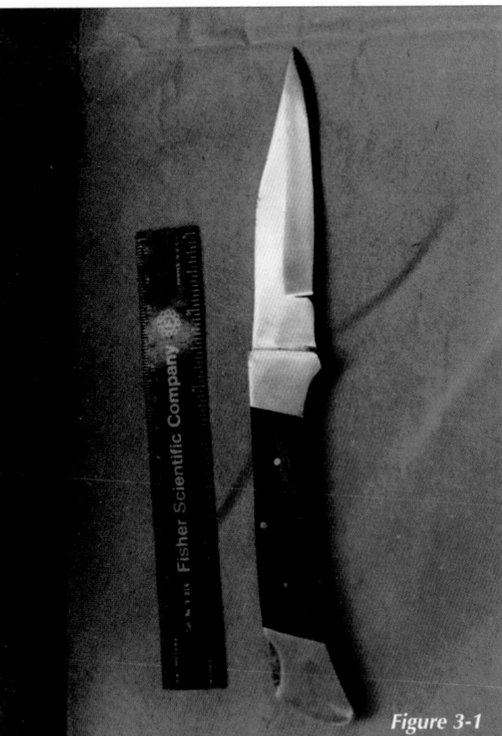

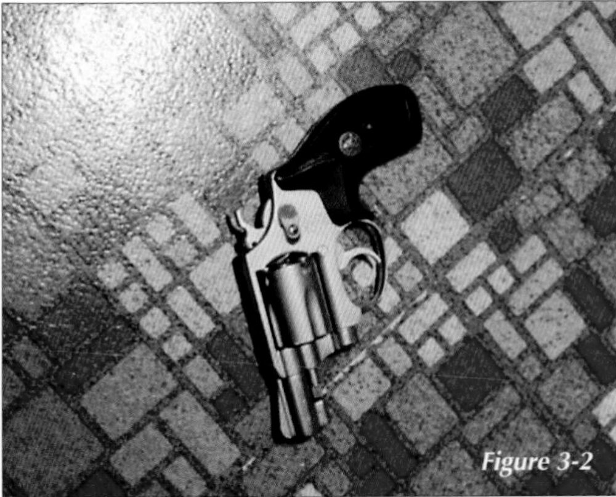

Figure 3-1. *Knife used as a weapon, shown alongside a ruler for measurement.*

Figure 3-2. *Gun used in an attack.*

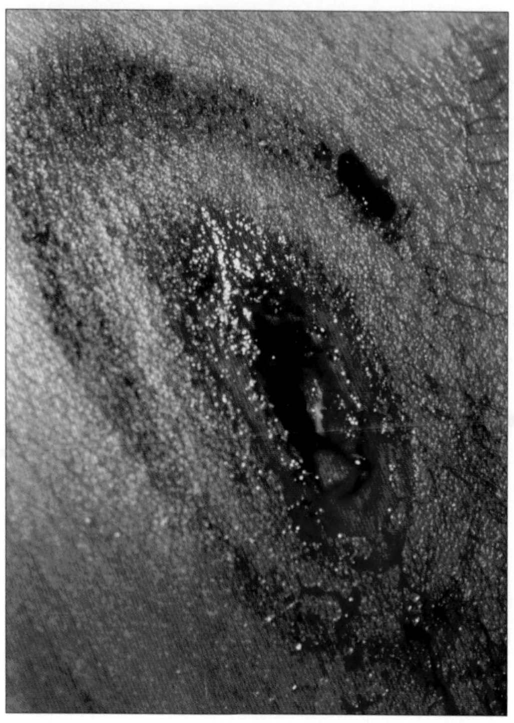

Figure 3-3. Contact gunshot wound.

Force

The use and amount of physical force in a rape attack are key determinants of offender motivation. The clinician should determine the amount of force, when it was employed, and the rapist's attitude before, during, and after the force was used. The clinician should elicit as precise a description of the physical force as possible. Four levels of force have been identified to assist clinicians in their description (**Table 3-1**).[5]

Substance Use

The offender may administer drugs or alcohol while the victim is completely unaware, through drink tampering. Alternatively, the offender may convince the victim to participate in consuming alcohol and/or drugs. While the victim is under the influence of drugs and/or alcohol, the offender can move him or her to where the assault will occur. It is not unusual for the offender to search for victims in settings where many people are using drugs and alcohol. It is easier to target a victim who is already under the influence with judgment impaired. In an impaired state, the victim can be convinced to go with the offender. An offender may also enlist the assistance of others to abduct a targeted victim from a setting and take him or her to a desired location for the sexual assault. Victims may be abducted from secluded roadways, alleys, or parking areas.

Table 3-1. Levels of Force

Levels of Force	
Minimal Force	Little or no physical force. The victim may be slapped, but it is not repetitive behavior; the force is employed to intimidate rather than punish. The rapist is typically nonprofane in his talk.
Moderate Force	The rapist repeatedly slaps or hits the victim in a painful manner, even without resistance. He typically uses profanity throughout the attack and is verbally abusive.
Excessive Force	The victim is beaten, has bruises and lacerations, and requires medical attention or hospitalization. The rapist is typically profane, directing derogatory remarks at the victim.
Brutal Force	Ultimate level of force; victim is subjected to an extreme amount of violence, including torture. Injuries demonstrate the offender intends to inflict serious physical trauma. Victim requires long-term hospitalization and may die of her injuries. The offender's verbal behavior reflects anger and hostility.

Reaction of the Victim

The victim basically has 2 options in reaction to the rapist's behavior: to comply or to resist. ***Resistance*** is defined as any action taken by the victim to preclude, delay, or reduce the effect of the attack, and the following describe different types of resistance.

— *Passive Resistance.* In passive resistance, the victim does not physically or verbally oppose the rapist but does not comply with his demands. For example, if ordered to disrobe, she does not and the rapist must remove her clothes. Simply not obeying the rapist's commands is a form of resistance.

— *Verbal Resistance.* Verbal resistance is demonstrated when the victim screams, pleads, refuses, or attempts to negotiate with her attacker. While crying is a verbal act, it is not considered to be resistance.

— *Physical Resistance.* Hitting, kicking, gouging, and running are examples of physical resistance.

Motivational Intent of the Offender

The intent of the offender becomes clear only by viewing the crime from his motivational position. The crime usually makes no sense from the perspective of the victim, a police officer, or a prosecutor. Behavior reflects personality and is the basis from which investigators and profilers attempt to form opinions about an unknown offender.

Early research for classifying the underlying motivational intent for sexual assault identified 3 domains: power, anger, and sexuality.[6] These primary motivations are frequently expressed in complex sexual fantasies that often begin to develop after puberty.[7] More contemporary classification typologies outline how various sex crimes are often fantasy driven.[8]

The amount of injury to the victim's body is often interconnected to the offender's fantasy. Some offenders view inflicting injury and pain onto the victim as an important part of the sexual fantasy. Physically hurting the victim, observing the victim's fearfulness, and seeing her in pain is sexually stimulating. Victims of these offenders who interfere with the sexual fantasy are more likely to suffer physical injury. For example, if the victim becomes physically aggressive toward the offender or tries to escape, physical injury may result.

Other offenders do not view inflicting physical injury as part of the sexual fantasy. However, these offenders can and will inflict injury to gain control of the victim or during the assault if the victim is not acting as the offender desires. For example, if the offender has a sexual dysfunction and cannot achieve or maintain an erection, the victim may be blamed and physically injured. If the victim does not say or do what the offender expects, physical injury may result.

When drugs and alcohol are part of the crime, the amount of injury to the victim varies. If the offender's fantasy is having nonconsensual sex with an unconscious or semiconscious victim, the victim may have no visible physical injuries. If the victim is too drugged to resist and the offender does not desire physical injury, the victim may escape physical harm entirely. If the offender desires that the victim be fearful and resist verbally and physically, but drugs and alcohol impair this process, the victim may be injured.

Ullman reported that drinking by the offender before the assault predicts victim injury.[9] Testa et al suggest that there may be 2 categories of rape[10]: forcible rape and incapacitated rape. The definition of incapacitated rape is rape when the victim is incapacitated by alcohol and/or drugs. Testa et al reported that high levels of alcohol in the perpetrator decreases the likelihood of penetration.[11] According to Testa, when the victim is highly intoxicated, penetration is more likely and victim injury is correlated with penetration. Physical injury to the victim was also correlated in Testa's study with perpetrator intoxication and a sober victim.

Some victims do not survive sexual assault. Health care providers must understand that if a victim survives the assault, whatever the victim said or did to preserve her or his physical integrity was correct at the time. Cooperating with offenders' fantasies can and does save victims' lives.

Exit Strategies

After the assault, the offender must remove himself from the situation and exit the crime scene. Various strategies are used for exiting, as follows:

— *Verbal threats.* The offender threatens the victim with physical violence of some type "if he or she tells." The offender may strike, kick, or hit the victim to reinforce the seriousness of the threat(s).

— *Using drugs and alcohol until the victim does not remember the assault.* Encouraging the victim to use drugs and alcohol or "slipping" a drug into a drink the victim consumes can affect his or her memory of the assault.

— *Confusing the victim by stating that the rape was not a rape and that the victim "wanted it."* This strategy is often coupled with telling a victim that "no one will believe you," "people will be angry with you," or "you will get into trouble for drinking and taking drugs" if the victim reports the assault. This combination of strategies is often successful in deterring victims of social-acquaintance rapes from reporting assaults.

— *Murdering the victim.* Homicide is a more common exit strategy when the victim is someone who is unlikely to be reported as missing (runaways and prostitutes). See **Figures 3-4** and **3-5**.

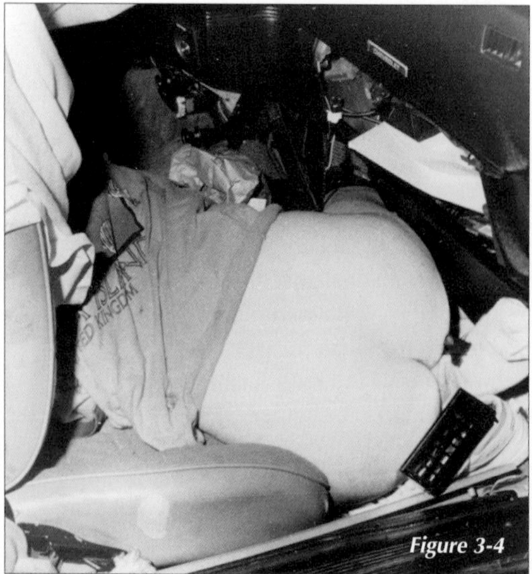

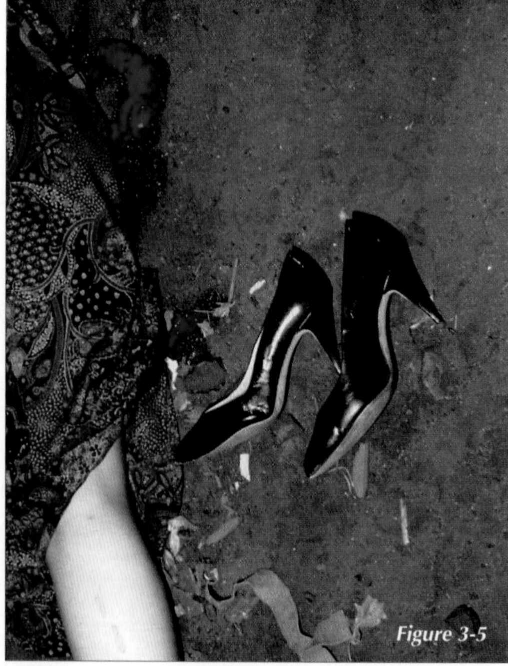

Figure 3-4. *This image displays the crime scene (inside a car) where this victim was raped and killed.*

Figure 3-5. *This image displays the crime scene of a rape and homicide.*

Mechanisms and Types of Injury

Identifying physical findings is not only a critical element in the treatment of the victim but also in the prosecution of most sexual assault trials. Although the law no longer requires proof of resistance, the public, including judges and jurors, still perceives physical injury, and especially genital injury, as the essential proof that the victim did not consent to intercourse. Although this perception is rooted in myth, physical evidence of injury, no matter how minimal, can corroborate a victim's account of the assault. For example, a circular pattern of bruising to the outer aspect of the upper arm can corroborate the victim's account that the assailant grabbed her by the arm to push her against a wall. With respect to genital injury, new techniques are enabling health care providers to identify and document injuries not visible to the naked eye, which will be discussed in subsequent chapters. To appreciate the impact that injury can have to a person's healing and recovery from sexual assault, it is also important to understand that the victim's entire body, not only the genital region, is a crime scene. As previously noted, the absence of physical injury does not indicate consensual sexual contact.

The mechanism of injury can explain how an injury occurred, dispel sexual assault myths, and corroborate the victim's account of the assault. Injuries are often classified by appearance and causation (if known). They are never classified by motivation of causation. The classification categories include abrasions, contusions or bruises, lacerations, and incised wounds, such as cuts (including stab wounds) and slashes. The different types of injuries are defined by the layers of tissue they affect.

Nonspecific findings can be related to circumstances other than sexual assault in adults as well as children. Many sexual assault victims have normal and nonspecific findings on exam. These findings can include but are not limited to the following: (1) hymenal tags, bumps or mounds, clefts or notches (if the hymen is present at all); (2) labial adhesions; (3) erythema of the genitalia or anus; (4) perianal skin tags; and (5) anal fissures. Findings specific to blunt force trauma in females resulting from forceful penetration include recent or healed lacerations or abrasions of the hymen and vaginal mucosa, posterior fourchette, perineum (**Figure 3-6**), labia minora, or labia majora. Exam findings can also be subjective. The victim's experience of pain and tenderness (with or without contact) cannot be documented by visual diagrams or photography. Only examiner observation, documentation, and victim statement can indicate the victim's pain; however, victims differ in how they perceive and tolerate pain, so this subjective finding may not be specific to forceful penetration in itself.

Figure 3-6. *Lacerations of the perineum.*

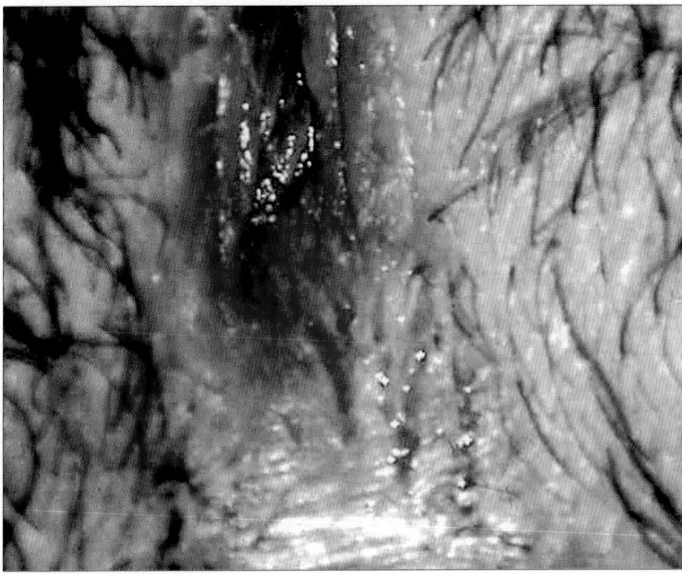

Any area of the body can be injured in sexual assault/rape. Offender aggression is the most significant predictor of victim injury.[12] If the offender is male and the victim female, the offender is usually larger and can use his body weight to restrain the victim in accomplishing the sexual assault.

Injury or tissue damage occurs when some quantity or quality of force is applied to the body. Force can be applied either by a moving object impacting the body or by the body contacting an object. Blunt force trauma refers to injury created by force applied with a blunt object and is divided into 4 types: contusions, lacerations, abrasions, and fractures.

The amount of force applied influences the trauma, but identical applications of force do not cause the identical injury in every person. The quality of the tissue subjected to blunt force trauma also influences the injury. A young person with pliable skin may show little injury because the force is easily diffused without overcoming the tissue's elasticity. On the other hand, an elderly person with thin, fragile skin may experience significant injury from a similar amount of force applied. Younger people also have more elasticity in their bones. The elderly victim may have osteoporosis and fracture more easily than a younger victim. Disease may also render the tissue more vulnerable. Any disease of the skin and/or any systemic disease will alter the body's response to blunt force trauma.

A patterned injury is a representation of the shape of the object that caused the injury. It is important to recognize and document patterns. The pattern can be represented by abrasions, contusions, lacerations, or all of these (see **Figures 3-7** and **3-8**).

The different types of injuries are defined by the layer of tissue affected. Skin anatomy includes 3 layers of tissue: the epidermis, which includes the stratum corneum (keratinized cells) and the basal cell layer; the dermis, which forms the greater part of the skin and contains blood vessels, hair follicles, cutaneous glands, and nerve fibers; and the subcutaneous or fatty layer. Deep fascia or connective tissue and muscle lie beneath these 3 layers. The mouth and vaginal vault are lined with mucosal tissue. These areas do not have the same protective layers as the epidermis (keratinized cells) or fatty tissue; therefore, mucosa is more vulnerable to injury. Victims do not demonstrate a set pattern of typical sexual assault injuries but some types of injuries are more indicative of forceful penetration. Injuries can be classified as abrasions, ecchymoses, erythema, lacerations, and swelling (**Table 3-2**).

Figure 3-7. *This image displays a patterned injury, shown with a ruler for measurement.*

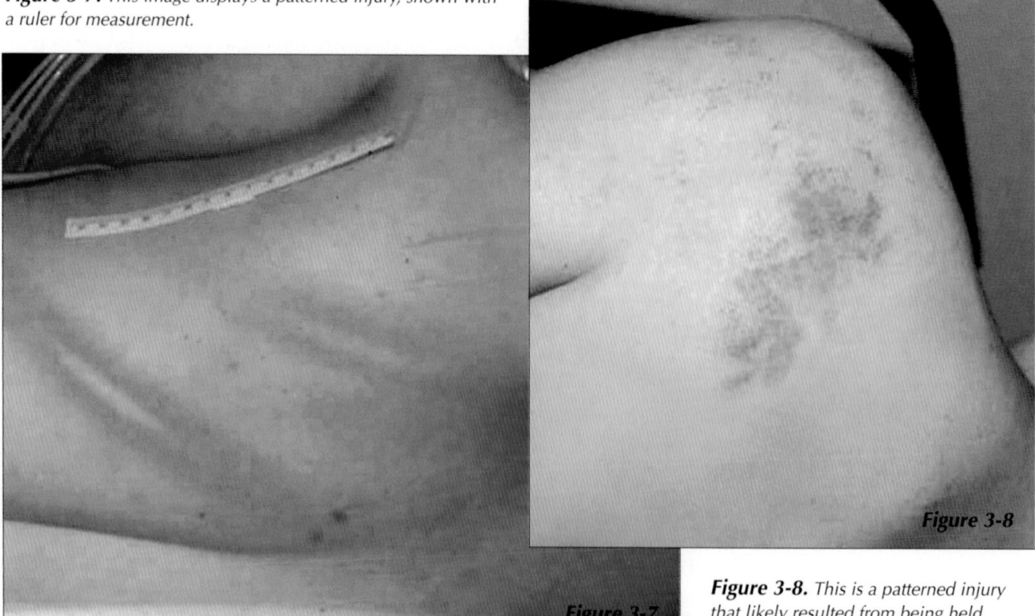

Figure 3-8. *This is a patterned injury that likely resulted from being held down.*

Abrasions

Abrasions are superficial skin injuries limited to the epidermis and superficial dermis (**Figure 3-9** through **3-12**). An abrasion is scraping and removal of the superficial layers of the skin. Small flaps of the uppermost layer of skin may remain attached to the area. These small flaps may indicate the direction in which the scraping occurred. Abrasions may also be called scratches when the injury is caused by a fingernail or brush burns if the injury is caused by frictional force against a rough surface or by dragging along coarse carpet. Rope burns are abrasions caused by the friction of a rope against the skin. Abrasions can be caused by handcuffs and by tying and binding. Such abrasions are usually found on wrists and ankles. Abrasions can have patterns that reflect abrasive clothing or a textured object.

Table 3-2. Acronym for Type of Injury: TEARS[13]

Acronym for Type of Injury	
T	**T**ear (laceration) or tenderness
E	**E**cchymosis (bruising)
A	**A**brasion
R	**R**edness (erythema)
S	**S**welling (edema)

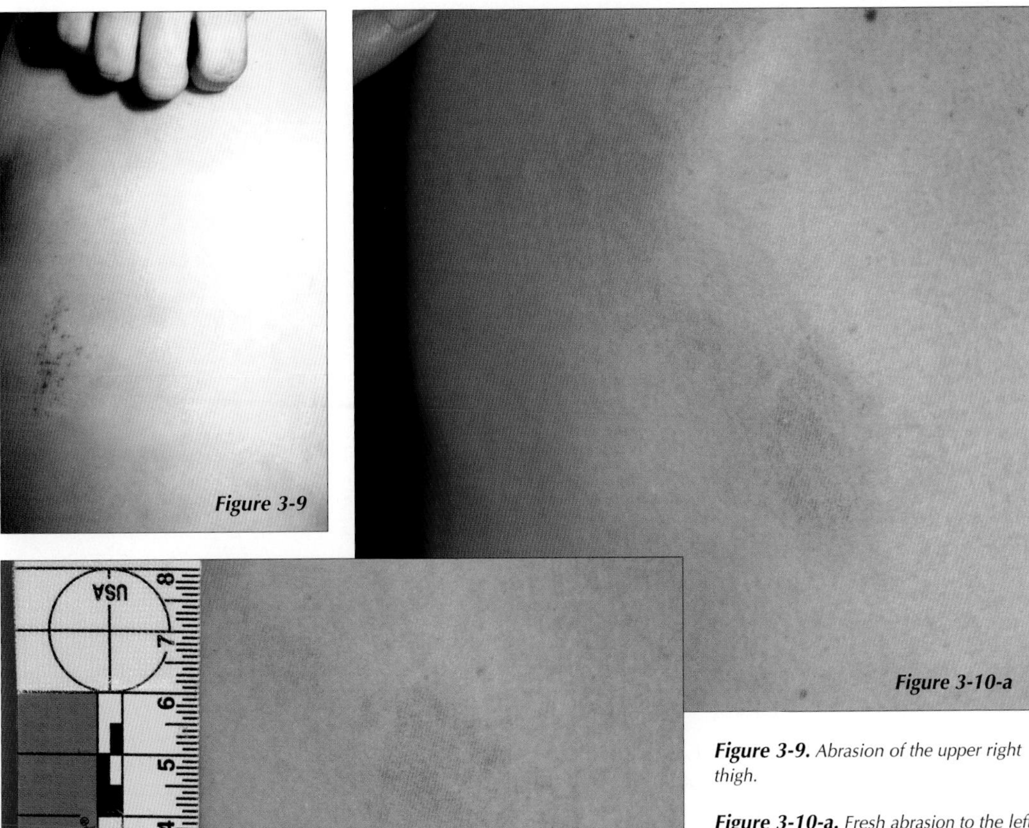

Figure 3-9. *Abrasion of the upper right thigh.*

Figure 3-10-a. *Fresh abrasion to the left upper back area. Patient stated that this area hurts.*

Figure 3-10-b. *In the same patient, this image focuses in on the injury with a ruler in place to measure the injury, which is 3 x 3 cm.*

Figure 3-11-a. Multiple abrasions to the left back area are visible in this image.

Figure 3-11-b. In the same patient, a ruler is in place to measure the fresh abrasion injury.

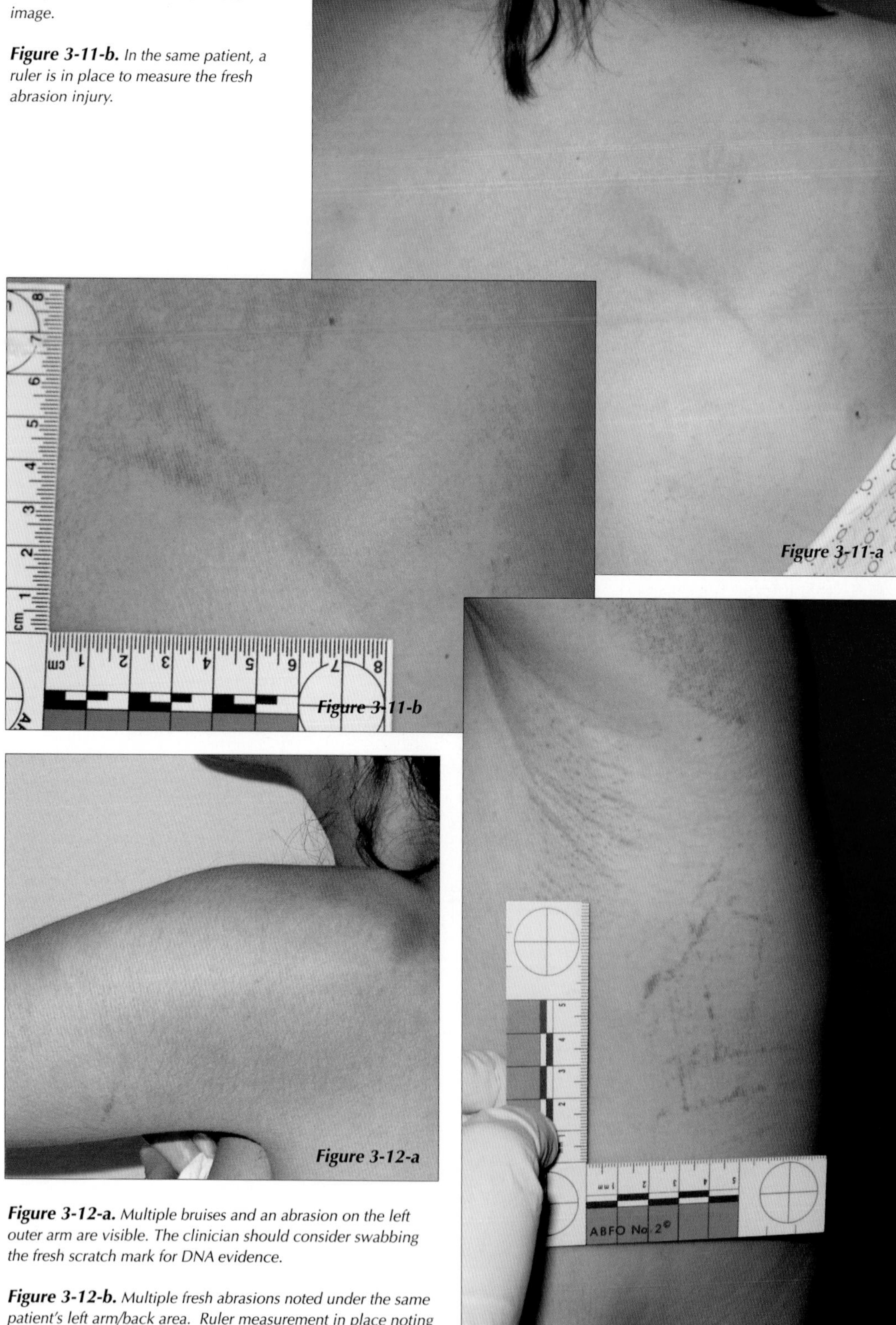

Figure 3-12-a. Multiple bruises and an abrasion on the left outer arm are visible. The clinician should consider swabbing the fresh scratch mark for DNA evidence.

Figure 3-12-b. Multiple fresh abrasions noted under the same patient's left arm/back area. Ruler measurement in place noting the cluster of abrasions, which is 5 x 5 cm. Patient stated she was injured when she was put on the floor in a garage.

Some materials used to restrain the victim are more likely to create abrasions than others. For example, abrasive clothing is more likely to cause an abrasion than a towel or smooth articles of clothing. Bleeding does not usually occur with an abrasion. The superficial nature of the abrasion precludes bleeding. Abrasions begin to heal within several hours of injury. A fresh abrasion usually oozes fluid from the tissues for a day or two. Gradually, the abrasion is covered with a crust or scab under which the healing proceeds until it is complete. The duration of healing depends on factors such as the extent of the injury and repeated trauma in the same area. Infection can also alter the healing of an abrasion.

Bite Marks

Human bites seldom cause tears in the skin, instead resulting in semicircular or crescentric-patterned abrasions. Bite marks create underlying hemorrhages. In sexual assault, biting is generally located on breasts and on or near genitalia. Forensic examiners should note that the skin could become twisted or distorted during the act of biting, thus distorting the pattern. Expert dental consultation is advised when the victim experiences biting.

Ecchymoses (Contusions and Bruises)

Bruises are also known as *ecchymoses* (**Figures 3-13** through **3-16**).[14] Bruises lie below the intact epidermis and consist of an extravascular collection of blood that has leaked from ruptured capillaries or blood vessels. A contusion or bruise is hemorrhage into the skin and the tissues under the skin or both. The bruise usually comes from a blow or a squeeze that crushes the tissue and ruptures the blood vessels. The quantity and quality of the force applied dictate the extent of the contusion. A contusion can occur in any tissue—skin, brain, or lungs. The following discussion will concern contusions of the skin, in which the blood is trapped under the skin because the skin does not break.

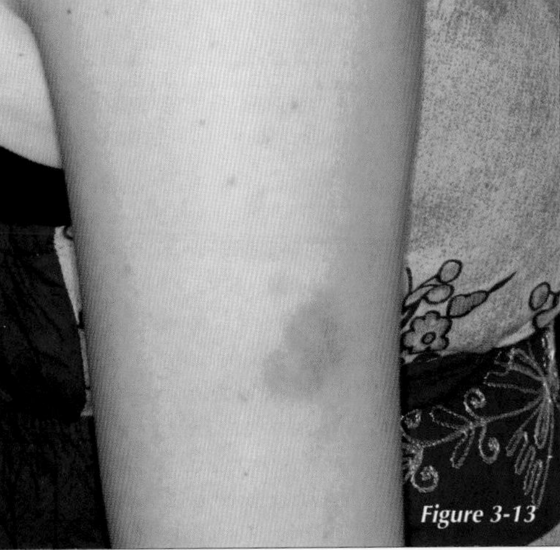
Figure 3-13

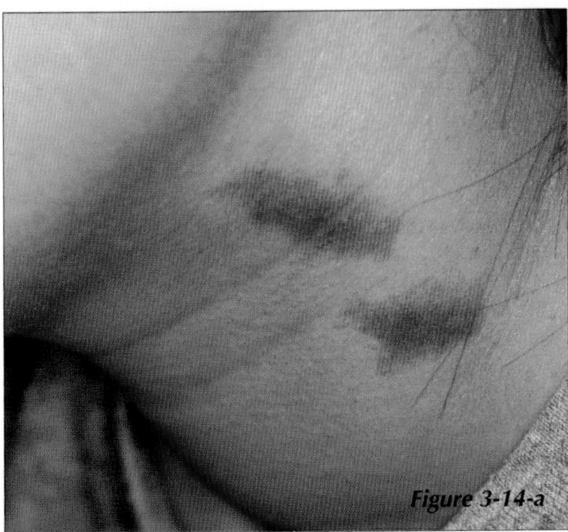
Figure 3-14-a

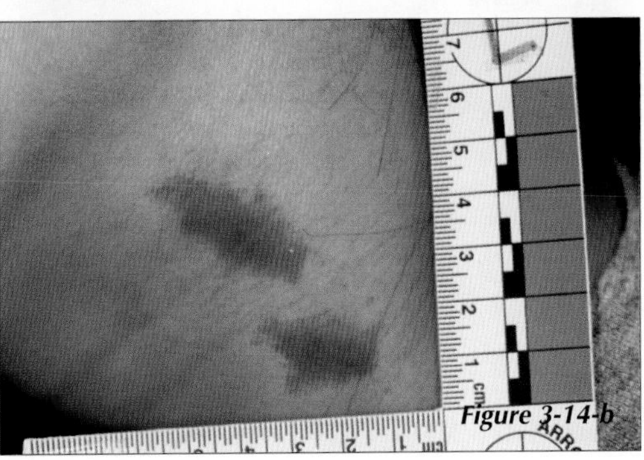
Figure 3-14-b

Figure 3-13. *Bruise to upper right arm.*

Figure 3-14-a. *Multiple bruises on the left neck area. The clinician should consider swabbing the bruises for DNA collection identification.*

Figure 3-14-b. *This image is a close up of the 2 bruises on the left side of the neck in the same patient. A ruler is in place for measurement, and both bruises are 1 x 2 cm.*

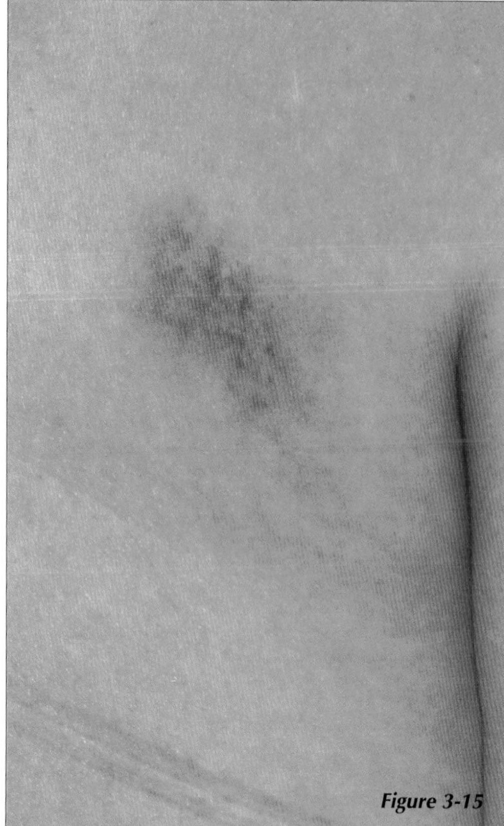

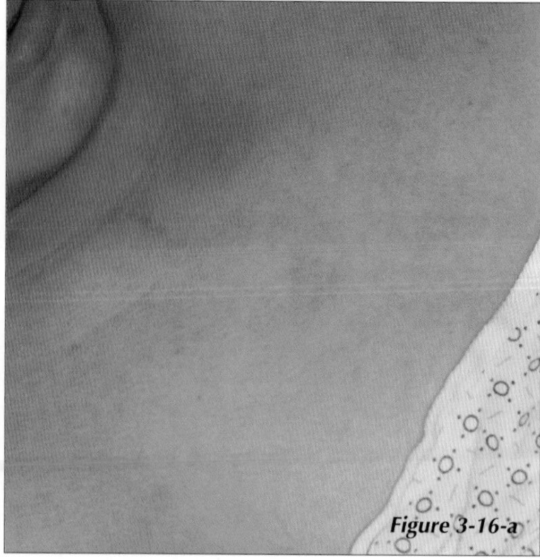

Figure 3-15. *Fresh bruise below the right scapula area. Patient stated she did not remember how this happened.*

Figure 3-16-a. *This is a series of three bruises on the upper chest. This image shows the upper chest area with blue bruises that the patient said were painful. Shape of bruise on the upper middle chest is the size of a fingertip. Another bruise is located along the clavicle area. Consider swabbing these areas for potential contact DNA. This is an orientation image noting the area is her chest, neck, and lower jaw and lips. It would be difficult to know the location of this bruise if the orientation image was not present.*

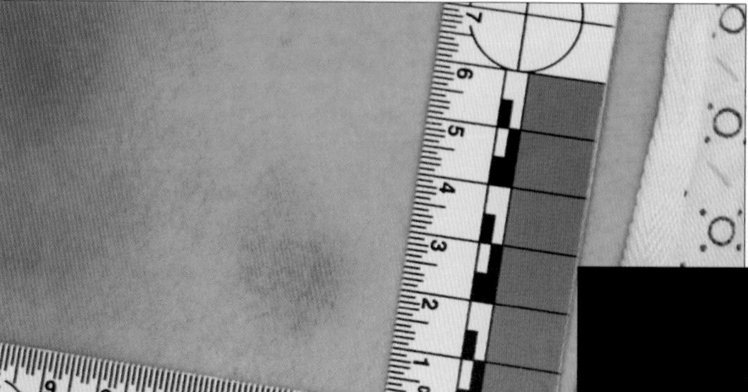

Figure 3-16-b. *In the same patient, this image shows a close-up view of the middle upper chest blue bruise with a ruler in place, showing that the injury is 2 x 2 cm.*

Figure 3-16-c. *This image is shown with a filter that was a global change per a computer software program highlighting the upper middle chest bruise in the same patient. This makes it easier to see under the skin. Using this filtered photograph with the global change to the picture can be presented in the courtroom. These images should always be presented side by side with a photograph with no filter used and a photograph with the global change. Federal Rules of Evidence do allow global photograph changes but do not allow for spot changes.*

Figure 3-16-c

Bruises can resemble the object that created the bruise, such as whips, shoes, boots, fists, hands, pipes, and gun handles. The forensic examiner should note any patterns within a bruise that may indicate the object used (**Figures 3-17-a** and **b**). Parallel track-like lines of hemorrhage result from a blow with a rod, a stick, or an object with a similar shape. The skin between the lines looks pale because the force of the blow displaces the blood sideways.

Bruises do not occur immediately, but may take hours or longer to develop. Several factors can influence the size, color, and appearance of a bruise: available space for blood to collect, weight of the force, vascularity of the area, fragility of the blood vessels, and the location of the bruise. Areas that do not have a hard structure such as a bone beneath may suffer less trauma.

The color of a bruise changes over time. Fresh injury ranges in color from light bluish red to purple. In time the bruise changes to green, yellow, and brown. This change proceeds from the periphery of the bruise toward the center. Light red usually becomes noticeable within a few hours. The change to purple occurs over time. Bruise color is affected by time, size and extent of the bruise, its depth, and the victim's circulatory efficiency and local circulation. No solid studies to date provide an accurate analysis related to age and color of bruising. Research must identify other factors influencing the color of bruising, such as impaired blood clotting, immunosuppression, certain diseases, diabetes, alcoholism, malnutrition, and age.[15] Even environmental temperature has been noted to influence the bruise's appearance.[16]

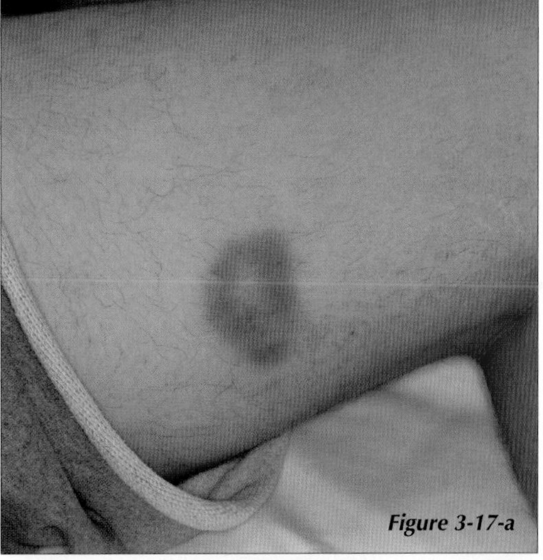

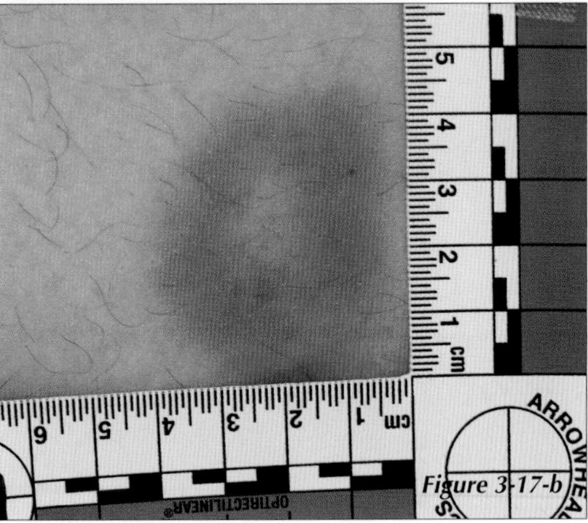

Figure 3-17-a. *Right inner thigh circular bruise with sparing in the middle of the bruise.*

Figure 3-17-b. *Patient is holding the ruler to measure the left inner thigh bruise, which is 4 x 4 cm.*

Bruising occurs when blunt force trauma is applied to an area of the body. However, a contusion or bruise does not necessarily indicate the exact point of force. Blood can shift under the skin due to gravity. For example, if the victim is in a recumbent position, the blood can gravitate to the posterior.

Petechiae are tiny red or purple spots on skin or other tissue. Petechiae less than 3 mm in diameter are pinpoint-sized hemorrhages of small capillaries in the skin or mucous membranes (**Figure 3-18**).

Petechiae, ecchymoses, and bruises do not blanch when pressed. Of special note to forensic examiners, superficial face and scalp wounds generally bleed more profusely than similar injuries elsewhere. Also, elderly people often get superficial hemorrhages in the skin after minor injury due to age-linked fragility of the small blood vessels. Kicking can create minimal bruising on the skin but deep organ damage under the bruise. Forensic examiners must carefully appraise bruising in the abdomen, back, and chest related to kicking.

All bruising must be noted in victims of rape/sexual assault (**Figure 3-19**). Documentation includes the bruise's appearance (including shape), and the location, distribution, and relationship of each bruise to every other. Recognizing a pattern in the bruising may be helpful in validating the victim's account of how the bruising occurred (**Figures 3-20-a** through **d**).

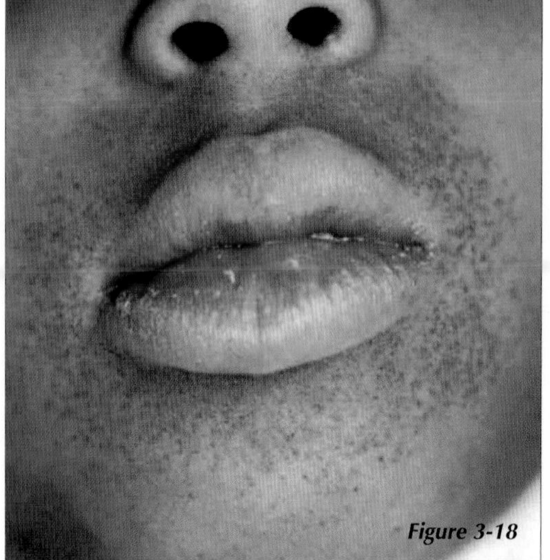

Edema is the swelling of tissues, a condition of abnormally large fluid volume in tissues between the body's cells (interstitial spaces) caused by pressure or trauma to a specific part of the body.

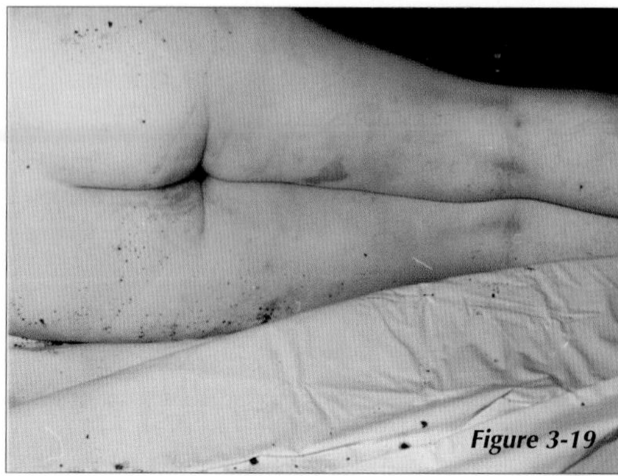

Figure 3-18. *Petechiae around the mouth and abrasions on the lips are visible.*

Figure 3-19. *Bruising and abrasions of legs and buttocks are visible in this patient.*

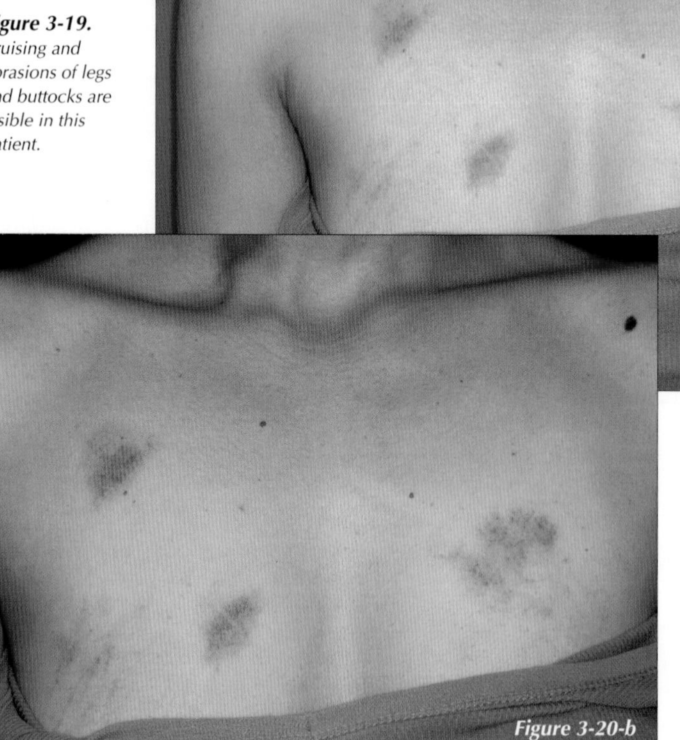

Figure 3-20-a. *Multiple bruises to the upper chest area are shown. Patient stated that the perpetrator was sucking on her chest. This area needs to be swabbed for potential DNA from him. This first image gives an overview of the upper chest and neck area.*

Figure 3-20-b. *In a closer view in the same patient, multiple bruises to the upper chest area are shown.*

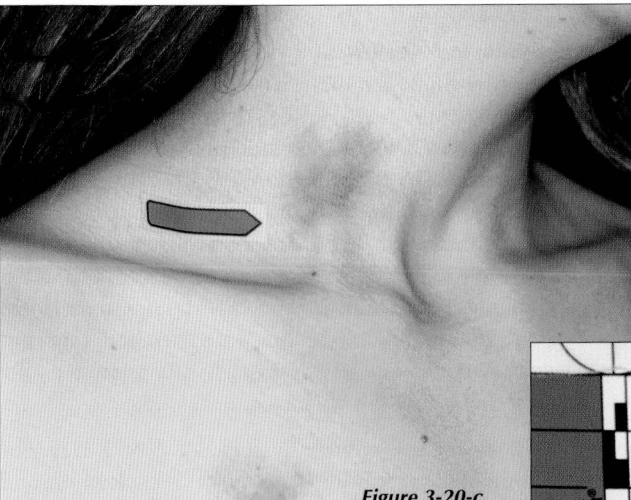

Figure 3-20-c. *This image of the same patient shows a close-up view of the bruise on the lower neck area. The injury itself does not indicate if it is the result of a consensual or nonconsensual action.*

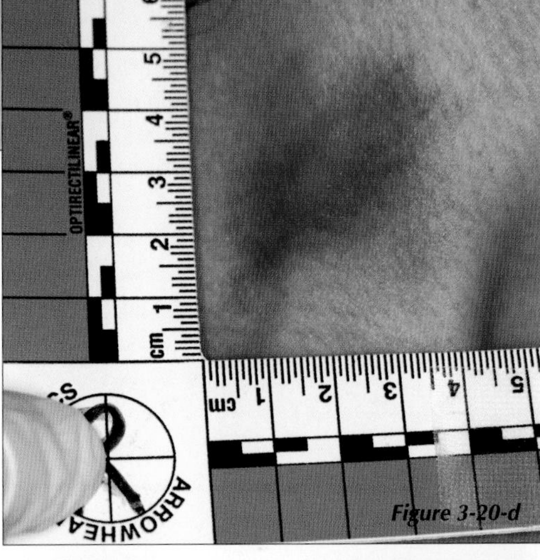

Figure 3-20-d. *This is a closer view of the bruise with a ruler in place. Note that the ruler has R on it denoting the right area. The bruise is 3 x 2 cm.*

Strangulation

Strangulation is often associated with a sexual motivation. The hallmarks of manual strangulation are fingertip bruising and fingernail marks on the neck (**Figure 3-21**). There may be extensive or minimal external injury. Fingertip bruising is circular and oval, produced by pressure from the fingertips on the skin of the neck. Underlying muscles are usually bruised. Fingernail marks appear as thin, linear, or crescentic marks.

Strangulation by ligature creates a mark resembling the ligature itself. Pinpoint and larger areas of hemorrhage are often noted on the face of the strangled victim, especially the conjunctiva and eyelids. The offender may employ a chokehold, placing a forearm across the front of the neck while pulling backward on the other hand. The chokehold compresses the airway. Chokeholds can cause serious damage and death, including hemorrhage in the eyes and face. Injury to the skin is usually absent.

Blockage of the nose and mouth can create asphyxia. This can occur by gagging the victim, holding a pillow over the victim's mouth and nose, or placing a hand over the mouth and nose.

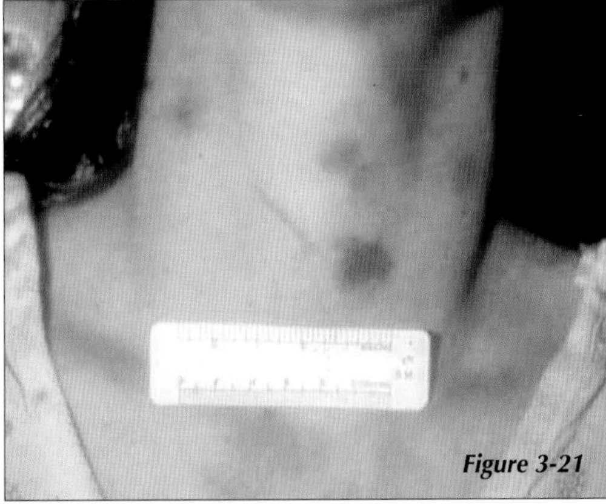

Figure 3-21. *Fingertip bruising of the neck.*

Erythema

Erythema, or redness of the skin, should not be mistaken for bleeding under the skin. Erythema blanches with gentle pressure, is usually diffuse, and does not form a pattern. The cause of redness can be a forceful slap or pressure to the skin. With sudden pressure, the blood is momentarily forced out of the capillaries in the area of contact. When the pressure is withdrawn, the blood returns to the capillaries, which may then dilate. The result is redness or flushing of the skin.

Lacerations

A ***laceration*** occurs when skin continuity is broken or disrupted by blunt force (**Figure 3-22-a** and **b**). It is a tear created by blunt trauma. Tissue opens because of force applied, with the amount of force and its direction creating the laceration's appearance. The impact creates crushing and tearing of tissue. Lacerations can occur in any tissue, but this discussion is confined to the skin. Between the sides of a laceration run multiple threads of tissue called tissue bridges, made up of fiber and blood vessels. The wound edges of a laceration are usually abraded. The abraded area may resemble what made contact with the impacting surface. Lacerations are not cut injuries, but rather breaks in tissue from blunt force trauma applied to tissue with enough force to overcome the strength of the tissue. Lacerations sustained by falling are generally located on protuberant areas such as knees, cheekbones, and jaws. In a fall, the eyes are typically spared and the rims of the eye socket are commonly abraded or torn.

A blow with a blunt object can produce a tear with finely abraded edges. Lacerations can indicate the point of force on the skin, so it is important to carefully examine and document all lacerations. Trace evidence from the crime scene such as dirt and fibers may be found in lacerations.

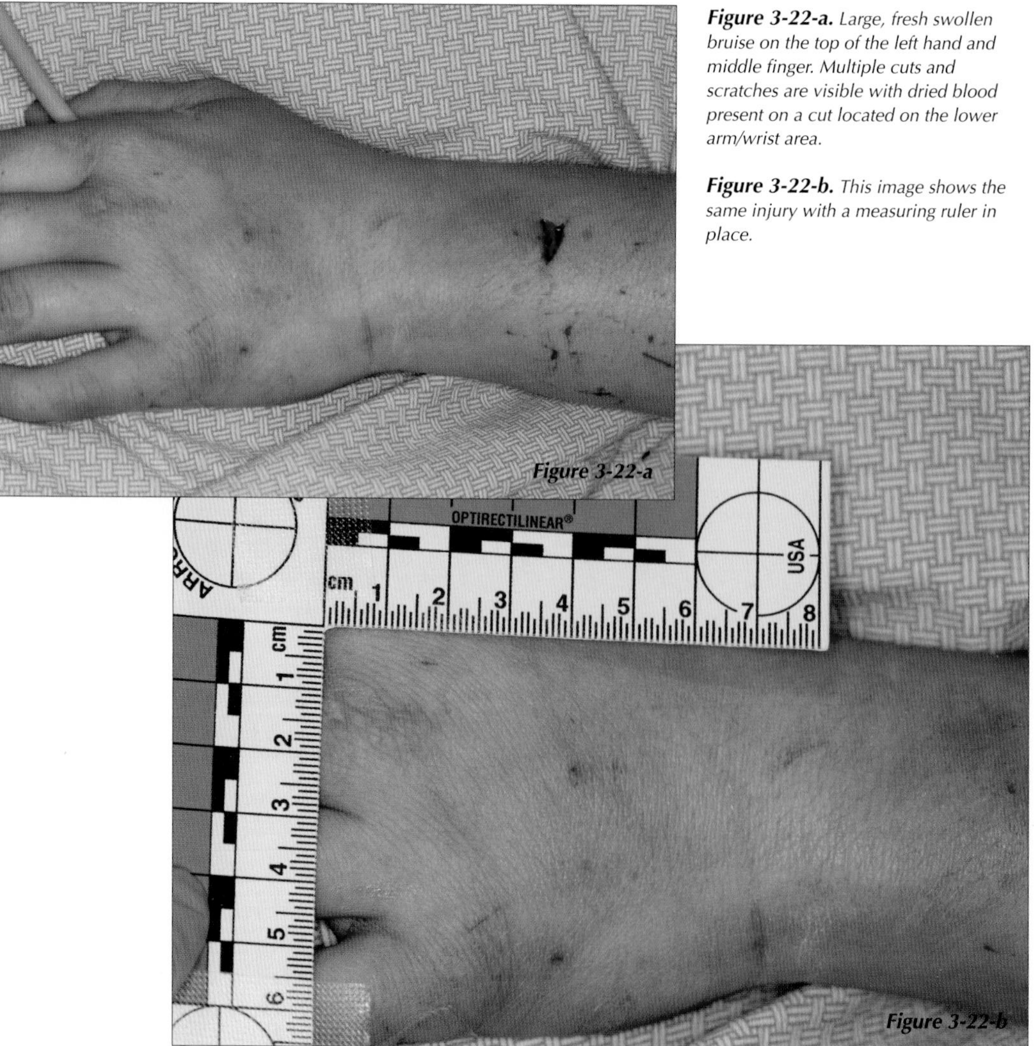

Figure 3-22-a. *Large, fresh swollen bruise on the top of the left hand and middle finger. Multiple cuts and scratches are visible with dried blood present on a cut located on the lower arm/wrist area.*

Figure 3-22-b. *This image shows the same injury with a measuring ruler in place.*

Cut Wounds and Stabs

A ***cut wound*** occurs whenever a sharp object is drawn over the skin with sufficient pressure to produce an injury (**Figure 3-23**). The wound edges can be straight or jagged, depending on the shape of the cutting instrument. The edges of a cut wound are not abraded and tissue bridging is not present. Cut wounds of the upper extremities, especially on the forearm and hands, are referred to as defensive wounds (**Figure 3-22-a**). These occur when the victim raises her arms to protect the face and chest from injury. Defensive wounds can also be found on the legs of a victim if she was on the ground during the sexual assault and was using the legs for defense.

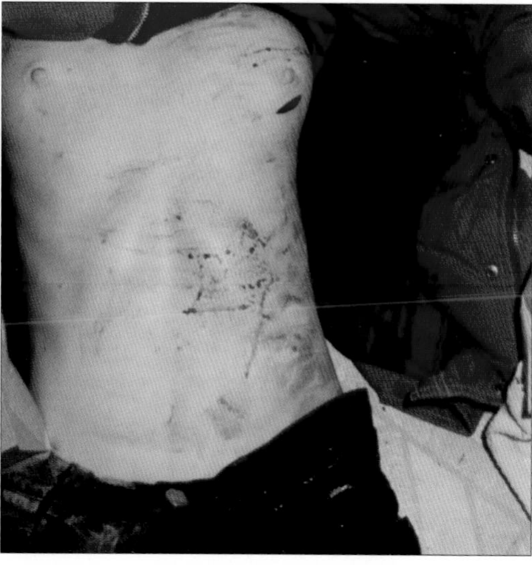

Figure 3-23. *Multiple cutting injuries are shown in this victim.*

Interruptions in cutting patterns usually indicate movement of the victim. Fingernails can create breaks or cuts in the skin. Fingernail marks are usually superficial, semi-circular, and irregularly shaped. These breaks in tissue are superficial, but gouges corresponding to fingernails can be noted. Bruising may accompany fingernail cuts.

A ***stab wound*** results from penetration by an instrument into the body. Any object that can be thrust into the body can create a stabbing injury. The edges of a stab wound are sharp, and the wound is deeper than the length on the skin. Wound edges may be abraded from the hilt of a knife. The amount of blood at the crime scene may be minimal because most bleeding is internal.

Sites of Injury

All areas of the body may be injured during a sexual assault, but there are some that are more likely to be injured and need careful attention. The areas for examination are as follows.

Genital Areas

Eckert et al reported that of 662 patients with a complaint of sexual assault, 21% had genital injury.[3] In a 1997 study, genital exams performed on victims of sexual assault were analyzed. The most common sites for genital injury were posterior fourchette, labia minora, hymen, and fossa navicularis. The most common injury per site was tearing of the posterior fourchette, labial abrasions, and hymenal ecchymosis.[17]

Physical or verbal resistance by the victim increases the risk for genitorectal injury.[18] Scott and Beaman report that injury correlates with a physical resistance strategy applied by the victim.[19]

By far, the most frequently observed genital injuries in adult women are tears and abrasions at the posterior fourchette. This is called a mounting injury where the penis first touches the perineum, usually between the 5 and 7 o'clock positions. The point of contact is often the area of greatest force, causing the tissue to stretch and ultimately tear.

In the labia minora, abrasions and bruising or ecchymoses may occur as a result of friction with repeated penetration or attempts to penetrate. Somewhat less frequent are tears and/or ecchymoses to the hymen or the fossa navicularis. The percentage of hymenal injuries may be increased in victims who have never been sexually active.

Cervical injury is less common, but it may be seen when the penetrating object is not a penis but something else, such as a finger with a sharp fingernail.

Adams, Girardin, and Faugno studied adolescent victims of sexual assault and reported finding tears in the posterior fourchette, erythema of the labia minora, hymen, cervix, and posterior fourchette, and swelling of the hymen, in descending order of prevalence.[20] Danielson and Holmes report adolescents as having more genital injury than adult victims of sexual assault.[21] Data on healing of adolescents is lacking.

HEAD

Sexual assault usually occurs when the victim's head is on the floor, on the ground, or on a couch or a bed. If the surface is hard, the likelihood of injury increases. During the attack, the victim is often pushed down and the head strikes a hard surface. Head injury can also occur during the assault if the victim's head hits a headboard, car door, or floor. Victims can also be struck in the head area with fists, a gun handle, or other objects.

Tenderness in the back of the head is a common complaint after a sexual assault. Swelling can occur in this area as well as bruising and lacerations. Heavy blows to the head can cause internal head injury that requires immediate medical intervention.

FACE

If the victim represents "hated" women, the face of a female victim is often a target for punching, hitting, slapping, and cutting. Black eyes can occur during sexual assault as well as cutting injuries and lacerations. Bruising of the face is common (**Figure 3-24**).

MOUTH AND THROAT

Victims frequently complain of sore throats after the assault from screaming and/or from forced oral sex. Offenders may also "stuff" something into the mouth and throat of the victim to ensure silence. Common injuries to the mouth and throat are bruises and abrasions (**Figure 3-18**). Punching the mouth can loosen teeth, lacerate the lips and mouth, and produce bleeding (**Figures 3-25-a, b,** and **c**). Stuffing cloth, paper towels, or rags into the mouth and throat can create airway obstruction and death.

NECK

Sex offenders often apply pressure to the victim's neck to achieve and maintain control. If the offender squeezes the victim's neck, the victim is likely to cooperate with the desires of the offender. If the victim resists instruction, the offender can apply more pressure until the victim cooperates or loses consciousness. Applying pressure to the neck can be done with one hand and arm.

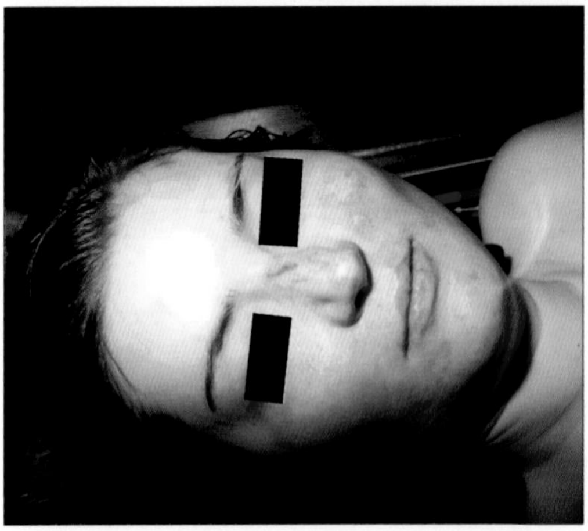

Fingertip bruising of the neck is also common in victims of sexual assault (**Figure 3-21**). The offender may apply a ligature to the neck of the victim, leaving ligature marks. Strangulation is the cause of death for many victims of sexual assault.

CHEST

The breasts of a female victim are considered sexual objects by many offenders and are therefore targeted for biting, punching, and bruising. Offenders may also slash the breasts and/or strike them with blunt objects. Common breast injuries are bruising, bite marks, cut wounds, and lacerations (**Figure 3-26**).

Figure 3-24. *Facial and neck injuries are visible in this victim.*

Figure 3-25-a. *This is a series of 3 pictures showing oral injury in a patient. This image shows multiple fresh bruises on the upper outer lip. Further inspection and photo documentation should follow showing the patient opening her mouth wider. Consider swabbing this area for contact DNA based on the history.*

Figure 3-25-b. *This image shows the patient pulling her lip up to show the injury located on the inner upper lip. Abrasions, bruises, and patterned injuries are visible on the upper inner lip. The pattered injury is the outline of her tooth on the inner upper lip tissue due to the force of the object smashing the lip and the inner upper lip hitting the tooth area leaving an imprint. Further inspection and assessment of this area is needed.*

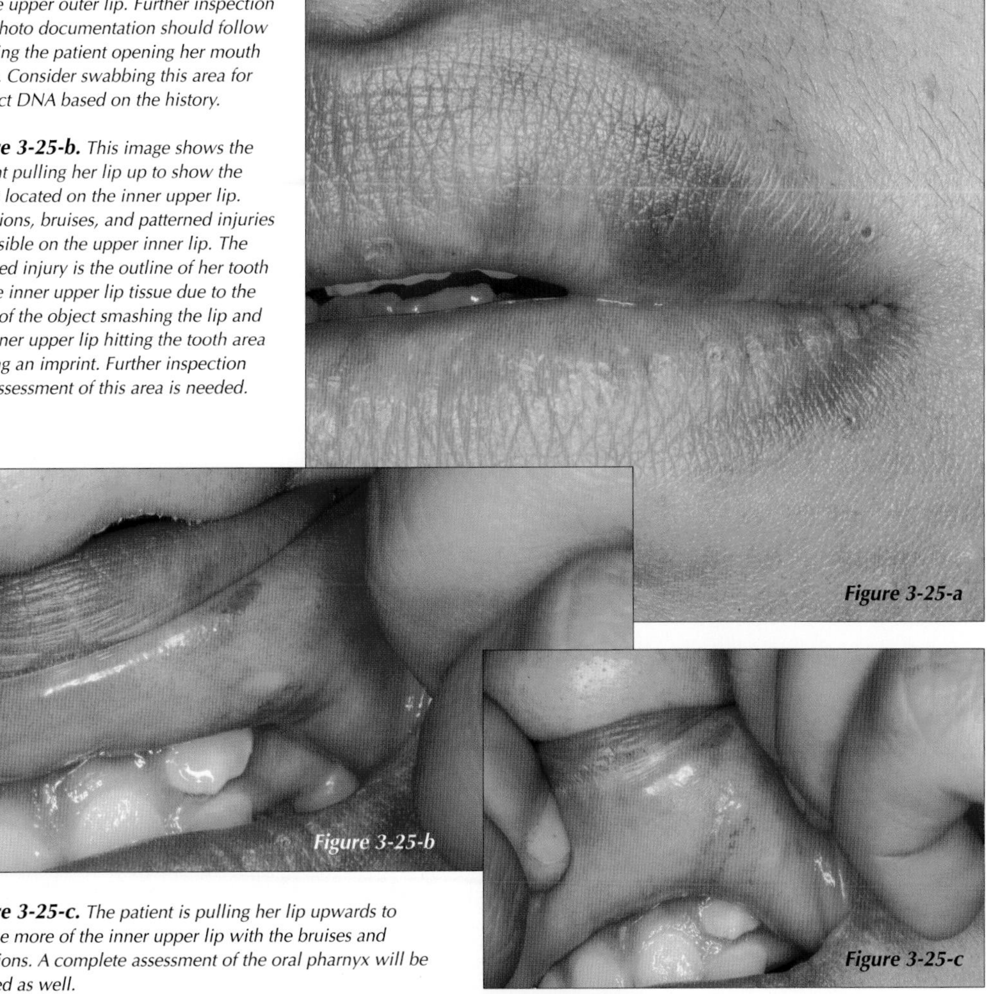

Figure 3-25-a

Figure 3-25-b

Figure 3-25-c

Figure 3-25-c. *The patient is pulling her lip upwards to expose more of the inner upper lip with the bruises and abrasions. A complete assessment of the oral pharnyx will be needed as well.*

Figure 3-26

Figure 3-26. *This patient is a 14-year-old female who reported that a male was sucking on her breast. A bruise is noted on her right upper breast area. A measurement ruler is in place noting the 2 x 1 cm bruise. The blue paper arrow is placed in the area to help the camera focus. This injury occurred when she was sitting up with her back against the wall. This area on her right breast should be viewed using an ALS or Woods light followed by swabbing for potential saliva containing the DNA of the male. Additional documentation of this injury should also be taken with a closer view.*

Back

Usually the victim's back is against the ground, floor, car seat, or bed. Abrasions can occur as the victim is dragged and/or pulled across a surface.

Extremities

Defensive wounds of the arms are common after sexual assault (**Figures 3-13** and **3-27**). If the offender comes toward the victim's face with a fist or a weapon, the victim will raise his or her arms up to protect the face; therefore, the back of the arms often shows bruising, lacerations, and cuts. Arms and legs may be tied during the assault, producing ligature marks. Arms and legs can also be punched, kicked, or slapped, creating bruising and/or lacerations (**Figures 3-28** through **3-30**).

Fingertip bruising can been seen on the inside of the thighs (**Figures 3-17, 3-28,** and **3-31**). If the offender forces the victim's legs apart, bruising of the inside of the thighs results. Bruising and laceration can also be located on the outside of the thighs, when the legs are forced apart and the outside of the leg strikes something hard (eg, a wall, car door handle, or headboard).

Examination Process

Subjective Report

Document any history of pain in the body. Palpate to reveal tenderness and document this also. Noting areas of pain and tenderness may help to validate the victim's account of what occurred during the attack.

Identify any injuries the victim sustains to provide appropriate treatment, assess the need for additional intervention, and determine the need for referrals. Because the victim's body is a crime scene, documenting injury can corroborate the victim's history of the assault. For example, the victim may report that the assailant grabbed her arm, pulled her into the living room,

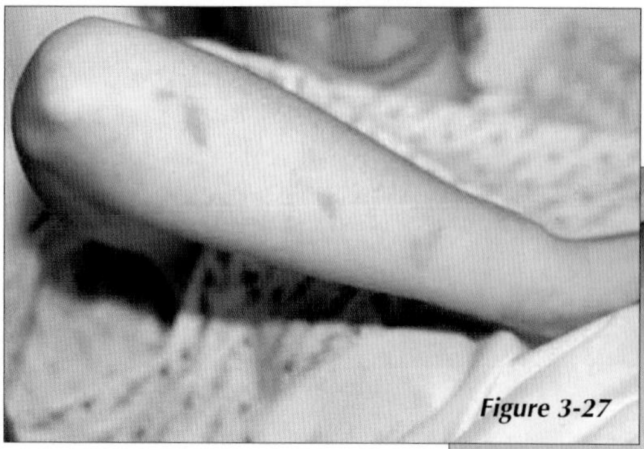

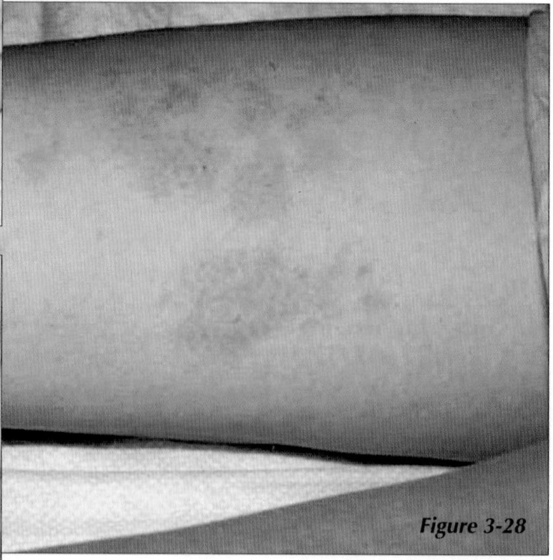

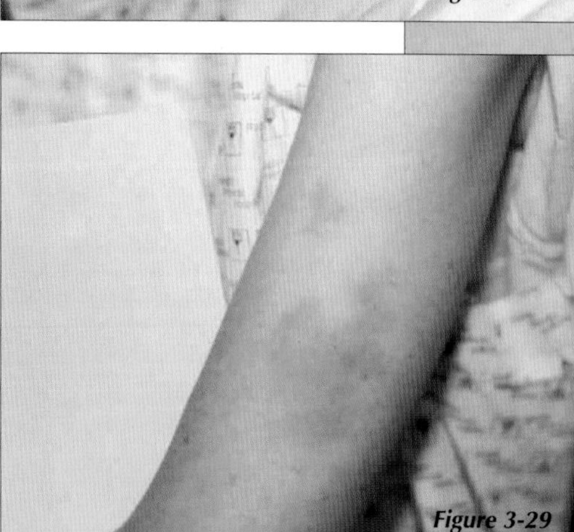

Figure 3-27. *This patient has defensive injuries on the arm.*

Figure 3-28. *Bruising of the thigh is visible on this patient.*

Figure 3-29. *Bruising of the arm is visible on this patient.*

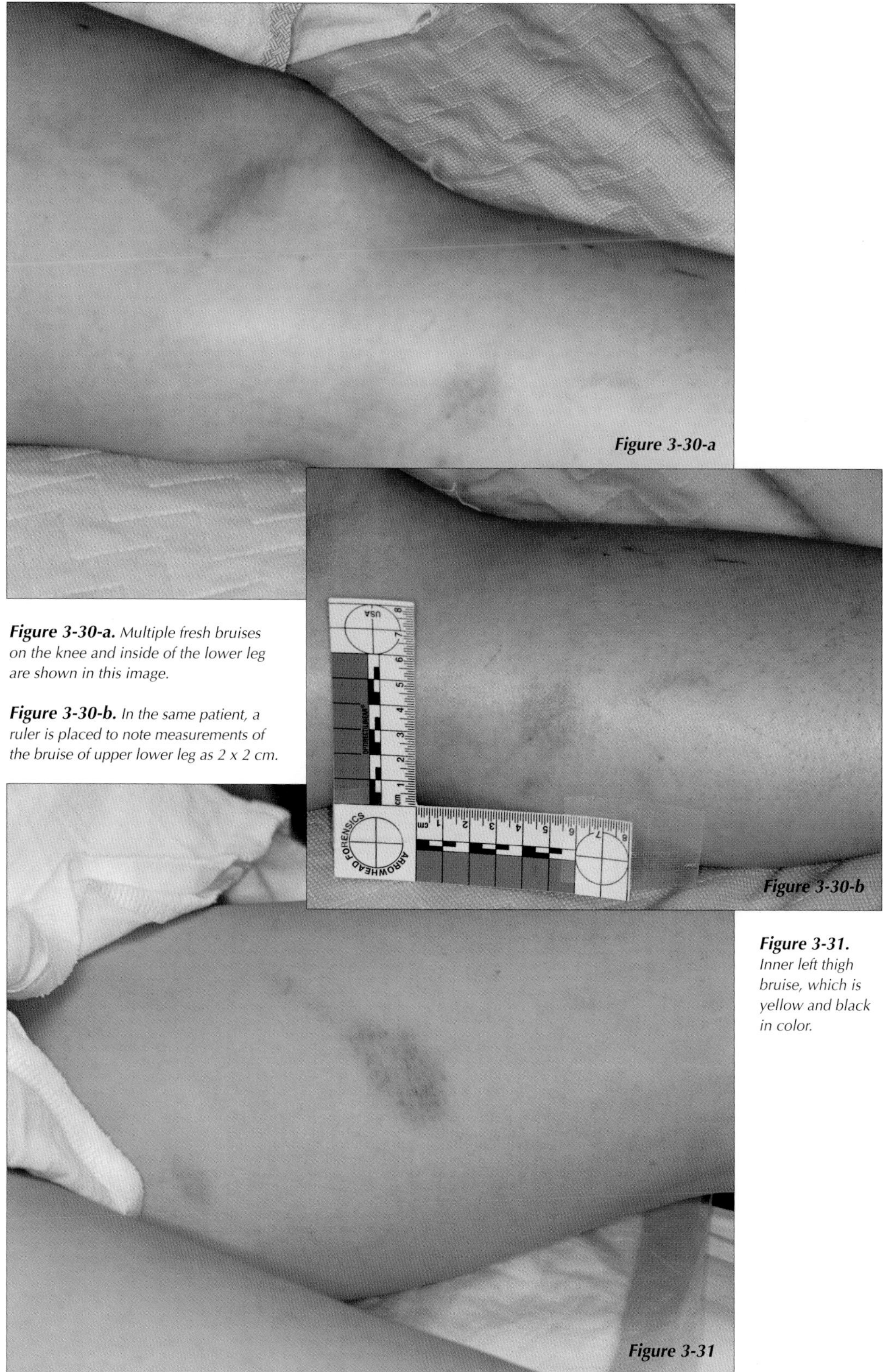

Figure 3-30-a. *Multiple fresh bruises on the knee and inside of the lower leg are shown in this image.*

Figure 3-30-b. *In the same patient, a ruler is placed to note measurements of the bruise of upper lower leg as 2 x 2 cm.*

Figure 3-31. *Inner left thigh bruise, which is yellow and black in color.*

threw her to the floor, and forced her legs apart. The assessment and examination may reveal bruising to the upper arm, shoulder, hip, and inner thighs, which is consistent with this history. It is critical to remember that the *absence* of such injuries does not mean that a rape did not occur. In addition, 2 victims with the same assault history may not have the same types of physical findings.

A complex relationship exists among the variables that can influence injury type and location. A comprehensive history is critical to understanding the presence or absence of injury. **Table 3-3** lists variables to be considered.

Factors Related to the Victim

Anatomy and Physiology of the Reproductive Organs

The vagina's anatomical structure is a key factor in understanding how the body may be protected from injury during sexual assault. The vagina is a muscular organ with 3 layers of tissue: an internal mucous lining, a muscular coat, and a layer of erectile tissue separating the other layers. The mucous membrane is continuous with the lining of the

Table 3-3. Variables Influencing Injury Type and Location

Factors Related to the Victim

— Anatomy and physiology of the reproductive structures

— Health and developmental status

— Condition of the genital structures

— Previous sexual experience

— Lubrication of the vaginal vault (natural or artificial)

— Partner participation

— Positioning and pelvic tilt

— Psychological response

Factors Related to the Assailant

— Object of penetration

— Lubrication

— Male sexual dysfunction

— Force of penetration

Factors Related to Circumstances

— Previous history with assailant

— Lack of communication

Factors Related to the Environment

— Location of the assault

— Materials and surfaces in surrounding area

uterus. The epithelium covering the mucous membrane is of the stratified squamous variety. The mucous membranes are similar to the lining of the mouth, but, unlike the smooth surface of the mouth lining, the vagina contains folds or wrinkles known as rugae. The submucous tissue is very loose and contains numerous large veins and mucous crypts, but no true glands. The muscular coat (tunica muscularis) consists of 2 layers: an external longitudinal layer, which is by far the stronger, and an internal circular layer.

The vagina resembles a flattened tube, the sides of which are collapsed on each other. It is not a continually open space, but a potential space. Because of its muscular tissue, the vagina can expand and contract, much like the cuff of a sweater or glove, allowing different-sized objects to pass through—a tampon, a penis, or an infant during childbirth.

The outer one-third of the vagina, especially the area near the vaginal introitus, contains nearly 90% of the vaginal nerve endings and is therefore much more sensitive to touch than the inner two-thirds of the vaginal vault. This means that penetration of the vaginal vault will cause more pain and discomfort as the penetrating object moves through the introitus into the lower third of the vaginal vault.

In theory, the vagina is designed to accept an adult penis without injury; therefore, it is possible that although force was used, there are no tears, lacerations, or abrasions to the vaginal walls.

Structures of the external genitalia may not be as immune to blunt force trauma as the vagina. The posterior fourchette, also known as the frenulum of the labia minora, is a short, flat fold of mucous membrane that forms the posterior border of the vestibule at the junction of the labia minora. This tissue is not elastic and is most prone to irritation and blunt force. In fact, the posterior fourchette is the site for episiotomies during childbirth. The posterior fourchette may also be where the penis first touches the female genitalia during attempted penetration.

Health and Developmental Status

The victim's health and developmental stage also play important roles in whether or not the victim suffers any injury. For example, injuries are observed less frequently in adolescents and younger adult victims, possibly because of the amount of estrogen produced in their bodies. In addition, younger individuals heal faster and have more resilient tissue, greater elasticity, and more adipose tissue supporting the dermis and epidermis. In older or postmenopausal victims, more injury can result from decreased estrogen levels and loss of tissue elasticity. The marked decrease in estrogen also directly affects normal cyclical lubrication of the vaginal surface. Injuries suffered by this population usually take longer to heal. A victim of any age who is ill may experience compromised tissue responses and ultimately become more vulnerable to traumatic forces.

Condition of the Genital Structures

Healing surgical procedures, such as a new episiotomy, renders the area less stable and more vulnerable to pressure and force. Even transsexual surgical procedures or female genital mutilation can contribute to injury in the genital area. Excessive scarring from a previous operation or lack of perineal elasticity in postmenopausal women can increase the possibility of tears and abrasions. Atrophic vaginitis, or urogenital atrophy, can result in changes to the external genitalia. The epithelium can appear pale, smooth, and shiny. Often inflammation with patchy erythema, petechiae, and increased friability may be present. External genitalia may have diminished elasticity, loss of skin turgor, sparsity of pubic hair, dryness of labia, vulvar dermatoses, vulvar lesions, and fusion of the labia minora. Introital stenosis may be apparent. These conditions put the individual at considerable risk of injury in sexual assault, insertion of the speculum, or intercourse.

In addition, there will be considerable pain. Vaginal epithelium that is friable with decreased rugae is much more prone to traumatic injury. Ecchymoses and minor lacerations at the peri-introital areas as well as the posterior fourchette may also recur after coitus or during a speculum examination.[21]

Any kind of introital lesion puts the victim at risk for significant injury after sexual assault. These lesions can result from inflammatory conditions such as vestibulitis or inflamed labial sweat glands. Abscesses of Bartholin's glands or any infection of the external genitalia can also contribute to tissue damage. Even using improperly fitted or inadequately lubricated condoms can cause irritation. Allergic reactions to the contents of contraceptive foams and jellies and to condoms; abnormalities of the female genital tract (eg, congenital septum, a rigid hymen); and dermatologic disorders (eg, lichen sclerosus) can further contribute to injury.

Previous Sexual Experience

After the onset of puberty, estrogen causes the hymen to be elastic and easily stretched (estrogenization). As a result, it is possible that a woman will have no tears or bleeding with intercourse, even for first-time intercourse or sexual assault. Myths about the hymen may especially impact sexual assault cases. Many jurors believe that the first time a woman has intercourse, there is always injury to the hymen and if the first intercourse is a sexual assault, the victim will have visible tears to the hymen. However, this is not necessarily the case.

Prior sexual experience is associated with different rates of genital injury. Biggs et al found that in a sample of 132 women examined within 10 days of their sexual assault, 65% of those without sexual experience exhibited genital injury whereas only 25% of those with prior sexual experience showed similar trauma.[22] Adams et al found that acute hymenal tears were more common in subjects who stated they were virgins before the assault (19% versus 3%).[23] Hymen injury, rupture, or transection as a result of first-time intercourse is very common, but not inevitable. The elasticity of the hymenal tissue may allow for penetration of a fully erect penis.[24] If the sexual assault victim has not had any previous sexual experience, physical findings may include rupture or hymenal tears. The incidence is higher than the 9% noted by Biggs et al[22]; however, the Adams study examined 87% of the victims within 72 hours using colposcopy, while the Biggs study examined the victims without magnification within 10 days of the reported sexual assault.

Lubrication

Lubrication can be artificial or natural. The menstrual cycle affects the vaginal environment and the secretions within the vagina. The vagina is lined by nonkeratinizing stratified squamous epithelium, which undergoes hormone-related cyclical changes.[25] Estrogens stimulate the proliferation and maturation of the epithelium with an accumulation of glycogen in the cells. Both increased vaginal secretions and altered consistency are seen at ovulation. The pH balance of the vagina fluctuates during the cycle and is least acidic just before and during menstruation. Although the vaginal tissue does not contain any secretor glands itself, it is rich with blood vessels.

Vaginal lubrication typically declines as women age. After menopause, the body produces less estrogen, which, unless compensated for with estrogen replacement therapy, causes the vaginal walls to thin out significantly.[26] The vaginal vault also tends to become slightly shorter and narrower, and the time needed to produce even a reduced amount of lubrication is prolonged. Sometimes a woman who is using a birth control pill that is high in progesterone can experience lessened vaginal lubrication.

Lubrication can also result from vasocongestion, which is an increase in blood volume to the genital area. The blood vessels become engorged with blood and pressure inside these blood vessels forces cellular fluid through the vaginal lining into the vaginal vault. The mucosal surface becomes coated with the liquid in *transudation*. Researchers once believed lubrication was the hallmark of the human sexual response, protecting both partners from injury during coitus. Studies now show that lubrication can be an element of sexual response, but it can also occur as a purely genital response. A genital response is an involuntary, autonomic body response to a sensory stimulus that results in increased blood flow to the pelvic area. The stimulus is most often tactile and can be anything from the slight brushing of underwear to forceful pushing against the perineum to effect penile penetration. Even in nonconsenting intercourse there is a certain degree of lubrication.[24] It is important to recognize that a sexual response includes both physical and psychological components. A genital response is only physiologic in nature.

Lubrication does not instantly disappear if the sexual response ends in fear. If a stranger breaks into a woman's home, attacks her, and begins to touch or press her genitals, her body automatically responds to that tactile stimulus. Blood begins to move to the pelvic vessels, engorgement is initiated, and she starts to lubricate. During sexual assault the genital response is affected by the activities of the sympathetic nervous system, which is in the survival mode, sending increased blood to the pelvis and increasing vasocongestion. In times of fear and threat of bodily harm, the sympathetic nervous system becomes activated and mobilizes the fight, flight, or freeze responses, putting the individual in survival mode. When this happens, neurochemicals are released, stimulating the body to send blood to the large muscle groups and pelvis. Nonessential body functions cease; heart rate, blood pressure, and respirations increase. In fact, the increased blood flow to the lower part of the body can further increase vasocongestion, causing more lubrication,[27] but this lubrication has nothing to do with sexual response.

Partner Participation

In consensual situations when both partners are participating, there is little or no discomfort or injury because of partner cooperation and assistance. The situation is relaxed and the partners assist each other with insertion. However, in the absence of cooperation, the muscles may become tense and insertion of the penetrating object is not facilitated. This risks pulling the labia minora into the vaginal vault and causes repeated attempts at insertion, prolonging contact and increasing tissue friction. In addition, there is the possibility of creating a less flexible surface against which the penetrating object forces itself.

Positioning and Pelvic Tilt

Protective positioning facilitates penile insertion. The use of a pelvic tilt aligns the penetrating body part with the receiving body orifice. If the pelvic tilt is not maintained, as when a woman pulls her body away from the penetrating object, the penis will not enter the vaginal introitus on a parallel plane. The perineum posterior to the vaginal introitus and the posterior fourchette will be subject to overstretching, causing a mounting injury. In addition, leg positioning can facilitate insertion and lessen muscle tension in the lower body and legs.

Psychological Response

The victim may not have any identified injuries because she offered no resistance to the assailant. When faced with a life-threatening situation, a victim's brain and body enter survival mode. The victim reacts with fight, flight, or freezing. ***Freezing***, or tonic immobility, is recognized in the animal kingdom as a deer in the headlights or the mouse lying lifeless in the cat's mouth. Levine describes this response as having an analgesic quality.[28] The victim's terror may also put her into a dissociative mental state. Victims can become totally passive as they literally separate their consciousness from the horror of reality.[29]

Sometimes victims make a deliberate decision not to fight back or resist the assailant. They follow the advice of law enforcement experts and other groups who make recommendations on survival strategies. A victim may follow her own immediate reaction not to fight back because she might suffer far greater injury or even death. It is appropriate for the clinician to explore what the victim felt during the attack. For example, victims frequently say, "I thought I was going to die." The victim also may explain that she did not scream or try to run away because "my children were in the next room, and he said he would kill them if I did not do what he wanted."

Factors Related to the Assailant

Object of Penetration

The penetrating object, perpetrator's finger, or penis may be very large, potentially injurious, or not lubricated. This can cause abrasions from increased friction, lacerations from overstretching, or cuts from sharp or jagged surfaces.

Lubrication

The assailant can supply artificial lubricants, including K-Y Jelly, lubricated condoms, or saliva to decrease friction between the penetrating object and the vaginal vault.

Sexual Dysfunction

It is not uncommon for the perpetrator to suffer some type of sexual dysfunction. Groth and Burgess and other authors suggest that about a third of offenders show clear evidence of sexual dysfunction at the time of the offense.[6,29-31] This leads to prolonged duration of the penetrating object within the vagina or anus, with increased tissue friction, and resulting abrasions.

Force of Penetration

Increased force and prolonged contact can increase the chance of injury, especially in anal penetration. This type of contact may be consistent with the victim's account of the incident.

Factors Related to Circumstances

The relationship between the victim and the perpetrator should be factored into evaluating the victim's account of the assault. If the parties were in an intimate relationship, they may have a history of consensual contact with each other. The history of intimacy can influence current, nonconsensual situations. A sexual overture from one partner may cause the other partner's body to respond as it has in the past. If there were objects, props, or tools used during the assault, these may contribute to nongenital injuries as well as anogenital injuries.

Patterned injuries may also corroborate the victim's account of the assault. The shape, size, and pattern of the injury can show the type of instrument used as a weapon.

Factors Related to the Environment

The environment in which the crime took place may increase the likelihood of both genital and nongenital injury to the victim. For example, if the sexual assault occurred in a wooded area, the victim may have pieces of wood or leaves embedded in the creases of her buttocks or labial folds. An assault on a gravel-filled street could result in small pieces of stone embedded in the soft tissue of the victim's back and arms. Debris from these environments can further increase friction between the penetrating object and the victim's body, resulting in abrasions or lacerations. In addition, these materials can be collected as physical evidence and corroborate the victim's history of the assault.

When Physical Findings Are Not Observed

All of the factors mentioned so far can explain lack of injury as well as presence of injury. The clinician must be aware of the complex relationship among the factors. The anatomy of the reproductive structures, delayed reporting, presence of lubrication, and health and age of the victim can all serve to protect her from injury. Many forms of sexual abuse do not cause physical injury. Although the lay public and law enforcement representatives may be fixated on vaginal penetration, sexual abuse may be nonpenetrating contact and may involve fondling; oral-genital, genital, or anal contact; and genital-genital contact without penetration.

Finally, there is also the possibility that a victim may be treated in a hospital where health care providers are not specially trained in conducting sexual assault exams. The examining health care provider may not recognize certain injuries. An inexperienced health care provider may mistakenly believe that too much time has elapsed from the time of the attack and decide not to do an exam. Today most sexual assault protocols recommend that evidentiary exams are completed within 72 hours after a sexual assault. After 72 hours, exams are sometimes conducted when there are injuries that can be documented or when the victim has not changed clothes or showered. Naturally, if the victim wants an exam at any time, the clinician should respond accordingly.

Treatment and Documentation of Physical Injury

Collection of evidence and documentation of injury take a backseat to identification and treatment of injury. Survivors of sexual assault are triaged in an emergency department setting before a forensic examiner is introduced. Any injury or illness that can be treated should be managed before a forensic evaluation. If a forensic examiner is present during the treatment of injury via trained medical personnel, nonobtrusive photography can be employed for later reference in court. Evidence may be collected before medical stabilization if the process does not interfere with treatment given. Triage in an emergency department typically evaluates cardiac function, systemic circulation, airway function, blood and plasma loss, and presence of fractures. Immediate medical attention is required if the triage process dictates that necessity. The health and safety of the victim are the highest priorities for victims of sexual assault.

Injury that results from sexual assault must be accurately and carefully documented. Injuries to the body, carefully documented, can provide an account of the victim's experience. The nature and location of injuries can assist in verifying the victim's account of the assault. Each injury is evidence of application of force during the assault and must be preserved as a piece of evidence.

Preservation of this evidence occurs in writing, drawing, and photography. Three methods of documenting injury are recommended: a text description, diagrammatic illustration, and, if available, photography (colposcopy). A labeled diagram or traumagram, as well as the photographs taken at the time of the forensic exam, can show relevant genital areas and injury location. Indicating location, size, shape, and color of any injury is imperative. Use of a measuring standard, such as the photomacrograph, allows exact measurements of the injury. To effectively communicate injury site to the reader of the medical record, the hours on the face of a clock are used as a locator. By using the clock as a locator, descriptive words such as left or right, anterior or posterior, or quadrants do not have to be used, thus ensuring that there will be no confusion or misinterpretation of the injury location. Even if photographs are taken, it is still appropriate to use the clock transparency for courtroom testimony.

Written Documentation

Accurate written descriptions of each injury are charted. Medical terminology may be used, depending on the education and experience of the examiner. Injuries may also be described by color, location, size, and appearance using lay language. Injury to genitalia is usually described using the guidelines of TEARS (see **Table 3-2**).[17]

Describing Physical Findings

Physical findings may be normal, nonspecific, or specific indicators of forceful penetration. Although these terms have been used in discussing child sexual abuse injuries, they are also useful for evaluating the adult victim. Adams has built on the classification approach developed by Muram et al and combined it with information from other elements of the sexual abuse assessment.[32,33] These investigators proposed a 5-category classification system for anogenital findings in children, as follows:

Class 1: Normal

Class 2: Nonspecific findings (may be related to conditions other than sexual abuse)

Class 3: Suspicious for abuse (should prompt examiner to question about sexual abuse)

Class 4: Suggestive of abuse and/or penetration

Class 5: Evidence of penetrating injury

Diagrams

Each injury should be entered into a trauma diagram using a diagram and a written description. Multiple blank drawings are required, specifically diagrams of a front and back view of the victim, drawings of genitalia both internal and external, a mouth drawing, and a drawing of the anal area.

Photographs

Injuries to the body are photographed with a digital camera. Those involving the genitalia are photographed with a digital camera or a colposcope. Forensic examiners need not be professional photographers. The purposes of forensic photography after sexual assault are to record injury postsexual assault and to provide photographic evidence. Trauma to the body is of importance to legal proceedings, making it critical that evidence of injury be documented via color photographs. If the victim is suffering from injury that will heal in time, injuries must be accurately preserved photographically. It takes months or years until any evidence is presented in a court of law and injuries may be minimal or completely healed by that time. Photographs are all that will remain.

Digital photography is advantageous in forensic work for several reasons. Images are recorded on a removable disk or memory card or memory stick, simplifying chain of custody. Images can be transmitted instantly. Federal Rules of Evidence allow the admission of digital photography. The authenticity of color in digital photographs can be assured by using a gray scale. Scales that include reassurance of a 90-degree angle are also recommended.

The colposcope is an instrument consisting of a light source, magnification, and a camera. It was developed for use by gynecologists, but was adopted by forensic examiners to assist in the documentation of sexual assault/abuse.

Consent for photography must be obtained from the patient or guardian. In urgent cases where a signature is unobtainable, consent is implied. "Patient consents to treatment and documentation of injury with photographs" is a typical statement found on a consent form given to sexual assault victims.

There are 2 kinds of light important to photography: ambient and artificial. Indoor artificial light must be added to the natural or ambient light in the room to get clear photographs of injury. Fluorescent light commonly found in hospitals tends to give photos a washed out or yellow or green hue. This can be eliminated by adding more artificial non-fluorescent light and by using a flash.

A full-body photograph should be taken first ensuring that the face is included. This full body photo identifies the victim and demonstrates the presence or absence of any overall injury. It often serves as documentation of the demeanor of the victim. Modesty must be considered in taking this first photo, so the victim should be provided with something to cover the body.

After the overall photo, a far away, midrange, and close-up photo of each injury should be taken (**Figures 3-32-a** through **d**). For example, a back injury is documented first with an overall photo of the entire back, then a midrange picture in a context of other body parts such as buttock, shoulder, or waist, and finally a close-up of each injury. One close-up photo of each injury is taken with a scale and one without.

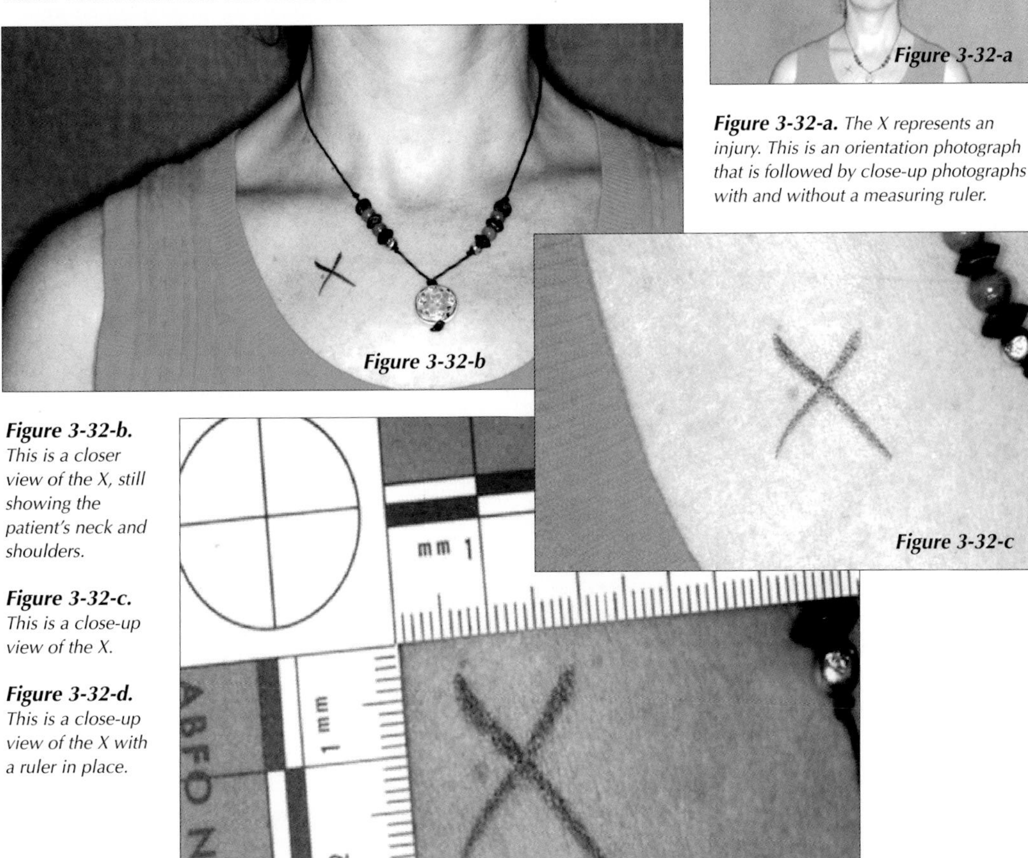

Figure 3-32-a. *The X represents an injury. This is an orientation photograph that is followed by close-up photographs with and without a measuring ruler.*

Figure 3-32-b. *This is a closer view of the X, still showing the patient's neck and shoulders.*

Figure 3-32-c. *This is a close-up view of the X.*

Figure 3-32-d. *This is a close-up view of the X with a ruler in place.*

The recommended background for forensic photos is uncluttered and of a soothing color. White tends to be stark and does not demonstrate injury well. Black and red are also poor choices. Light blue and light green, however, make excellent backgrounds for photographing injury.

Flat surfaces are better backgrounds than shiny surfaces, which reflect backlight. A blue pad with the shiny side down and the dull side under the victim would be excellent for photographing injuries. Forensic nurses should cover or remove clutter from the workspace to enhance photographs, placing emphasis on the injury and not on the clutter. A 90-degree angle is also recommended because it eliminates distortion of the size of the injury.

The photographic set represents a record of the event experienced by the victim. The full body photo is the introduction to the photo log and is listed as number one. Each photo of every injury is then listed in order, including all midrange and close-up shots (**Table 3-4**).

Chain of custody or chain of evidence must be followed for photographs as for all evidence. Photographs should be turned over to law enforcement along with all other evidence collected. If photographs are saved to a computer, they must be encrypted so that only the sexual assault response team has access. Law enforcement must sign the chain-of-custody forms, including the photography log.

Follow-up photographs of injury may be required to document the progress of an injury. Photographs of healing may be desired, sometimes those that heal without scarring, are photographed over time. Sexual assault exams may be performed within hours of the event. At times, injury is not seen at early intervals. For example, fingertip bruising of the neck may not be evident in the first few hours after an assault. Depending on the amount of pressure applied to the neck, the bleeding from the ruptured vessels may only become visible with time.

Jones et al emphasizes the importance of using *toluidine dye* after the insertion and removal of the speculum.[34]

Table 3-4. Steps in Photographing Injuries

Steps in Photographing Injuries
1. Take a before and after cleaning-up-the-victim photograph, especially in cases with bleeding, blood spatter, gunshot residue, and excessive dirt.
2. Take a full-length photo of the person that captures the face and overall injuries.
3. Respect the patient's privacy and allow her or him to cover up for this photograph.
4. Take faraway, midway, and close-up photographs of each injury.
5. Take close-up photos with and without a scale.
6. Label each photograph with date and time, medical record or case number, name of the hospital, and the photographer's name.

Conclusion

It is critical that clinicians have both an advanced knowledge of anatomy and physiology and an understanding of the dynamics of victimization. These dynamics include the relationships between victim and offender, method of approach, control of the victim, mechanism of injury, use of threats and force, substance use by both victim and offender, reaction of the victim, and motivation of the offender.

References

1. Saltzman L, Mahendra R, Ikeda R, Ingram E. Utility of hospital emergency department data for studying intimate partner violence. *J Marriage Fam.* 2005;67(4):960-970.

2. National Violence Against Women Survey. *Full Report of the Prevalence, Incidence, and Consequences of Violence Against Women from the National Violence Against Women Survey* (NCJ 183781). Washington, DC: US Dept of Justice; 2000.

3. Eckert L, Sugar N, Fine D. Factors impacting injury documentation after sexual assault. *Am J Obstet Gynecol.* 2004;190(6):1739-1743.

4. Read K. Population based study of police reported sexual assault in Baltimore MD. *Am J Emerg Med.* 2005;23(3):273-278.

5. Hazelwood RR, Burgess AW. *Practical Rape Investigation.* 4th ed. New York, NY: Elsevier; 2009.

6. Groth AN, Burgess AW. Male rape: offenders and victims. *Am J Psychiatry.* 1980;137(7):806-810.

7. Prentky R. *Human Sexual Aggression.* New York, NY: New York Academy of Sciences; 1988.

8. Douglas JE, Burgess AW, Burgess AG, Ressler RK, eds. *Crime Classification Manual.* 2nd ed. San Francisco: Jossey-Bass; 2006.

9. Ullman S. Factor structure of PTSD in a community sample of sexual assault survivors. *J Trauma Dissociation.* 2008;9(4):507-524.

10. Testa M, Vanzile-Tamsen C, Livingston J. The role of victim and perpetrator intoxication and sexual assault outcomes. *J Stud Alcohol.* 2006;65(3):320-330.

11. Testa M. The role of substance use in male to female physical and sexual violence. *J Interpersonal Violence.* 2004;19(12):1494-1505.

12. Ullman S, Brecklin L. Sexual assault history and health related outcomes in a national sample of women. *Psychol Women Q.* 2003;27:46-57.

13. Girardin B, Faugno D, Seneski P, Slaughter L, Whelan M. *Color Atlas of Sexual Assault.* St. Louis, MO: Mosby; 1997.

14. Lee GR, Foerster J, Lukens J, Wintrobe MM, eds. *Wintrobe's Clinical Hematology.* 9th ed. Philadelphia, PA: Lea & Febiger; 1993.

15. Rabkin M. HIV in primary care. General Medicine Clinic. http://www.columbia.edu/~am430/HIV.htm. Accessed January 27, 2010.

16. Besant-Matthews PE. Blunt Force Trauma. Unpublished paper. Dallas, TX; 2001.

17. Slaughter L, Brown C, Crowley S, Peck R. Patterns of genital injury in female sexual assault victims. *Am J Obstet Gynecol.* 1997;176:609-616.

18. Sachs C, Chu L. Predictors of genitorectal injury in female victims of suspected sexual assault. *Acad Emerg Med.* 2002;9(2):146-151.

19. Scott H, Beaman R. Demographic situational factors affecting injury, resistance, completion and charges brought in sexual assault cases: what is best for arrest. *Violence Victims.* 2004;19(4):479-494.

20. Adams JA, Girardin B, Faugno D. Signs of genital trauma in adolescent rape victims examined acutely. *J Pediatr Adolesc Gynecol.* 2000;13(2):88.

21. Danielson C, Holmes M. Adolescent sexual assault: an update of the literature. *Curr Opinion Obstet Gynecol.* 2004;16:383-388.

22. Biggs M, Stermac L, Divinsky M. Genital injury following sexual assault of women with and without prior sexual intercourse experience. *Can Med Assoc J.* 1998;159:33-37.

23. Adams J. Evaluating children for possible sexual abuse. *Am Fam Physician.* 2001;63(5):883-892.

24. Paul D. Medico-legal examination of the living. In: Mant K, ed. *Taylor's Principles and Practice of Medical Jurisprudence.* 13th ed. London: Churchill Livingstone; 1984.

25. Berman J, Adhikari S, Goldstein I. Anatomy and physiology of sexual function and dysfunction: classification, evaluation and treatment options. *Eur Urol.* 2000;38:20-29.

26. Cardozo L, Bachmann G, McClish D, Fonda D, Birgerson L. Meta-analysis of estrogen therapy in the management of urogenital atrophy in postmenopausal women: second report of the Hormones and Urogenital Therapy Committee. *Obstet Gynecol.* 1998;92:722-727.

27. Basson R. The female sexual response: a different model. *J Sex Marital Ther.* 2000;26:51-65.

28. Levine P. *Waking the Tiger.* Berkeley, CA: North Atlantic; 1997.

29. Bowker LH. Marital rape: a distinct syndrome? *Soc Casework.*1983;64(6):347-352.

30. Groth N. *Men Who Rape.* New York, NY: Plenum; 1979.

31. Rosenbaum A, O'Leary KD. Marital violence: characteristics of abusive couples. *J Consult Clin Psychol.* 1981;49:63-71.

32. Adams JA, Girardin B, Faugno D. Signs of genital trauma in adolescent rape victims examined acutely. *J Pediatr Adolesc Gynecol.* 2000;13(2):88.

33. Muram D, Arheart K, Jennings S. Diagnostic accuracy of colposcopic photographs in child sexual abuse evaluations. *J Pediatr Adolesc Gynecol.* 1999;12:58-61.

34. Jones JS, Dunnuck C, Rossman L, Wynn BN, Nelson-Horan C. Significance of toluidine blue positive findings after speculum examination for sexual assault. *Am J Emerg Med.* 2004;22(3):201-203.

Chapter 4

THE SEXUAL ASSAULT EXAM COMPONENTS AND DOCUMENTATION

Linda E. Ledray, RN, SANE-A, PhD, FAAN
Colleen O'Brien, RN, MS, SANE-A, SANE-P

The goal of this chapter is to summarize the process of the sexual assault evidence collection exam and to recommend best practices. It is important to remember that there are 2 primary goals of the forensic examination: to provide the victim with the best medical care possible and to collect forensic evidence in order to identify and prosecute the offender. To best accomplish these goals, it is recommended that the medical forensic examiner function as a member of a sexual assault response team that typically also includes an advocate, prosecutor, law enforcement officer, and crime laboratory specialist. All members of the team will not be present at the time of the exam, but rather they need to collaborate and facilitate the best medical care for the victim of sexual assault and prosecution of the offender.

In 1987, California became the first state to standardize their sexual assault protocol statewide.[1] Not everyone has followed their example, and today there is still significant variation among states, as well as within states, regarding what evidence is collected and how it is collected. The first attempt to standardize protocols throughout the United States came from the American College of Emergency Physicians[2] and the Association of Genitourinary Medicine, in conjunction with the Medical Society for the Study of Venereal Diseases[3] when they established guidelines for the management of sexual assault survivors.

The most recent attempt at standardization of the sexual assault exam came from the Office on Violence Against Women. In September 2004, they released *A National Protocol for Sexual Assault Medical Forensic Examinations: Adult/Adolescent.*[4] This protocol is meant as a guide for suggested practice (not a requirement) and to supplement (not supersede) existing protocols. While the development of this protocol was indeed a monumental task and it has certainly added substantially to the sexual assault field, it was immediately criticized by many experts and organizations for the way it addressed sexually transmitted infections (STIs) and for the lack of information or attention to emergency contraceptive issues.

EXAM OVERVIEW

A number of articles explain the specific components of the evidentiary exam, some step-by-step.[2-7] Collectively, all of the articles and protocols recommend the following components: obtain written consent; complete an assault history including orifices where contact occurred or penetration resulted; and note the object and method used.

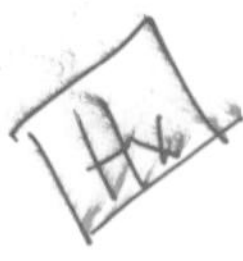

They also recommend a pertinent limited medical history including allergies, current pregnancy status, and menstrual cycle, as well as a physical exam for trauma and areas of tenderness. In addition, they direct that skin surfaces and orifices involved in the assault are examined for trauma and collection of body fluids; combing the pubic hair for foreign hair and matter hair; complete fingernail scrapings or swabs if the victim reports scratching the assailant; collecting a DNA standard from the victim; and collecting the victim's clothing.

The areas of variation in these protocols include the amount of documentation; prophylactic treatment for STIs versus culturing, or both; what clothing is saved as evidence (all as opposed to only torn or soiled clothing); the type of victim DNA standard that is collected (saliva, whole blood, blood stains, or buccal swabs); and the collection of urine and blood for drug and alcohol analysis. A few programs still require pulling 15 to 25 head hairs and pubic hairs, others allow cutting hairs rather than pulling. Most experts today, however, do not recommend the collection of head or pubic hair in the evidentiary exam. Hair evidence is seldom needed from the survivor, and, if needed, it is retrievable at a later time. Some state crime labs still request this evidence, however, and it is essential that the sexual assault nurse examiner (SANE) or sexual assault forensic examiner (SAFE) be aware of local standards.

Use of Evidence

Evidentiary exam of the sexual assault survivor includes the collection of evidence for 4 purposes:

1. To confirm recent sexual contact
2. To confirm that force or coercion was used
3. To help identify the suspect(s)
4. To corroborate the survivor's account of the assault[5,6,8]

Time Frame

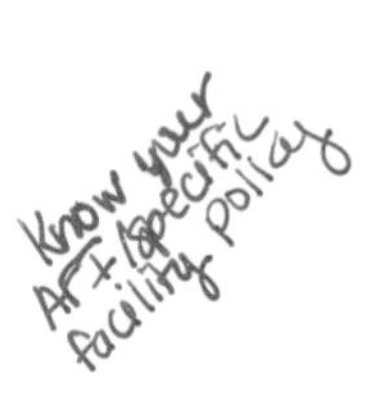

Many areas have extended the recommended time for evidence collection to 96 or even 120 hours after the assault based on advances in DNA recovery techniques.[2,5,8,9] Even areas that have not extended their routine evidence collection period beyond 72 hours typically recommend evidentiary exams be completed in cases, such as when injuries can be documented or when the survivor has not changed clothes or showered, as evidence may still be available for collection. An uncomplicated exam, without injury, can take 1 to 5 hours to complete. It will more likely take 2 to 4 hours.[10]

In regards to the time frame for the SANE/SAFE's response, the SANE/SAFE on call is usually expected to be able to meet the victim and begin the exam 60 minutes after being paged.[2,5] A few programs use a 30-minute response time.[11]

Forensic Evidence

One of the first studies to examine the likelihood of obtaining positive forensic medical evidence after a sexual assault was conducted in the late 1980s, prior to the utilization of DNA. This study was designed to gather information about the likelihood of finding positive sperm and acid phosphatase (an enzyme found in seminal fluid) as a function of the time lapsed between the assault and the evidentiary exam and the orifice involved in the assault. This information is important for court testimony, especially to explain cases where no positive evidence is found. In 1007 cases, including 919 vaginal assaults, 34% were positive for sperm and 62% for acid phosphatase (indicating the presence of semen). Most (88%) of the positive specimens were collected within 12 hours of the assault, with only 7 collected over 20 hours after the assault.[12] In a similar, more recent study of 273 child sexual assault cases the researchers looked for evidence of semen and sperm up to the recommended 72 hours after a suspected sexual assault.[13] Forensic evidence was identified in only 25% of all cases, and 90% of the positive evidence was collected in less than 24 hours after the assault. Unfortunately, these studies did not look at the impact of cleaning methods used by the victims, such as bathing, or brushing teeth.

DNA Evidence

Today, the most common procedure for substantiating a sexual assault is still through the collection of swabs (oral, anal, vaginal, or skin) that are analyzed for sperm and seminal fluid; however, there is often no ejaculate collected or there was no ejaculation, so no semen is identified.

With the recent advances in DNA recovery, crime labs also look for DNA on these same swabs. In fact, today the identification of acid-phosphatase is typically used by the crime lab to suggest that there is sufficient sample available to complete DNA analysis. The DNA can be used to identify a perpetrator in stranger cases or corroborate a victim's claim regarding the identity of a perpetrator in nonstranger cases. Typical sources of DNA obtained from the survivor's body or clothing include hair, blood, skin cells, saliva, perspiration, and semen from the assailant. Based on recent advances in DNA recovery, more and more programs are extending the time for evidence collection from 72 to 96 or 120 hours or more after the assault.

Nuclear STR amplification using the core 13 CODIS loci is probably the most typical form of DNA testing used by state crime labs whenever semen, saliva, sweat, or blood samples are recovered. It has been used at the Minnesota Bureau of Criminal Apprehension (BCA) Laboratory since January 1999. This polymerase chain reaction (PCR) based testing performs well with single source samples, allowing detection of DNA that is present in quantities as low as 250 pg. This change has allowed labs to improve their ability to detect low levels of semen in sexual assault cases. This technique has been accepted in dozens of cases in the Minnesota court system and upheld by the Minnesota Supreme Court, and it has also been accepted in courts around the United States.[9]

An additional type of DNA testing, also accepted by courts, Y-STR amplification has been used in forensic casework at the Minnesota BCA Laboratory since 2003. This type of testing is not used routinely, but it is used in cases where the goal is to detect male DNA in a mixture sample with an overwhelming amount of female DNA. This is common in cases where samples are not collected right after a sexual assault, and in cases where no semen is left behind and samples such as saliva from a male are present.

Recent published papers discuss Y-STR testing on postcoital samples up to 72 hours, regardless of the presence of identifiable sperm. In one study, evidence from 26 child sexual assault cases collected 6 to 72 hours after the suspected assault were examined.[14] Nuclear STR did not detect signs of DNA in any of the cases, whereas Y-STR DNA markers were detected in a remarkable 24 of the 26 cases; however, as the postcoital time is extended beyond 48 hours, there is dramatic loss in the ability to identify the male donor with most Y-STR technology. In another study using cervicovaginal collection techniques (as opposed to lower or mid-vaginal tract specimens) and carefully selected Y-STR loci subset typing strategies, male samples were recovered up to 4 days postcoitus.[15] Also Y-STRs were detected in all postcoital samples tested (up to 90 hours) at the University of Central Florida (J. Ballantyne, personal communication, December 2006).

Unfortunately, all these studies of Y-STR testing focus on vaginal specimens, not oral or anal specimens, even though these represent 15% (anal) and 35% (oral) of reported sexual assault cases.[16]

It is important to collaborate with your local SART team, especially the crime laboratory, as these additional exams represent an added expense *per case* of $1000 to $2000 for the hospital exam and an additional $2000 on average *per case* for the lab analysis to the state, county, or law enforcement department. If the crime laboratory has the resources to conduct the additional analysis, it can be a valuable investigative tool and well worth the additional expense. However, since the research has only identified additional positive DNA in vaginal swabs, it may make sense to only extend the evidence collection time for vaginal samples. Using these STR testing techniques described above, the West Virginia State Patrol Forensic Laboratory has never identified DNA beyond 2 hours in an oral assault. While they have intended their protocol to allow for evidentiary examination for up to 96 hours after a reported assault based on the evidence in oral cases, they have taken the bold step to reduce the time for oral evidence collection to 24 hours (T. Smith, personal communication, December 2006). Clearly, more research is needed not only about the ability to recover DNA, but also about DNA recovery from sites other than the vaginal site.

DNA Evidence Collection

Potential DNA evidence is obtained by collecting any possible biological specimen that the assailant could have left on the clothing or body of the survivor, such as saliva (from a bite mark or any other oral contact), perspiration, hair, or blood. Skin specimens are best collected by slightly moistening a cotton swab with a couple of drops of sterile water, then firmly swabbing the suspected area in a circular motion. Most evidence collection protocols require 2 swabs from each site that are equally saturated. One swab will be analyzed by the crime lab, and the other stored for possible analysis by a defense expert.

If the survivor reports that she scratched the assailant, wet swabs from under the fingernail or clippings should also be collected. DNA can also be obtained by swabbing the involved orifices with a standard size cotton tip swab for sperm and seminal fluid or skin cells.[17] In addition, when the SANE/SAFE completes the evidentiary exam, clothing that could contain useful specimens should also be collected. All specimens should be properly labeled, indicating why it was collected, such as "swab of breast area where suspect had oral contact with the victim." Areas the perpetrator might have touched or exerted pressure (eg, while holding the victim down) should also be swabbed for epithelium cells to recover DNA. The forensic examiner should always err on the side of collecting skin specimens when the survivor reports there was oral contact or possible semen deposits, even with a negative alternate light source reading. Buccal swabs (or saliva or blood stains) are always collected from the survivor for a known DNA analysis to distinguish her DNA from that of the assailant.[8]

Alternate Light Source

The alternate light source (ALS) most commonly used in sexual assault evidence collection is the Wood's lamp, which emits ultraviolet light. It causes sperm to fluoresce, identifying areas with secretions that can be collected. Recent studies have, however, determined that sperm will not always fluoresce with the use of an ALS, and examiners cannot always distinguish between sperm and other substances, such as hand cream, ointment, and petroleum jelly using the Wood's lamp.[18,19] The important thing for the forensic examiner to remember is that the history provided by the victim is the most accurate guide for specimen collection.

Seminal Fluid Evidence

Semen on the victim's body can be useful both to prove there was recent sexual contact and to identify the assailant through DNA recovery. However, the absence of positive sperm or seminal fluid findings does not prove there was no recent sexual intercourse.[12] Studies have shown that 34% or more rapists are sexually dysfunctional,[20] and as many as 40% wear condoms.[21] Seminal fluid evidence is usually analyzed for sperm, whether it is motile (alive and moving when observed under the microscope) or nonmotile, and for prostatic specific antigen (p30 or PA), which is indicative of the presence of semen. Cases are typically negative for sperm and positive for PA when the assailant had a vasectomy, but this is also possible in cases of chronic alcoholism.[22] Unfortunately, few studies address the results of sexual assault exams and the likelihood of getting specimens positive for sperm or PA.

Nongenital Injuries

Significant nongenital injury requiring treatment or hospitalization from a sexual assault is rare, occurring in only 3% to 5% of rape survivors. Even minor injury is usually documented in only about one-third of the reported rapes.[12] Injuries, when they do occur, are more common in stranger rapes and rapes by someone the survivor knows intimately, such as a domestic partner, than in date rape or acquaintance rape situations.[23] In one study of 351 rape survivors, the rate of physical injury for male rape survivors (40%) was higher than for female survivors (26%). While 25% of the men and 38% of the women in this study sought medical care after the rape for their physical injuries, only 61% of them told the treating physician they had been raped. The women expressed a strong preference for medical treatment and counseling by a woman. The male survivors were less likely to express a gender preference.[24]

In a study of 1076 sexual assault survivors, nongenital trauma was found more often than in previous studies—67% of the time.[25] The forensic examiner must be aware of the likely pattern of injuries from violence so that she knows what to ask and where to look for injuries. Intentional injuries tend to be more central, and accidental injuries more toward the extremities. In domestic violence situations, injuries are usually inflicted where the survivor can easily hide them. The most common injuries are broken eardrums from slapping and head and neck petechiae, scratches, and bruises from strangulation. Voice changes and difficulty swallowing are also common with strangulation. Significant airway injury can be done to the neck without leaving any visible marks. Examiners should always pay close attention to a history of strangulation, punch bruising to the upper arm, and "defensive posturing" injuries to the outer mid-ulnar areas of the arms. Also common are whip- or cord-like injuries to the back; punch or bite injuries to the breasts and nipples; punch injuries to the abdomen, especially in pregnant women; punch and kick injuries to the lateral thighs; and facial bruises, abrasions, and lacerations.[26]

The literature cautions the forensic examiner against trying to date the age of a bruise by its color. While it is known that in people with light skin that recent bruising is red or dark blue in color, and older bruising may be green-blue or yellow-blue, and even older bruising may be barely visible, people vary greatly in their rates of healing. Medications may affect bleeding and healing response as well. Experts suggest that the size and color should be documented without further interpretation (eg, "2 cm x 3 cm, deep blue-purple bruising").[5] It is also important to remember that it can be very difficult to even identify bruising in individuals with dark skin if an ALS is not available. Unfortunately, since these light sources are very expensive, most medical facilities do not have them available.

Physical injuries are probably the best proof of force and should always be photographed, described on body drawings, and documented in writing on the sexual assault exam report.[5] Specific consent to photograph is necessary but may be included as a standard part of the exam consent. Two sets of images are generally obtained. One set remains with the chart, while the second set is given to law enforcement personnel with the other sexual assault evidence; these are usually the pictures used in court. The rule of threes should be followed, meaning a full body orientation shot first, then a midrange view, and then a close-up, following a systematic order including front to back. Pictures are taken first without a scale to show nothing is being hidden, then with a scale to document size. A measuring device should be used; even a coin such as a quarter is sufficient. A gray photographic scale also assists with color determination. Each picture should include a label with the victim's name and/or case number in the picture. (Note: Within the first 72 to 120 hours, the term *victim* is generally used as opposed to *survivor*.) On every picture, the SANE/SAFE should label the date, time, client number and/or name, and the examiner's name or initials and title.

Use of digital cameras is standard today in SANE programs. Ease of training staff to use this equipment, no waiting time to see if the photographs are satisfactory, and the ability to retake photos immediately if needed make this technology attractive. The cost of taking and developing pictures is also greatly reduced and much less space is needed to store and archive cases. Digital photography is also generally well accepted by the courts today. Care must be taken to store photos in an unaltered state, but the ability to enhance photos is allowed in court as long as the steps for enhancement can be duplicated and the original is retained.[27]

Some examiners have been hesitant to take pictures of survivors' breasts and genitals, but not properly documenting injuries with pictures may result in liability for failure to document.[28] The survivor's dignity can be maintained and proper evidence made available by taking close-up pictures of the injury and by properly draping other areas. While genital photographs are rarely used in the courtroom, photo documentation of all injuries is still the norm and useful for expert review. While important, photographs are not meant to take the place of other forms of documentation.[28]

Anogenital Trauma

Finding anogenital trauma can help determine that recent sexual contact occurred and that force was used. It can also corroborate a reported history of sexual contact by the survivor. Anogenital trauma is identified using direct observation, magnification, examination with a colposcope/camera or anoscope and staining the tissue with a substance such as toluidine blue. It is important that the forensic examiner is aware that injury may not be as easily detected in women with darker skin color. In a study comparing anogenital injury identification in 120 white and black women following consensual intercourse using visual inspection, colposcopy with digital imaging, and toluidine blue, injury was identified in 55% of the total sample. However, while the percentages significantly differed for white (68%) and black (43%), when the specific anogenital region of injury was considered, this difference was only significant for the external genitalia (white =56%, black=24%) and not for the internal genitalia (white =28%, black=24%). The authors concluded that darker skin color was the significant variable, not race.[29]

Colposcopic anogenital exam is extremely useful to visualize and document genital abrasions, bruises, and tears, as they are sometimes so minute they are difficult to see with the naked eye.[4,8,30] When a colposcope is used in the forensic exam of the sexual assault survivor, its purpose is to magnify microtrauma in the anogenital area that is not readily visible with the naked eye, and to photograph the trauma. The colposcope is not being used by the forensic examiner to identify pathology. The use of the colposcope is an accepted practice in the forensic exam of adults and children,[31] and colposcopy for this purpose is within the scope of the SANE/SAFE practice.[30] The colposcope is an essential tool in the examination of children.[32] When a colposcope is used, it is important to always document the magnification, the patient's position during the exam, and the dimensions of the injury.[32]

Most research on sexual assault without the use of colposcopy documents the likelihood of genital trauma identification at about 1% for severe injury and 10% to 30% for minor injury.[5] In a study without using colposcopy, Riggs et al found genital trauma in 52% of the cases reviewed.[25] With colposcopy, genital trauma has been identified in up to 87% (N=114) of sexual assault cases.[33]

Rape survivors often fear vaginal trauma and are concerned that their genital area has been permanently damaged. Since this is rare, it is helpful and reassuring to a traumatized survivor to have the extent of the trauma, or the lack of trauma, explained to her after the forensic exam is completed.[5] When a video colposcope or camera is available it may be helpful to discuss the findings with the patient or to let her view the pictures.

In an older study in which a colposcope was not used for examination, vaginal injuries represented only 19% of the total injuries, and they were always accompanied by complaints of vaginal pain, discomfort, or bleeding.[34] Another study found only 1% of rape survivors have genital injuries so severe they required surgical repair, and 75% of these are upper vaginal lacerations. Lacerations in the superior vaginal vault usually present with profuse bleeding and pain.[35] In another study that used a colposcope for the exam, 311 sexual assault survivors were compared to a group of 75 women who had consenting sexual contact, researchers identified genital trauma in 68% (N=213) of the rape survivors, while only 11% (N=8) of the women had injuries from consenting sex.[33] While this study had several methodological problems, including moving rape victims who recanted to the consensual group, it was one of the first studies that compared rape and nonrape victims.

In studies using both colposcopy and toluidine blue,[33,36] sites of genital injury were found on the posterior fourchette, fossa navicularis, labia minora, labia majora, and perineum. Further studies found injuries in the vaginal vault, the cervix, clitoral hood, and periurethral areas. In another study, 73% of a consensual group of women had anogenital injuries, while the nonconsenusal group had a rate of 85% anogenital injuries. In a study by Smugar, 52% of the women age 15 or older who presented for a sexual assault exam had nongenital injuries, 20% had anogenital injuries, and 41% were without injuries.[37] This same study found that general body injuries were twice as frequent as anogenital injuries. Also found in this research were data that general body trauma was associated with victim reports of being hit, kicked, penetrated orally or anally; attempted strangulation; and stranger assault. Anogenital injury was found related to victim age (more frequent in victims less than 20 years of age and older than 49 years). Another study by Rosay and Henry concerning 813 rape victims also found significantly more anogenital injury when there was also nongenital physical injury and in victims 12 to 17 years of age when compared to older victims 18 to 69.[38] This study also found anogenital trauma was not related to alcohol consumption, and there was less genital trauma in victims who had been sexually active in the past 96 hours prior to the assault.[38] Similarly, Jones, Rossman, Wynn et al, reported significantly more anogenital injury in victims who had been virgins prior to the assault when compared to those who were sexually experienced.[39]

Anderson et al, in 102 women, found no statistical difference in the presence of injury between a consensual group (21.4%) and a nonconsensual group (23.9%) who came for a sexual assault exam.[40] Their findings specific to the nonconsenting group found that lubricant was used less frequently, that participants with abrasions were 4.2 times more likely to be in the nonconsenting group, and that participants with 2 or more injury types present were 9.7 times more likely to be in the nonconsenting group.

In a study by Crane, both body and genital injury were found in 53.9% of women seeking a sexual assault exam. Injury of the body only was found in 14.4%; genital injury only was found 20.5% of the time.[41] This study suggests that 88.7% of women (age 13 to 87 years) had an injury documented during an exam.

Both the colposcope and anoscope improve the identification of anal trauma. In a study of 67 male rape survivors, all examined by experienced forensic examiners, 53% had genital trauma identified with the naked eye alone. This number increased only slightly (an additional 8%) when the colposcope was used; however, the positive findings increased a significant 32% when an anoscope was used. The combination of naked eye, colposcope, and anoscope resulted in a total positive finding in 72% of the cases.[42]

Blood Evidence

Most states are moving toward the use of dry kits that do not require refrigeration for storage. Because of this, they no longer include the collection of whole blood. Most evidence collection kits today use buccal swabs or blood stains cards for known (victim) DNA standard. In cases of suspected drug-facilitated sexual assault (DFSA), however, the examiner should also collect urine and a tube of blood to be refrigerated until it is analyzed by the crime laboratory for alcohol or drugs.[5]

Urine Evidence

While alcohol has long been used to facilitate sexual assaults, today additional memory-erasing drugs are also employed. The agents used in DFSA include flunitrazepam (Rohypnol), other benzodiadepines, ketamine, gamma hydroxybutyrate (GHB), and gamma butyrolactone (GBL) as well as numerous other substances. Symptoms include a history of having only a couple of alcoholic beverages but quickly feeling and looking extremely intoxicated. The survivor can often remember very little of the incident other than flashes, sometimes referred to as "cameo appearances" after she awakens. She may then find herself undressed, or partially dressed, with vaginal or anal soreness, making her believe she has been raped.[5]

Whenever a survivor of a potential DFSA is seen within 96 hours of the likely assault, a urine specimen should be collected for a drug screen analysis.[2] While 96 hours is the recommended time limit because most substances cannot be detected beyond that time, newer techniques of drug analysis are being developed, and the time frames may change. While the technique is still under study, a new process of analysis can now detect a 2 mg dose of flunitrazepam for up to 28 days after ingestion.[43]

Even though there is little memory and perhaps no certainty of a sexual assault, whenever the survivor's report is consistent with a DFSA or is suspicious, the forensic examiner should collect a urine specimen and blood for DFSA analysis as a part of the sexual assault evidentiary exam. If the victim calls prior to the exam, she should be encouraged to void at the hospital/clinic; if she must void sooner, have her collect the urine in a clean container and bring it with her.[6,44]

Debris Collection

If the assault occurred in an area the victim does not normally frequent, the collection of debris may be useful in placing her at the crime scene. Debris on the body, clothes, or shoes may include fibers from carpet or clothing, leaves, dirt, sand, gravel, asphalt, or other trace evidence. Having the victim undress over a paper sheet, with a barrier (another sheet) under it may be useful. A clean sticky note can be used to collect debris stuck to the skin. With this method, the piece(s) of debris can be contained, and then the paper can be labeled with where it was collected on the body. This evidence is processed with the evidentiary kit.

Male Evidence Collection

The same principles apply to evidence collection in the male victim of sexual assault. Any possible biological or trace matter from the scene found on the victim should be collected. The penis shaft and scrotum should always be swabbed separately for saliva or vaginal fluids, being careful to avoid the urethra, so as to avoid collecting biological fluid from the victim.

Chain of Evidence Issues

Maintaining proper chain of evidence is as important as thoroughly collecting all evidence. Establishing meticulous documentation, with the signature of every person who had custody of the evidence, from the individual who initially collected it to each person who handled it until the time the evidence arrives in the courtroom, is essential or the evidence may be inadmissible in court.[5]

If the SANE/SAFE must leave the room for any reason during the exam, the evidence must go with her.[8] It is inappropriate to ask the advocate or anyone else to "watch" the evidence. The advocate should never be included in the chain of custody for the forensic medical evidence.

It is not necessary, nor is it appropriate, for the police officer to be in the exam room when the evidence is collected to maintain proper chain of evidence. The police can leave the area and the nurse can call when the exam is completed so that the evidence can be picked up. Signatures on the chain of evidence document, from the nurse who collected to the officer who received the kit, are all that is necessary. When the police cannot immediately return, the SANE/SAFE can place the evidence in a locked storage area, preferably a refrigerator with limited access. When the police arrive, any available nurse can sign that the kit was turned over to an officer.

Maintaining Evidence Integrity

All specimens should be air-dried before packaging. These samples can last indefinitely if kept dry in a room with even temperature and when they are packaged in paper. While it is suggested that whole blood and urine specimens be refrigerated for long-term storage to prevent deterioration of the specimens, it is essential that the evidence be kept in an area of less than 75°F. Whole blood, if included in the evidence kit, must not be frozen. This means that storage in an air-conditioned room is sufficient for short-term purposes.

Documentation

Many authors caution against the forensic examiner collecting detailed investigative information and suggest that the SANE/SAFE should ask only for information needed to guide her exam, identify possible injuries and collect the proper medical evidence, deal with the immediate physical and psychological needs of the survivor, and collect and interpret the physical and lab findings. The SANE/SAFE must remember they are conducting a medical forensic interview that centers on the survivor and not other assault details or investigative information, such as the height or weight of the assailant. Details reported by the nurse that differ from the police report may be used by the defense attorney to show discrepancies in the survivor's story.[5,45]

Basic documentation should include the following:

— Place(s) and time of assault

— Nature of physical contacts

— Race and number of assailants

— Relationship to assailants(s)

— Weapons or restraints used

— Actual penetration and attempted penetration of which orifice by penis, objects, or fingers

— Ejaculation, if known, and where

— Use of condom

— Statements made by the victim that explain threats or other actions of the assailant that made her afraid to resist

— Activities of the survivor after the assault that may have destroyed evidence, such as changing clothes, bathing, douching, having bowel movement, brushing teeth, or using mouth wash

— Consenting sex within the last 72/96/120 hours

— Use of tampon

— Change of clothes

— Contraceptive use

— Current birth control or pregnancy

— Allergies

— Survivor's emotional response during exam

— Survivor's appearance

— Survivor's cognitive state

— Physical injuries

In addition to the SANE/SAFE assault exam report, the entire chart is a part of the legal record and may be admitted as evidence if the case goes to court. All statements, procedures, and actions must be accurately, completely, and legibly recorded. It is important to accurately and completely document the emotional state of the survivor and quote important statements, especially "excited utterances" made by the survivor, such as threats made by the assailant.[5] Since victims rarely fight back and are rarely injured, it is important to document things the victim reports that will help explain why she was afraid to resist or try to get away from the assailant.

When appropriate, qualifying statements such as "patient states..." or "patient reports..." should be used. Since physicians do not record "alleged chest pain" or "alleged shortness of breath," examiners should not record "alleged sexual assault or rape" either. These terms are legal, not medical, and have negative connotations that may be interpreted by judges and juries as indicating that the examiner does not believe the survivor.

Nonforensic Exam Components

Sexually Transmitted Infections

In the past, forensic examiners tested for STIs during the acute exam and then again at follow-up. An attempt was made to link the disease status of the victim on follow-up testing with that of the suspect to show that she contracted an STI from the assailant. Research on the variability of disease transmission and clinical expression does not support this practice, and victim/suspect testing is no longer used to prove intimate contact. A further disadvantage was the use of the victim's STI status at the time of the initial exam to discredit the victim; therefore, the Centers for Disease Control (CDC) guidelines allow the clinician the option of providing disease prophylaxis without testing. Initial testing is, however, recommended for ongoing child sexual abuse.[2,5,8,46] In a survey of 61 SANE programs, 90% offered STI prophylactic care.[47]

The fear of contracting an STI is a common concern for survivors. Ledray reported that 36% of rape survivors cited STIs as the primary reason for seeking medical care. However, the risk of contracting an STI during sexual assault is rather low. The CDC estimates the risk of rape survivors contracting gonorrhea is 6% to 12%, chlamydia 4% to 17%, syphilis 0.5% to 3%, and HIV less than 1%.[48] STI testing is expensive and time-consuming for the survivor, who must return 2 or 3 times and, unfortunately, most survivors do not return.[49] Ledray reported that only 25% of the survivors seen in the emergency department returned for STI follow-up. In an earlier study, only 15% returned. The researchers were able to contact 47% of those who had not returned for follow-up. While 11% of these patients did seek medical care elsewhere, only 14% disclosed a history of recent sexual assault to that provider.[34]

Adult/adolescent prophylaxis recommends coverage for chlamydia, gonorrhea, trichomoniasis, and hepatitis B. Nonimmunized patients may receive the first dose of the hepatitis B vaccine at the initial visit. Hepatitis immune globulin is no longer recommended, except in the case of a known hepatitis B–infected assailant. Chlamydia and gonococcal infections in women are of particular concern because of the possibility of ascending infections that lead to pelvic inflammatory disease.[46] Medication counseling should be provided to the patient so that an informed consent may be given before administration. Pediatric cases have very different guidelines for testing and treatment, as described by the CDC in 2006.

Postexposure prophylaxis for HIV depends on the HIV status of the assailant, type of exposure to blood or body fluids, risk of transmission, medical status of the victim, and available medications. The CDC has published guidelines for postexposure prophylaxis for persons seeking care within 72 hours of exposure via sexual assault.[46] The following factors should be considered when determining if a sexual assault could be considered high risk:

— Anal penetration

— Ejaculation on mucous membranes

— Multiple assailants

— High local HIV rate

— Mucosal lesions

— Assailant is a suspected or known intravenous drug user

— Assailant is suspected or known to be HIV positive[48]

Since the early 1980s, HIV has been a concern for rape survivors even though the actual risk is 1 in 500 nationally.[50] A study of 412 Midwest rape survivors with vaginal or anal penetration tracked HIV testing results at the initial visit, 3 months postassault, and 6 months postassault. No patients developed an HIV infection in this time period. Patients described anxiety about the issue of acquiring an infection. Even if the survivor did not ask about HIV at the initial visit, within 2 weeks it was a concern reported by either the patient or her partner. Based on these findings, the SANE/SAFE should provide patients with information about HIV risk, testing, confidentiality considerations, and safer sex options. Informed consent will help patients make decisions based on facts, not fear.[51] If antiretroviral postexposure prophylaxis is being considered, medical consultation by a trained expert is recommended.

SANE/SAFE must be knowledgeable about rates of HIV in local communities so they can counsel patients with accurate risk information. The CDC recommends that if antiretroviral postexposure prophylaxis is offered, the SANE/SAFE should discuss the following with the survivor:

— Unknown efficacy of the drugs

— Known toxicities of the drugs

— Essential, frequent follow-up visits

— Importance of strict compliance with the complete recommended course of therapy

— Necessity of immediately initiating treatment to maximize the effectiveness of the drugs[39]

Pregnancy

The risk of pregnancy from a rape is the same as the risk of pregnancy from a one time sexual encounter, only 2% to 4%; however, pregnancy is a concern of many sexual assault survivors and must be addressed at the initial exam. Oral contraceptives such as Ovral or Lovral have been used for postcoital contraception for many years.[52] This Yuzpe regimen reduces the risk of pregnancy by 60% to 90%. Today, however, clinicians primarily use a progestin-only contraceptive, Levonorgestrel 0.75 mg (Plan B). Plan B is slightly, but not significantly, more effective in reducing the risk of pregnancy. In one study, when Plan B was started within 72 hours of unprotected intercourse, 85% of pregnancies were prevented, compared to 57% using the Yuzpe regimen.[53] While Plan B is usually offered for up to 5 days after a sexual assault, the effectiveness decreases as the time between the assault and the first dose of emergency contraception (EC) increases. When given within the first 24 hours, Plan B reduced the risk of pregnancy by 95%, but only by 61% when given between 48 and 72 hours after unprotected intercourse. The most significant advantage is the decreased side effects of nausea and vomiting, significantly reduced from 50% with the Yuzpe method to 23.1% with Plan B.[53]

Even if the treating medical personnel or the medical facility does not support termination of an existing pregnancy, issues brought by sexual assault survivors must be addressed.

The National Conference of Catholic Bishops has agreed, "A female who has been raped should be able to defend herself against a potential conception from the sexual assault. If, after appropriate testing, there is no evidence that conception has occurred, she may be treated with medication that would prevent ovulation, or fertilization."[54] Because of the controversy around this issue, even in cases of sexual assault, Dr. Ronald P. Hamel—senior director of ethics for the Catholic Health Association—published an opinion supporting the prevention of pregnancy through EC.[55]

According to a national study, only 20% of rape survivors nationally receive EC.[56] The situation is much improved when SANE programs are evaluated separately. A Canadian study found 45% of rape victims seen by a SANE program received EC.[57] Because this was a retrospective chart review, the number of victims offered EC who declined was not documented and is not known. Ciancone et al found 97% of sexual assault victims seen in the 61 SANE programs they surveyed were offered both pregnancy testing and EC.[47] The number who chose to take the EC was not reported. Since the US House and Senate have not been successful in passing a bill to require sexual assault survivors be offered EC in the United States, many states have tried to require that victims of sexual assault be informed about the option of EC and also be provided with the medication if they decide it is the best option for them.

To date, several states have passed legislation requiring sexual assault victims be informed about EC or given the medications when they are requested. The first state to do so was Washington. Other states to follow their example include California, Illinois, Massachusetts, New Jersey, New Mexico, Minnesota, and New York, and fortunately, the list is growing rapidly. Even though providing EC after a sexual assault to victims who request it is still not legislated in most states and is noticeably absent as a recommendation in the *National Protocol for Sexual Assault Medical Forensic Examinations*,[4] nearly all SANE programs recognize that the best medical practice is to inform the rape victim about the option of EC. If she is at risk of becoming pregnant, is being seen within 5 days of the rape, and has a negative pregnancy test, then it is up to the victim to decide if she wants to take EC to lower her risk of a pregnancy resulting from the sexual assault.

Patient rights of justice, autonomy, and self-determination are recognized as key concepts in the ethical provision of health care. Failure to provide pregnancy protection may result in censure, legal action, or civil liability. Chivers reports a New York City hospital was fined for failing to provide postcoital contraception to a victim of sexual assault in addition to other errors in conducting the evidentiary exam.[58]

Crisis Intervention and Counseling

Among the basic components of the evidentiary exam are crisis intervention, mental health assessment, support, and referral for follow-up counseling. While crisis intervention will be the primary role of the rape crisis center advocate, when one is present, the SANE/SAFE, or forensic examiner is also responsible to provide the patient crisis intervention and ensure follow-up counseling services are available.[4,11,59] When domestic violence is suspected or substantial drug/alcohol abuse appears to be an issue, it is important to have a protocol in place for screening and/or referral. Many medical facilities have domestic violence advocates available who can be called to the hospital, similar to the concept of support from a rape crisis center/advocate. It is also important to provide information on the availability of shelters for survivors of domestic violence so they have a safe place to go after the exam.

Continued fear and anxiety resulting from the rape can significantly affect the survivor's life, including her work, school, and relationships with others, for the rest of her life.[5] Trauma work after the assault can help prevent long-term posttraumatic stress disorder (PTSD). The emotional impact and treatment needs of the survivor are addressed extensively in the psychological literature.[60] Self-help books, such as Ledray's *Recovering From Rape,* are also available both to help the victim and to help those working with the victim provide the victim support and better understand their own feelings and reactions to doing this work.

After the Exam

Many medical facilities now have a place for the survivor to shower, brush her teeth, and change clothes after the exam. SANE programs often provide clothes as well.[4,8,10] It is not unusual for the survivor to be afraid to return home alone, so the advocate or forensic examiner should offer to call a friend or relative to be with the survivor during the exam and to take her home.[6] Alternative safe housing, perhaps with a friend or family or in a shelter, may be required and referral sources should be available.

Since the survivor may be in a state of shock in the ED, it is important to provide her with written information to take home with her.[11] Follow-up phone calls within 24 to 48 hours to check on her status, address medical concerns, and provide assistance with follow-up referrals are also recommended. Most advocate programs will provide this follow-up support and counseling.[5]

Conclusion

Significant advances in the medicolegal exam of the sexual assault survivor have occurred in recent years. Much improvement can be credited to the development of SANE/SAFE programs and the sexual assault response team (SART) (see Chapter 12). By working together, members of the SART have improved services to the survivor, increased both reporting and prosecution rates, improved medicolegal evidence collection, and facilitated a seamless system response. The continued collaboration among professionals working with the survivor of sexual assault is essential to advance our knowledge and to support recovery for survivors.

References

1. Arndt S. Nurses help Santa Cruz sexual assault survivors. *California Nurse.* 1988;84(8):4-5.

2. American College of Emergency Physicians (ACEP). *Evaluation and Management of the Sexually Assaulted or Sexually Abused Patient.* Dallas, TX: ACEP, US Dept of Health and Human Services; 1999.

3. Association for Genitourinary Medicine, Medical Society for the Study of Venereal Disease. *2002 National Guidelines on the Management of Adult Victims of Sexual Assault.* London: Association for Genitourinary Medicine, Medical Society for the Study of Venereal Disease; 2002.

4. US Department of Justice. *A National Protocol for Sexual Assault Medical Forensic Examination: Adult/Adolescent.* Washington, DC: US Dept of Justice, Office on Violence Against Women; 2004.

5. Ledray LE. *Sexual Assault Nurse Examiner (SANE) Development & Operation Guide.* Washington, DC: US Dept of Justice, Office for Victims of Crime; 1999.

6. Ledray LE. The sexual assault resource service: a new model of care. *Minn Med J Clin Health Aff.* 1996;79(3):43-45.

7. Littel K. Sexual assault nurse examiner programs: improving the community response to sexual assault victims. *Office Victims Crime Bull.* 2001;4:1-19.

8. Frank C. The new way to catch rapists. *Redbook.* December 1996:104-120, vi.

9. Ledray LE. Expanding evidence collection time: is it time to move beyond the 72-hour rule? How do we decide? *J Forensic Nurs.* 2010;6:60-63.

10. Sandrick K. Tightening the chain of evidence. *Hospitals Health Networks.* 1996;70(11):64, 66.

11. Speck P, Aiken M. Twenty years of community nursing service. *Tenn Nurse.* 1995;58(2):15-18.

12. Tucker S, Claire E, Ledray L, Werner JS. Sexual assault evidence collection. *Wis Med J.* 1990;89:407-411.

13. Christian C, Lavelle J, De Jong A, Loiselle J, Brenner L, Joffe M. Forensic evidence findings in prepubertal victims of sexual assault. *Pediatrics.* 2000;106(1): 100-106.

14. Delfin FC, Madrid BJ, Tan MP, Ungria MCA. Y-STR analysis for detection and objective confirmation of child sexual abuse. *Int J Leg Med.* 2005;119:158-163.

15. Hall A, Ballantyne J. Novel Y-STR typing strategies reveal the genetic profile of the semen donor in extended interval post-coital cervicovaginal samples. *Forensic Sci Int.* 2003;136(1-3):58-72.

16. National Database. http://www.sane-sart.com. Accessed March 29, 2009.

17. Ledray LE, Netzel L. Forensic nursing: DNA evidence collection. *J Emerg Nurs.* 1997;23(2):182-186.

18. Santucci KA, Nelson DG, McQuillen KK, Duffy SJ, Linakis JG. Wood's lamp utility in the identification of semen. *Pediatrics.* 1999;104(6):1342-1344.

19. Nelson D, Santucci K. An alternate light source to detect semen. *Acad Emerg Med.* 2002;9(10):1045-1048.

20. Groth A, Burgess AW. Sexual dysfunction during rape. *N Engl J Med.* 1977; 297(14):764-766.

21. Larkin H, Paolinetti L. Pattern of Anal/Rectal Injury in Sexual Assault Victims Who Complain of Rectal Penetration. Presented at: IAFN Sixth Annual Scientific Assembly; October 1998; Pittsburgh, PA.

22. Enos WF, Beyer JC. Prostatic acid phosphatase, aspermia, and alcoholism in rape cases. *J Forensic Sci.* 1980;25(2):353-356.

23. Kilpatrick D, et al. *Rape in America: A Report to the Nation.* Arlington, VA: National Victim Center; 1992.

24. Petrak J, Clayton E. The prevalence of sexual assault in a genitourinary medicine clinic: service implications. *Genitourin Med.* 1995;71:98-102.

25. Riggs N, et al. Analysis of 1,076 cases of sexual assault. *Ann Emerg Med.* 2000;35(4):358-362.

26. Polsky S, Markowitz J. Injury patterns and patterned injuries. In: Polsky S, Markowitz J, eds. *Color Atlas of Domestic Violence.* St. Louis, MO: Elsevier; 2003: 17-56.

27. Kreeger L, Weiss D. *DNA Evidence Policy Considerations for the Prosecutor.* Washington, DC: American Prosecutors Research Institute; 2004.

28. Pasqualone GA. Forensic RNs as photographers. Documentation in the ED. *J Psychosoc Nurs Ment Health Serv.* 1996;34(10):47-51.

29. Sommers M, Zink T, Fargo J, Baker R, Buschur C, Schambley-Ebron D, Fisher B. Forensic sexual assault examination and genital injury: is skin color a source of health disparity? *Am J Emerg Med.* 2008;26(8):857-866.

30. Ledray LE. Is the role within the scope of nursing practice? On "pelvics," "colposcopy," and "dispensing of medications." *J Emerg Nurs.* 2000;26(1):79-81.

31. International Association of Forensic Nurses Statement. Utility of the colposcope in the Sexual Assault Examination. Presented at: Fourth Annual Scientific Assembly of Forensic Nurses; November 1996; Kansas City, MO.

32. Soderstrom RM. Colposcopic documentation: an objective approach to assessing sexual abuse of girls. *J Reprod Med.* 1994;39(1):6-8.

33. Slaughter L, Brown CR, Crowley S, Peck R. Patterns of genital injury in female sexual assault victims. *Am J Obstet Gynecol.* 1997;176(3):609-616.

34. Tintinalli J, Hoelzer M. Clinical findings and legal resolution in sexual assault. *Ann Emerg Med.* 1985;14(5):447-453.

35. Geist R. Sexually related trauma. *Emerg Med Clin North Am.* 1988;6(3):439-466.

36. Jones JS, Dunnuck C, Rossman L, Wynn BN, Nelson-Horan C. Significance of toluidine blue positive findings after speculum examination for sexual assault. *Am J Emerg Med.* 2004;22(3):201-203.

37. Smugar SS, Spina BJ, Merz JF. Informed consent for emergency contraception: variability in hospital care of rape victims. *Am J Public Health.* 2000;90(9):1372-1376.

38. Rosay AB, Henry T. *Alaska Sexual Assault Nurse Examiner Study* (NCJ 224520). Washington, DC: US Dept of Justice.

39. Jones J, Rossman L, Wynn G, Dunnuck C, Schwartz N. Comparative analysis of adult versus adolescent sexual assault: epidemiology and patterns of anogenital injury. *Acad Emerg Med.* 2003;10(8):872-877.

40. Anderson S, McClain N, Riviello RJ. Genital findings of women after consensual and nonconsensual intercourse. *J Forensic Nurs.* 2006;2(2):59-65.

41. Crane P. Predictors of injury associated with rape. *J Forensic Nurs.* 2006;2(2):75-83, 89.

42. Ernst A, Green E, Ferguson M, Weiss S, Green W. The utility of anoscopy and colposcopy in the evaluation of male sexual assault victims. *Ann Emerg Med.* 2000;36:432-437.

43. Negrusz A, Moore CM, Stockham TL, Poiser KR, Kern JL. Elimination of 7-aminoflunitrazepam and flunitrazepam in urine after a single dose of Rohypnol. *J Forensic Sci.* 2000;45(5):1031-1040.

44. Anglin D, Spears KL, Hutson HR. Flunitrazepam and its involvement in date or acquaintance rape. *Acad Emerg Med.* 1997;4(4):323-326.

45. Slaughter L, Brown C. Colposcopy to establish physical findings in rape victims. *Am J Obstet Gynecol.* 1992;176(3):83-86.

46. Centers for Disease Control and Prevention. Sexually transmitted diseases guidelines, 2006. *MMWR Recomm Rep.* 2006;55(RR-11):1-94.

47. Ciancone AC, Wilson C, Collette R, Gerson LW. Sexual assault nurse examiner programs in the United States. *Ann Emerg Med.* 2000;35(4):353-357.

48. Centers for Disease Control and Prevention. Sexually transmitted diseases guidelines. *MMWR Recomm Rep.* 1993;42(RR-14):1-102.

49. Blair T, Warner C. Sexual assault. *Topics Emerg Med.* 1992;14(4):58-77.

50. Centers for Disease Control. NCHHSTP-Division of HIV/AIDS Prevention, Statistical Projects and Trends; 1999.

51. Ledray LE. Sexual assault. In: Lynch VA, ed. *Forensic Nursing.* St Louis, MO: Elsevier Mosby; 2006: 279-291.

52. American College of Obstetricians and Gynecologists. Practice patterns: evidence-based guidelines for clinical issues in obstetrics and gynecology. *Am Coll Obstet Gynecol.* 1997;4:947-954.

53. Task Force on Postovulating Methods of Fertility Regulations. Randomized controlled trial levonorgestrel verses the Yuzpe regimens of combined oral contraceptives for emergency contraception. *Lancet.* 1998;352(9126):428-433.

54. National Conference of Catholic Bishops. *Ethical & Religious Directives for Catholic Health Care Services.* 4th ed. http://www.usccb.org/bishops/directives.shtml. Published in 2001. Accessed March 22, 2010.

55. Hamel R, Panicola M. Emergency contraception and sexual assault. Assessing the moral approaches in Catholic teaching. *Health Progress.* 2002;83(5):12-19, 51.

56. Amey A, Bishai D. Measuring the quality of medical care for women who experience sexual assault with data from the National Hospital Ambulatory Medical Care Survey. *Ann Emerg Med.* 2002;39(6):631-638.

57. Stermac L, Dunlap H, Bainbridge D. Sexual assault services delivered by SANE practitioners. *J Forensic Nurs.* 2005;1(3):124-128

58. Chivers CJ. In sex crimes, evidence depends on game of chance in hospitals. *The New York Times.* August 6, 2000:1-6.

59. Ledray LE, Faugno D, Speck P. SANE: advocate, forensic technician, nurse? *J Emerg Nurs.* 2001;27(1):91-93.

60. Burgess A, Holmstrom L. Rape trauma syndrome. *Am J Psychiatry*. 1974;131(9): 981-986.

Chapter 5

Biological Evidence: Identification, Collection, Preservation, and Use in Courtroom Testimony

Anjali R. Swienton, MFS, JD
Robert D. Laurino, JD

The realm of forensic evidence can involve every member of a sexual assault response team (SART). *Advocates* and *first responders* must be aware of the need for evidence preservation so that nothing is disturbed before collection. *Sexual assault forensic examiners* (SAFEs) and *law enforcement personnel* must be skilled in techniques of collection, packaging, and preservation to properly obtain items for testing. The *forensic lab analyst* performs the DNA testing and must be able to convey to a jury the power of the technology when examined by the *prosecutor*. Working together, the various team members can advance the use of this valuable evidentiary tool.

Types of Biological Evidence Found in Sexual Assault

In the early 20th century, the French scientist Dr. Edmond Locard developed what is known as the Locard exchange principle.[1] The theory is that when 2 objects come into contact with each other, there will be an exchange of material from one object to the other. This transfer of evidence is not only applicable to contact between 2 people but can also include contact between a person and an object, or a person and a location.

Sexual assault cases by their very nature can yield significant sources of biological evidence, since there is often intimate body contact and the exchange of bodily fluids. In every sexual assault case, at least 3 crime scenes may yield biological evidence: the victim's body, the suspect's body, and the physical location where the offense was committed. The SAFE and law enforcement personnel should look for semen, saliva, blood, skin, hair, body excretions, and products of conception as warranted by the facts of the case.

Semen

Semen is the primary source of biological evidence in sexual assault cases. The lab analyst extracts DNA from spermatozoa present in the semen. Sexual assault kit swabbings attempt to recover semen from the vaginal, anal, and oral cavities. Some programs use oral rinses or floss to try to recover samples in cases of oral sexual assault. Clothing, particularly the underwear worn by the victim immediately after the sexual assault, may contain the suspect's semen. Semen can also be recovered from items used for personal hygiene, including tampons, sanitary pads, wiping objects such as tissues or towels, and, of course, condoms. Other evidence collected from the scene, such as bedding or swabs from a vehicle, may contain semen as well.

Saliva

Saliva may be transmitted through oral sexual contact or acts such as licking, biting, or sucking on a part of the body. The analyst does not actually extract DNA from the liquid portion of the saliva, but rather from the skin or epithelial cells of the mouth contained in the saliva. Saliva may also be transmitted to items that contact the mouth, such as partially eaten food, drinking containers, chewing gum, and cigarettes.

Blood

Bleeding may have resulted from an injury caused to the victim, or a wound to the suspect caused by the victim in self-defense. In blood, the DNA is found within the nuclei of white blood cells.

Skin

Fingernail scrapings or swabbings are routinely taken from victims (especially if there was a struggle) to try to obtain skin cells of the suspect. Epithelial cells may also be transferred. Epithelial cells can be found on clothing items that contact the skin, such as gloves, hats, or masks, or on items used to bind or gag the victim.

Hair

When hairs are forcibly removed from the body, as in a struggle, they often contain a skin tag or clump of cells at the root end. A hair sample containing a root may be a good source for nuclear DNA. If a hair is cut or shed naturally and only the shaft is present, nuclear DNA may not be present, but the sample may still yield mitochondrial DNA. Hairs may be obtained in combings from the body, or may be on the victim's or suspect's person or clothing. If the victim was bound, hairs may be recovered from ligatures, tapes, or similar objects. Hairs may also be recovered from the physical location of the crime on such items as furniture, bedding, carpeting, or vehicle interiors.

Bodily Excretions

Excretions include perspiration, vaginal secretions, expectorants, urine, fecal material, or even vomitus. Epithelial cells may be analyzed from these substances excreted from the body.

Products of Conception

When a sexual assault results in pregnancy, DNA testing can be performed on the products of conception or on a child brought to term. While DNA can determine who the biological father is, the other elements of assault must still be proved.

Other Evidence

The forensic examiner and law enforcement officer are only limited by their imagination as to items from which biological evidence may be recovered. DNA is not always recoverable. Environmental factors can cause degradation or contamination of a sample. Even with the best efforts at recovery, an area containing DNA may be missed during the collection process, or an insufficient sample may be recovered.

When there is contact and transfer between 2 or more individuals, there is the possibility a *mixture* of the biological samples will occur. In a mixture of sperm and another type of biological specimen (such as blood or saliva), the forensic lab analyst attempts to separate the samples into distinct DNA profiles. This is possible because of the unique chemical properties of the sperm cell membrane. If separation is accomplished, the analyst may designate a *major* and *minor contributor* based on the amount of DNA contributed by each party. Sometimes, as in the case of multiple donors of blood or blood/saliva mixture, the separation is not possible. In these cases, the analyst reports an *irresolvable mixture.*

Finding the Biological Evidence

Some types of biological evidence, such as blood, are characterized by a deep red or brown color and metallic smell, making it often quite evident. However, many body fluids encountered in sexual assault, including semen, saliva, and perspiration, may not be visible to the naked eye. Knowing where to look and what tools are available to help locate these stains assists the SAFE in maximizing the potential evidence collected.

When blood is present in large amounts, either wet or dried, it is easily seen. DNA can be recovered, however, even if attempts have been made to wash an item or area where blood was deposited. If no visible stain exists but investigators suspect blood was present, luminol or other chemiluminescent chemicals, such as fluorescein, can be used. Luminol can reveal traces of blood through its light-producing chemical reaction with hemoglobin, an oxygen-carrying molecule in blood. Investigators spray a suspicious area with liquid luminol and turn off all lights. Any traces of blood present fluoresce (**Figures 5-1** through **5-2**). The location of the stains is recorded immediately as the chemical reaction does not last long. Common household substances, such as bleach, can cause a false-positive result; therefore, luminol is used only as a screening or presumptive test for blood. The chemicals in luminol do not interfere with the lab's ability to recover DNA evidence. However, since it is a liquid, its use can dilute any biological stains present. For this reason, luminol should only be used when no stain is visible.

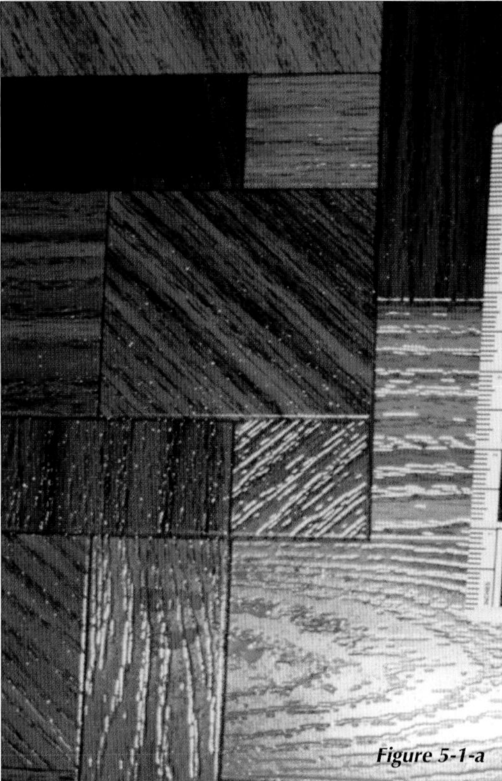

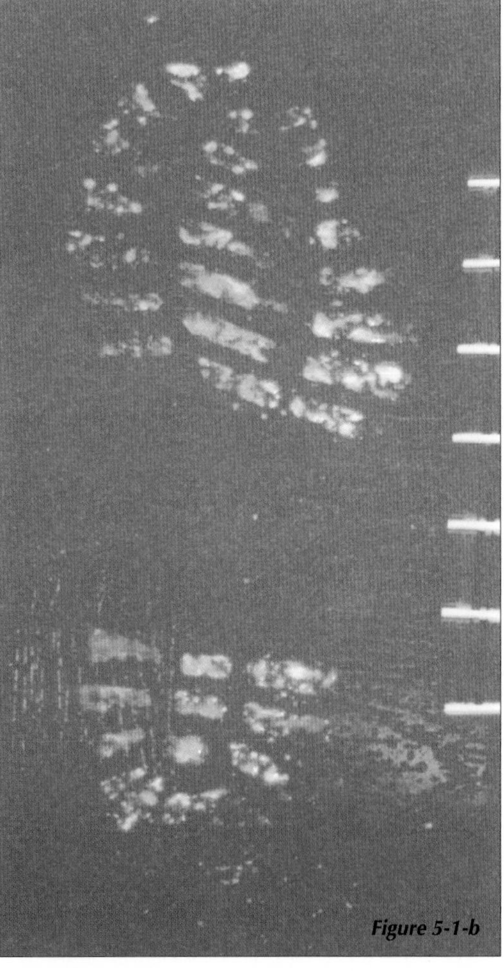

Figure 5-1-a. *Blood is suspected to be present on this floor, though no stain is visible.*

Figure 5-1-b. *Luminol is sprayed onto the floor to detect the presence of blood, and the lights are turned off, revealing a bloody shoe print.*

Figure 5-2-a. *This bandage may have blood on it, though it is not visible.*

Figure 5-2-b. *Luminol is sprayed onto the bandage, and the lights are turned off, revealing the presence of blood.*

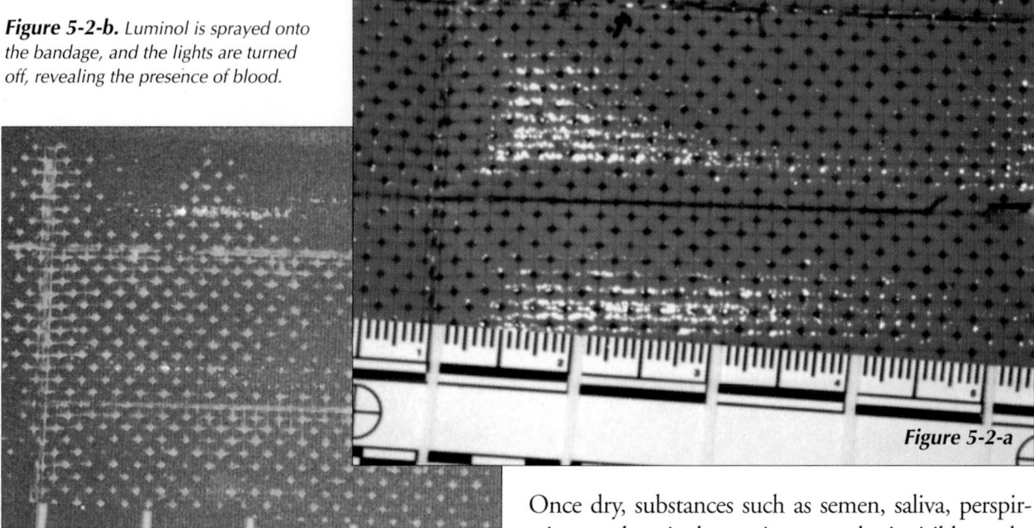

Once dry, substances such as semen, saliva, perspiration, and vaginal secretions may be invisible to the naked eye. Such substances may be found on the victim's or suspect's body, clothing, bedding, vehicles, condoms, towels, etc. Such stains on a dark background can be readily visible, but they can disappear against a patterned or light background. Body fluids like semen, saliva, and vaginal secretions are naturally fluorescent. Light sources, such as a Wood's lamp or an alternate light source (ALS), can be used to reveal the stains in a dark environment (eg, with the lights off and windows covered). These tools operate at a frequency of light outside the visual spectrum. Special goggles or glasses may be needed along with the light source to see the stains. This method is also only presumptive, since some nonbiological substances may cause a positive reaction.

Hairs are often found in sexual assault cases but can be easily lost. They may be or become stuck to other items, be prone to static, or simply be overlooked. Depending on how many hairs are present and where they are located, they may be readily visible. When they are not visible, oblique or parallel lighting of a surface, such as a floor or carpet, with a strong white light reveals these samples. Some hairs and fibers may also be detectable because they glow under ultraviolet (UV) or visible light.

Every case involving forensic evidence requires the collection of "known" or reference samples for analysis and comparison. Buccal swabs from the inside of the mouth are routinely taken to serve as a DNA standard or known sample. The *buccal swab* is used to obtain the individual's own DNA; an *oral swab* is used to obtain material foreign to the individual. Buccal swabs are easier to store than glass vials of whole blood. However, dried blood cards can also be used as a known sample. If the victim was orally assaulted and the exam is being conducted within 24 hours of the assault, an alternative known sample such as blood (venous or finger prick) should be taken, or the buccal swab can be taken after all evidence is collected and the mouth has been vigorously rinsed.

Obtaining Biological Evidence from the Victim

Victims of sexual assault are usually examined by a medical professional, such as a SAFE, who is skilled in identifying and obtaining biological or other types of evidence related to the crime. In addition to ensuring that all needed medical treatment is given, the SAFE documents any evidence present as dictated by organizational and jurisdictional policies. The evidence is then properly collected and preserved before being turned over to law enforcement for safekeeping or transportation to the crime lab.

Factors that Influence the Amount of Biological Evidence

The amount of visible biological evidence present on a victim or her clothing depends on various factors.

Amount of Time Since the Assault

The longer the interval between the assault and the exam, the less likely usable DNA samples will be recovered. The current guideline is to conduct an exam within the first 72 hours postassault. Beyond that time frame, guidelines vary from agency to agency. With the increased sensitivity of DNA testing methods, viable sperm and other DNA samples have been recovered beyond the conventional 72-hour cutoff, so many agencies conduct exams up to 120 hours (5 days) postassault and may even collect and submit the samples for testing if a victim reports beyond that time frame. Victims may have delayed reporting the crime because of embarrassment, lack of memory for the event because of alcohol or drugs (taken voluntarily or involuntarily), lack of understanding that the act legally constitutes a crime, or only being convinced by family or friends to report much later after the occurrence.

Actions Taken by the Victim in the Interim

A victim who is very active after the assault (engaging in exercise or "busy work" around the home to try to forget what happened or remain distracted) may inadvertently contribute to the loss of evidence. A victim who remains inactive (remaining at home and failing to immediately report) may maintain much of the original evidence on or around her body. Showering, douching, going to the bathroom, using mouth wash or brushing the teeth, and eating and drinking may eliminate much physical evidence; therefore, refraining from these activities may preserve much evidence.

Amount of Biological Material Originally Deposited

If little or no biological material was deposited during the assault, little or no evidence may be recovered, regardless of the time interval between assault and collection. The victim's perception of what occurred could also be mistaken (eg, if assaulted from behind or blindfolded, the victim could assume that she was assaulted with a penis when in fact an object was actually used, leaving no semen or other biological substances).

Collection of Biological Evidence During the Sexual Assault Exam

Programs differ on exactly what should be collected during a sexual assault exam. A victim may not be comfortable in relaying everything that happened, or simply be unaware or unable to remember all the facts. Some programs routinely collect vaginal, rectal, and oral swabs, regardless of what the victim says occurred. Others may only collect the body swabs relevant to the victim's account. Victims are often more forthcoming with the examiner than with law enforcement and will reveal more details about the assault during the exam. This information can help shape the scope of the exam and what evidence is ultimately collected.

All injuries are photographed and documented. Body cavity swabs are taken according to protocol and air-dried before packaging. The swabs are taken to look for DNA foreign to the victim. When taking vaginal, rectal, and oral swabs, be aware that the victim's own DNA will inevitably be included. The foreign sources will likely not be visible or readily distinguishable from the victim's, so adequate sampling techniques that comply with departmental policies must be followed to ensure the best chance that the lab will receive a representative sample to test. Collection of foreign material in the mouth may be accomplished with dental floss. This technique is somewhat controversial because it may break the skin in the mouth, potentially exposing the victim to diseases the perpetrator may carry.

Pubic hair combings should be attempted to recover any hairs foreign to the victim. In addition, exemplar or known samples may be taken from the victim for comparison purposes. These should be packaged separately from any evidence hairs that may be removed from the victim's pubic or other areas and may belong to the assailant.

If the victim claims a struggle occurred, fingernail scrapings should be collected. Even with no apparent blood, a victim may have scratched the assailant in self-defense, resulting in skin cells from the suspect being lodged underneath the victim's fingernails. Rather than clip the fingernails, which often results in obtaining mostly the victim's own DNA, commercial kits exist to collect fingernail scrapings. These include a wooden or plastic tool, flat at one end, and collection paper and envelopes. Any foreign material from each of the 5 fingers from one hand is gently scraped (**Figure 5-3**) into the paper and packaged together into a druggist's fold (a clean piece of paper folded over onto itself with the foreign material inside) to ensure no particles are lost, then packaged in evidence envelopes and sealed. Alternatively, any foreign material under the nails may be removed by swabbing with a sterile cotton swab moistened with sterile or deionized water (**Figure 5-4**).

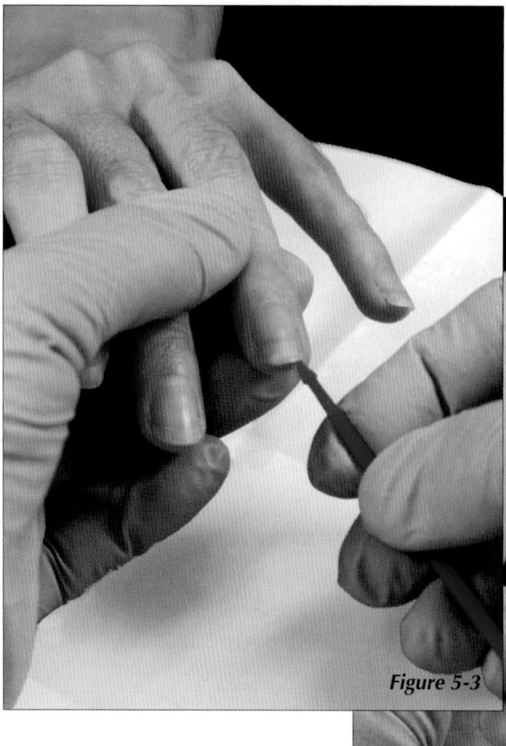

Figure 5-3. *A plastic tool is used to take fingernail scrapings as part of a sexual assault evidence collection. Reprinted with permission from TRITECHFORENSICS.*

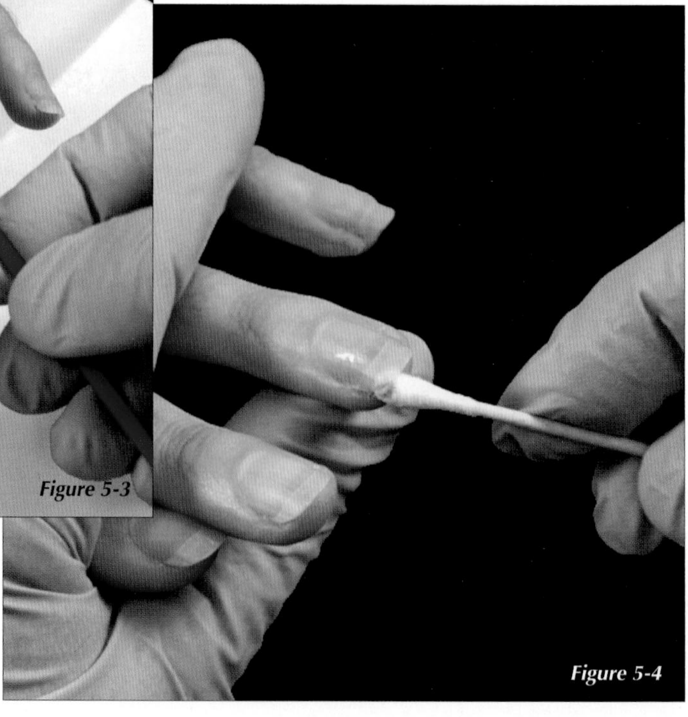

Figure 5-4. *A sterile cotton swab is used to take fingernail swabbings as part of a sexual assault evidence collection. Reprinted with permission from TRITECHFORENSICS.*

Figure 5-3

Figure 5-4

In addition to all biological evidence taken from the victim's body, evidence may be found in or on the victim's clothing. If the victim arrives at the exam in the clothes worn during the assault, the clothes should be carefully removed, collecting any hairs or fibers adhering to them and packaging these separately. At the least, these should be preserved with the clothing for further analysis at the lab. When the clothing is wet, it should ideally be allowed to air-dry before packaging and sealing. If the victim has already changed clothes, the original clothes should be located and inventoried, and the clothing worn to the exam should also be processed.

Obtaining Biological Evidence from the Suspect

SART members are often focused on obtaining biological evidence from 2 distinct crime scenes: the physical location where the assault took place and the body of the victim. There is, however, a third equally important crime scene that is often overlooked: the body of the suspect.

The body of the suspect may be the repository for various types of forensic evidence, including blood, hair, saliva, and/or epithelial cells from the victim. The suspect's body may also contain trace evidence such as fibers or environmental specimens from the victim and/or location of the crime. Courts have routinely allowed law enforcement officers to seize a suspect's clothing upon arrest. When taken contemporaneously to the crime, these articles can be an important source of biological evidence.

A buccal swab should be obtained from the suspect by a trained law enforcement officer or SAFE. The SAFE or other health care provider may also examine the suspect's body, according to local protocol, especially if the victim injured the suspect during the assault, and to otherwise document physical markings (tattoos, moles, etc) or physical abnormalities the victim observed on the suspect. Findings can corroborate the victim's account, including substantiating items that the victim could only have observed through close personal contact with the suspect's body. If penile penetration was alleged, a penile swabbing may be useful to detect the victim's epithelial cells. If the suspect may have used a lubricant to attempt penetration, a swabbing may detect such a substance. Since these items are considered evidence, and for the examiner's personal safety, law enforcement officers often must be present when suspect samples are taken.

A suspect may permit biological samples to be taken by giving voluntary and knowing consent. Some jurisdictions further require that the suspect be advised of his right to refuse consent. If a suspect refuses to give consent for a biological sample, the prosecutor must be prepared to apply to the court for a search warrant, court order, or other court-authorized means for obtaining the specimens. Ordinarily, the prosecutor must demonstrate to the court that there is probable cause to believe that the requested sample will assist in linking the suspect to the crime. The law enforcement officer and forensic examiner should work closely with the prosecutor to assure that all samples are obtained according to the laws of their jurisdiction. A sample obtained illegally may be inadmissible at trial and may taint other evidence subsequently collected by law enforcement.

Obtaining Biological Evidence from Other Items or Places

Often biological evidence taken from locations other than the victim or suspect can be instrumental in tying a particular individual to a location or crime. Although this may not fall under the responsibility of the SAFE, knowing where additional evidence may be found and how it may fit into the bigger picture of the investigation can be useful.

If a victim was transported from one location to another and assaulted, or transported after being assaulted, biological evidence consistent with the victim may be found in the vehicle. If the victim was assaulted inside the vehicle, even more probative evidence may be recovered. When the victim is found somewhere other than where the assault occurred or brought to the hospital for examination, information about where she was assaulted can assist investigators in recovering vital evidence that can place her at the scene (such as a dwelling or outdoor locale). Likewise, a suspect who claims to have never before seen the victim or been at the scene of the crime may be tied to the location through DNA evidence left on items at the scene. Thinking outside the conventional box in these circumstances can be useful. In addition to sources such as blood, saliva, and semen, DNA from skin cells may be found on items the victim or suspect may have used or touched, such as computers, phones, ransom notes, weapons, brushes, or food or drink items.

Packaging Evidence

Because it tends to degrade, biological evidence should be packaged to preserve its integrity. All evidence should first be photographed or otherwise documented before its removal. Since there is a high probability that evidence collected during a sexual assault examination will be used in court, the chain of custody must always be maintained.

Samples should always be air-dried. This is done either in an evidence-drying cabinet or an area separate from the other items of evidence before they are packaged and sealed. Items are packaged individually in paper containers to minimize potential cross-contamination between samples. A limited exception to this rule applies to packaging particles from underneath a victim's 5 fingernails on one hand in a single package, or packaging several hairs found together in one envelope. Once dried, wet stains should be packaged in paper evidence or coin envelopes, sealed with tamper-resistant evidence tape, and signed across the seal with the appropriate information. The mode of documentation varies between agencies, but usually includes the initials or name of the person collecting the sample, case number, date, item number, and any other identifying information. Once dried, swabs taken from the victim's body or scene can either be packaged in paper envelopes or in special swab boxes. Packaging items in plastic containers introduces the possibility of bacterial invasion, since the environment inside the container can become warm and moist. Paper bags allow airflow and prevent bacteria from settling in. However, if an item is too saturated to effectively dry before transportation, it should be packaged in a sealed plastic bag or container, refrigerated if possible, and immediately transported to the lab for drying and repackaging.

Clothing from the victim should be inventoried and packaged individually, taking care not to lose any trace evidence that may be stuck to or on the items. If dry, each item should be placed in a separate paper bag and sealed. In addition to biological stains, there may also be hairs, fibers, soil, plant material, pet hairs, glass, or other trace evidence that could link the suspect to the crime. If weapons or tools were used, cuts or tears in the clothing may be useful for future comparison should the weapon be found.

Hairs removed from the victim that appear to be foreign should initially be documented, then packaged in paper envelopes. Collection can be accomplished with a gloved hand, metal or plastic forceps or tweezers (taking care not to crimp the hairs), or lifting tape. Because hairs are often subject to static electricity, they can be difficult to collect. If lifting tape is used, the tape should be packaged along with the hairs. To ensure the hairs are not lost when the package is opened, they can be packaged inside a druggist's fold, and then placed into an envelope and sealed. If substances adhere to the shaft of the hair, such as blood or semen, attempts should be made to dry the hairs before packaging.

Large volumes of liquid (such as urine) or anything else that cannot be dried (generally anything that has some "substance," such as organs or tissue, vomit, feces, or products of conception) should be placed in an airtight plastic container, refrigerated or frozen, and transported to the laboratory. If liquid blood is collected as a known sample, the glass tubes should be refrigerated but never frozen. Special attention should also be paid to evidence samples suspected to contain semen, since a repeated series of freezing and thawing cycles can have a negative impact on the lab's ability to separate sperm DNA from other DNA during testing.

Storage and Transportation of Evidence

Storage policies may differ between agencies. If it is customary to hold evidence at a centralized location for increased efficiency so that multiple cases can be transported to the laboratory together, the type of evidence and the manner of storage should be considered. Adequate space and appropriate temperature for various types of biological specimens should be ensured. Although some items of evidence may be transported in the trunk of a vehicle, this is not optimum for long-term storage because temperature and humidity cannot be controlled, especially in certain climates.

Evidence may be transported in person or via one of many acceptable overnight services. This can be especially useful if the evidence is being sent out of state for rush testing at a private lab or for specialized testing unavailable at the local lab. Chain of custody is usually considered intact while the evidence is in transit as long as it reaches its destination undamaged and still sealed. While it is customary to mail evidence, in the case of damage, destruction, or loss, carriers usually accept no liability.

Once received in the testing lab, the condition of the package should be noted and all items received should be inventoried and photographed according to lab policy. If testing will not be started immediately, all items must be stored appropriately. If the items are opened numerous times for testing and/or resampling throughout the testing process, each instance should be separately noted in the case file. Evidence envelopes or containers should never be reopened across an existing seal, so that it will be apparent how many times the item was accessed. Containers should always be resealed with a new seal and appropriately labeled.

Once testing is complete, arrangements for the final disposition of the evidence should be made according to jurisdictional policy. Items created during the testing process, such as any remaining DNA extracts, are also considered evidence. Evidence items may remain at the lab, be returned to the submitting law enforcement agency, or be sent directly to the prosecutor. Long-term storage should be considered. In light of advances in DNA testing methods, extended statutes of limitations for some crimes, and potential postconviction litigation, less evidence is being destroyed after conviction. More jurisdictions require evidence be kept for longer periods of time, or even indefinitely, in case retesting is requested or newer advances permit previously untestable samples to be tested. Although this may create space problems, where statute requires, evidence must be maintained.

Chain of Custody and Admissibility Issues

In a criminal trial, the judge decides what evidence may be brought in and what evidence must be excluded. Two types of evidence may be admissible at trial: testimonial evidence and physical or demonstrative evidence. *Testimonial evidence* is the actual verbal testimony of the witness under oath on the witness stand. The prosecutor must show that the testimony is both relevant and material for the witness to offer it at trial. *Physical* or *demonstrative evidence* is nontestimonial and may take the form of physical objects, reports, records, and other similar items. Because an object cannot be administered an oath, the evidence must not only be relevant and material to be admitted, but the prosecutor must also demonstrate its integrity. To demonstrate the integrity of demonstrative evidence, courts have developed the concept of *chain of custody*. To assure the integrity of evidence, protocols have been established for both law enforcement officers and SAFEs concerning the recovery, packaging, and documentation of evidence collected. As in the case of a chain that is composed of many links, many people may handle a piece of evidence, from its initial recovery to its examination and analysis. The person who collects the evidence should always initiate the chain of custody documentation. If turned over to another individual for temporary holding or transportation to the testing lab, all persons having custody of the evidence should be included on the documentation. For a prosecutor to introduce such evidence at trial, the prosecutor must be prepared to show every person who came into contact with the evidence, as documented on a continuous form. The evidence must be accounted for at all times, to prove that it was not subject to any form of tampering or alteration.

In a sexual assault case, the most common, and often the most important, type of forensic evidence collected is the sexual assault kit (**Figures 5-5** and **5-6**). At a minimum, there will be at least 3 links in the chain of custody: the SAFE who collected the evidence, the law enforcement officer who took receipt of the kit from the examiner, and the forensic laboratory analyst who examined the kit for DNA evidence.

There could, however, be many other individuals who handled the kit, including police officers or evidence technicians who may have taken possession of the kit and logged it into evidence or hand-delivered it to the lab; postal workers, couriers, or express mail personnel who may have routed the kit for delivery; or even lab technicians who may have prepared the evidence for analysis but not actually conducted the testing themselves.

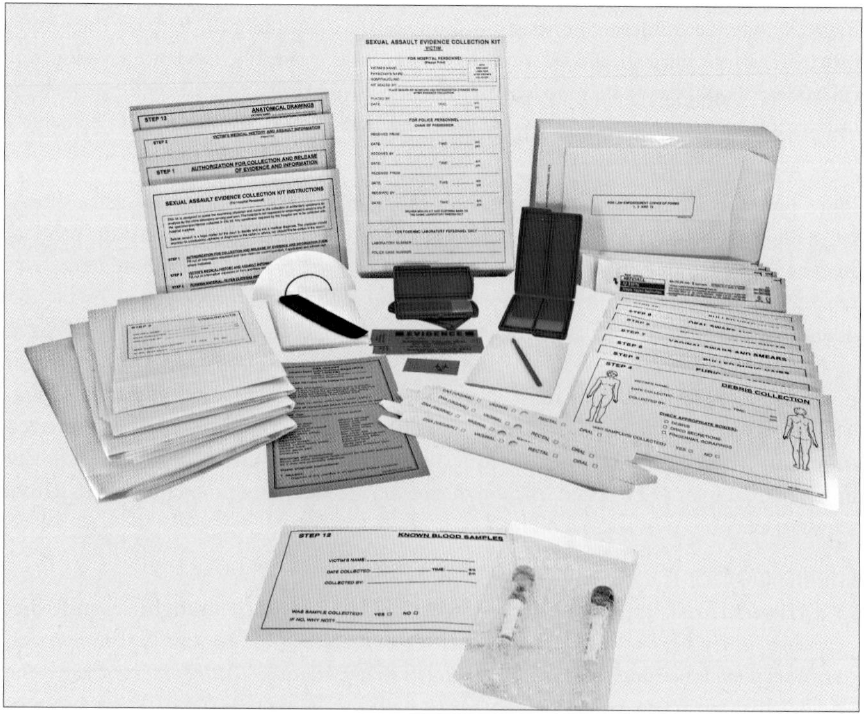

Figure 5-5. *Components of a sexual assault evidence collection kit. Kit includes an authorization form; medical history and assault information form; foreign material, undergarments, and outer clothing bags; envelopes and tools for collection of debris, pubic hair, and head hair; envelopes and tools for collection of vaginal, rectal, and oral swabs and smears; envelopes for collection of saliva and blood samples; anatomical drawings; police evidence seals; and a law enforcement forms envelope. Reprinted with permission from TRITECHFORENSICS.*

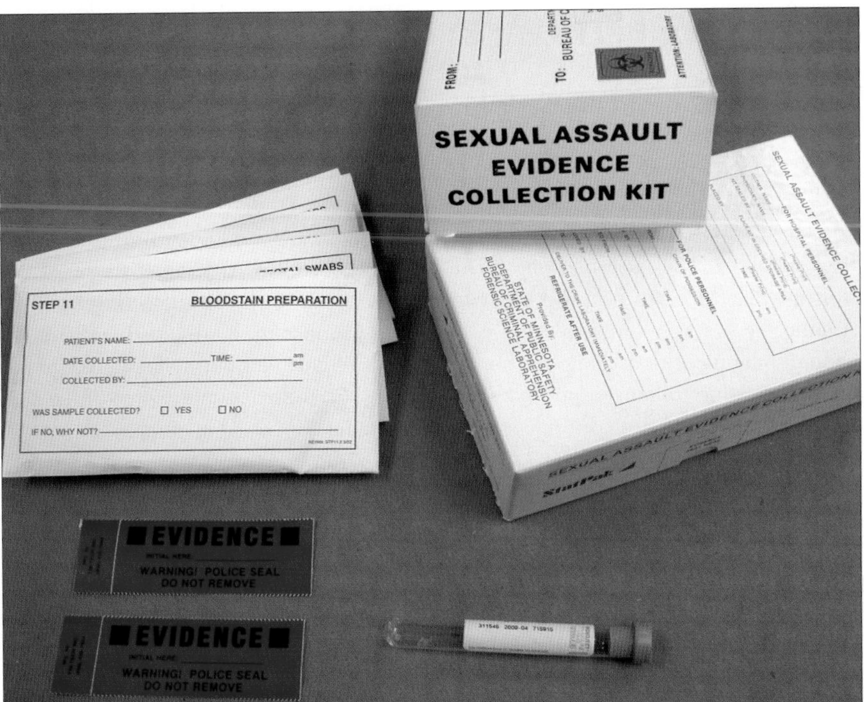

Figure 5-6. *Components of a sexual assault evidence collection kit. Reprinted with permission from the Minnesota Bureau of Criminal Apprehension Laboratory.*

In some jurisdictions, everyone on the chain of custody form may be called to court to document an unbroken chain. In other jurisdictions, only the people who actually had access to the evidence (versus those who may have merely transported or inventoried the sealed containers) will be called. By coming into contact with the kit, each has potentially become a witness who could be called to testify at trial. Fortunately, the prosecutor usually does not have to call all of these individuals due to a crucial final step taken by the examiner: the sealing of the kit.

By sealing and initialing the kit, the SAFE is vouching for the evidence she or he personally collected. It is presumed that if the seal is not broken, the evidence has not been compromised. The next important link in the chain is the analyst who opens the kit for analysis. For the prosecutor to introduce the DNA results into evidence, ordinarily only the examiner who collected the evidence and sealed the kit and the analyst who opened the kit and performed the DNA analysis must testify. Other items of demonstrative evidence produced by the SAFE are also scrutinized to assure trustworthiness. The report produced by the examiner, together with anatomical drawings and photographs, must be properly retained to be admissible at trial. The report is signed by the examiner, verifying findings. It should be placed in a secure location, as local protocol dictates, to prevent tampering. Drawings must accurately depict the locations of trauma or other abnormalities observed by the examiner. Photographs should be initialed or signed by the examiner, dated, and maintained for safekeeping. For the photograph to be admissible at trial, the examiner must verify to the court that the photo accurately depicts what he or she observed when the picture was taken.

Since those individuals who may have had contact with the evidence can be called into court to testify under oath, under no circumstance should an advocate assist the forensic examiner in collecting forensic evidence. The advocate, having become a witness, would lose any privilege she or he may have protecting the otherwise confidential relationship with the victim.

Deoxyribonucleic Acid (DNA)

Basics

All body cells except red blood cells have a nucleus. Deoxyribonucleic acid (DNA) is found on the 46 chromosomes residing inside the nuclei. Nucleic acids, including DNA, are made up of nucleotide units consisting of 3 parts: a sugar, a phosphate, and a nucleobase. There are 4 nucleobases in DNA: adenine (A), thymine (T), cytosine (C), and guanine (G) (**Figure 5-7**). In DNA, 2 strands of bases combine to form a double helix or ladder. The sugar and phosphate molecules form the backbone or sides of the ladder, while the bases, held together by hydrogen bonds, form the rungs (**Figure 5-8**). Among the bases, A can only bind with T, and C can only bind with G. There are about 3 billion positions along the human DNA molecule that must contain one of the 4 bases, creating trillions of possible combinations. Scientists examine these differences in the crime laboratory to distinguish among individuals involved in crimes.

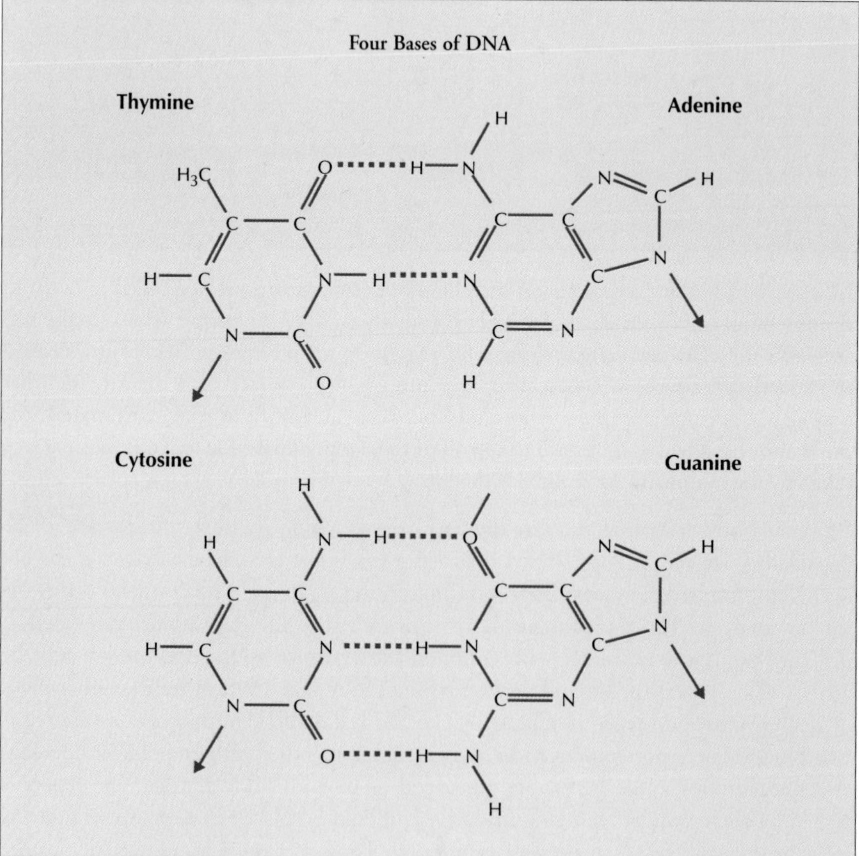

Figure 5-7. *This image displays the 4 bases that make up DNA: adenine (A), thymine (T), cytosine (C), and guanine (G).*

Sperm and egg cells each contain only 23 chromosomes. Upon fertilization, the chromosomes from the egg and sperm combine to create the full complement of 46 chromosomes (22 pairs plus the sex chromosomes X and Y). The result is that we obtain half of our DNA from our mother and the other half from our father.

At each location or locus on the DNA molecule, we have one trait from each parent. In short tandem repeat (STR) testing, the conventional 13-marker test used by most labs in the United States, these traits are denoted by numbers that indicate the number of times a particular DNA sequence is repeated. For example, if an individual possesses 3 copies of the repeat sequence, he or she has a type 3, and if an individual possess 6 copies of the repeat sequence, her or she would have a type 6, and so on. If by coincidence each parent contributed the same type at a particular location (eg, 3, 3), that person would be called *homozygous* for that location, possessing 2 copies of the same gene but expressing only one visible type. If each parent contributed a different type at that location (eg, 3, 6), the person would be called *heterozygous* and would possess and express 2 different types. Since we inherit only one type from each parent, there should only be 2 types at any given location. If at any particular location 3 or more types are detected, this would be indicative of a mixture of DNA samples from 2 or more people. The mixture may have occurred either when the samples were deposited or, less often, through contamination when the evidence was collected, packaged, or tested.

Conventional DNA testing looks at 13 different locations along the DNA molecule across various chromosomes. The specific 13 loci are often referred to as the Combined DNA Index System (CODIS) loci, and they form the basis for the Federal Bureau of Investigation's (FBI's) national DNA database. In the testing process, each type detected by the forensic laboratory analyst is recorded. Databases of all the possible DNA types for each locus show the distribution of the various types and the frequency of

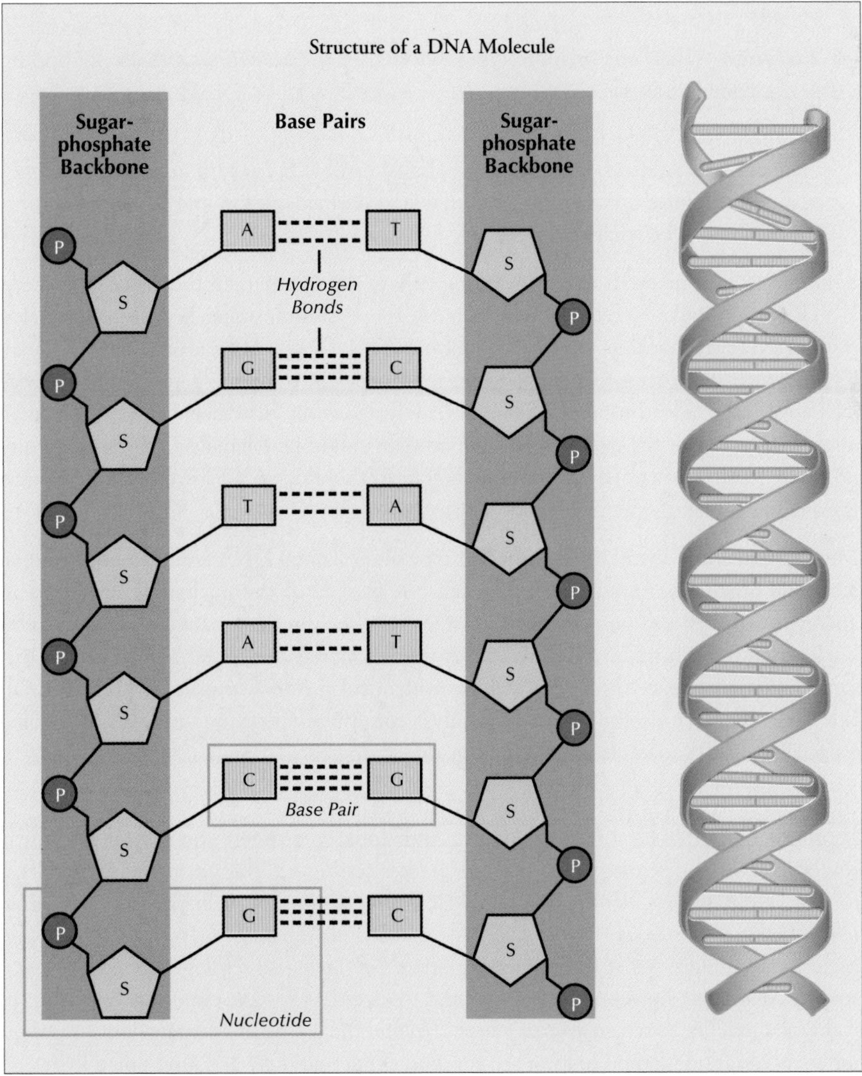

Figure 5-8. *This image illustrates the structure of a DNA molecule. The sugar and phosphate molecules form the backbone, while the bases (held together by hydrogen bonds) form the rungs.*

occurrence of each particular type. Since the particular 13 loci tested have been found to be independently inherited from one another, a scientific principle called the *product rule* applies. The frequency of the first type can be multiplied by the frequency of the next and the next to generate statistical estimates of how common or rare a particular 13-locus DNA profile would be expected to be found at random. These numbers help put a "match" into perspective when DNA evidence from a crime scene is found to be consistent with DNA taken from a victim or suspect.

Conventional DNA testing can be used in sexual assaults when conception occurs. If the fetus is aborted, the products of conception can be subjected to DNA testing. At each location tested, one type should match a type from the mother. The remaining type at each location must match the purported father. If any of the types cannot be attributed to the alleged father, he is not the biological parent.

Crime scene evidence is tested for all 13 genetic loci, and the types detected are compared to all relevant parties (eg, victims, suspects, consensual partners). The possible results include the following:

— ***Inclusion.*** When all types detected in the known sample appear in the evidence sample.

— ***Exclusion.*** When one or more types detected in the known sample do not appear in the evidence sample.

— ***Inconclusive.*** When the evidence sample is either too degraded to get a profile, there are other factors inhibiting the ability to obtain readable results, or there is such a convoluted mixture of types that it is deemed irresolvable and no scientific conclusion can be reliably drawn.

Some specialized methods of DNA testing behave differently than those just described. Y-STR testing looks at DNA found only on the Y chromosome. Because only males possess a Y chromosome, only males have Y-STR DNA. Also, unlike conventional STRs, which differ from person to person, all males in the same paternal lineage will have identical Y-STR profiles. Y-STR DNA testing can be extremely valuable in sexual assault cases where the evidence sample contains abundant female DNA that would normally mask a lesser quantity of male DNA. In those cases, Y-STR testing may allow the analyst to identify the male suspect's profile.

Mitochondrial DNA (mtDNA) is another type of specialized DNA testing. Mitochondria are small organelles found within the cell but outside of the nucleus. They produce energy for the cell and possess their own DNA. Mitochondria are inherited maternally, but everyone (both male and female) has mitochondrial DNA. All relatives from the same maternal lineage, however, will have identical mtDNA profiles. Mitochondrial DNA can be very useful when the analyst cannot obtain a nuclear DNA profile, especially when the sample may have been subject to degradation.

Serology and Other Protein Marker Testing

Serology encompasses a variety of tests that look at antigen and serum antibody reactions. Forensic serology and protein marker testing are the precursors to modern forensic DNA testing. While most serological tests are merely preliminary or screening tests, they can help steer an investigation in the right direction or provide conclusive exclusionary results. Most labs today no longer routinely use serology. Serological tests may be conducted, however, if there is a need to identify a specific biological fluid, or if it is the lab's practice to screen evidence items beyond the use of an alternate light source or other visualization method to locate where a potential stain may be found on an item.

Amylase is an enzyme found in high concentrations in saliva. Although also found in other fluids such as vaginal secretions, concentrations are usually higher in saliva. With the exception of feces, no other body fluid contains comparable amylase levels; therefore a positive test result for amylase is a presumptive positive finding for saliva.

Acid phosphatase (AP) is an enzyme secreted by the prostate gland. Although found in other body fluids as well, its levels are 400 times greater in semen. A simple colorimetric chemical test can indicate the presumptive presence of semen with a positive AP test result.

P30 is a protein once thought to be unique to semen. However, it is also detected in breast milk and other fluids in lower concentrations. A positive p30 test also presumptively indicates the presence of semen.

Microscopy may provide a more definitive result. The microscopic identification of sperm cells (from a slide prepared from an evidence sample) is considered a confirmatory test for the presence of semen.

The ABO blood group system was the first genetic system used to distinguish among individuals. However, there are only 4 possible types: A, B, AB, and O. There is an uneven distribution among the types, ranging from approximately 16% of the population being type B, to 60% of the general population being type O.[2] Because of this, ABO testing can be useful for exclusion, but is no longer considered strong enough evidence for an inclusion alone.

Phosphoglucomutase (PGM) typing was another early protein marker system used to distinguish between individuals. When combined with ABO typing it could provide useful information, although nowhere near the degree of discrimination found in today's DNA testing using the CODIS 13 loci. PGM typing is no longer routinely performed in forensic laboratories.

DNA Testing of Sexual Assault Evidence

Most labs in the United States currently use STR testing of the standard CODIS 13 loci. This enables all states (and some labs outside the United States) to participate in a searchable online database of DNA profiles to help identify suspects in unsolved cases. STR testing uses the polymerase chain reaction (PCR) to amplify or copy small amounts of DNA so the analyst can visualize the particular types present and compare those found in evidence samples to those from known victim or suspect samples. PCR can be performed on miniscule amounts of biological material, as low as a single nanogram (one billionth of a gram). However, to be able to actually visualize the types present, more of the target or template DNA must first be synthesized.

PCR is a 3-step process (**Figure 5-9-a, b,** and **c**). The first step involves extracting the DNA from the evidence or known item. In single source samples, such as buccal swabs taken from suspects or saliva stains from a cigarette, the procedure is fairly straightforward. Sexual assault samples, however, often contain mixtures of at least 2 contributors (the victim and suspect or suspects). When these mixtures come from multiple sources of different types of body fluids such as blood, blood and saliva, or saliva and perspiration, it can be difficult to fully resolve the different contributors. The mixture most often encountered in sexual assault involves semen and blood, or semen and vaginal or rectal secretions. Because of a special property of sperm cells, using a process called *differential extraction,* analysts are usually able to separate the sperm donor's DNA from the victim's DNA to better answer the question, "Who contributed the sperm to the sample?"

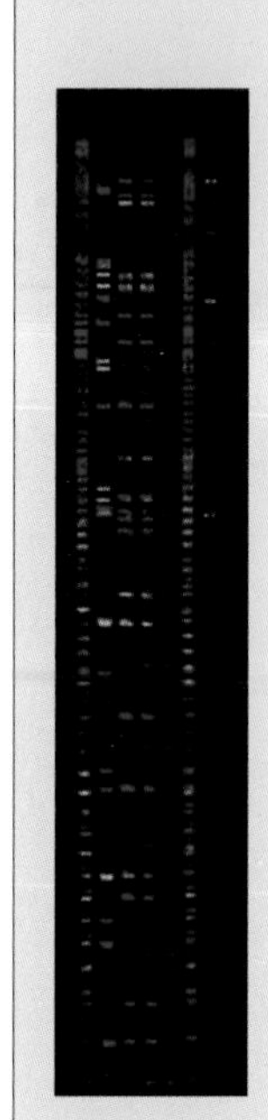
Figure 5-9-a

Figure 5-9-a. *Scanned gel image showing multiple markers being made visible in various fluorescent dyes.*

Figure 5-9-b. *Depiction of 2 loci with the genotypes 8, 10, and 8, 9 respectively denoted by the presence of 8 and 10 repeats and 8 and 9 repeats of the target sequence.*

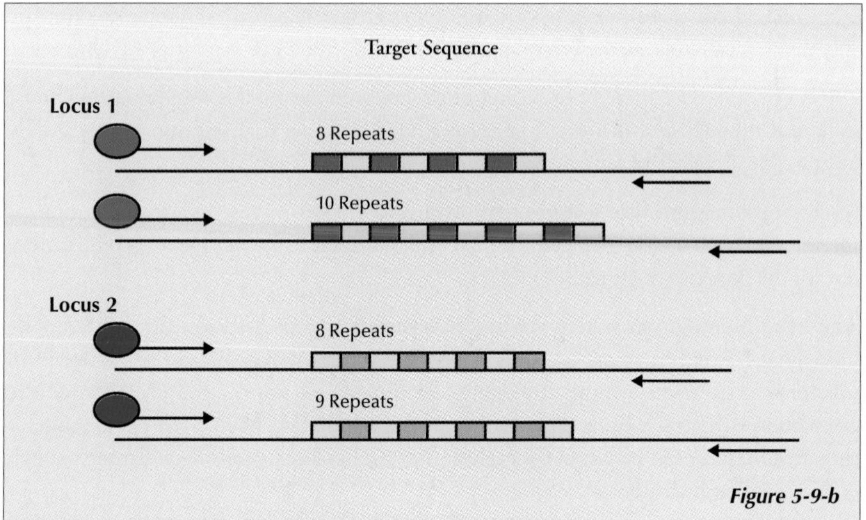

Figure 5-9-b

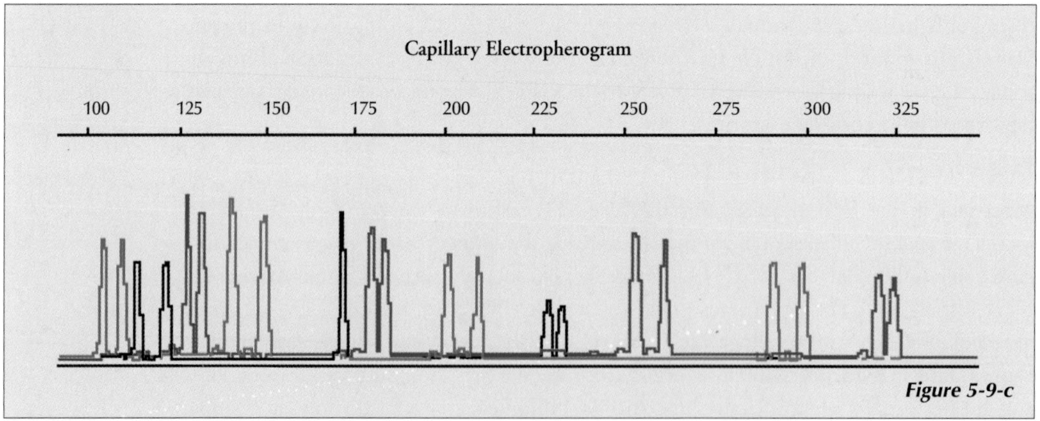

Figure 5-9-c

Figure 5-9-c. *Capillary electropherogram showing the automated printout of the peaks corresponding to the alleles detected.*

Since the cell membrane around a sperm cell is particularly robust, adding chemicals to a test tube containing a mixed sample, such as a vaginal swab from a rape kit, will cause all cells other than the sperm cells to rupture, thus giving up the DNA from their nuclei. Sperm cells remain intact and are the largest components in the test tube. The sperm can then be separated from the other cellular components in the tube by spinning them down to a small pellet at the bottom of the tube. The DNA from the other broken cells is transferred to a second tube with a pipette. Harsh chemicals are added to the tube containing the sperm to finally burst open the sperm cell membranes. When this process is successful, what began as a single sample (the vaginal swab) will result in 2 separate test tubes with one containing the DNA from the male suspect and the other containing the DNA from the victim. Both tubes are subjected to the rest of the testing process in tandem, and processed and reported as unique samples, often called fraction one and fraction two, or sperm and non-sperm fractions. The process is the same if the suspect sperm donor and victim are both male and the evidence item is a rectal swab.

The second step of the PCR process is amplification or copying. Although only a small amount of DNA is required to obtain results, it is necessary to generate more DNA for the analyst to detect the present types. The original sequence of DNA is not altered in any way; it is merely duplicated in the lab. A simplified way to think of this is to imagine a copying machine. Placing an original single sheet document on the platen glass and programming the machine to make 100 copies begins the process. Unless the machine runs out of ink or gets a paper jam, at the end of the process there should be 100 exact replicas of the original document. The original, however, should remain intact and will not be changed by the process. Similarly, in the lab, once extracted, the template DNA is put into a test tube. Additional components needed to make more DNA (eg, the nucleotides A, T, C, and G as well as enzymes and other chemicals) are added to the tube. The tube is placed in a machine and subjected to controlled temperature fluctuations optimal for the creation of more DNA. The double strand of DNA will break apart, leaving 2 single strands. The added chemical agents (called primers) then attach to each of the single nucleotides to create a new pair: A binds with T, and C binds with G. New bonds are now formed, creating a new double strand of DNA identical to the one split into two. Each time this process takes place, the amount of DNA generated is doubled exponentially. A standard test goes through 30 to 33 cycles, potentially generating about a billion copies of the original template DNA. Several commercial kits enable all 13 loci to be copied by running only 2 tests, with some loci being repeated in each of the 2 tests for comparison purposes as a quality control measure. Newer testing methods can allow up to 15 loci to be tested at a single time.

The last step in the PCR process is the detection step, when the types present at each of the 13 loci tested are reported and recorded. When PCR testing first became prevalent in crime labs, this step was fairly labor intensive and hands-on. Current technology has almost fully automated this step. Analysts must load the amplified DNA into a machine that performs a process called electrophoresis, which separates the DNA fragments by their size. This can be done either on a slab gel or, most recently, a capillary system. A computer, using software specifically designed for DNA STR genotyping, provides the actual fragment sizes that correlate to the types obtained. The computer program prints out a series of peaks corresponding to each of the loci tested and notes the size or height of each peak (**Figure 5-10**). Because of mutations, variants, and potential artifacts or anomalies inherently detectable with the PCR testing process, an analyst must still confirm the types or alleles called by the computer and import them into his or her analytical report for the case. If a match is obtained between items of evidence and known samples, a statistical frequency of the genetic profile may be calculated from existing databases and included in the report.

Figure 5-10. *Raw DNA Data. A computer program prints out a series of peaks corresponding to each of the loci tested and notes the size or height of each peak, which should be sharp and well-defined.*

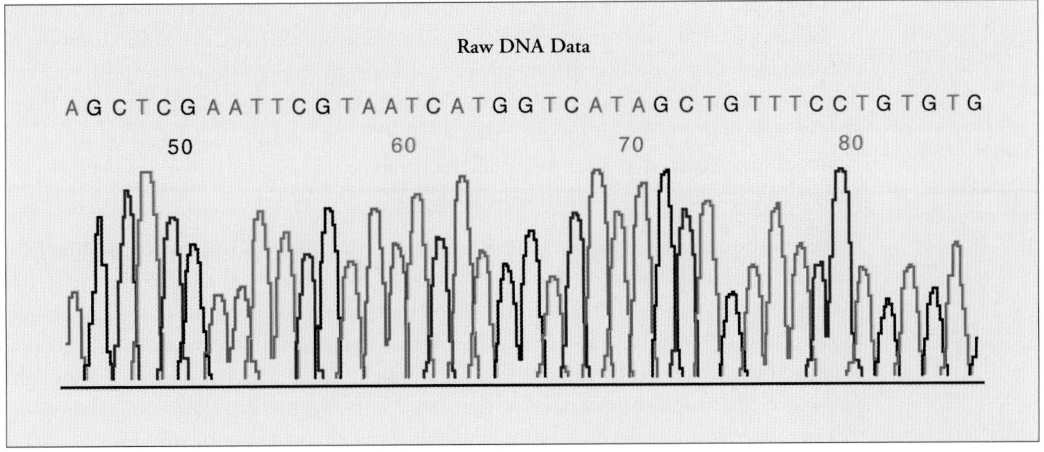

Unlike earlier versions of DNA testing (restriction fragment length polymorphism [RFLP]), which required large starting amounts of DNA to get a readable profile, the PCR process generally starts with a small amount of DNA. However, contamination at any point in the process (at collection, packaging, or testing) is carried forward into the final results and may confound the ability to resolve the profiles. Although contamination may result in the analyst obtaining only a partial profile or no profile at all, it will not change one person's DNA profile into that of another. To minimize contamination, protective measures should always be taken when dealing with biological specimens. Personal protective equipment, such as masks and gloves, should be worn. Quality assurance and quality control measures such as changing gloves between samples, using disposable collection and testing tools, or ensuring that tools and workspaces are thoroughly cleaned between samples, help to ensure that any DNA detected with these testing procedures came from the evidence and nowhere else. Throughout the PCR process, controls ensure that all machinery and chemical components are behaving properly. Any outcome that varies from expected ones indicates a potential problem with equipment, reagents, or analyst error. The usual course of action is to document the variation and repeat the test.

Genetic Markers

Except for fingerprints, which are thought to be unique even between identical twins, a 13-locus DNA profile match is perhaps the most uniquely discriminating method of identifying individuals. However, with current technology, identical twins share the identical DNA profile and would therefore be indistinguishable by their DNA. This is logical, since identical twins are derived from one fertilized embryo, with the full complement of 46 chromosomes from the mother's egg and the father's sperm dividing after fertilization, thus creating 2 identical offspring. By contrast, fraternal twins result from the separate fertilization of 2 sperm and 2 eggs within the same womb. Since each carries slightly different variations of the parent's genetic information, they will share a large amount of DNA but will be distinguishable from one another by physical appearance and by DNA testing. Fraternal twins can also be different genders if the 2 sperm cells fertilizing the 2 eggs carry different sex chromosomes.

First-degree relatives (parent/child) share 50% of their DNA. Siblings from the same sets of parents share about 25% of their DNA, statistically more than 2 unrelated individuals chosen at random.

Sometimes when DNA testing is attempted, a full 13-locus profile is not obtained. Instead, information from only some of the markers is detected. Partial profiles may be obtained for a variety of reasons, including slightly or badly degraded DNA, inhibitors in the sample that prevent the PCR reaction from optimizing, or allelic dropout, a phenomenon that can occur where alleles that are truly present do not amplify and are therefore not detected. To upload a DNA profile to CODIS, the FBI requires data from at least 10 of the loci. Although a partial profile may result in a larger number of potential hits returned from a query of the database, these can still be reviewed by an analyst and provide leads for further investigation.

A new, although not widely used variation on this theme involves low stringency searches, commonly referred to as kinship-based DNA. Based on the fact that relatives share a larger amount of DNA than unrelated individuals, investigators have used partial matches through CODIS as investigative leads. For example, if an individual in the database matches an evidence sample from an open case at 10 of the 13 loci, although that individual would be excluded as the donor, investigators may seek out relatives of that person (not in the database) using the partial match as an investigative lead.

Y-STRs and/or mtDNA may be performed when conventional DNA testing is inapplicable or simply as additional information for use at trial. However, in both the Y-STR and mtDNA systems, all relatives through the patrilineal and matrilineal lines, respectively, share identical DNA profiles and are therefore indistinguishable.

Statistical Frequency of Individual DNA Profiles

The matching DNA profiles scientifically derived from the evidence and control samples are virtually meaningless and may even be inadmissible without a statistical interpretation of how frequently they are found in the general population. The forensic lab analyst must therefore perform a statistical analysis from which a *frequency estimate* can be given. To estimate its frequency of occurrence, the profile generated from the evidence or crime scene sample is compared against an existing allele frequency database. Such databases comprise the genetic profiles of randomly selected, unrelated individuals. Databases need only contain about a 100 samples to be considered statistically reliable. The databases most often used in the United States are those compiled by the FBI, although individual states or labs may use their own databases. The databases are often further broken down into racial/ethnic groups, the most common of which are those for the Caucasian, African-American, and Hispanic populations.

The *product rule* and *Theta correction* are also used. The Theta correction is a factor by which certain allele frequencies are multiplied to account for slight differences among various subpopulations. Since the effect is to increase the overall number reported, thereby making the statistical occurrence less rare, there is no adverse impact to the suspect. The resulting number is the *random match probability*, a statistically conservative estimate of the expected occurrence of this specific combination of alleles.

The random match probability is generally stated as a rate of inclusion. This expresses the statistical frequency that the evidence profile would be randomly found in a population of unrelated individuals; for example, the frequency that the profile from the evidence sample is randomly found in a population of unrelated individuals is one in a quadrillion. Some analysts may give the figure as a rate of exclusion, particularly where there is a mixture or partial profile. Here the analyst would describe the percentage of unrelated persons randomly found within a general population that could be excluded as a contributor to the evidence sample; for example, X% of the population may be excluded as a possible contributor to the evidence sample.

Prosecutors and defense attorneys have been known to make incorrect assumptions or improper extrapolations of the data. For example, assume that the random match probability on a partial profile is one in a million. In the case of the prosecutor's fallacy, the prosecutor infers that since there are a few other people in the population that may have that same partial profile, there is only a one in a million chance that the defendant is actually innocent. The fatal flaw with this logic is that the random match probability does not project odds or likelihood of the defendant's guilt; it is simply the likelihood that someone in the general population would have the same genetic profile as that found in the evidence sample. Similarly, in the case of the defense fallacy, the defense attorney also assumes that since there are a few members of the population who may have the same partial profile, each of those individuals has an equal likelihood of guilt. The reasoning here is flawed because it ignores all the other evidence in the case (eg, physical characteristics of the suspect, access to the victim, geographic location of the crime) that changes the odds in favor of the defendant actually being the guilty party. Thus, to avoid a mistrial or reversal of conviction, both parties must state the statistical outcomes accurately and precisely.

DNA Role in Legal Proceedings

DNA has revolutionized the investigation and trial of sexual assault cases. There have traditionally been only 3 basic defenses that defendants have relied on in sexual assault prosecutions. The primary defense was that of identification. Today, DNA can identify those individuals who may have participated in the offense. The second major defense was that of nonoccurrence. A defendant would maintain that the incident was a case of victim fabrication, where no sexual act actually took place. Once again, DNA has given investigators the ability to corroborate a victim's account and identify individual participants. With the diminished use of these 2 common defenses, defendants have turned to a third: consent. Although DNA cannot determine whether 2 parties consented to a sexual act, the power of DNA to identify and corroborate may have a significant impact on the case by bolstering the victim's credibility.

DNA is often extraordinarily compelling evidence when presented against a defendant. DNA is extremely discriminating and therefore able to single out a potential offender from the population at large. Presently, the FBI laboratory will identify an individual as the source of the sample analyzed if the likelihood of randomly finding an unrelated person having the same DNA profile as that obtained from the evidence sample is less than or equal to 1 in 6 trillion—that is, essentially 1000 times greater than the world population. Many state crime labs follow the lead of the FBI, with their analysts testifying to identity when the statistics associated with the genetic profile meet the FBI guidelines. States may, however, employ different threshold levels. Using these guidelines, the forensic lab analyst can state with a reasonable degree of scientific certainty that the defendant was the source of the evidence sample recovered in the crime. This is commonly referred to as *source attribution*. Thus the defendant's biological evidence in or on the victim is highly probative of who committed the act.

The analyst may, however, take a more conservative approach to describing the match between evidence and control samples. The forensic lab analyst could testify to the expected statistical frequency of the genetic profile generated from the evidence, which, in the case of a match, would be the same genetic profile found in the defendant's known sample. A statement would be made that the 2 profiles are consistent, and that the defendant could not be excluded as the source of the DNA. The implication of identity would ultimately be left for the prosecutor to make.

Even when the defendant's identity is not in question, DNA can be a powerful means of corroboration. As in the case of identity, DNA can link the defendant to the victim. In a sexual assault case where the defense is consent, the defendant's DNA would be expected to be found. Finding the defendant's DNA under the victim's fingernails, however, may corroborate her account that force was used and she tried to fight off her assailant. The defendant's DNA on her body where the victim claimed the defendant licked her, or even the defendant's DNA on a towel the victim maintained the defendant used to wipe himself after the sexual act, can all lend credence to the victim's account. DNA from the location where the assault took place—vegetative debris from the environment, animal hair where a pet may have been housed, or the defendant's own DNA left at the location of the crime—can powerfully corroborate and support details revealed by the victim.

Conversely, DNA can be used to refute a matter. For example, the suspect may maintain that he never had sex with the victim, yet his DNA is found in samples taken from the sexual assault kit. Confronted with such evidence, the suspect may be compelled to admit complicity. If the suspect changes his testimony and now alleges consent, the consent defense is severely compromised.

The power of DNA to identify and/or corroborate can be an essential tool of the prosecutor in proving to the jury beyond a reasonable doubt the defendant's involvement in the crime. Faced with such compelling evidence, many defendants may opt to enter a plea of guilty in hope of obtaining a lesser charge and/or sentence. Forensic science may spare the victim from being subjected to a criminal trial and recounting the harrowing details of the assault.

Presenting DNA Evidence in Court

When presenting forensic evidence in court, prosecutors should keep it simple, for less is truly more when dealing with DNA. The prosecutor must always be aware of the intended audience: a lay judge and/or jury. As with any witness, the prosecutor must present the testimony in a simple, direct fashion so as not to confuse or bore the listeners.

The trial is actually the culmination of a lengthy legal process. After formal charges are brought in a criminal case, the parties engage in *discovery*. As the name implies, the prosecution and defense seek to learn about each other's case through the exchange of information. In a case involving DNA evidence, this can include information concerning the testing lab, the background and qualifications of the forensic lab analyst, and the analyst's lab report. Expert witnesses may be interviewed by opposing counsel and, in some states, may even be subject to a sworn deposition.

During this pretrial period, the prosecution and defense may file motions with the court to have certain legal issues resolved. As the proponent of the forensic evidence, the prosecutor must be prepared to defend any objections to the admissibility of the evidence. The very science of DNA may be subject to attack. Over the years the federal courts have established legal standards for the admissibility of scientific evidence. The older method, called the Frye standard, requires the proponent of the evidence to prove that the scientific method employed is generally accepted in the scientific community.[3] A newer method, referred to as the Daubert standard, requires a showing of the validity of the underlying scientific theory, the reliability of the scientific testing, and the usefulness of the scientific evidence to the jury.[4] Various states have adopted either one of the methods, or a hybrid of the two. Although today the admissibility of the 13-loci STR DNA test is fairly well settled, newer forms of DNA testing may be subject to ongoing legal scrutiny.

After all pretrial issues have been resolved and plea negotiations completed, the case can go to trial. The SAFE and forensic lab analyst both play key roles in the prosecutor's case. Through these witnesses the prosecutor will seek to introduce the medical and scientific evidence. If the prosecutor is seeking to have the witness testify as an expert, the witness will be subject to an examination outside the presence of the jury for the judge to determine the witness' qualifications and expertise. At this point the prosecutor will elicit the witness' knowledge, skill, experience, training, and education for the court's consideration. If the judge qualifies the witness as an expert, the witness can then not only testify to her or his actions, but also offer a medical or scientific opinion on a fact that is in issue (eg, the forensic examiner opining that an injury to the victim was caused by blunt force trauma or the lab analyst declaring that the suspect was detected as the source of the crime scene evidence sample).

In the direct examination of the laboratory analyst, the prosecutor should seek to show the broad nonforensic application of the 13-loci STR DNA technology. The witness may explain that this technology is used daily in paternity testing; medical applications in genetic research, diagnostics, and tissue typing, where accuracy can mean the difference between life and death; identification of the missing and dead, including the victims of mass disasters; and wildlife management, for the protection of endangered species. It may also be noted that this test, which is used to solve crimes, is the same test used to exonerate those who have been wrongly accused or convicted.

The analyst should next give a brief explanation of DNA, emphasizing its uniqueness and discriminating power. The testing procedures should then be summarized, including how and where the DNA was extracted, how it was amplified or copied, the testing process where the DNA profiles were generated, and the computer analysis or interpretation of the testing data. A simple exhibit could include an enlarged copy of the analyst's report showing the allele tables where there was a match at each and every locus between the crime scene or evidence sample and the defendant's known sample (**Figure 5-11**). If a mixture was found, an analysis should be given, if possible, of the major and minor contributors to the sample. Finally the witness is asked to provide the statistical frequency of the genetic profile found in the evidence and the defendant's known sample. If qualified as an expert, the witness may further be able to offer an opinion with a reasonable degree of scientific certainty that based on a comparison of the profile obtained from the defendant's known sample and the evidence sample, the defendant was the source of the DNA found in the evidence sample.

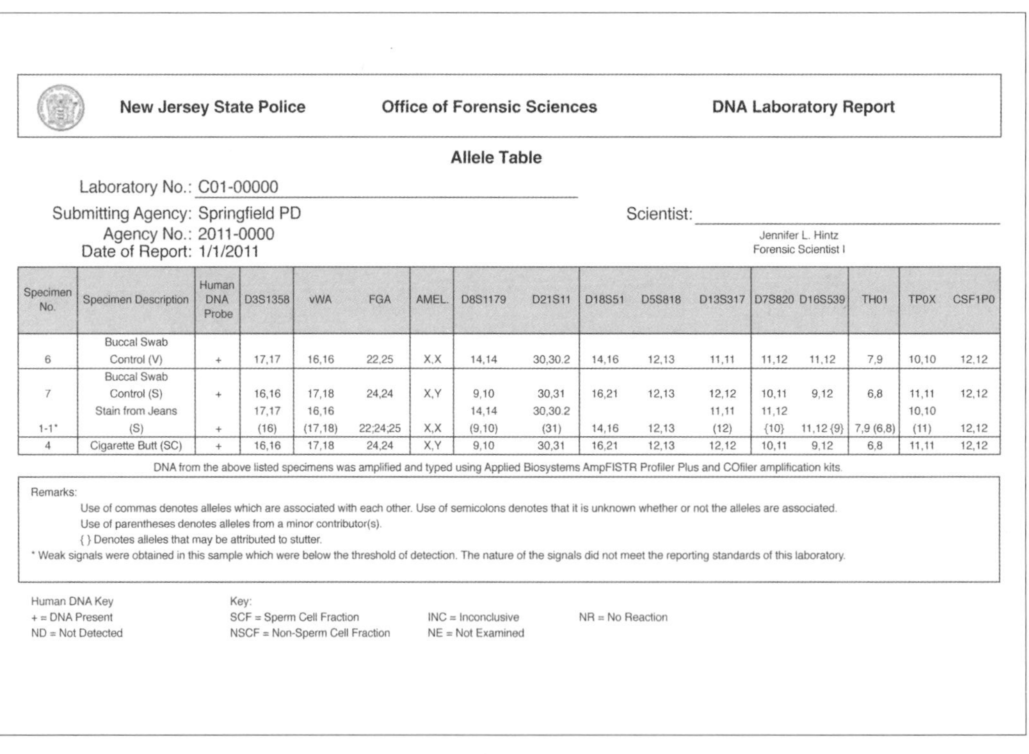

New Jersey State Police **Office of Forensic Sciences** **DNA Laboratory Report**

Allele Table

Laboratory No.: C01-00000
Submitting Agency: Springfield PD
Agency No.: 2011-0000
Date of Report: 1/1/2011

Scientist: ____________
Jennifer L. Hintz
Forensic Scientist I

Specimen No.	Specimen Description	Human DNA Probe	D3S1358	vWA	FGA	AMEL.	D8S1179	D21S11	D18S51	D5S818	D13S317	D7S820	D16S539	TH01	TPOX	CSF1PO
6	Buccal Swab Control (V)	+	17,17	16,16	22,25	X,X	14,14	30,30.2	14,16	12,13	11,11	11,12	11,12	7,9	10,10	12,12
7	Buccal Swab Control (S)	+	16,16	17,18	24,24	X,Y	9,10	30,31	16,21	12,13	12,12	10,11	9,12	6,8	11,11	12,12
1-1*	Stain from Jeans (S)	+	17,17 (16)	16,16 (17,18)	22;24;25	X,X	14,14 (9,10)	30,30.2 (31)	14,16	12,13	11,11 (12)	11,12 {10}	11,12 {9}	7,9 (6,8)	10,10 (11)	12,12
4	Cigarette Butt (SC)	+	16,16	17,18	24,24	X,Y	9,10	30,31	16,21	12,13	12,12	10,11	9,12	6,8	11,11	12,12

DNA from the above listed specimens was amplified and typed using Applied Biosystems AmpFISTR Profiler Plus and COfiler amplification kits.

Remarks:
Use of commas denotes alleles which are associated with each other. Use of semicolons denotes that it is unknown whether or not the alleles are associated.
Use of parentheses denotes alleles from a minor contributor(s).
{ } Denotes alleles that may be attributed to stutter.
* Weak signals were obtained in this sample which were below the threshold of detection. The nature of the signals did not meet the reporting standards of this laboratory.

Human DNA Key
+ = DNA Present
ND = Not Detected

Key:
SCF = Sperm Cell Fraction
NSCF = Non-Sperm Cell Fraction
INC = Inconclusive
NE = Not Examined
NR = No Reaction

Figure 5-11. *This is a sample DNA laboratory report, which shows an allele table. Reprinted with permission from the New Jersey State Police Office of Forensic Sciences.*

CODIS

The CODIS national DNA databank allows its participants to exchange and compare DNA profiles electronically. Today all 50 states, the FBI, and the United States Army participate in the system.

CODIS is composed of 2 major indexes that can be of great assistance to law enforcement in solving crimes. The first is the *forensic index*, which contains DNA profiles recovered from crime scenes. This can include such evidence as the results obtained from the processing of sexual assault kits. The second major index is the *offender index*. This index includes the DNA profiles of known offenders, whose DNA samples were taken pursuant to various federal and state collection laws on their conviction of a criminal offense. The federal government and some states have now expanded their collection laws to permit taking a DNA sample from a suspect upon his arrest. This allows the suspect's profile to be entered into CODIS as soon as possible to search against those profiles recovered from unsolved crime scenes. Provisions are also in place to require the removal of the sample if the suspect is not convicted. CODIS is also an instrumental component of the FBI's National Missing Person DNA Database program, wherein biological samples can be entered into the database to identify missing persons or unidentified human remains.

CODIS is set up in a hierarchical manner, consisting of 3 levels. The base of the system is the Local DNA Index System (LDIS), which covers local, municipal, or county forensic labs. Crime scene DNA profiles or convicted offender DNA profiles obtained at this level are forwarded to the State DNA Index System (SDIS). The state system permits local labs within the state to compare their results. Only the state system, however, is allowed to upload DNA profiles into the National DNA Index System (NDIS). To do so, the submitting agency must have attempted to develop a 13-loci profile, with at least 10 loci having been found. Although private forensic labs are not participants in CODIS, profiles generated from those labs may be submitted to the state lab for inclusion in the system. At the national level, all samples that have been submitted are routinely run against each other to determine whether there is a match or "hit" in the system.

A hit within the system can occur in one of 2 manners. A *forensic hit* occurs when the DNA profile from the evidence sample(s) taken from one crime scene matches the DNA profile taken from another crime scene. This may provide invaluable investigative leads to law enforcement concerning the operation of a serial offender. An *offender hit* occurs when a DNA profile taken from a crime scene matches that of a known convicted offender whose profile is contained in the offender database. The offender will then have to be located, and a new control sample taken from the suspect to confirm the results.

To be identified through the database, an offender must commit at least 2 qualifying offenses. On commission of the first offense, the defendant's genetic profile is entered into the database either from the evidence sample recovered (through the forensic index) or from a sample required to be provided on his conviction of a qualifying offense (through the offender index). After the second offense, the evidence sample can be uploaded to the system to begin searching against the other casework and offender samples already online.

If a hit is not obtained immediately, the uploaded samples will continue to search against all current and future uploaded samples. Often, samples uploaded on a certain date may not hit against other samples until months or years later, depending on when the second sample is uploaded to the system. CODIS is especially helpful with sexual offenders because of the high tendency for these types of crimes to involve biological evidence and the high recidivism rate of sexual offenders.

CODIS has assisted law enforcement in solving crimes that were decades old. As states continue to modify their laws to permit the collection of samples from a growing list of criminal offenses, the convicted offender database will continue to increase, and more crimes will be effectively solved.

Explaining the Absence of DNA Evidence

One unanticipated byproduct of the explosion in the use of forensic DNA analysis is the expectation that every crime will have DNA evidence as a component of the case.

Popular television shows have spawned what is commonly referred to as the *CSI Effect*, wherein jurors who have observed the use of DNA technology in fictional entertainment expect the same to hold true in reality. In the world of television entertainment, evidence samples are gathered and analyzed before the first commercial break, and the crime has been solved and a jury verdict rendered before an hour has passed. High-tech equipment depicted may not even be commercially available or of general acceptance in the scientific community. Faced with such unrealistic expectations, the prosecutor must use the SAFE and forensic lab analyst to debunk such popular myths. The use of such testimony is often referred to as *negative evidence*, which is evidence that explains why DNA is not involved in a particular case.

Savvy criminals have often sought means to prevent detection in sexual assault cases. The suspect may use gloves to prevent leaving fingerprints at a scene; use a condom to prevent recovery of his semen from the victim; or force the victim to bathe, douche, or rinse her mouth to remove any of his biological material from her body. Sophisticated criminals today use chlorine bleach to destroy residual DNA left at the location of the attack or on the body of the victim.

Prosecutors must be prepared to educate the jury through expert witnesses why the lack of DNA evidence does not mean that a crime has not been committed; essentially, that the absence of evidence is not evidence of absence. Straightforward explanations may include that there was simply no DNA deposited, or the evidence sample was collected from a location where DNA was not present. A delayed reporting of the incident may have also diminished the possibility of recovering a sample. DNA may have been collected, but it could have been in such a small quantity that it was insufficient for analysis, or it was so degraded that no DNA profile could be generated.

In sexual assault cases, there may be many medically explainable reasons why DNA was not recovered or a profile was not generated. Semen may not have been recovered because the defendant failed to ejaculate; the assailant had a vasectomy or was aspermatic; or the offender has a sexual dysfunction, thereby resulting in a premature or retarded ejaculation. With regard to the victim, if a female was on her menses, a sample may not have been collected by the forensic examiner, or there may be such an abundance of the victim's DNA that it masked that of her assailant. It is also possible that the cleansing actions of the victim's own vaginal secretions may have purged any semen from her vaginal cavity.

Even if DNA has been recovered in a case, it may be of no consequence depending on the nature of the case being prosecuted. DNA can be irrelevant in a case where the defense of consent is being offered. In the case of spousal or intimate partner sexual assault, where the sample was found may render it of no probative value. For example, semen stains recovered from the marital bed are generally irrelevant, since it is expected that such biological material would be found there. Unfortunately, current testing methods cannot tell when the sample was deposited.

Emerging DNA Technology

PCR testing has revolutionized the forensic identification arena so that testing minimal samples, often referred to as low copy number (LCN) or "touch" DNA, is being attempted in criminal and even civil cases. Even when body fluids are not left behind, mere contact with an item such as the gear shift or steering wheel of a vehicle, or holding a book or a glass, may leave enough DNA for emerging technologies to detect.

Of course, the ability to do this is a double-edged sword—any other sources of DNA on these items will likely be detected as well. Whether or not mixed or contaminated samples can be reliably interpreted remains to be seen.

When only partial or no results are obtained using conventional STR testing, 2 other powerful tools exist that are becoming more routinely used by the nation's crime labs: mtDNA and Y-STRs.

MtDNA is very robust, and enough mtDNA can often be recovered to test even in badly degraded samples. It can also be used on samples that would not otherwise yield good nuclear DNA results, such as bones, teeth, and hair shafts. In addition, it has been used on ancient samples such as Egyptian mummies to document the maternal lineage of the royal dynasties, and more recently on some of the remains entombed at Arlington National Cemetery in the Tomb of the Unknown. MtDNA is maternally inherited and, therefore, less discriminating than conventional STR testing. It originates during conception when the sperm's nucleus enters the egg and combines with the egg's nucleus. Once the fertilized egg begins to divide, all other cellular components derive from the mother's original egg cell and are passed down to her children. In cases such as the Tomb of the Unknown, or in missing persons cases where there may be other factors leading investigators to suspect a particular identity, obtaining comparison samples from relatives can provide conclusive exclusionary results or, when combined with other evidence, strong inclusionary results.

Because they are paternally inherited, Y-STRs also provide less discriminating information than conventional STRs, but can still be quite useful in certain circumstances. When a sexual perpetrator has been vasectomized or is aspermatic for some other medical reason, detecting DNA foreign to the victim with conventional STRs may not be possible because of the overwhelming amount of victim DNA compared to a relatively small amount of male DNA. In the case of a female victim and male assailant, using Y-STRs should still offer some identifying information because the test would only detect contributions from a male and would virtually ignore any DNA present from a female donor. Likewise, when a man may be abusing his daughter, with conventional DNA testing they would share at least 50% of their DNA. Y-STRs, however, would only detect DNA on the victim or evidence items from a male. This type of testing would not be useful when a man was abusing his son, as they would both share the same Y-STR sequence.

New testing techniques and testing instruments are constantly being developed. One promising form of DNA testing is the use of single nucleotide polymorphisms (SNPs). SNPs are single base sequence variations between individuals at a particular point along the DNA molecule. Advantages to SNPs include their ability to get results with very badly degraded samples. This type of testing was employed to help identify the remains of many of the victims of the September 11, 2001 attacks on the World Trade Center and Pentagon. When DNA degrades, it gets cut into smaller and smaller fragments. If a particular test is looking for a fragment of a specific length, and the degraded DNA is already smaller than that length, the test will not work and no result will be obtained. SNPs are already so small they are still likely to be detected when all other testing methods fail. However, to be forensically significant, a large panel of SNPs (anywhere from 25 to 45) must be examined.[5] For certain circumstances, such as a plane crash or a mass disaster, SNPs can provide valuable information. However, because such a high number is required to get an acceptable degree of discrimination, it is unlikely that this type of testing will make its way into the mainstream crime laboratory.

Another type of DNA testing gaining acceptance that may provide more information is mini-STRs. Mini-STRs are short tandem repeats with smaller target lengths than the 13-CODIS STR loci. Because of this, degraded DNA that may give only partial or no results with conventional STR testing may still yield interpretable results with mini-STRs. There are, however, disadvantages to this system. For example, unlike the 13 CODIS loci, where numerous loci can be amplified in one reaction, only a few mini-STR loci can be amplified together, increasing the number of reactions that must be performed to obtain meaningful results. However, mini-STRs are promising for use in highly degraded samples where conventional testing is simply not possible. Even telogen hair shafts, previously only tested with mtDNA, have been successfully typed using mini-STRs.[6]

Sometimes evidence in cases comes not from human biological material but from plants, animals, or even germs. DNA from pet hair transferred to a suspect or victim or DNA from plant material found on a victim's body can be typed, often providing a useful link to a location or person key to solving the crime. In addition, as the threat of biological warfare agents becomes increasingly real, viral or microbial DNA testing is becoming more widespread. Research is ongoing on ways to trace a particular strain of a virus through its DNA.

Existing DNA testing methods are constantly being reviewed and revised in order to deliver results more quickly, cheaply, and efficiently. As more law enforcement and medical personnel are educated about where potential DNA evidence can be found, more evidence is collected and submitted for testing. This has proved to be both a blessing and a curse. While more evidence is now available to help solve crimes, the additional samples also contribute to increased bottlenecks at the lab, resulting in longer turnaround times for the delivery of test results. Research is ongoing to miniaturize many of the instruments used in PCR testing for potential transportation to crime scenes. Development is underway on several portable devices (eg, the "lab-on-a-chip") that would allow a partial or possibly full DNA screening test to be done on the spot, and provide investigators with preliminary leads much more quickly than having to wait for the lab to issue a report. Additionally, new methods are being investigated to decrease turnaround time for large-scale sample testing such as convicted offender samples. Time-of-flight mass spectrometry is a technique that can accommodate large numbers of samples and can work with STR analysis. When combined with robotic sample preparation, this technique may be able to process thousands of DNA samples in a day.[7]

Preserving Jurisdiction

DNA evidence that has been properly preserved can last indefinitely and can be used today to solve cases that are decades old. Advancements in technology, however, have run into legal barriers. Statutes of limitations have traditionally limited how long a case may remain active, so as to give finality to criminal proceedings. Once a statute of limitations has expired, a criminal case cannot go forward.

Many states have recognized the dilemma presented by a finite statute of limitations versus the power of DNA to identify and hold accountable offenders many years after the occurrence of a crime. To remedy the situation, a number of states have modified their laws to either abolish the statute of limitations completely for cases involving sexual assault, or to create a tolling provision for those cases where biological evidence has been collected but no suspect has yet been identified. The extended statute of limitations can only apply to cases where the present statute has not expired; to do otherwise would constitute an ex post facto law and therefore be unconstitutional.

Thus, the law can be used to extend the statute of limitations of an active case pending at the time of the new statute's inception, but it cannot revive a case whose statute of limitations has already expired.

In jurisdictions where the statute of limitations has not been extended, prosecutors have found a creative means to keep the criminal case from expiring. As a general rule, if a suspect is charged in a criminal matter but has absconded, the statute of limitations is tolled and the case remains open until the defendant is taken into custody. This could be problematic with unknown offenders, since a defendant must be sufficiently identified to have criminal charges filed against him or her. To remedy this problem, prosecutors have devised the John Doe warrant, wherein the otherwise unidentified suspect is charged by specifying his or her DNA profile in papers filed with the court.[8] Unlike names, which can be changed or falsified, DNA is unique to the individual. Courts have held that a DNA profile sufficiently identifies the person being sought, so that the case may remain open pending the actual identification of the person by name.[9]

Conclusion

The use of biological evidence is now considered to be a routine matter in sexual assault cases. Although routine, the members of a SART must never become complacent, because a proper analysis of the evidence depends on the team's ability to appropriately identify, collect, and preserve the evidence at hand. All team members must be cognizant of the evidentiary power of DNA and carefully adhere to the protocols of their local jurisdictions to assure that such evidence will be admissible in court. Evidence collected today may be of use for years to come. Ultimately, the greatest value of the technology may not merely lie in its ability to identify and bring an offender to justice, but rather its ability to give a victim of sexual assault the closure he or she has long been seeking.

References

1. Locard E. Manual of Police Techniques. In: Brahney K, trans. *An Exchange in Locard's Own Words*. 3rd ed. Paris, France: Payot; 1939, Parts 1, 2, 3. Modern Microscopy Web site. http://www.modernmicroscopy.com/main.asp?column=3. Accessed February 24, 2010.

2. O'Neil D. Distribution of blood types. *Modern Human Variation: An Introduction to Human Biological Diversity*. http://anthro.palomar.edu/vary/vary_3.htm. Updated July 21, 2006. Accessed February 24, 2010.

3. *Frye v United States*, 54 App DC 46, 293 F 1013, (1923).

4. *Daubert v Merrell Pharmaceutical*, 509 US 579 (1993).

5. Butler JM. *Forensic DNA Typing, Biology, Technology and Genetics of STR Markers*. 2nd ed. Burlington, MA: Elsevier Academic Press; 2005.

6. Coble MD, Vallone PM, Butler JM. *Genotyping of Nuclear Loci from Telogenic Hair Shafts Using Mini-STRs*. Paper presented at: the 57th Annual Conference of the American Academy of Forensic Sciences; February 2005; New Orleans, LA.

7. Butler JM, Becker CH; Office of Justice Programs, National Institute of Justice. Improved analysis of DNA short tandem repeats with time-of-flight mass spectrometry. Final Report for NIJ Grant 97-LB-VX-0003; 2001 (75 published pages); http://www.ojp.usdoj.gov/nij/pubs-sum/188292.htm. Accessed August 27, 2009.

8. *State of Wisconsin v Dabney*, 663 NW2d 366 (2003).

9. Delaney CE. Seeking John Doe: the provision and propriety of DNA-based warrants in the wake of *Wisconsin v. Dabney*. *Hofstra L Rev*. 2005;33:1091.

Chapter 6

COMPLICATIONS OF SEXUAL ASSAULT: SEXUALLY TRANSMITTED INFECTION AND PREGNANCY

Margaret L. Simpson, MD

In addition to the serious psychological and physical trauma that occurs with a sexual assault, the complications of sexually transmitted infection (STI) and pregnancy must be evaluated after a sexual assault. Sexual assault programs must delineate their approach to STI and pregnancy testing as well as prophylactic therapy. Genetic testing for *Neisseria gonorrhoeae* as well as *Chlamydia trachomatis* are now available and may replace culture. Increasing *N. gonorrhoeae* resistance may change the prophylactic regimens in some areas of the United States. Because of the significant rate of asymptomatic infection, prophylactic therapy of bacterial STIs is highly recommended. Human immunodeficiency virus (HIV) postexposure prophylaxis (PEP) is recommended in known high-risk HIV exposures. With easier regimens and less toxicity, HIV PEP may be offered more frequently in cases when the risk of HIV exposure is lower or unknown. With the wide availability of emergency contraception (EC), this must be offered as a part of the sexual assault visit for all women of childbearing age at risk of becoming pregnant, including women taking contraceptive measures. A recent review of sexual assault evaluation revealed that 66% of women did not receive any medications for STIs, and less than half of those at risk for pregnancy received EC.[1]

EPIDEMIOLOGY

The Centers for Disease Control Sexually Transmitted Diseases Treatment Guidelines now state "the decision to obtain genital or other specimens for STI diagnosis should be made on an individual basis."[2] This particularly refers to the immediate postassault evaluation. Evidence of previously acquired STI is theoretically restricted from evidentiary use in all 50 states. Serology results for syphilis, hepatitis, and HIV at the time of the assault will reflect prior infection. Culture, smears, or genetic testing for *Neisseria*, *Chlamydia* (**Figures 6-1** and **6-2**), and *Trichomonas* with positive results may reflect residual secretions from the man or prior infection in the woman. Testing at follow-up visits can reflect acquisition from the assault or

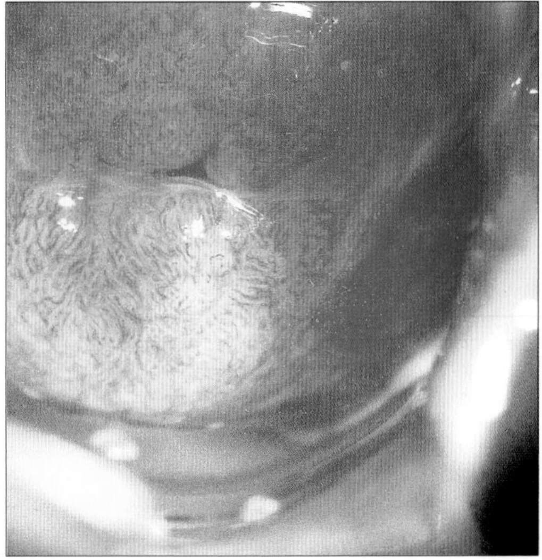

Figure 6-1. *This cervix has a vascular pattern on the cervix inferior to the os. Vaginal cultures revealed* Chlamydia trachomatis.

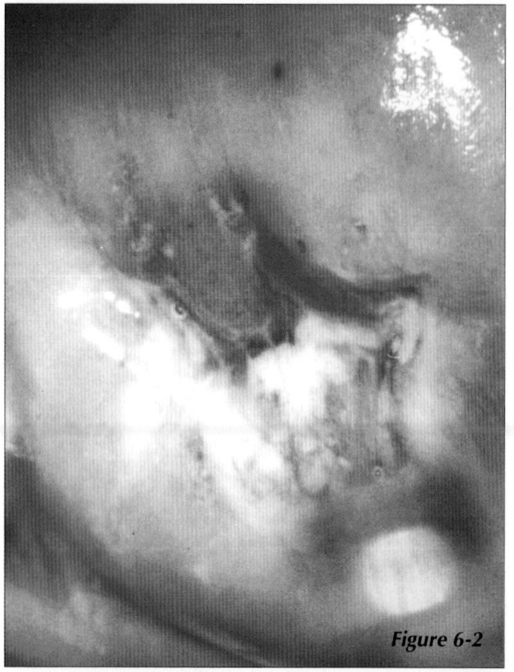

from resumption of sexual activity. Regardless of the use of diagnostic tests, an empiric regimen to treat *Chlamydia*, gonorrhea, *T. vaginalis*, and bacterial vaginosis is recommended.[2] Emergency contraception for women at risk is also recommended as well as evaluating the need for hepatitis B vaccination and HIV PEP. Positive tests for gonorrhea and *Chlamydia* provide assistance in partner notification and treatment of other persons who may be at risk. Many states have clinics that offer free HIV testing, counseling, and treatment.

Historically, *N. gonorrhoeae* has been the most frequently diagnosed STI related to sexual assault evaluations. Now *C. trachomatis*, *T. vaginalis*, bacterial vaginosis, as well as human papillomavirus (HPV) are identified increasingly after sexual assault. See **Figures 6-3** through **6-7** for examples of *Condyloma acuminata*, which are a symptom of HPV. **Table 6-1** defines these STIs and their prevalence from reviews of studies.

Figure 6-2. *This female is negative for gonorrhea and positive for* Chlamydia trachomatis, *which are commonly found together. Thick, white mucous is visible in the cervix. The drainage would need to be removed for a complete evaluation of the cervical os.*

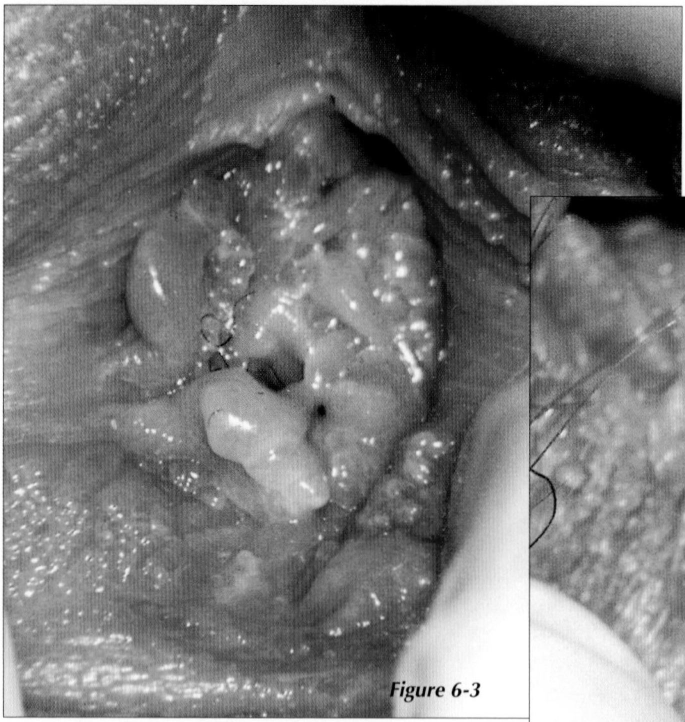

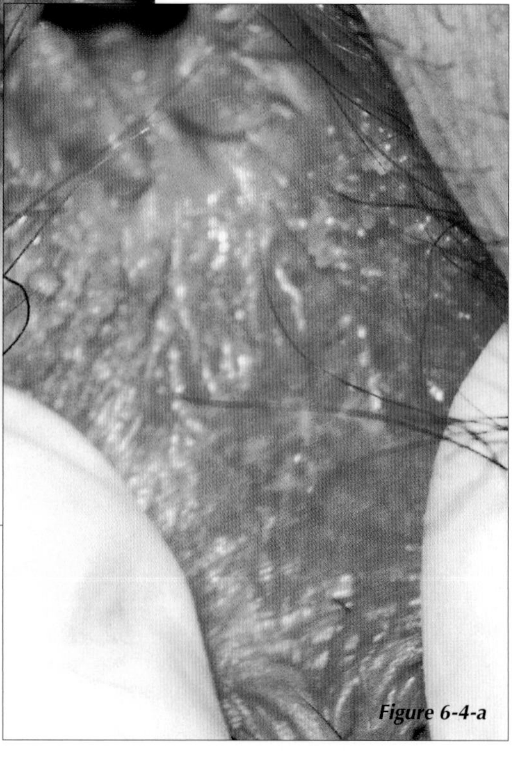

Figure 6-3. *This female is being treated for* Condyloma acuminata. *The hymen is fragmented with caruncula at 6 and 9 o'clock and multiple condylomatous lesions. There is focal erythema on the hymen at 11, 12, and 1 o'clock, and a dark hair at 9 o'clock.*

Figure 6-4-a. Condyloma acuminata *are visible. Her hymen has an old transection at 6 o'clock.*

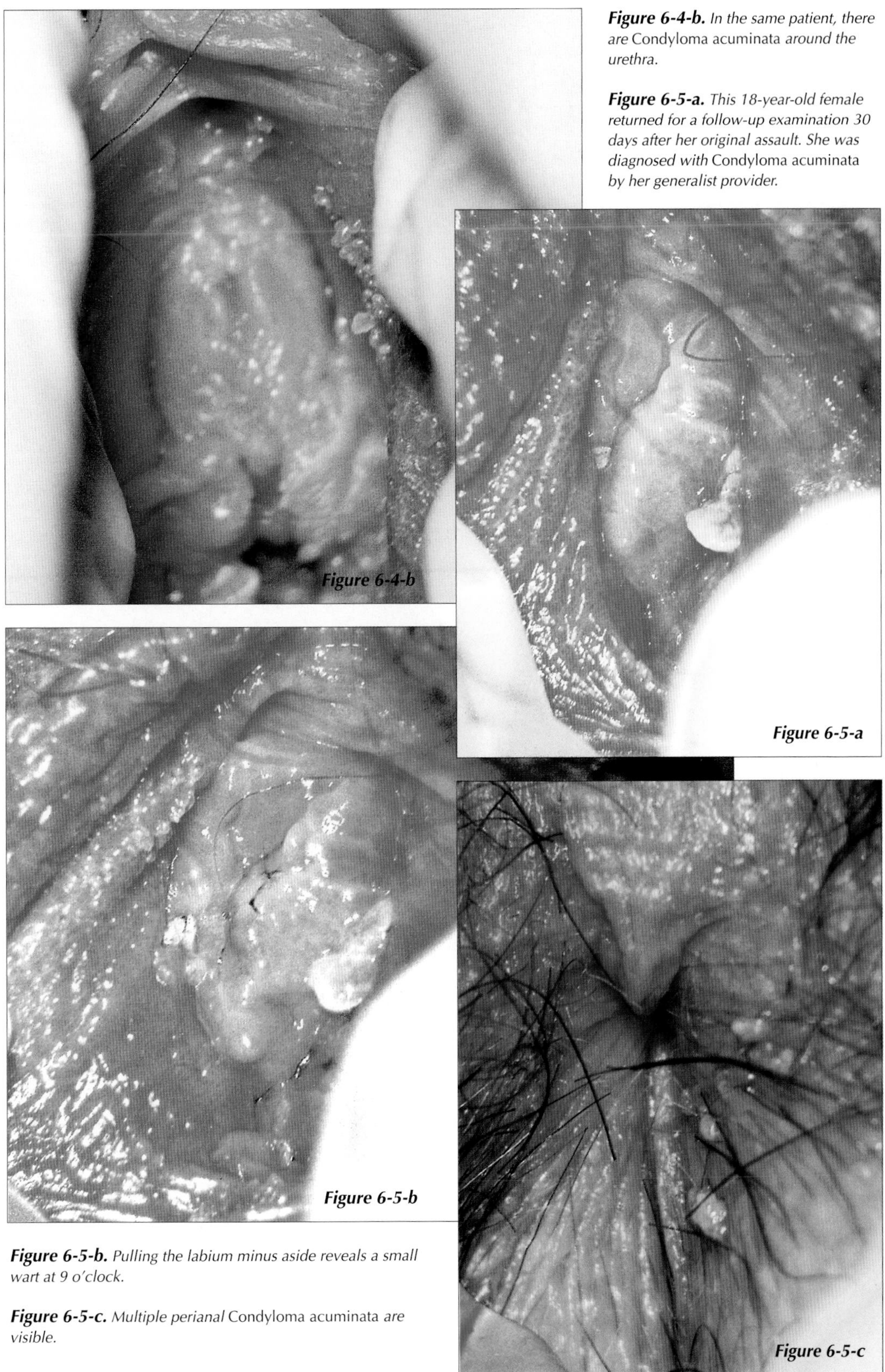

Figure 6-4-b. *In the same patient, there are* Condyloma acuminata *around the urethra.*

Figure 6-5-a. *This 18-year-old female returned for a follow-up examination 30 days after her original assault. She was diagnosed with* Condyloma acuminata *by her generalist provider.*

Figure 6-5-b. *Pulling the labium minus aside reveals a small wart at 9 o'clock.*

Figure 6-5-c. *Multiple perianal* Condyloma acuminata *are visible.*

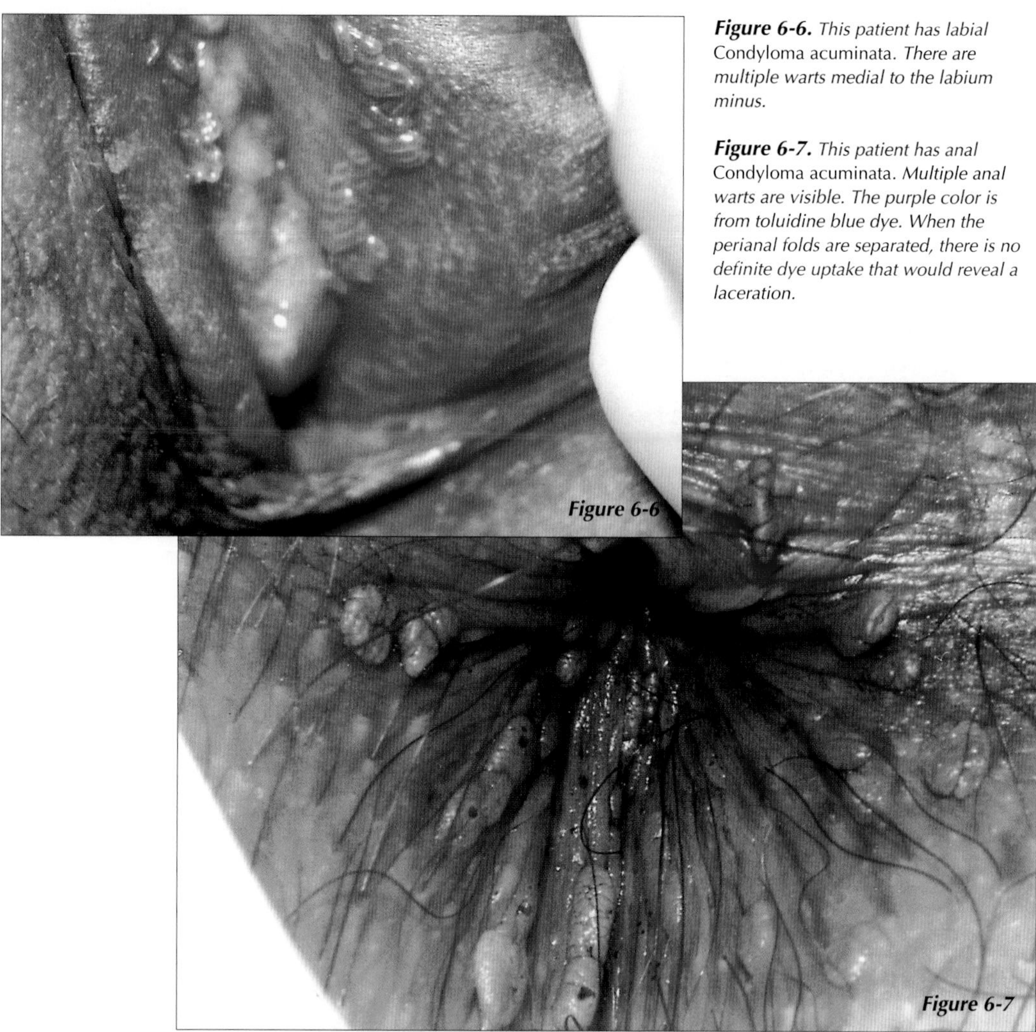

Figure 6-6. *This patient has labial* Condyloma acuminata. *There are multiple warts medial to the labium minus.*

Figure 6-7. *This patient has anal* Condyloma acuminata. *Multiple anal warts are visible. The purple color is from toluidine blue dye. When the perianal folds are separated, there is no definite dye uptake that would reveal a laceration.*

Table 6-1. STI Prevalence in Sexual Assault

Prevalance	(%)
Neisseria gonorrhoeae	1.8-13.3
Chlamydia trachomatis	2.0-17
Trichomonas vaginalis	2.0-13
Bacterial vaginosis	2.0-19
Human papillomavirus	1.8-9
Syphilis	0-2.9

Adapted from Reynolds MW, Peipert JF, Collins B. Epidemiologic issues of sexually transmitted diseases in sexual assault victims. Obstet Gynecol Survey. *2000;55:51-57 and Beck-Sague CM, Solomon F. Sexually transmitted diseases in children and adolescent and adult victims of rape. Review of selected literature.* Clin Infect Dis. *1999;28(suppl 1):PS74-83.*

Less information is available regarding hepatitis B, herpes simplex (**Figures 6-8** through **6-11**), and HIV. With the prevalence of hepatitis B in the community decreasing and universal vaccination of children increasing, the need to address this as part of the postsexual assault evaluation will diminish in the next decade. In one study there was no seroconversion for herpes simplex for any women.[5] In consensual sex, the risk of HIV transmission is from 0.1% to 0.2% per episode for vaginal intercourse and 0.5% to 3.0% for receptive rectal intercourse.[6] This risk could increase with the physical trauma of a sexual assault, particularly in children and adolescents.

The risk of pregnancy after sexual assault is estimated to be 2% to 4% if a woman is not protected by some form of contraception at the time of the attack. Surveys have suggested that up to 55% of women between ages 15 and 44 years are not at risk for pregnancy by actively using contraception, being pregnant, or being infertile.[1]

Although the risks of acquiring most STIs from a sexual assault are low, and many can be effectively prevented, victims are very concerned about the risk of an STI and pregnancy (see Case Study 6-1). In the National Women's Study, over 40% of survivors said they feared contracting an STI, particularly HIV.[7] This fear contributes to the significant stresses relating to the mental health aspects of recovery. Follow-up testing and counseling, particularly for HIV, will provide some assurance for the victims.

Case Study 6-1

A 22-year-old woman presents to a walk-in clinic requesting testing for sexually transmitted infections. As the care provider begins to ask questions, the patient bursts into tears. She relates that 24 hours ago she was at a party and mildly intoxicated. When a man attending the party offered to drive her home, she accepted. He then sexually assaulted her. She calms down with assistance from the provider and accepts a sexual assault exam.

Since she has not been sexually active for 4 months, she is not on active birth control. Her last menstrual period was 2 to 3 weeks ago and she is very concerned about being pregnant. During a women's health evaluation 1 year ago, she had a negative HIV test as well as normal PAP and pelvic exams. She denies any history of sexually transmitted infections.

The general examination reveals a distraught young woman, intermittently tearful. A nurse from the sexual assault services is called and performs the examination. There is mild trauma at the introitus of the vagina. No other significant vaginal or cervical abnormalities are noted. Following protocol, emergency contraception is provided as well as treatment with ceftriaxone, azithromycin, and metronidazole. An antiemetic was also given because of the gastrointestinal toxicities of the medications given. No testing for sexually transmitted infections is being performed since coverage or prophylaxis for the major sexual transmitted infections is being provided. Information was also given to the patient about HIV postexposure prophylaxis. She was told to return if any further genitourinary symptoms developed. Extensive counseling and legal resources were also provided to her.

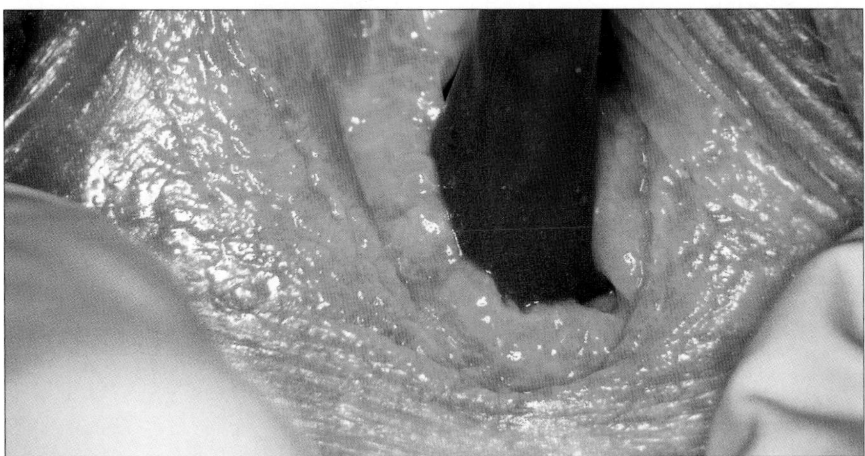

Figure 6-8-a. *This victim has a history of genital herpes. There is an old hymenal transection at 5 o'clock. No acute injury is noted.*

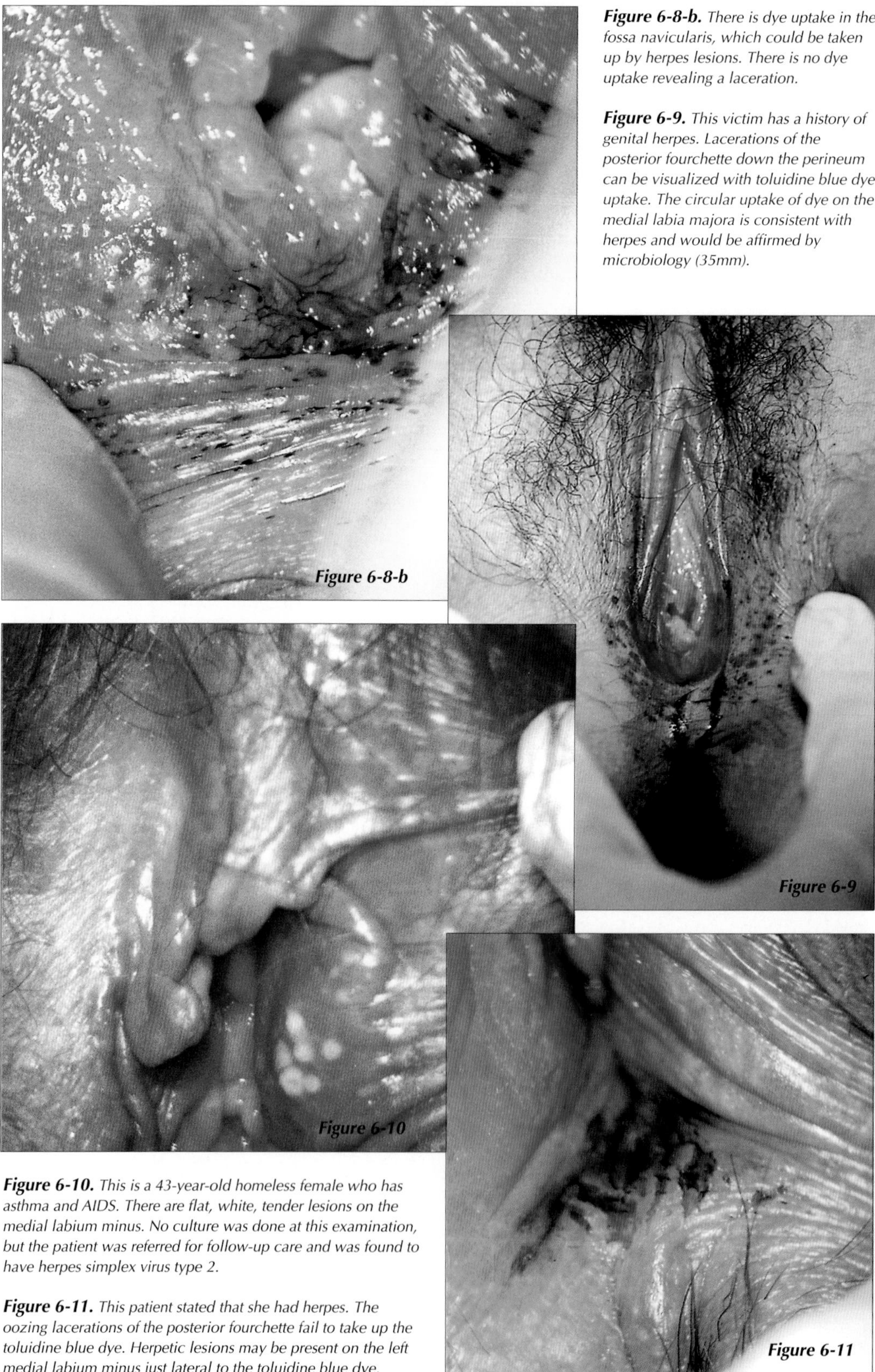

Figure 6-8-b. *There is dye uptake in the fossa navicularis, which could be taken up by herpes lesions. There is no dye uptake revealing a laceration.*

Figure 6-9. *This victim has a history of genital herpes. Lacerations of the posterior fourchette down the perineum can be visualized with toluidine blue dye uptake. The circular uptake of dye on the medial labia majora is consistent with herpes and would be affirmed by microbiology (35mm).*

Figure 6-10. *This is a 43-year-old homeless female who has asthma and AIDS. There are flat, white, tender lesions on the medial labium minus. No culture was done at this examination, but the patient was referred for follow-up care and was found to have herpes simplex virus type 2.*

Figure 6-11. *This patient stated that she had herpes. The oozing lacerations of the posterior fourchette fail to take up the toluidine blue dye. Herpetic lesions may be present on the left medial labium minus just lateral to the toluidine blue dye.*

STI and Pregnancy Testing

Nucleic acid amplification tests (NAAT) can now be used to make the diagnosis of a *N. gonorrhoeae* or *C. trachomatis* infection. With the NAAT tests, up to 80% more *Chlamydia* infections may be identified as compared to culture.[8] In addition, these tests (depending on type and FDA approval) can be used on urine, vaginal swabs (self-collected), endocervical swabs, and urethral swabs. For evaluating *N. gonorrhoeae* at other sites that have been penetrated (pharynx and rectum), cultures are required. The sensitivity of diagnosing *N. gonorrhoeae* from a Gram's stain of the endocervix showing gram negative intracellular diplococci is only 50%, so a more sensitive test should also be performed.

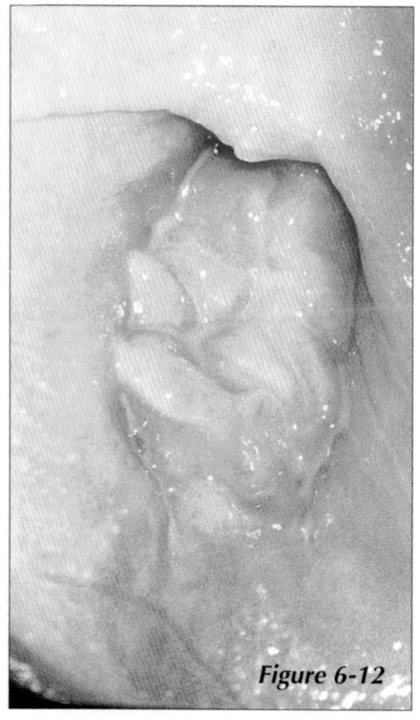

Figure 6-12. *This image displays a 49-year-old victim's pale, pink hymen and labia minora. There is white vaginal discharge present.* Gardnerella vaginalis *was seen in the vaginal culture.*

A wet prep of vaginal secretions may be useful in identifying *T. vaginalis*, bacterial vaginosis (**Figures 6-12** through **6-14**), and candida (**Figures 6-15** and **6-16**). Baseline serology for HIV, hepatitis B, and syphilis (**Figure 6-17**) are also recommended. A repeat exam for STIs should occur 1 to 2 weeks after the assault, particularly if no prophylaxis treatment was provided.[2] If preventative treatment was provided, only victims with symptoms will need an exam and repeat testing. Serology follow-up for HIV and syphilis should occur 6 weeks, 3 months, and 6 months after the assault, particularly if an infection in the assailant cannot be ruled out.

Before EC is administered, a preexisting pregnancy must be excluded. A serum pregnancy test is more sensitive, but a urine pregnancy test may be used if it is the only screening test available. Because EC should be given within 72 hours of the assault, either test can be used.

Even with established programs aimed at assisting victims of sexual assault, follow-up rates are low (rate of 31%). Many decline a repeat pelvic exam but desire laboratory results and counseling.[9]

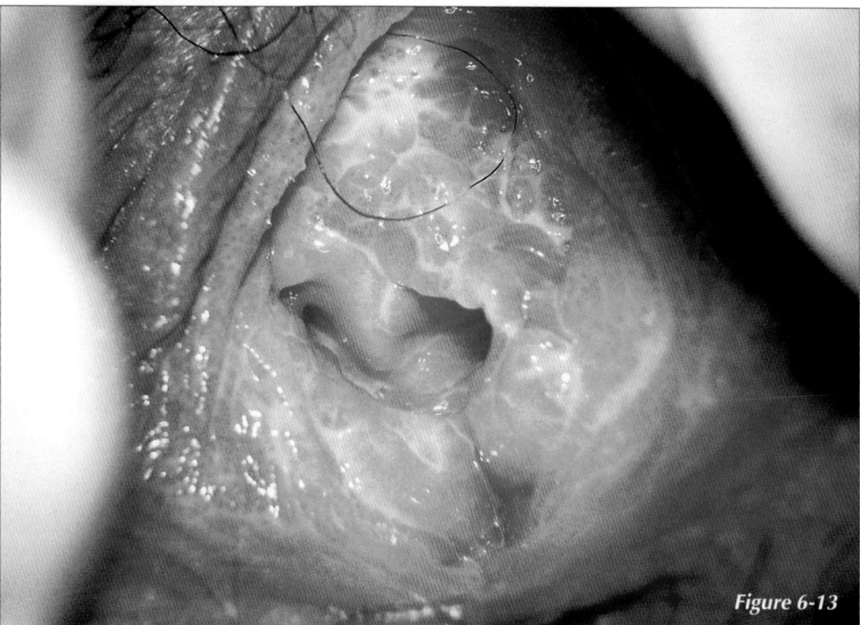

Figure 6-13. *Milky white discharge is visible on the surface of the hymen. Vaginal cultures revealed* Gardnerella vaginalis. *Erythema is present from 2 to 3 o'clock and also at 6 o'clock.*

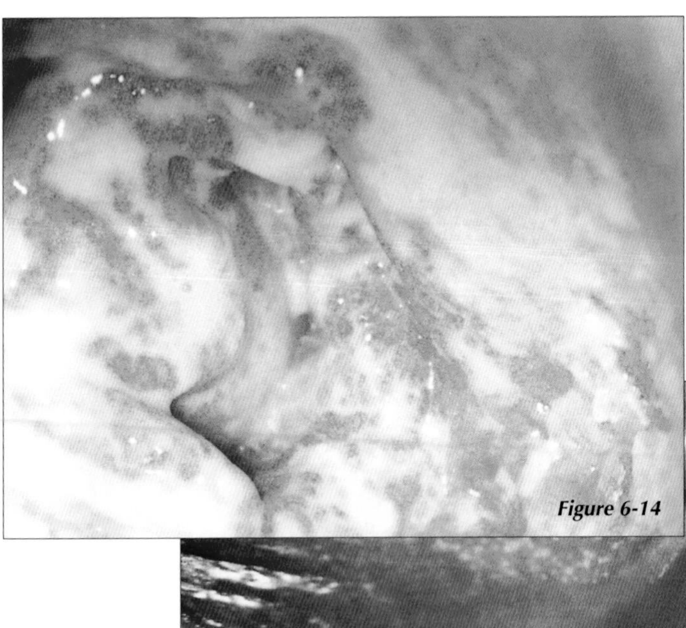

Figure 6-14. *This female presented for dysuria. The photo shows her external genitalia. There is a thick, white malodorous discharge on the external genitalia, positive for* Candida albicans *and* Gardnerella vaginalis.

Figure 6-15. *White discharge is present on the external genitalia. The vaginal culture revealed* Candida albicans.

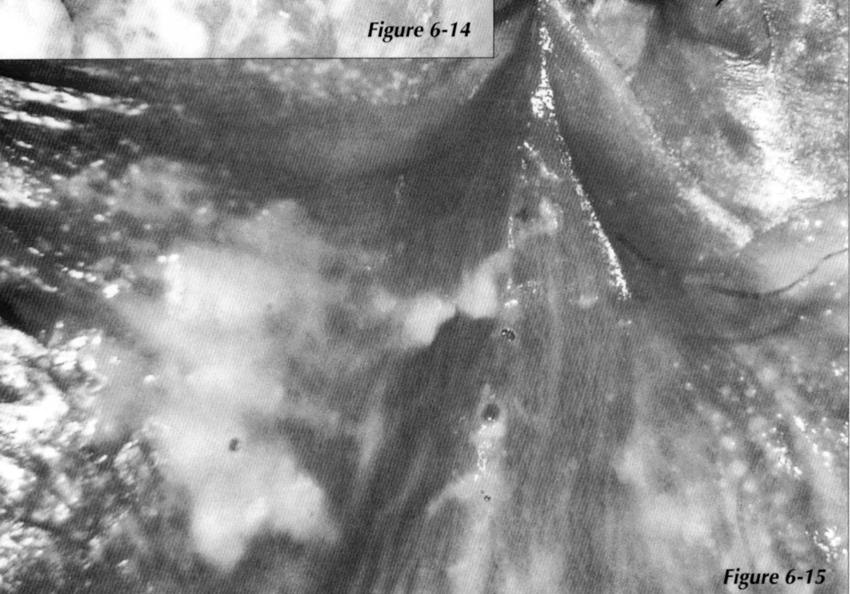

Figure 6-16. *This patient presented with curd-like lesions on the labium minus that are consistent with* Candida albicans.

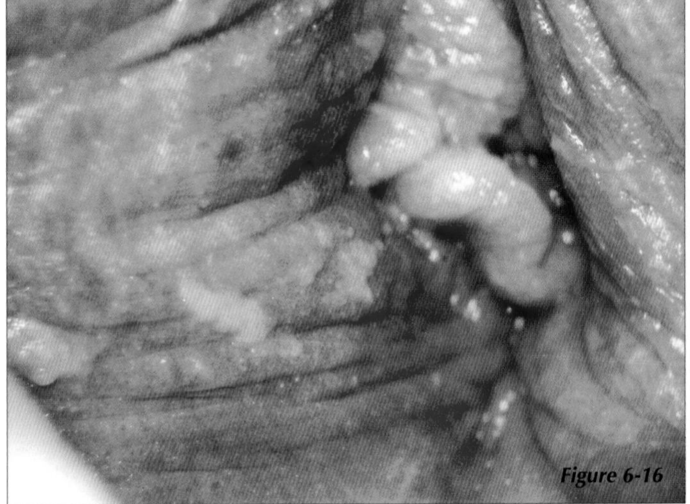

Figure 6-17

Figure 6-17. *There is a syphilitic chancre visible on the upper lip of this patient.*

STI Prophylaxis

Considering the STIs that have been most associated with sexual assault, the CDC guidelines provide recommendations regarding preventive treatment.[2] As a part of the evaluation, a pelvic exam should be performed to assess trauma and pelvic inflammatory disease (PID), as this will not be treated by the single-dose antimicrobial regimen suggested. Because significant nausea and/or vomiting may occur with the administration of the 3 antimicrobials and EC, an antiemetic is recommended.

Recommendations for STI preventive therapy are given in **Table 6-2**. Ceftriaxone or ciprofloxacin will treat *N. gonorrhoeae*. Single-dose azithromycin is being used with increasing frequency to treat *C. trachomatis*, and doxycycline for one week is an alternative. Metronidazole will treat *T. vaginalis* as well as bacterial vaginosis. Single-dose treatment for bacterial vaginosis is less efficacious, and if a diagnosis of it is made, a longer course of treatment may be needed. Incubating syphilis is usually covered by ceftriaxone, azithromycin, or doxycycline.

Quinolone-resistant *N. gonorrhoeae* (QRNG) are becoming more prevalent in the United States. They are already very common worldwide. Presently, the quinolones (ciprofloxacin, levafloxacin, and ofloxacin) are not recommended for use in men who have sex with men (rates of QRNG of 23.9% is 2.9% in heterosexual men). In addition, with the high rates of QRNG in California and Hawaii, the quinolones are not used in these 2 states for gonococcal treatment.[2]

An evaluation of any prior history of hepatitis B vaccine should be a part of the protocol. If the sexual assault victim has not been vaccinated previously, the vaccine series should be initiated. Written instructions for follow-up injections at 1 to 2 months and 6 months should be provided. If the vaccine series is initiated promptly, hepatitis B

Table 6-2. STI Preventative Treatment

Preventative Treatment
— Ceftriaxone 125 mg in a single dose intramuscularly OR Ciprofloxacin 500 mg orally PLUS Metronidazole 2 g orally in a single dose PLUS Azithromycin 1 g orally in a single dose OR Doxycycline 100 mg orally twice a day for 7 days
— Hepatitis B vaccine series after evaluation
— Tetanus booster if more than 10 years since last vaccination or after physical injury
— HIV postexposure prophylaxis (see remaining chapter).

Adapted from CDC. Sexually transmitted diseases treatment guidelines. MMWR. *2006;55:RR-11; Holmes MM, Resnick HS, Frampton D. Follow-up of sexual assault victims.* Amer J Obstet Gynec. *1998;179:336-341; and Patel M, Minshall L. Management of sexual assault.* Emerg Med Clin North Am. *2001;19:817-831.*

immune globulin does not need to be administered and has been removed from recommendations.[2] A tetanus booster should be administered with significant physical injury or if it has been greater than 10 years since last given.

HIV Postexposure Prophylaxis

Antiretroviral therapy to prevent HIV infection has been well documented in 2 circumstances. It is now routinely used to interrupt maternal-fetal transmission. Use of a single agent reduces transmission from 25% to 8%.[11] Use of multiple antiretrovirals has reduced this to a rate less than 2%. In addition, PEP is offered after a significant blood and body fluid exposure in the health care setting, particularly with known HIV-infected exposures. The use of HIV PEP in health care has decreased the risk of HIV acquisition from 0.4% to 0.1% after a needlestick injury from a known HIV-infected source.[12]

As antiretrovirals become easier for people to take, there may be an expanded role after sexual exposures including sexual assault. Guidelines are available for the use of HIV PEP in the health care setting.[13] Animal studies as well as human clinical and observational studies confirm that antiretroviral therapy initiated within 48 to 72 hours of sexual relations or injection drug use exposure might reduce the likelihood of transmission.[14] Although suggested by guidelines, presently PEP is not widely used after sexual assault.[14] Limitations to the use of HIV PEP include medication cost ($600 to $1000 for the 28-day course), medication side effects, and monitoring for toxicities. Follow-up with the use of HIV PEP has been poor, with only 12% completing the 4 weeks of therapy in a postsexual assault program.[15] It should be considered in some higher risk assault, including male-to-male sexual assault, known HIV-infected assailant, and physically traumatic sexual assaults (particularly in children and adolescents).[2]

When evaluating for the use of PEP, optimal initiation should occur within a few hours of the risk exposure. It is rarely used more than 72 hours after exposure unless there is a very high HIV risk. Because early initiation of this prophylaxis is needed and to address concerns of victims of assault, an initial short course of 3 to 5 days may be given with follow-up by a sexual assault program to reassess. In a high-risk assault, when it is unknown if there was an HIV exposure, 2 drug combinations may be used. Truvada (tenofavir/emtricitabine) once daily or Combivir (zidovidine/lamividine) twice daily are frequent regimens used for PEP. In a known HIV exposure, more aggressive therapy would include the addition of a protease inhibitor with one of the listed medications. If PEP is used, consultations with an infectious disease or HIV provider should be done to assist with side effects and medication monitoring. In addition, a baseline complete blood count and renal/liver function must be performed. Postexposure prophylaxis is usually administered for 4 weeks, and follow-up should include appropriate monitoring for the toxicities of these medications.

Emergency Contraception

Women who are at risk for pregnancy should be counseled about options for pregnancy prevention. All women should be offered EC. Pregnancy testing is indicated in the acute setting to rule out a preexisting pregnancy. EC regimens are 97% to 98% effective if started within 24 hours of the sexual assault and are generally recommended within the first 72 hours.[16,17] Counseling must include the discussion of a 2% to 3% failure rate with the small potential for teratogenic effects if the pregnancy continues after using EC.

The side effects of EC include nausea in up to half of patients and emesis in 10% to 20%. These toxicities are decreased with the use of antiemetics one hour before the first contraceptive dose. The gastrointestinal side effects of the progestin-only (levonorgestrel)

Table 6-3. Emergency Contraception

Brand Name	Generic Name	Dosage	Dosage Instructions
Plan B	levonorgestrel	0.75mg	One dose now, repeat in 12 hours (in the future may be modified to a single 1.5 mg dose)
Preven	ethinyl estradiol levonorgestrel	0.05mg 0.25mg	One dose of each now, repeat in 12 hours

Note: Antiemetics one hour before each dose strongly recommended.

Adapted from: American Medical Association. Strategies for the Treatment and Prevention of Sexual Assault. *Chicago, IL: American Medical Association; 1995 and ACOG Practice Bulletin. Emergency oral contraception.* Int J Gynecol Obstet. *2002;78:191-198.*

regimen are significantly less, and efficacy is improved.[17] Breast tenderness may also be noted after EC. Up to 98% of women will menstruate within 21 days of treatment. If given before ovulation, menstrual bleeding may start 3 to 7 days earlier than expected but may be delayed if given after ovulation. This should be reviewed at the follow-up visit. If menses has not begun within 21 days, a patient should seek immediate medical care.

The two most used regimens are listed in **Table 6-3**. Plan B is now available over the counter without a prescription. Other combinations of oral contraceptives can be given, but the pill burden is greater. If the postsexual assault evaluation is occurring 72 to 120 hours after the event, the insertion of a copper intrauterine device can prevent unwanted pregnancy.[18,19] If any menstrual irregularities are occurring at the follow-up visits, repeat pregnancy testing should be performed.

Male Sexual Assault

Before the 1970s, nearly 100% of sexual assaults in the nonincarcerated population were reported by women. Now male sexual assaults constitute 2% to 10% of the sexual assaults reported.[20] Because of the increased prevalence of HIV, hepatitis B, QRNG infection, and syphilis in men who have sex with men, postsexual assault prophylaxis treatment may need modification (**Figure 6-18**). The rate of isolating QRNG in men who have sex with men in the United States is 23.9% compared to heterosexual men where the isolate-resistant rates are 1.4% to 2.9%.[2] Because the prevalence of syphilis is up to 11% in men who have sex with men,[21] serological testing is of particular importance as a baseline and in follow-up.

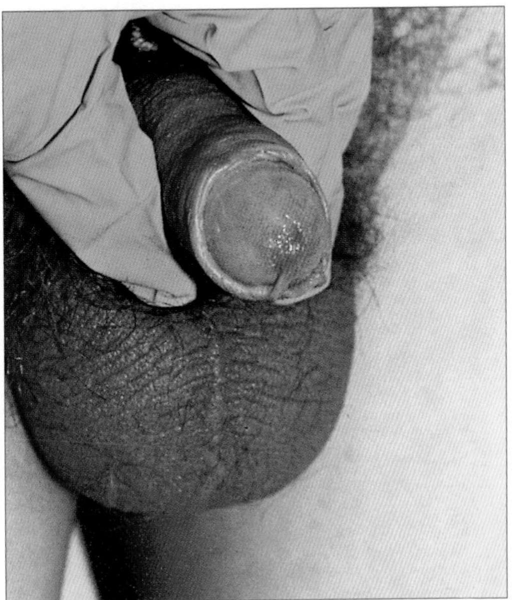

Figure 6-18. *This patient has* Neisseria gonorrhoeae. *The periurethral erythema and dripping from the urethra are secondary to gonorrhea (35mm).*

Postsexual assault treatment with ceftriaxone (**Table 6-2**) will cover QRNG as well as incubating syphilis. To cover *Chlamydia*, which is less common in men who have sex with men, azithromycin or doxycycline might be used. Doxycycline may be a better option because it covers proctitis if anal insertion has occurred. However, if a single-dose regimen is preferred, azithromycin should be chosen. Hepatitis B vaccination should be offered if an assault victim has not previously received it. Careful follow-up exams should be performed to assess the development of viral infections (herpes simplex, HPV) also (**Figures 6-19** through **6-20**).

HIV PEP should be offered to every male sexual assault victim if receptive anal exposure has occurred. This activity has one of the highest percentage rates of HIV transmission. Appropriate follow-up for medication adherence and repeat HIV testing should be instituted along with referral to an HIV-specific care provider.

More research is required in this increasingly common type of assault.

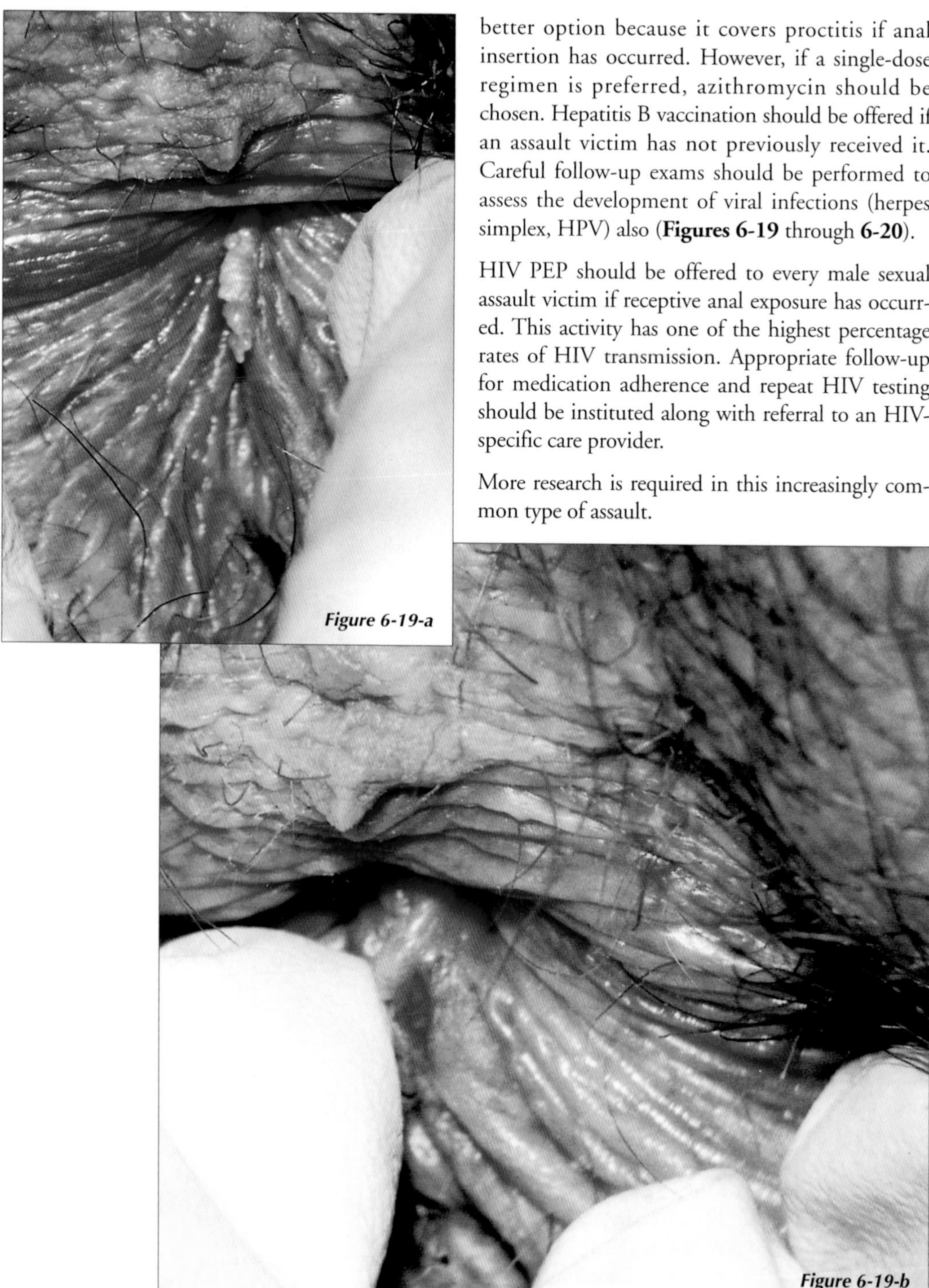

Figure 6-19-a. *This victim was examined 5 hours after the assault.* Condyloma acuminata *on the anus at 6 o'clock. The victim stated that he was unaware of the warts.*

Figure 6-19-b. *There is a laceration at 6 o'clock on the side of the wart. This is an example of the necessity of magnified examination around the side of warts and tags for injury.*

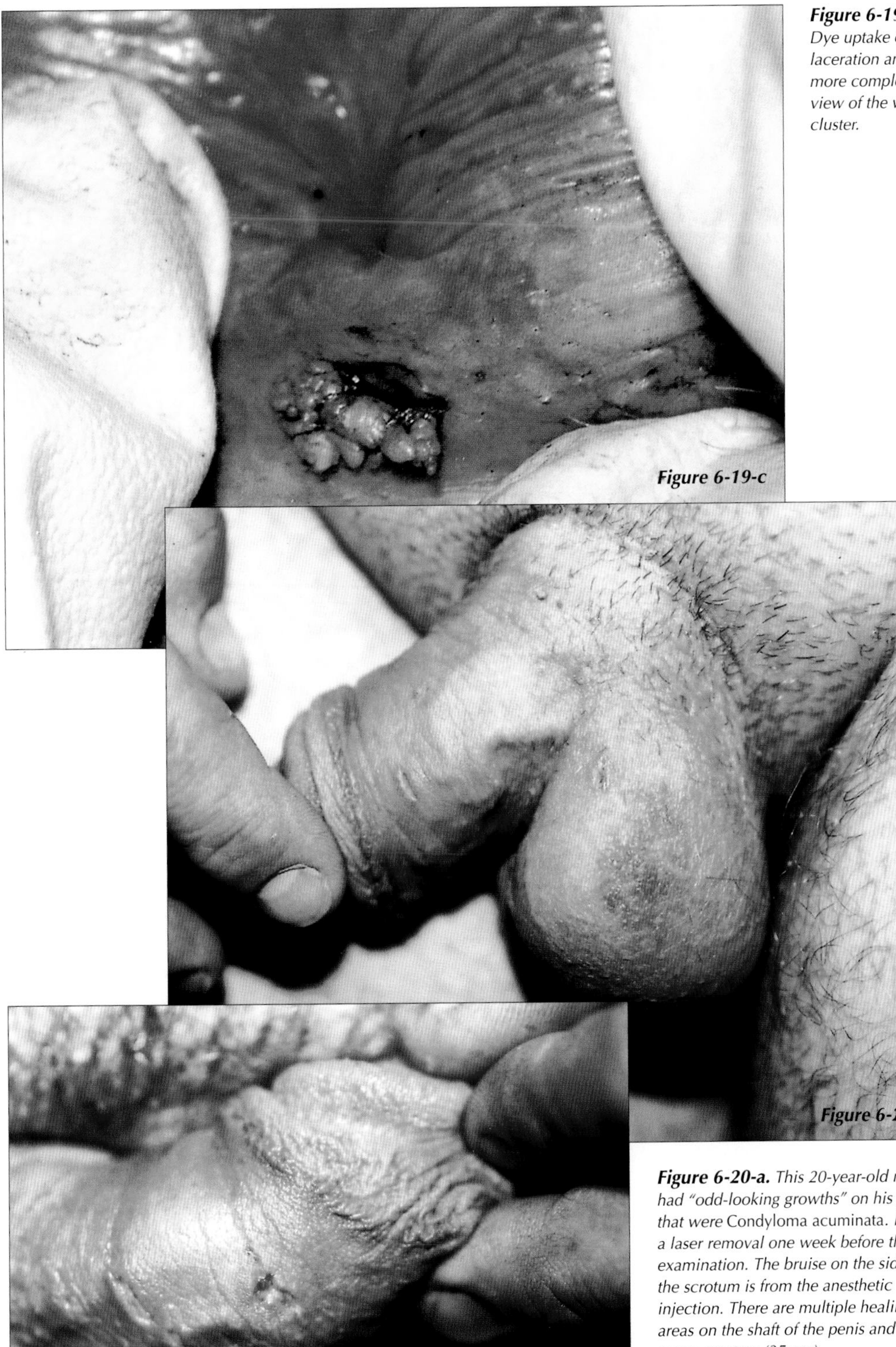

Figure 6-19-c. *Dye uptake on the laceration and a more complete view of the warty cluster.*

Figure 6-20-a. *This 20-year-old male had "odd-looking growths" on his penis that were* Condyloma acuminata. *He had a laser removal one week before this examination. The bruise on the side of the scrotum is from the anesthetic injection. There are multiple healing areas on the shaft of the penis and the upper scrotum (35mm).*

Figure 6-20-b. *A closer view of 2 sites where warts have been removed (35mm).*

Conclusion

Excellent guidelines have been developed to manage STI prevention and pregnancy prevention after sexual assault.[2,16,17,22] Studies reviewed the National Hospital Ambulatory Medical Care Survey of diagnostic codes in emergency departments in the late 1990s to assess for STI prophylaxis, as well as EC, after sexual assault.[1,23] No medications were administered for STI prevention in approximately 50% of reviewed charts. Only 20% to 24% of women received 2 medications for STI prevention, and a much lower number received 3 medications. The rate of administered EC was 20%. However, no review of prior pregnancy prevention methods could be found. HIV PEP was not well reviewed in these studies because no overt guidelines existed. A study at a sexual assault clinic[9] reported that 96.6% of victims were provided antibiotic prophylaxis, and 73% received EC. More recent studies of emergency department practices have delineated a rate of 60% to 90% of victims being administered STI prevention. Up to 43% of victims at risk for pregnancy receive EC.[24] In a survey of sexual assault nurse examiner (SANE) programs, 82% of programs provide STI prophylaxis to every patient, and 14% provide it most of the time. Emergency contraception was provided by 66% of the programs to every patient and by 29% most of the time. Catholic hospitals may not present EC discussion. HIV PEP is provided to every patient by only 14% of SANE programs.

In many states, minors are granted the status of emancipation after a sexual assault. As an emancipated minor, the victim can consent to an exam and treatment without the presence of a parent or guardian.

Increasing use of the STI prophylaxis and EC are assisted by the development of SANE programs as well as guideline development by specialty societies. The use of HIV PEP remains an evolving standard for multiple reasons. Over time, a guideline for HIV PEP in a female sexual assault victim may be developed and is now strongly recommended for male sexual assault victims. With improved implementation of STI prophylaxis and EC, ongoing studies should continue to assess efficacy and adverse outcomes.

References

1. Amey AL, Bishai D. Measuring the quality of medical care for women who experience sexual assault with data from the National Hospital Ambulatory Medical Care Survey. *Ann Emerg Med.* 2002;39:631-638.

2. Centers for Disease Control. Sexually transmitted diseases treatment guidelines. *MMWR.* 2006;55:RR-11.

3. Reynolds MW, Peipert JF, Collins B. Epidemiologic issues of sexually transmitted diseases in sexual assault victims. *Obstetrical and Gynecological Survey.* 2000;55:51-57.

4. Beck-Sague CM, Solomon F. Sexually transmitted diseases in children and adolescent and adult victims of rape: review of selected literature. *Clin Infect Dis.* 1999;28(suppl 1):S74-83.

5. Jenny C, Hooten TM, Bowers A, Compass MK, Krieger JN, Hiller SL, et al. Sexually transmitted diseases in victims of rape. *N Engl J Med.* 1990;322:713-716.

6. Varghese B, Maher JE, Peterman TA, Branson BM, Steketee RW. Reducing the risk of sexual HIV transmission: qualifying the per-act risk for HIV on the basis of choice of partner, sex act, and condom use. *Sex Transmit Dis.* 2002;29:38-43.

7. Kilpatrick DG, Edmunds CN, Seymour AK. *Rape in America: A Report to the Nation*. Arlington, VA: The National Victim Center and the Medical University of South Carolina; 1992.

8. Gaydoc CA. Nucleic acid amplification tests for gonorrhea and chlamydia: practice and applications. *Infect Dis Clin N Amer*. 2005;19:367-386.

9. Holmes MM, Resnick HS, Frampton D. Follow-up of sexual assault victims. *Amer J Obstet Gynec*. 1998;179:336-341.

10. Patel M, Minshall L. Management of sexual assault. *Emerg Med Clin North Am*. 2001;19:817-831.

11. Connor EM, Sperling RS, Gelber R, et al. Reduction of maternal-infant transmission of human immunodeficiency virus type I with zidovudine treatment. *N Engl J Med*. 1994;331:1173-1180.

12. Cardo DM, Culver DH, Cieselski CA, et al. A case-control study of HIV seroconversion in health care workers after percutaneous exposure. *N Engl J Med*. 1997;337:1485-1490.

13. Centers for Disease Control. Updated U.S. Public Health Service guidelines for the management of occupational exposures to HIV and recommendations for post exposure prophylaxis. *MMWR*. 2005;54:RR09.

14. Centers for Disease Control. Antiretroviral postexposure prophylaxis after sexual, injection drug use, or other nonoccupational exposure to HIV in the United States. *MMWR*. 2005;54-RR02.

15. Wiebe ER, Comay SE, McGregor M, Ducceschi S. Offering HIV prophylaxis to people who have been sexually assaulted: 16 months' experience in a sexual assault service. *CMAJ*. 2000;162:641-645.

16. American Medical Association. *Strategies for the Treatment and Prevention of Sexual Assault*. Chicago, IL: American Medical Association; 1995.

17. ACOG Practice Bulletin. Emergency oral contraception. *Int J Gynecol Obstet*. 2002;78:191-198.

18. Cantu M, Coppolo M, Linder AJ. Evaluation and management of the sexually assaulted women. *Emerg Med Clin North Am*. 2003;21:737-750.

19. Glasier A. Emergency postcoital contraception. *New Engl J Med*. 1997;337:1058-1064.

20. Pesola GR, Westfal RE, Kuffner CA. Emergency department characteristics of male sexual assaults. *Acad Emerg Med*. 1999;6:792-798.

21. Centers for Disease Control. *Sexually Transmitted Disease Surveillance, 2005*. Atlanta, GA: Centers for Disease Control and Prevention, US Dept of Health and Human Services; 2006.

22. ACOG Educational Bulletin. Sexual assault. *Int J Gynecol Obstet*. 1998;60:297-304.

23. Rovi S, Shimoni N. Prophylaxis provided to sexual assault victims seen at US emergency departments. *J Am Med Women's Assoc*. 2002;57:204-207.

24. Campbell R, Townsend SM, Long SM, Kinnison KE, Pulley EM, Adames SB, Wasso SM. Respond to sexual assault victims' medical and emotional needs: a national study of the services provided by SANE programs. *Res Nurs Health.* 2006;29:384-398.

Chapter 7

Male Sexual Assault Victims

Diana Faugno, MSN, RN, CPN, SANE-A, SANE-P, FAAFS, DF-IAFN
Jenifer Markowitz, ND, RN, WHNP-BC, SANE-A, DF-IAFN

A 2006 report from the National Institute of Justice estimates that 1 in 33 men will be sexually assaulted in his lifetime. This figure translates into approximately 2.8 million men in the United States alone.[1] Men account for a relatively small percentage of reported sexual assaults each year but have specific needs related to medical care, evidence collection, follow-up, and referrals. Unfortunately, they are often invisible to the health care establishment, resulting in fewer appropriate services and a general lack of recognition of the scope of the issue of male sexual assault. This chapter will examine the reported experiences of male sexual assault victims and discuss methods for providing comprehensive and compassionate medical-forensic care to this victim population.

Barriers to Reporting

Male sexual assault is often underreported due to a cultural resistance to the belief that men can be victims of sexual violence. Sable et al found that male college students identified the same barriers to reporting sexual assault as had been identified 30 years ago in women, before the efforts of the rape reform movement.[2] These barriers include shame, guilt, embarrassment, not wanting friends and family to know, concerns about confidentiality, and fear of not being believed. Both men and women perceived a fear of being judged as gay as a significant barrier for male victims.

The issue of homosexuality remains significant for male victims of sexual assault. Men who have erections and ejaculate during forced sexual contact may believe they unconsciously enjoyed or invited the assault, potentially calling into question their own sexual identity.[3] This issue of culpability is also shared by society. Several studies have found that people assign more blame to homosexual men assaulted by another man, while discounting the level of trauma the assault caused.[4-6] Even professionals working with victims hold attitudes about male sexual assault victims that can prevent or otherwise dissuade disclosure. Donnelly and Kenyon's study of gender stereotypes and services to male sexual assault victims found that law enforcement professionals frequently expressed opinions that men could not be raped or were only raped because they wanted to be raped.[7] Other professionals, including health care professionals, expressed the belief that the small number of men coming forward as victims meant the crime was not occurring. The public and professional awareness of men as sexual assault victims has increased since this study was published, but fallacies that have been somewhat overcome for female sexual assault victims still remain for male victims.

Males are also vulnerable to assault by women. These victims may face an even greater challenge in obtaining support and services. Struckman-Johnson and Struckman-Johnson examined the issue of male victimization by women and found a commonly held belief that men cannot be coerced or forced to have unwanted sexual contact, particularly if the woman is attractive.[8] Often female-perpetrated assaults of males, particularly adolescent males, are simply dismissed as "initiations" or "rites of passage." These types of attitudes are frequently illustrated in the public discourse surrounding assaults of male students by female teachers.[9]

Sexual assault remains vastly underreported, but some factors make reporting more likely. Data from the National Crime and Victimization Survey indicate that, although men were less likely to report sexual assault than women, reporting was more likely when the rape was committed by a stranger, when injuries were sustained, and when medical treatment was required. In fact, men were 5 times more likely to report when bodily injuries were sustained, and more than 8 times more likely to report when medical treatment was necessary.[10]

Characteristics of Male Sexual Assault Victims

Many studies cited in this chapter relate to the prevalence and characteristics of male sexual assault victims, but these findings must be regarded with an appropriate perspective. Sexual assault, in general terms, is a vastly underreported crime, and the sexual assault of men even more so. Therefore, the data cited should be interpreted within the framework of cases reported and not as cases in total.

Age

The age for male sexual assault victims does not appear to deviate significantly from that of female sexual assault victims, with a range between 18 and 30 years, although a recent study of men in Virginia indicates significant numbers of sexual assaults in men under the age of 18.[11-14] In men coming to San Diego, California hospitals for medical-forensic examinations, the largest percentage were between ages 18 and 25 years (**Figure 7-1**).

Vulnerability

Stermac et al examined the characteristics of sexual assault victims and divided male subjects into stranger and acquaintance assault victims.[15] Compared to female victims, men exhibited greater levels of homelessness and unemployment, particularly among those assaulted by strangers. Males also had higher rates of physical disability, cognitive disability, and mental health diagnoses than female victims. Alcohol use, so often a

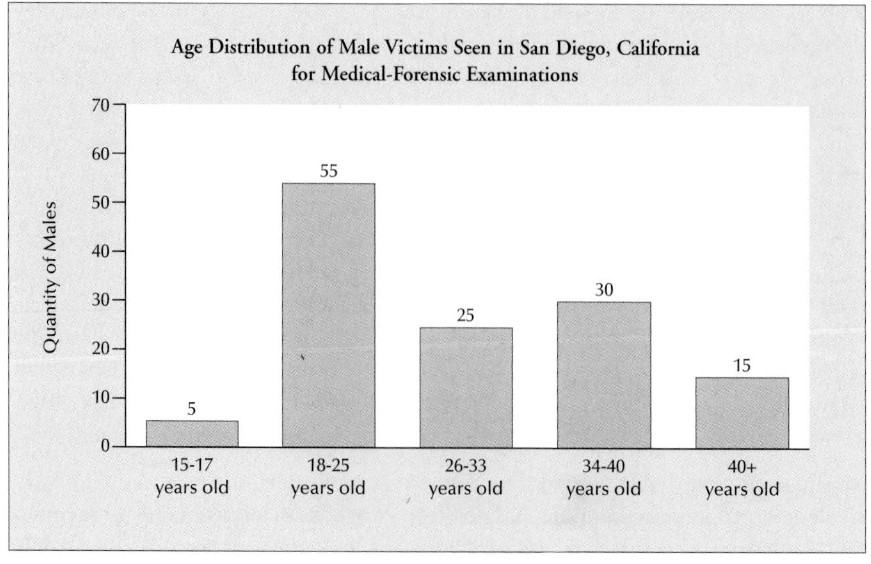

Figure 7-1. *Data provided from San Diego County Sexual Assault Response Team.*

component of sexual violence against women, did not appear to differ significantly for male victims of acquaintance sexual assault, although reported usage was lower in men sexually assaulted by a stranger. As with women, vulnerable men appear to be at increased risk for sexual assault.

Prior Victimization

Recent studies of female sexual assault victims point to prior sexual violence victimization as a risk factor for future sexual violence victimization.[16-19] There is evidence that this is also true for men. In Frazier's study of males coming to a hospital-based sexual assault program, she found more than 1 in 3 reported a prior instance of sexual assault, and more than 1 in 4 reported prior incest.[13] This was echoed in a 1996 study by Stermac et al, who reported that 34% of male sexual assault victims disclosed childhood sexual abuse and 14% disclosed prior adult sexual assault victimization.[20] King and Woolett studied men seeking counseling for sexual assault victimization and found that 61% of participants who had been assaulted at age 16 years or older had also been assaulted at an earlier age.[21]

Assault Characteristics

Assailant-Victim Relationship

As with female victims, male sexual assault victims typically know their assailants, even if only for a brief period of time. A study of 8 communities across the United States found only 16% involved an unknown assailant.[22] For a further breakdown of suspect-victim relationships, see **Figure 7-2**.

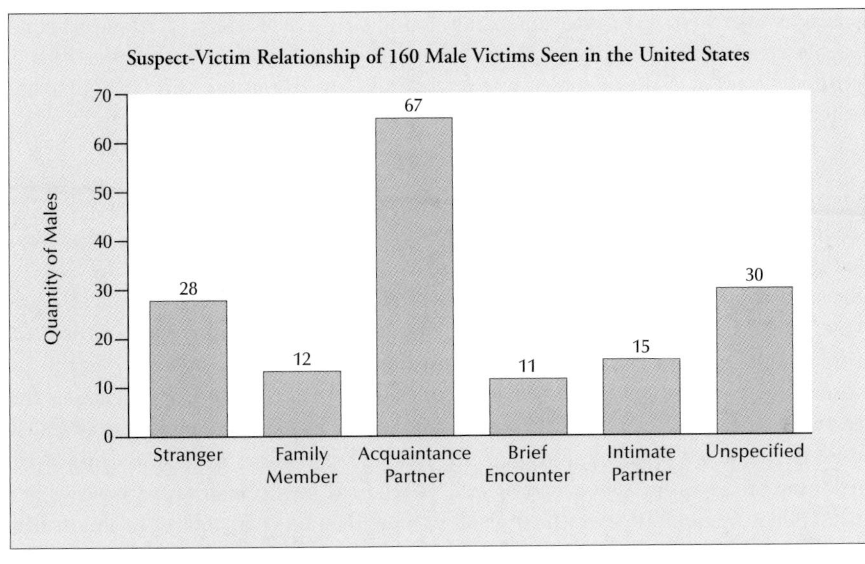

Figure 7-2. *2005 MAD Data: 160 male victims from 8 communities in the United States. Data provided from End Violence Against Women (EVAW) International.*

Number of Assailants

Males appear more likely to be sexually assaulted by multiple assailants. This includes both multiple male assailants, as well as mixed male-female pairs and groups. Several studies found that about one-fourth to one-third of males were victimized by multiple assailants, with one[8] reporting that among male stranger assault victims, more than 6% disclosed both male and female assailants.[10,13,20] Corrections facilities report lower incidents of multiple assailant sexual assaults than is found among males in the general population.[23]

Type of Assault

The type of assault also differs in male victims, with men experiencing a far greater number of fondling-type assaults than women. Although penetration is reported by many male victims, Stermac and colleagues found more than twice as many men reported touching or fondling assaults than women in the study (21.5% in both the male stranger and acquaintance assaults versus 10.4% in the female assaults).[15] Not surprisingly, anal assaults were also more frequently reported, with 7 to 8 times the numbers reported for male stranger and acquaintance assault victims than female victims. This figure becomes significant when clinicians consider the availability of clinical services such as anoscopy and human immunodeficiency virus (HIV) prophylaxis in the routine care of sexual assault patients.

Injury and Treatment

Several studies have found that male victims of sexual assault are more likely to have a weapon used as a component of the crime.[10,15,20] The amount of injury suffered by males is inconsistently reported. Several studies documented a greater amount of physical injury, including perianal and anal injury, but others found no difference between male and female victims. However, in studies focused on hospital admission data, males were more frequently admitted after the sexual assault medical-forensic examination than females.[11,15]

Few studies examined the frequency with which male sexual assault victims come for health care after sexual assault and how long they delay before seeking care. Pesola et al reviewed the medical records of male sexual assault patients in an urban emergency department and reported a mean presentation time after the sexual assault of 13.5 hours, with the greatest delay being 3 days.[11] Stermac et al found that male victims of stranger sexual assault delayed seeking care less than either male or female victims of acquaintance sexual assault.[15] However, the same study found that male victims of stranger sexual assault were less likely to have a physical exam or evidence collection than the other 2 groups. Overall, 65% of male stranger sexual assault victims and 71% of male acquaintance sexual assault victims received a physical examination in this study.

Sexual Assault in Corrections Facilities

Overcrowding and insufficient staffing are key contributors to prisoner rape. Recent changes in criminal justice policy have exacerbated the problem by swelling prison and jail populations beyond capacity. More than 2 million people are now serving time in the United States, and millions more pass through the criminal justice system every year.[24] In 2003, the US Congress passed the Prison Rape Elimination Act (PREA), which, among other things, created a zero-tolerance standard for sexual assault in corrections facilities and mandated data collection concerning sexual violence in the corrections system. Since PREA, there has been a 21% increase in the number of sexual violence incidents reported, although this may be explained, in part, by improved reporting processes. In 2006, there were 2.91 reported incidents of sexual violence per 1000 inmates, about 10% of which involved more than one perpetrator. In almost half of all occurrences, the victims were under age 25 years, and almost 90% were under age 40 years.[25] A recent study of prisons in 4 Midwestern states found that about 1 in 5 male inmates reported a pressured or forced sex incident while incarcerated. About 1 in 10 male inmates reported that that they had been raped.[26]

Studies of male victims of prison rape document that fewer victims in this setting receive health care or evidence collection after sexual assault than in the general population. US Department of Justice statistics reported more than 6000 cases of prison sexual assault known to correctional authorities in 2005. Of the cases of inmate-on-inmate sexual violence substantiated by corrections authorities, only 53% of victims received any type of medical care; 19% had an evidence collection kit completed; and 12% received testing for HIV and/or other sexually transmitted infections (STIs). These numbers decreased across the board in substantiated cases of staff-on-inmate sexual violence.[23] It is worth noting, however, that newly published PREA Commission standards "require facilities to offer the victim a forensic exam by a specially trained professional" in cases of acute sexual assaults.[27]

Sexual violence in the corrections setting contributes to the spread of STIs, with HIV and acquired immunodeficiency syndrome (AIDS) being of particular concern. According to a fact sheet published by Stop Prisoner Rape, between 12% and 18% of the US HIV-positive population pass through the nation's jails and prisons each year. Prison populations have an HIV rate 4 times higher than the general population.[28] In a 1999 bulletin, the US Department of Justice reported that between July 1, 1998 and June 30, 1999, 1 in 12 deaths among jail inmates were from AIDS-related causes.[29]

The Medical Forensic Examination

Victims of sexual violence coming to the health care arena for medical forensic care after sexual assault should receive consistent, compassionate, and victim-centered care regardless of their gender. In fact, the examination and evidence collection for male victims deviate very little from what is typically completed for female victims (**Figure** 7-3). **Table** 7-1 provides an overview of the examination process.

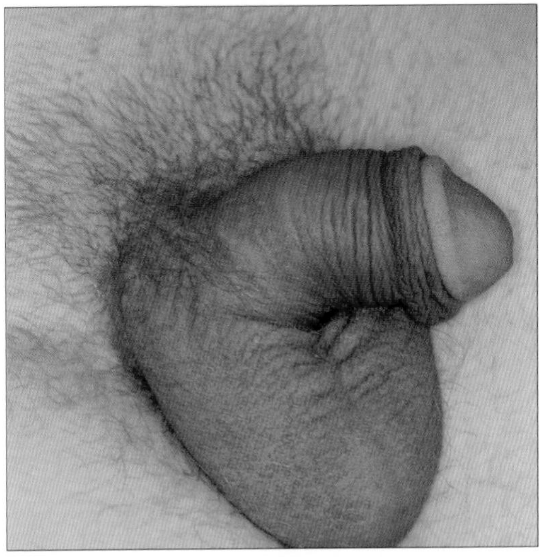

Figure 7-3. Genital area of male victim exposing the penis and scrotal area. No acute injury is noted here, but the examiner should follow the evidence collection protocol for swabbing and evidence collection.

Physical examination should be methodical and thorough, looking for signs of trauma (**Figure** 7-4), general physiologic changes, and foreign materials, such as debris or fibers. For patients who report forced receptive oral copulation (patient's mouth to assailant's genitals), a thorough inspection of the oral cavity is particularly important. Residual signs of oral penetration (**Figure** 7-5), such as frenal tears, palatal contusions (**Figure** 7-6), and petechiae should be documented and photographed according to jurisdictional policies. Consider using creative techniques, such as a patient-held speculum or oral retractors, to better visualize the oral cavity (**Figure** 7-7 and **Table** 7-2).

Table 7-1. Examination Components[30]
General Physical Examination
— Vital signs
— Physical appearance
— Demeanor
— Behavior and orientation
— Injury and trauma identification
— Physiologic changes
(continued)

Table 7-1. Examination Components[30] *(continued)*

Anogenital Examination

- External and perineal area for injury identification and physical evidence
  - Abdomen
  - Buttocks
  - Thighs
  - Foreskin
  - Urethral meatus
  - Penile shaft
  - Scrotum
  - Perineum
  - Glans
  - Testes
- Anal examination
- Rectal examination using anoscope (if appropriate)
- Oral examination (if appropriate), looking for injury such as frenal tears or palatal bruising following forced receptive oral copulation

(Physical evidence, including foreign materials, fluids, etc, should be completed per protocol throughout the examination process)

Documentation

- Narrative documentation of examination findings
- Diagramming of findings on body maps or traumagrams
- Photography, including genital photography, per jurisdictional policy

Adapted from US Department of Justice, Office of Violence Against Women. A National Protocol for Sexual Assault Medical Forensic Examinations: Adults/Adolescents. *Washington, DC: US Department of Justice; 2004.*

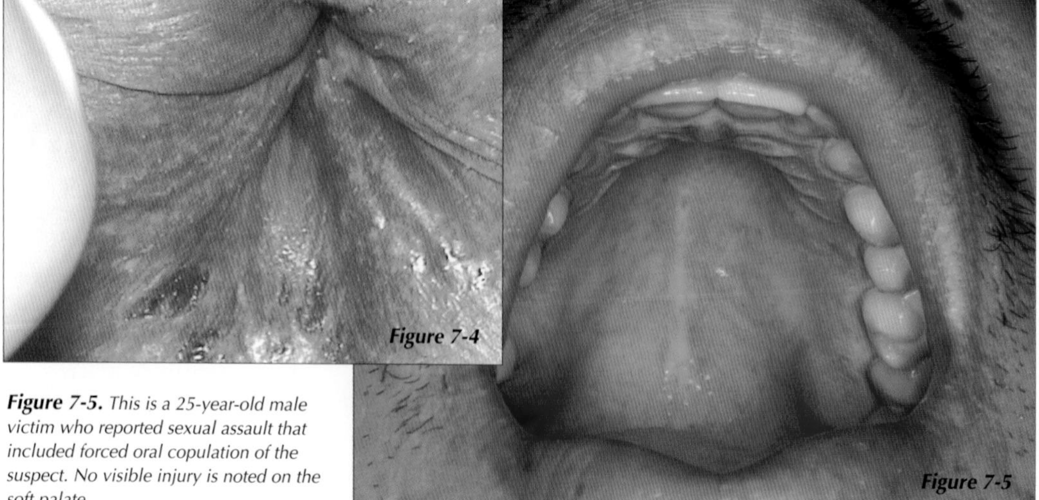

Figure 7-4. *Perianal contusion with lacerations. Reprinted with permission from The DOVE Program, Summa Health System.*

Figure 7-5. *This is a 25-year-old male victim who reported sexual assault that included forced oral copulation of the suspect. No visible injury is noted on the soft palate.*

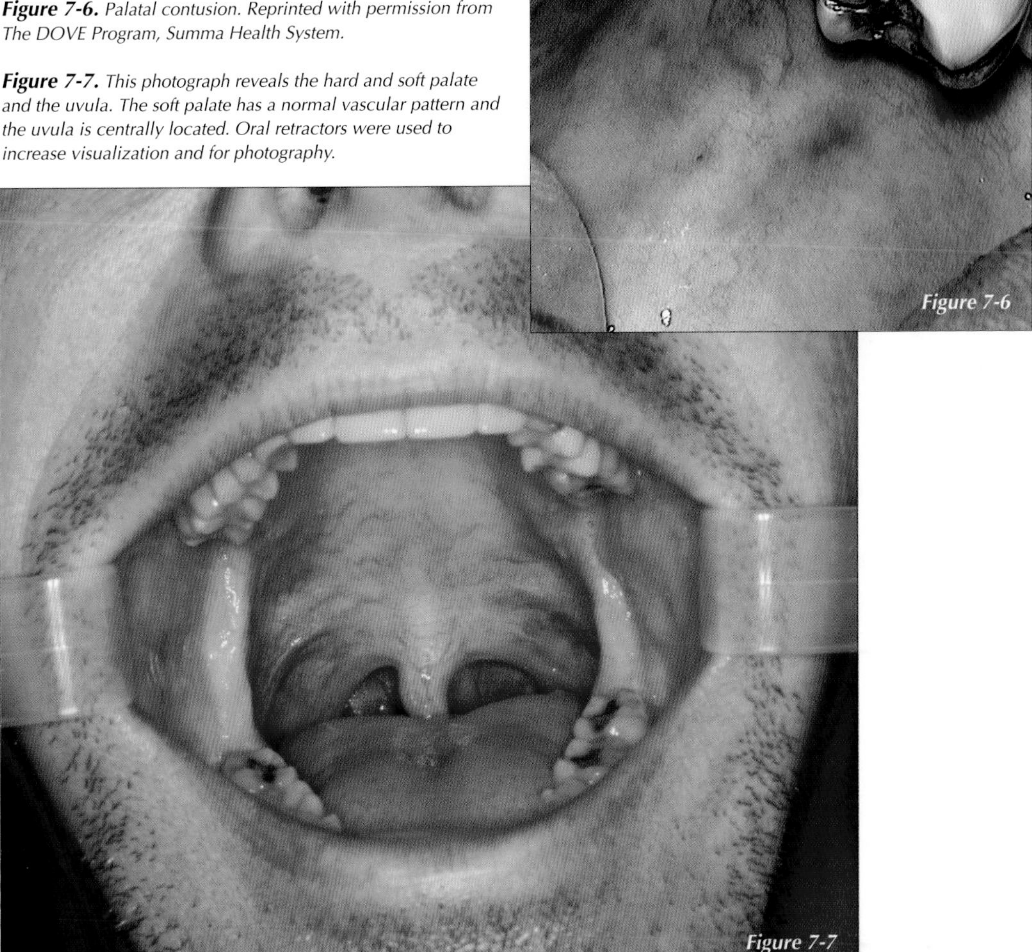

Figure 7-6. *Palatal contusion. Reprinted with permission from The DOVE Program, Summa Health System.*

Figure 7-7. *This photograph reveals the hard and soft palate and the uvula. The soft palate has a normal vascular pattern and the uvula is centrally located. Oral retractors were used to increase visualization and for photography.*

Table 7-2. Using a Speculum to Visualize the Oral Cavity*

Instruction
1. Obtain a small or medium plastic speculum with a place for light source attachment (such as those made by Wyeth).
2. Take the speculum apart, retaining only the bottom portion.
3. Insert the light source into the speculum.
4. Have patient sit on a chair or stool. Give him the speculum and have him use it like a tongue depressor. Sit facing the patient.
5. Inspect the oral cavity, gently guiding the patient's hand when the speculum must be moved to visualize other areas of the oral cavity.
6. Photograph according to jurisdictional policy.

* *Oral retractors are also an excellent tool for visualizing the oral cavity, although specula are more commonly found across SANE/SAFE units and emergency departments.*

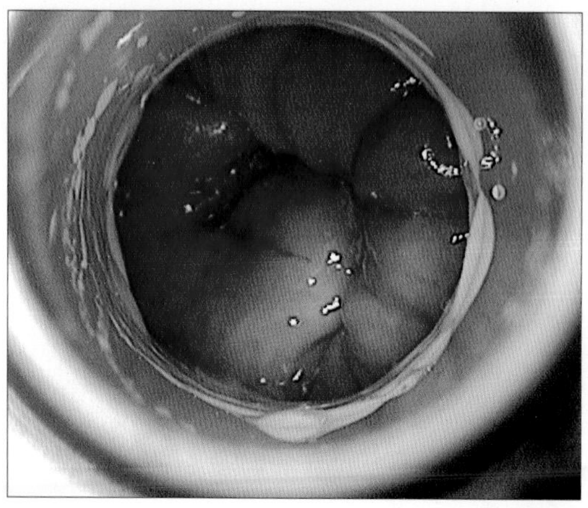

Figure 7-8. An abrasion on the rectal wall is visualized with anoscopy. Reprinted with permission from The DOVE Program, Summa Health System.

Patients who have experienced forced anal penetration may be offered anoscopy as another component of the examination. Although this procedure can be uncomfortable or even painful, particularly after sexual assault, it does provide the opportunity for greater documentation of injury and evidence collection (**Figure 7-8**). Patients should be fully informed of the benefits and drawbacks to having anoscopy performed before its use and allowed to withdraw consent at any point in the process if it becomes too uncomfortable.

Evidence collection kits differ between jurisdictions; however the *National Protocol for Sexual Assault Medical Forensic Examinations* contains general recommendations for inclusion, which can be seen in **Table 7-3**.

Evidence should be collected and packaged according to jurisdictional policies. Special attention should be paid to the integrity of the evidence, with all samples remaining under the control of the responsible clinician until they are packaged and turned over to law enforcement with a clear written chain of custody. Any specimens that are obtained solely for the purpose of medical treatment should be kept separate from forensic specimens and do not require chain of custody maintenance. These specimens should be collected and processed according to institutional policy.[30]

Table 7-3. Recommended Evidence Collection[30]
ITEMS TO BE COLLECTED
— Clothing evidence
— Debris — From patient's body — From under fingernails
— Foreign materials and swabs from body surface
— Hair combings — Head hair — Pubic hair
— Hair reference samples — Head hair — Pubic hair
— Oral and anogenital swabs — Penile sample: moistened swabs along shaft and glans — Anal sample: moistened swabs perianally and swabs in anus per patient history — Oral sample: swabs along gum lines with history of forced receptive oral copulation

(continued)

Table 7-3. *(continued)*

ITEMS ALSO TO BE CONSIDERED FOR COLLECTION

— Moistened swabs *around* mouth and chin with history of forced receptive oral copulation

— DNA standard from patient
  — Buccal swab
  — Dry blood (finger stick)
  — Drawn blood

— Toxicology samples, per history, patient presentation, or community protocol

Note: Evidence should be completed according to jurisdictional policies.

Adapted from US Department of Justice, Office of Violence Against Women. A National Protocol for Sexual Assault Medical Forensic Examinations: Adults/Adolescents. *Washington, DC: US Department of Justice; 2004.*

FOLLOW-UP AND DISCHARGE PLANNING

An integral component of the medical forensic examination is follow-up and discharge planning. Patients seen after a sexual assault should have individualized discharge plans based on their health and safety needs. Clinicians should consider that patients sexually assaulted by an intimate partner have very different discharge needs from those of patients sexually assaulted by a stranger. Likewise, patients who have been anally penetrated have very different follow-up needs compared to patients who were genitally fondled. The patient's medical and assault histories should guide the planning process. Information regarding discharge instructions and follow-up appointments should be provided in writing as well as orally reviewed with the patient.

HUMAN IMMUNODEFICIENCY VIRUS AND SEXUALLY TRANSMITTED INFECTIONS

Patients should be offered prophylaxis for STIs, as indicated, before discharge.[30] Information regarding postexposure prophylaxis for hepatitis B should be provided, if it is not available within the treating facility, with clear guidelines given to patients about the importance of receiving the treatment within 14 days of exposure. Prophylaxis for HIV should be determined on a case-by-case basis and provided according to jurisdictional and institutional policies, along with information about HIV testing and transmission. Clinicians should clearly review benefits and drawbacks of prophylaxis and obtain informed consent before treatment. More detailed information about STI and HIV treatment guidelines can be obtained from the Centers for Disease Control and Prevention: www.cdc.gov/std/treatment.

MENTAL HEALTH AND CRISIS INTERVENTION

Sexual assault victims express and handle trauma in a multitude of ways. In fact, there is no one single appropriate expression of trauma or coping strategy. Several studies find an increased amount of anger and hostility in many male rape victims after the assault.[13,31-33] However, a review of the literature by Rentoul and Appleboom uncovered a wide variety of reported reactions by male sexual assault victims, including those typically ascribed to rape trauma syndrome: anxiety, depression, irritability, somatic complaints, insomnia, and behavioral changes.[34] Masho and Anderson found that compared to men with no history of sexual assault, those who had been assaulted as children were 3 times more likely to be depressed and twice as likely to harbor suicidal ideations.[14] Posttraumatic stress disorder (PTSD) has also been exhibited in adult male sexual assault victims.[31]

In light of this development, working with various victim advocacy agencies and other community-based professionals can provide patients with individualized plans for assistance with coping and counseling as needed. Traditional crisis referrals should be expanded to include faith-based organizations and institutions, gay and lesbian organizations (if relevant), shelter programs, and other victim service organizations. Whenever possible, the services of advocates should be used during the medical-forensic examination process to provide support and allow patients to make contact with helping professionals face-to-face.

Patients who do not wish to have advocacy or other support services at the time of the medical-forensic examination should still be provided information about available resources, both orally and in writing. If possible, patients should be given the opportunity to make contact with agencies and organizations while still in the health care facility, rather than simply be given pamphlets or phone numbers.

Safety Planning

In a national crime victim survey, 16% of men reporting sexual assault state that they were raped, physically assaulted, or stalked by an intimate partner.[26] It is important to consider this as patients are prepared for discharge from the health care setting. As with female patients, a thorough discussion regarding safety planning is required, including information about shelter, protection orders, and other resources for any male patient coping with violence from a current or former intimate partner. Victim advocates can be a valuable source of support during the examination process and contribute to helping patients plan for safety after discharge.

Patients dealing with intimate partner violence are not the only ones who will benefit from individualized safety planning. All patients should be assessed for safety concerns as part of the discharge plan, knowing that concerns differ depending upon the circumstances of the assault. Assaults by known acquaintances on college campuses or places of employment; assaults that include theft of personal information, including a driver's license and other identifiers; and assaults by family members result in a variety of safety issues. A multidisciplinary approach to safety planning, utilizing victim advocates and other community service providers (**Table 7-4**), will help ensure an appropriate and comprehensive discharge plan.

Table 7-4. Resources

Organization	Web Site
Human Rights Watch	www.hrw.org
MaleSurvivor	www.malesurvivor.org
National Center for Victims of Crime	www.ncvc.org
National Gay and Lesbian Task Force	www.thetaskforce.org
National Sexual Violence Resource Center	www.nsvrc.org
Stop Prisoner Rape	www.spr.org

REFERENCES

1. Tjaden P, Thoennes N. Extent, nature, and consequences of rape victimization: findings from the national violence against women survey. http://www.ncjrs.gov/pdffiles1/nij/210346.pdf. Published January 2006. Accessed September 15, 2009.

2. Sable MR, Danis F, Mauzy DL, Gallagher S K. Barriers to reporting sexual assault for women and men: Perspectives of college students. *J Amer Coll Health.* 2006;55;157-162.

3. McMullen RJ. *Male Rape: Breaking the Silence of the Last Taboo.* London: Gay Men's Press; 1990.

4. Davies M, Rogers, P. Perceptions of male victims in depicted sexual assaults: a review of the literature. *Aggression Violent Behav.* 2006:11:367-377.

5. Mitchell D, Hirschmann R, Hall GCN. Attributions of victim responsibility, pleasure and trauma in male rape. *J Sex Res.* 1999;36:369-373.

6. Wakelin A, Long KM. Effects of victim gender and sexuality on attributions of blame to rape victims. *Sex Roles.* 2003;49:477-487.

7. Donnelly DA, Kenyon S. "Honey, we don't do men": gender stereotypes and the provision of services to sexually assaulted males. *J Interpers Violence.* 1996;11:441-448.

8. Struckman-Johnson C, Struckman-Johnson D. Men's reactions to hypothetical female sexual advances: a beauty bias in response to sexual coercion. *Sex Role.* 1994;31:387-406.

9. Stop Educator Sexual Abuse, Misconduct and Exploitation. Michael's Story. Stop Educator Sexual Abuse, Misconduct and Exploitation Web site. http://www.sesamenet.org/stories/mike.html. Accessed October 4, 2009.

10. Pino NW, Meier RF. Gender differences in rape reporting. *Sex Roles.* 1999;11/12: 979-990.

11. Pesola GR, Westfal RE, Kuffner CA. Emergency department characteristics of male sexual assault. *Acad Emerg Med.* 1999;6:792-798.

12. Walker J, Archer J, Davies M. Effects of rape on male survivors: a descriptive analysis. *Arch Sex Behav.* 2005;34:69-80.

13. Frazier PA. A comparative study of male and female rape victims seen at a hospital-based rape crisis program. *J Interpers Violence.* 1993;8:64-76.

14. Masho SW, Anderson L. Sexual assault in men: a population-based study in Virginia. *Violence Victims.* 2009;24(1):98-110.

15. Stermac L, Del Bove G, Addison M. Stranger and acquaintance sexual assault of males. *J Interpers Violence.* 2004;19:901-915.

16. Tjaden P, Thoennes N. *Full Report of the Prevalence, Incidence, and Consequences of Violence Against Women: Findings from the National Violence Against Women Survey.* Washington, DC: National Institute of Justice; 2000.

17. Elliott DM, Mok DS, Briere J. Adult sexual assault: prevalence, symptomatology, and sex differences in the general population. *J Trauma Stress.* 2004;17:203-211.

18. Rickert VI, Wiemann CM, Vaughan RD, White JW. Rates and risk factors for sexual violence among an ethnically diverse sample of adolescents. *Arch Pediatr Adolesc Med.* 2004;158:1132-1139.

19. Classen CC, Palesh OG, Aggarwal R. Sexual revictimization: a review of the empirical literature. *Trauma Violence Abuse.* 2005;6:103-129.

20. Stermac L, Sheriden PM, Davidson A, Dunn S. Sexual assault of adult males. *J Interpers Violence.* 1996;11:52-64.

21. King M, Woollett E. Sexually assaulted males: 115 men consulting a counseling service. *Arch Sex Behav.* 1997;26:579-588.

22. End Violence Against Women. Making A Difference grant project [unpublished data]; 2005.

23. Beck AJ, Harrison PM. *Sexual violence reported by correctional authorities, 2005.* Washington, DC: US Department of Justice, Bureau of Justice Statistics; 2006.

24. US Department of Justice, Bureau of Justice Statistics. Nation's prison and jail population exceeds 2 million inmates for the first time. http:// www.ojp.usdoj.gov/bjs/pub/press/pjim02pr.htm. Published April 6, 2003. Accessed September 15, 2009.

25. Beck AJ, Harrison PM, Adams DB. *Sexual violence reported by correctional authorities, 2006.* Washington, DC: US Department of Justice, Bureau of Justice Statistics; 2007.

26. Struckman-Johnson C, Struckman-Johnson D. Sexual coercion rates in seven midwestern prison facilities for men. *Prison J.* 2000;80;379-390.

27. National Prison Rape Elimination Commission. *National Prison Rape Elimination Commission Report.* Washington, DC: US Dept of Justice; 2009.

28. Maruschak LM; Bureau of Justice Statistics. HIV in prisons, 2006. http://bjs.ojp.usdoj.gov/content/pub/html/hivp/2006/hivp06.cfm. Updated April 22, 2008. Accessed October 4, 2009.

29. Maruschak LM; Bureau of Justice Statistics. HIV in prisons and jails, 1999. http://bjs.ojp.usdoj.gov/content/pub/pdf/hivpj99.pdf. Published July 2001. Updated October 25, 2001. Accessed September 15, 2009.

30. US Department of Justice, Office of Violence Against Women. *A National Protocol for Sexual Assault Medical Forensic Examinations: Adults/Adolescents.* Washington, DC: US Dept of Justice; 2004.

31. Huckle PL. Male rape victims referred to a forensic psychiatric service. *Med Sci Law.* 1995;35:187-192.

32. Groth A, Burgess A. Male rape: offenders and victims. *Amer J Psychiatry.* 1980;137:806-810.

33. Goyer P, Eddleman H. Same-sex rape of nonincarcerated men. *Amer J Psychiatry.* 1984;141:576-579.

34. Rentoul L, Appleboom N. Understanding the psychological impact of rape and serious sexual assault of men: a literature review. *J Psychiatr Ment Health Nurs.* 1997;4:267-274.

Chapter 8

THE SEXUAL ASSAULT SUSPECT EXAMINATION

Jenifer Markowitz, ND, RN, WHNP-BC, SANE-A, DF-IAFN
Diana Faugno, MSN, RN, CPN, SANE-A, SANE-P, FAAFS, DF-IAFN

When evaluating potential sources of evidence...always keep in mind that anything that could be transferred from the suspect to the victim may also be transferred from the victim to the suspect. Therefore, depending on the type of offense, the body of the suspect will often be the best source of probative evidence.[1]

Evidence collection from suspects of sexual assault can be vital in effectively investigating and prosecuting cases; however, there is little consistency from jurisdiction to jurisdiction in approaches to suspect evidentiary exams, with only a handful of states having standardized protocols and procedures for the process. Some jurisdictions do not routinely perform suspect exams at all, or do so infrequently. Furthermore, little research relates to best practices for the suspect evidentiary exam. This chapter will look at approaches to the suspect exam, barriers to conducting suspect exams, and legal issues related to the examination process.

THE SUSPECT EXAM

Suspect evidentiary exams are routinely performed in many sexual assault forensic examiner (SAFE) programs and hospitals across the United States, Canada, and abroad. This examination is important for many reasons:

- Evidence collection may aid in the thorough and successful investigation and prosecution of a case by law enforcement professionals.
- Discovery of compelling evidence may contribute to a suspect pleading guilty before trial, thereby sparing the victim the trial process.
- Evidence collection may result in the exoneration of a suspect who has been falsely accused or misidentified.
- Addition of suspect services can be an ideal presentation of objective forensic medical examiners, particularly when qualifying as an expert witness in the courtroom.
- Aside from the benefit to the legal system, offering suspect services may be a source of revenue for SAFE programs.[2]

In discussing suspect services, it's critical to clarify the specifics of the encounter. Clinicians may gather limited samples at the behest and direction of law enforcement, (such as buccal or penile swabs), without obtaining a patient medical history or conducting a physical examination. Alternatively, clinicians may complete full examinations comprised of assessment, diagnosis, planning, implementation, and evaluation (recognizable as the nursing process). Exploring such distinctions may serve to clarify the role being assumed in working with suspects and assist in creating policies and procedures for these types of interactions. For the purpose of clarity, this chapter will begin by discussing the suspect examination (including, for registered nurses, the full nursing process), before moving on to more limited types of suspect services.

The suspect exam may follow a similar process to the victim exam when completed. Therefore, a medical history should be considered an initial component of the evidentiary exam. As with the victim exam, information in the medical history can assist with interpreting physical findings and document the existence of preexisting conditions or injuries (**Figures 8-1** and **8-2**). While assault histories are not typically garnered from the suspect by the clinician conducting the exam, spontaneous statements made by the suspect may be recorded in the forensic record.[2] The extent to which other information is gathered from the suspect related to statements made by the victim or about the origin of potentially relevant injuries appears to be of some debate—some advise that the forensic examiner undertake a complete interview of the suspect.[2] Examiners should adhere to local protocols regarding this and all other aspects of the suspect exam. Regardless, the clinician should not draw conclusions as to the consistency of the exam with the history provided by the patient.[3]

Most states do not have suspect-specific evidence collection kits, leaving many examiners to adapt kits used for victim evidentiary exams. Private companies such as TRITECHFORENSICS make designated suspect kits (www.tritechusa.com); however, these may be cost-prohibitive depending on the manufacturer, the frequency of use, and the program's reimbursement stream. Physical evidence should be collected from the suspect according to state or local protocols with an approved evidence collection kit. For general guidelines, consider the *National Protocol for Sexual Assault Medical Forensic Examinations*, published by the US Department of Justice.[4] Although the protocol is written for the care of victims, the sections on evidence collection remain relevant for the suspect exam as well.

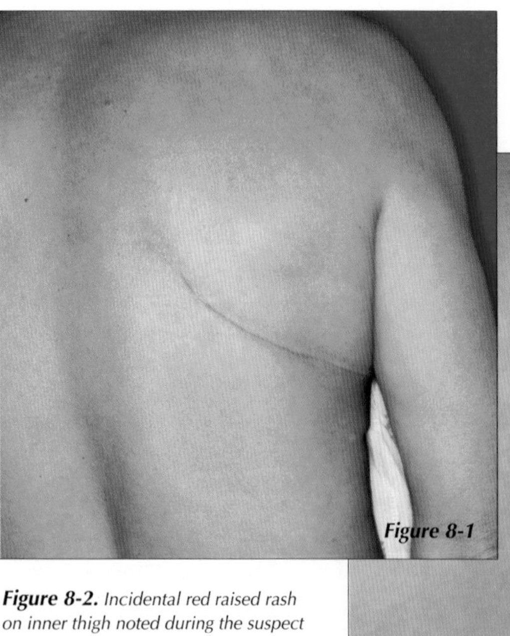

Figure 8-1. *Suspect has had surgery 4 weeks prior to the taking of this photograph. This scar is not related to the time frame for this suspect evidentary examination and is an incidental finding. The scar, however, might be a point of identification by the victim if identify is questioned.*

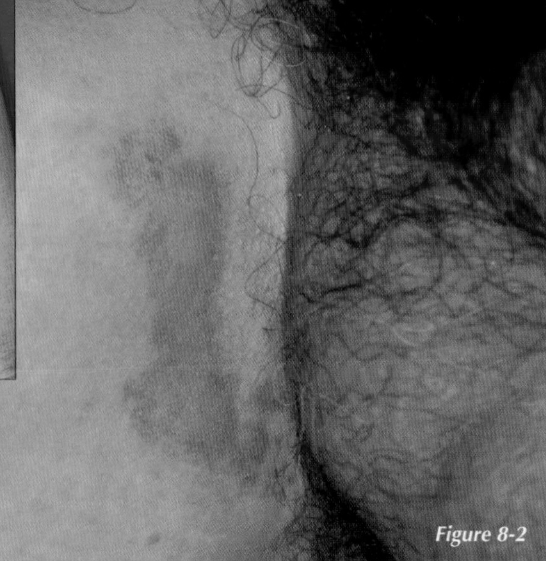

Figure 8-2. *Incidental red raised rash on inner thigh noted during the suspect examination. Patient was referred back to the prison infirmary for treatment and follow-up.*

Time frames for conducting suspect exams vary in the literature. Jurisdictions should turn to sexual assault response team (SART) members, including area crime labs if they are not already participating as members of the SART, to determine appropriate time parameters for conducting exams. Some jurisdictions set time limits according to whether the exam is conducted with voluntary consent versus search warrant.[5] According to the *National Training Manual for Law Enforcement*, in a section on investigating nonstranger sexual assaults,[6] "If the suspect is not arrested for several days following the assault, a full forensic examination is not recommended, but an abbreviated exam should still be obtained to collect a DNA reference sample." Law enforcement agencies may contract with clinicians to collect reference samples or may choose to obtain samples themselves.

Before undertaking the suspect exam, forensic examiners must ensure that law enforcement remains with the suspect throughout the process (**Figures 8-3** and **8-4**). At no time should a clinician take custody of a suspect.[6,7,8] Consideration must also be given to avoid cross-contamination if the facility has also examined the victim. Precautions such as having different examiners conduct the victim and suspect exams and using different examination suites for the two can reduce the likelihood of accusations of cross-contamination.[1,2,5] Whenever possible, suspects and victims should not be cared for in the same facility to avoid confrontation between the two.

Physical exam of the suspect should be undertaken to document injuries that may indicate signs of struggle or use of force. All injuries or pertinent remarkable findings should be photographed according to agency policy (**Figure 8-5**). An anogenital exam can be useful in identifying indicators of sexually transmitted infections (STIs), including penile lesions and discharge, as well as signs of friction and dried or crusting fluids.

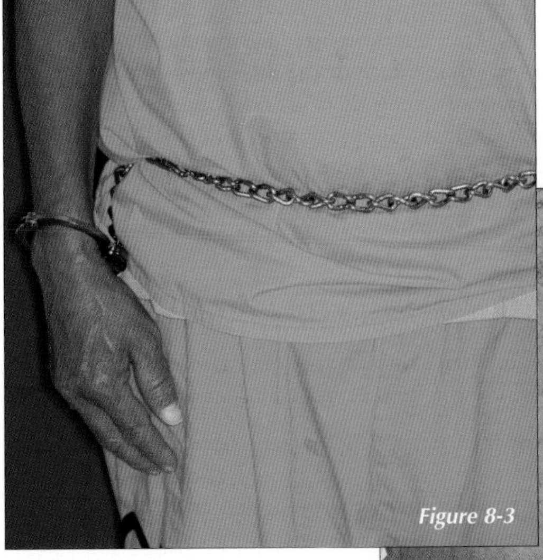

Figure 8-3. *This is a suspect who was presented with law enforcemnt for an evidentary examination. Two officers remain with the suspect and the examiner during the examination.*

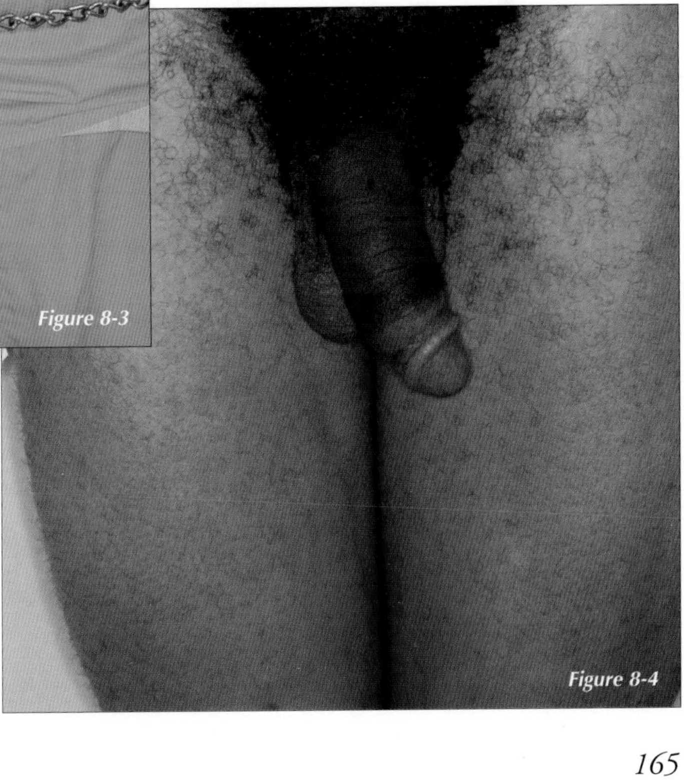

Figure 8-4. *This picture displays the length of the penis and size of the nonerect genital area. Some examiners may be asked to put a measurement ruler or tool in the picture that might be used later in the courtroom for understanding the size of the penis; this all depends on the agency policy.*

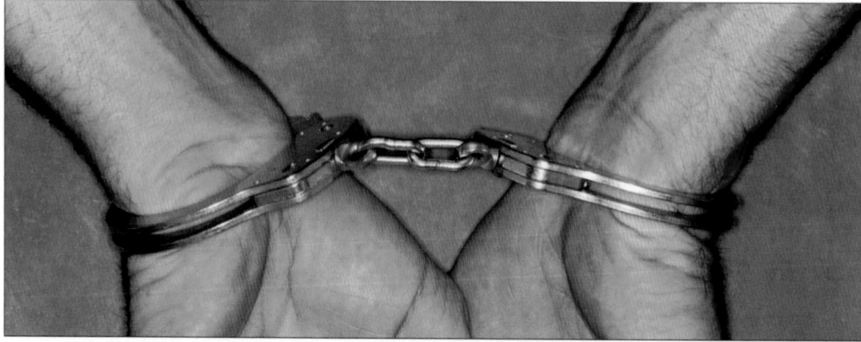

Figure 8-5.
This suspect was presented to the SANE nurse for a suspect examination. Handcuffs are in place, and, typically, the handcuffs leave a red mark on the wrists. This is due to the handcuffs and not an injury sustained during the assault.

Evidence collection may be guided by the details of the assault or search warrant or may be uniformly conducted per protocol. Basic evidence collection consists of the following, with allowances for differences in jurisdictional protocols, policies, and procedures:

— *Oral swabs* obtained as a reference sample or in cases where there is suspected orogenital contact by the suspect (clinicians may choose to swab areas of the face surrounding the mouth in cases where this is suspected as well).

— *Fingernail scrapings, swabbings, or clippings* can contain the victim's epithelial cells (clipping and swabbing appear to yield best evidence per Keel et al[9]). Clinicians should also consider swabbing the suspect's hands, including around rings and other jewelry, when digital penetration is suspected.[5]

— *Hair samples* (pulling or cutting) may include head, facial, chest, and pubic hair.[10]

— *Genital swabbing* includes penis, scrotum, vulva, vagina (and potentially, perineum/perianus, per history). Penile swabbing should include the shaft and scrotum, whether done as different swabbings or as one swabbing (P. O'Donnell, personal communication, December 2006) (**Figure 8-6**). If the suspect is uncircumcised, the clinician should swab beneath the foreskin (**Figures 8-7** and **8-8**).

— *Debris collection*

— *Dried fluid samples*

— *Urine samples* should be taken for toxicology, per jurisdictional protocol.

— *Blood samples* are obtained as reference samples and may also be obtained for toxicology (along with urine) or STI testing per suspect's consent or search warrant.

Chain of custody must also be maintained when sending samples to hospital labs or outside labs for STI and toxicologic testing. Examiners should also collect clothing, particularly underwear or clothing worn next to the genitalia, from suspects as a component of the exam process. Undergarments should be collected regardless of whether the suspect is believed to have changed since committing the assault. Examiners should note any stains, tears, or other alterations to collected garments. Caain writes,[11] there is a "frequent failure to seize the suspect's clothing, which again could be a terrific source of probative evidence [and] could be a better source of evidence than the forensic examination of the victim." Examiners should consider the following when obtaining suspects' clothing:

— Avoiding cutting through bullet or stab wounds

— Drying clothing when possible (hang in plain view)

— Packaging evidence in paper bags

— Maintaining chain of custody, as with any other components of the evidentiary exam

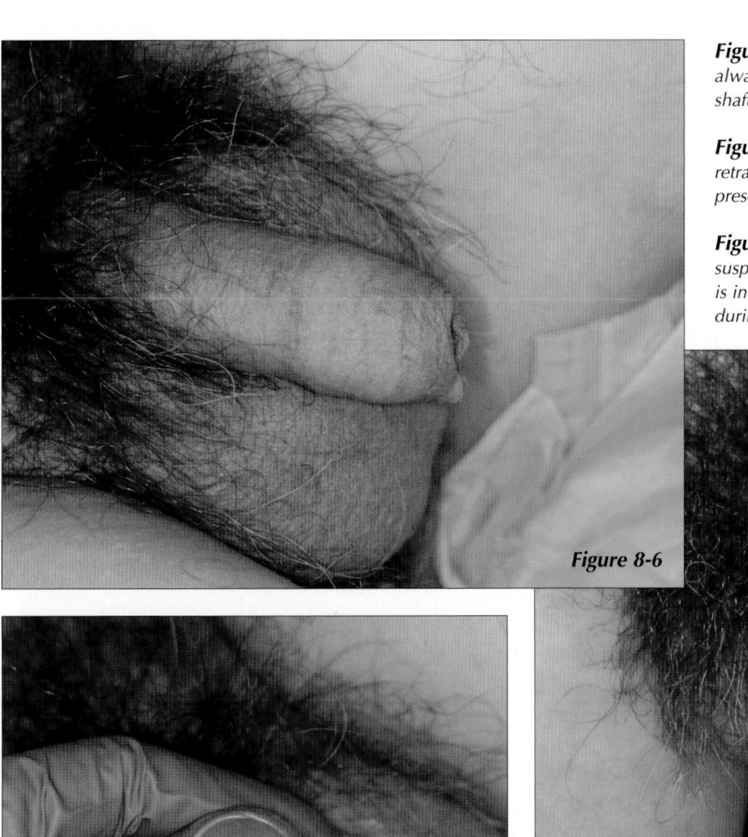

Figure 8-6. *The scrotal area should always be swabbed as well as the penis shaft with 2 moistened cotton swabs.*

Figure 8-7. *The foreskin has been retracted, and no redness or discharge is present at and around the urethra.*

Figure 8-8. *This image displays a suspect's uncircumcised penis while he is in standing position as photographed during the suspect examination.*

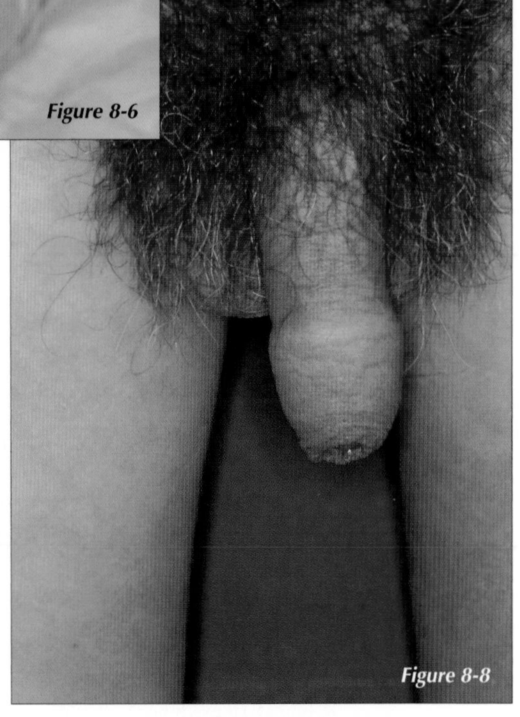

If there is a suspicion or knowledge that the suspect used a condom during the assault, take extra care to collect an appropriate number of penile swabs. While many evidence collection kits provide only 2 swabs, a third may assist with identifying condom trace evidence that could be potentially lost with fewer swabs:

> With sexual offenders using condoms, however, forensic laboratories should use three swabs: one to save for the defense and two to conduct examinations. With the potential for positively identifying a suspect, most laboratories first look for traces of seminal fluids, vaginal cells, blood, and the like. Unfortunately, the solvents used to conduct this examination also remove any condom traces present, thus losing potentially valuable evidence. Although examiners feasibly could divide each swab in half, providing an additional swab in kits for each condom trace examination easily could solve the problem.[12]

Basic treatment protocols should also be adhered to during the exam process. Immunizations for tetanus should be provided if warranted. Wound care; antibiotic treatment for penetrating wounds, including bite wounds; pain management; and postdischarge care should all be included as dictated by the exam.

Suspect exams should not be ruled out if penile penetration was not a component of the assault. Cases involving oral or digital penetration can also yield important evidence on the exam:

> Fingernail scrapings have proven critical in digital penetration cases. Some laboratories may prefer to take cuttings. We have found that there are real performance differences with the type of toothpick. Also, with toothpicks it really helps if you can tell one side of the toothpick from the other as otherwise sometimes it is hard to figure which side was used in the scraping. You may also find some laboratories that take swabbings of the fingers. I am not sure there is any good publication that shows whether cuttings, scrapings, or swabbing gives the best result, and there are probably a number of variables that would influence which yields the best result (P. O'Donnell, personal communication, December 2006).

Although much of the exam focuses on the collection of samples for DNA evidence, the suspect exam is useful for more than just DNA identification. Suspect exams can elicit information about the specific acts committed, which can be helpful in cases where the victim has impaired memory (due to alcohol or drug facilitation). It can clarify the participation of a particular suspect in cases where multiple suspects exist. It can also corroborate victim statements related to events of the assault or the victim's sensory experiences of the suspect.[8] Archambault wrote in her article on suspect exams:

> [One] of the most important reasons for conducting a suspect examination is to document evidence of force, resistance, and injury. As you know, most sexual assault cases result in a consent defense these days—even when the suspect is a stranger to the victim. Therefore, biological and trace evidence may not be as critical for establishing the identity of the suspect as one might initially think. Yet many investigators assume this means a suspect examination will not be particularly useful, and that is not necessarily true.[8]

Documenting the suspect evidentiary exam can be challenging for programs without dedicated recording forms. To date, only a few states, such as North Dakota and California, have statewide forms for documenting the exam. Most sexual assault evidence collection kit paperwork requires significant alteration to be useful for the suspect exam, particularly regarding the sections for consent and assault history. For an example of a suspect documentation form, see **Appendix 8-1**.

As mentioned earlier in the chapter, there is great variation in how suspect encounters may occur. This has led to debate among forensic examiners about whether the clinician is engaged in a therapeutic patient encounter when working with suspects or acting solely as an evidence collector. Although clinicians are licensed professionals accountable to state boards of nursing and medicine, the perception of the role pertaining to suspect encounters varies greatly, within both health care and collaborating professions. The International Association of Chiefs of Police specifically refers to the examiner as an agent of law enforcement.[3] The extent to which the process is clinically driven also contributes to this ambiguity. While states such as North Dakota have a protocol that outlines a standardized approach to every suspect exam and encourages clinicians to consult with law enforcement to determine appropriate evidence collection within the context of the full exam, other jurisdictions have protocols that speak to a range of suspect evidence collection services, ranging from site-specific collection (buccal swabs, penile swabs, injury photographs) to completion of the full sexual assault evidence collection kit.[13] The latter approach may not involve any aspect of the nursing process, include basic medical services, or even take place in a clinical setting, placing the examiner in a position of being more forensic technician than health care provider. This does not absolve clinicians from their duties as dictated by their licensure; however, it does contribute to confusion about the role of the clinician in the suspect exam process.

To be clear, the debate of whether the clinician is acting as a health care provider versus evidence collector is not limited to sexual assault suspect encounters. One could also pose this argument in a situation such as alleged driving under the influence (DUI) in which the suspect requires nothing more than a blood draw at the local jail for toxicology purposes. Is the nurse, contracted by law enforcement to draw blood on the suspect, engaged in a patient encounter? While it may be difficult to come to consensus on this point, it is vital that all programs providing any level of suspect services have clear protocols guiding practice, ideally reviewed by agency risk management to ensure limited liability and exposure.

Suspect Exam Protocols

Protocols for suspect evidentiary exams may be statewide, community-specific, or exclusive to a particular agency. Some protocols include the suspect exam information within the larger, victim-focused sexual assault medicolegal protocol.[5,14] For jurisdictions that have no existing protocol, consider working with local or regional SARTs to develop appropriate guidelines for conducting the exam. As with victim exams, the multidisciplinary approach to protocol development will yield a more nuanced and useful tool. For an example of a multidisciplinary, hospital-based protocol, see **Appendix 8-2**.

Case Study 8-1

A 27-year-old male grabbed a woman in a park and threw her down behind the bushes. She screamed and struggled. He attempted to put his penis in her mouth several times. When he finally penetrated her mouth, she bit his penis, breaking the skin. He pulled out and ran away. Later, he sought treatment for the penile injury at a local hospital. Police had already notified emergency rooms to call if this type of injury presented to them, and the triage nurse called law enforcement after the suspect entered the facility for treatment.

The suspect was arrested at the hospital and charged with sexual assault. After his arrest, he had a suspect exam and complained of pain with his penile injury. He did not voluntarily disclose anything else nor was he asked any history. He was cooperative with the nurse examiner and voluntarily consented to the exam. The sheriff's officers remained on site for the suspect exam. Handcuffs had to be removed to swab the suspect's hands and for the nurse to note any injuries on the hands relating to the history given to her by law enforcement. The suspect was also examined by an emergency room physician due to the nature of the bite mark on his penis, and follow-up treatment instructions and medical referrals were given to the sheriff for the jail medical staff.

Several weeks later, the DNA from the victim's mouth (obtained during her own evidentiary exam) positively identified the suspect. Although the victim's exam also took place in the same facility, no cross-contamination occurred. Separate rooms were used and the examiner changed outer coverings between patients. The suspect pled guilty to the charge and is currently serving time in a state prison.

Barriers to Suspect Exams

Suspect exams are not routinely completed in many jurisdictions for the following reasons:

— *Lack of protocols:* As mentioned earlier in this chapter, many jurisdictions lack specific protocols for suspect exams or are unaware of existing protocols at the state level. More frequent discussion regarding the importance of suspect exam protocols within forensic clinician professional organizations, such as the International Association of Forensic Nurses (www.iafn.org) and the American College of Emergency Physicians' Forensic Section (www.acep.org), can help highlight their importance.

— *Lack of standardization:* Few states have suspect-specific evidence collection kits or documentation forms. Jurisdictions may struggle with modifying existing tools typically used for victims.

— *Lack of training:* Few clinicians receive specific training related to suspect exams. Most SAFE education programs only focus on victim exams and do not cover issues such as areas for optimal suspect evidence collection or avoidance of cross-contamination between the victim and suspect exams. Training also needs to be conducted on the legal issues around consent-driven versus search warrant–driven exams.[15]

— *Lack of funding:* Law enforcement agencies may lack funds to pay for exams of suspects, or may choose to use police personnel for aspects of evidence collection rather than engage clinicians to complete full exams.

— *Disinclination of clinicians to perform exams:* Examiners may be reluctant to work with suspects based on concerns for safety or because of personal victimization history.

Agreed upon jurisdictional policies and procedures help mitigate barriers. SARTs or other coordinated community responses (where they exist) can work collaboratively to ensure members agree on process issues to further overcome potential barriers.

Legal Issues

On forensic examinations of sexual assault suspects, Archambault says "Essentially, there are three ways that a suspect exam may take place: (1) The suspect may consent to a forensic examination; (2) An examination may be conducted incident to an arrest,* or; (3) A warrant or court order may be obtained."[8]

As with obtaining consent from any patient, it is critical that forensic examiners feel confident in the abilities of the suspect to give consent for the exam. Suspects who have developmental disabilities, who are intoxicated, or who have some type of cognitive impairment may still require a search warrant, regardless of willingness to consent to the exam. Examiners completing exams as a result of a search warrant should ensure that they comply with the parameters of the search warrant and not exceed its limits. However, there may be instances where deviations from the search warrant occurs based on the medical needs of the suspect.

Conclusion

The International Association of Forensic Nurses has standards for Sexual Assault Nurse Examiner (SANE) practice available online (www.iafn.org). The standards address care of victims, suspects, and perpetrators of sexual violence. Examiners should refer to this document, revised and updated in 2007, for additional information related to issues about the suspect exam and the role of the forensic clinician.

Although there is a wide disparity regarding the suspect exam process and the role of the forensic examiner, clinicians should, at a minimum, consider the following:

— Maintaining currency as information becomes available regarding best practice for suspect evidence collection

— Encouraging area crime labs to review the evidence collection kit contents and procedure for suspect exams based on the current literature for best practice

— Developing state or regional protocols and standardized forms for suspect exams to ensure consistency of approach and documentation

— Engaging SARTs in creating a unified approach to suspect exams in individual communities

* *This practice will be dependent on jurisdiction. Some states, such as California, "...allow the exam based on exigent circumstances—because the evidence may no longer be available if too much time elapses."*[5]

Appendix 8-1: Sample Sexual Assault Suspect Examination Documentation Form

FORENSIC MEDICAL REPORT:
SEXUAL ASSAULT SUSPECT EXAMINATION
STATE OF CALIFORNIA
OFFICE OF CRIMINAL JUSTICE PLANNING
OCJP 950

Confidential Document **Patient Identification**

A. GENERAL INFORMATION (print or type) **Name of Medical Facility:**

1. Name of patient			Patient ID number	
2. Address	City	County	State	Telephone (W) (H)

3. Age	DOB	Gender M F	Ethnicity	Arrival Date	Arrival Time	Discharge Date	Discharge Time

B. AUTHORIZATION **Jurisdiction** **(❑ city ❑ country ❑ other):**

1. Name of Law Enforcement Officer	Agency	ID Number	Telephone

2. I request a forensic medical examination for suspected sexual assault at public expense.

Law enforcement officer signature	Date	Time	Case number

C. MEDICAL HISTORY

1. **Any recent (60 days) anal-genital injuries, surgeries, diagnostic procedures, or medical treatment that may affect the interpretation of current physical findings?** ❑ No ❑ Yes
   If yes, describe: ____________
2. **Any other pertinent medical condition(s) that may affect the interpretation of current physical findings?** ❑ No ❑ Yes
   If yes, describe: ____________
3. **Any pre-existing physical injuries?** ❑ No ❑ Yes
   If yes, describe: ____________

D. RECENT HYGIENE INFORMATION ❑ **Not Applicable if over 72 hours**

	NO	Yes		NO	Yes
Urinated	❑	❑	Bath/shower/wash	❑	❑
Defecated	❑	❑	Brushed teeth	❑	❑
Genital or body wipes	❑	❑	Ate or drank	❑	❑
If yes, describe: ____			Changed clothing	❑	❑
Oral gargle/rinse	❑	❑	If yes, describe: ____		

E. GENERAL PHYSICAL EXAMINATION

1. Blood Pressure	Pulse	Respiration	Temperature	2. Exam Started		Exam Completed	
				Date	Time	Date	Time
3. Height	Weight	Hair color	Eye color	❑ Right-handed ❑ Left-handed			

4. **Describe general physical appearance**
5. **Describe general demeanor**
6. **Describe condition of clothing upon arrival.**
7. **Collect outer and under clothing, if indicated.** ❑ **Not indicated**

DISTRIBUTION OF OCJP 950

❑ Original - Law Enforcement ❑ Copy within evidence kit - Crime Lab ❑ Copy - Medical Facility Records

E. GENERAL PHYSICAL EXAMINATION
Record all findings using diagrams, legend and a consecutive numbering system

8. **Conduct a physical examination. Record scars, tattoos, skin lesions, and distinguishing physical features.** ❑ Findings ❑ No Findings
9. **Collect dried and moist secreations, stains, and foreign materials from the body. Scan the entire body with a Wood's Lamp.** ❑ Findings ❑ No Findings
10. **Collect fingernail scraping or cuttings according to local policy.**
11. **Collect chest hair reference samples according to local policy.**

Patient Identification

Diagram A

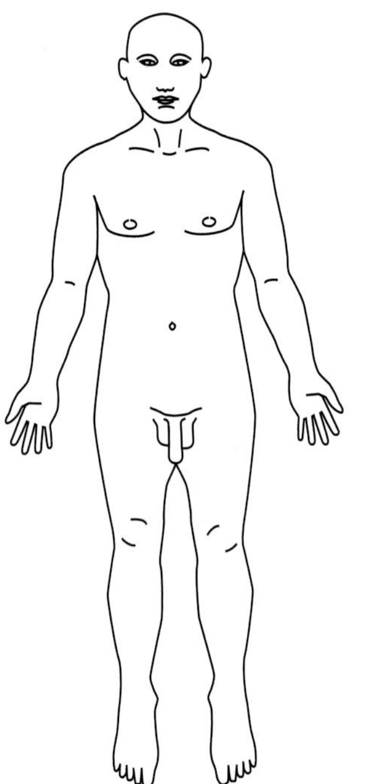

Diagram B

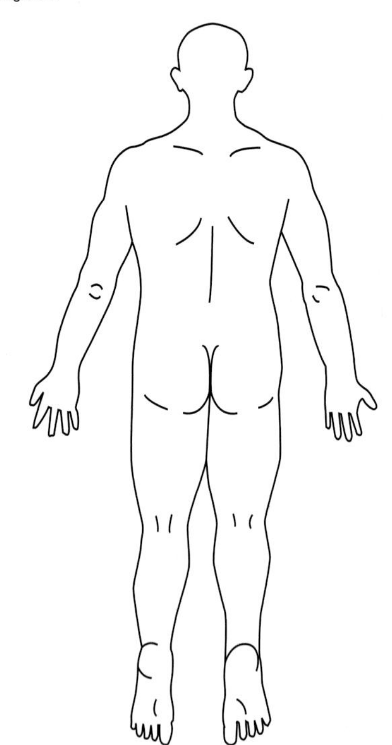

LEGEND: Types of Findings

AB	b	**DE**	eb	**F/H**	be/h	**OF**	OtheeMte (ecbe) I	**SC**	Sc	**TA**	Tt t
BI	Bte	**DF**	ef ty	**IN**	Iut			**SHX**	Splepe Hty	**TB**	Tl ueBe+
BP	Byec	**DS**	ySec et	**IW**	IceW u	**OI**	Othelju y(ecbe)			**TE**	Te ee
BU	Bu	**EC**	Ecchy(b ue)	**LA**	Lcet	**PE**	Peteche	**SI**	Suctljuy	**V/S**	Ve ett/SI
CS	CtlSwb	**ER**	Eythe(ee)	**MS**	MtSecet	**PS**	Pt etlSlv	**SW**	Swell	**WL**	W 'Lp+

Locator #	Type	Description	Locator #	Type	Description

RECORD ALL CLOTHING AND SPECIMENS COLLECTED ON PAGE 5

2

F. HEAD, NECK AND ORAL EXAMINATION
Record all findings using diagrams, legend and a consecutive numbering system

1. **Examine the face, head, hair, scalp and neck for injury and foreign materials.**
   ❑ Findings ❑ No Findings
2. **Collect dried and moist secreations, stains, and foreign materials from face, head, hair, scalp, and neck.**
   ❑ Findings ❑ No Findings
3. **Examine the oral cavity for injury and foreign materials (if indicated by assault history). Collect foriegn materials.**
   Exam done: ❑ Not applicable ❑ yes ❑ Findings ❑ No Findings
4. **Collect 2 swabs from the oral cavity up to 12 hours post assault and prepare one dry mount slide from one of the swabs.**
5. **Collect head and facial hair reference samples according to local policy.**

Patient Identification

Diagram C

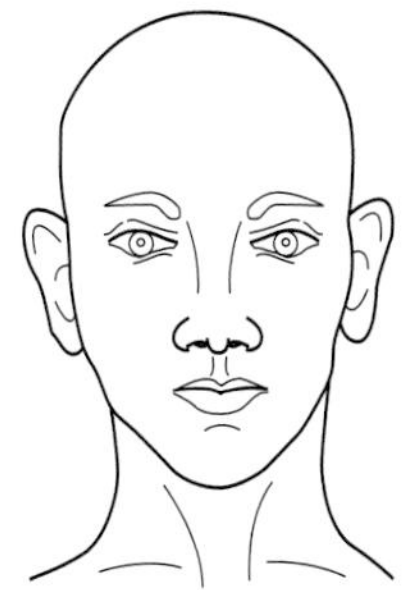

Diagram D

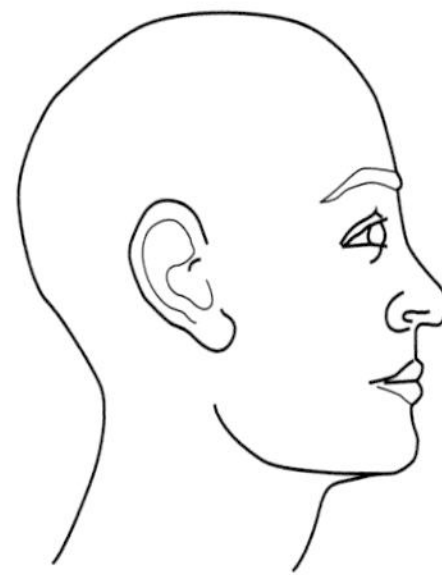

Diagram E

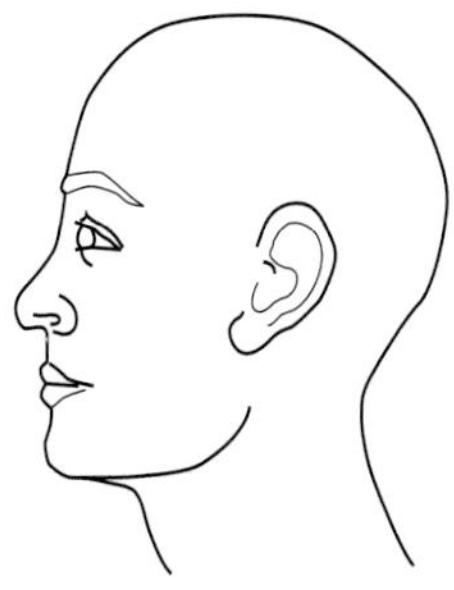

Diagram F

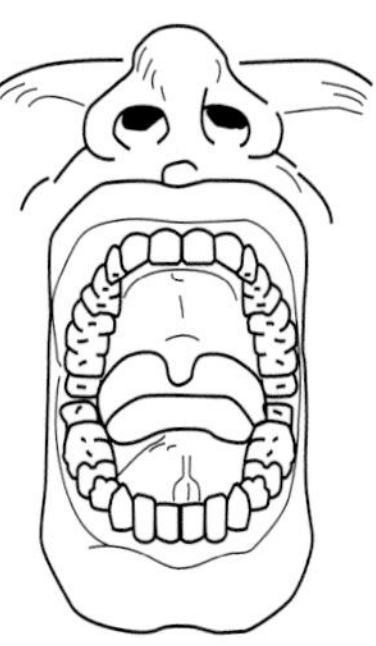

LEGEND: Types of Findings

AB	Abrasion	**DE**	Debris	**F/H**	Fiber/hair	**OF**	Other Foreign Materials (describe)	**SC**	Scars	**TA**	Tattoos
BI	Bite	**DF**	Deformity	**IN**	Induration			**SHX**	Sample per History	**TB**	Toluidine Blue +
BP	Body Piercing	**DS**	Dry Secretion	**IW**	Incised Wound	**OI**	Other Injury (describe)			**TE**	Tenderness
BU	Burn	**EC**	Ecchymosis (bruise)	**LA**	Laceration	**PE**	Petechiae	**SI**	Suction Injury	**V/S**	Vegetation/Soil
CS	Control Swab	**ER**	Erythema (redness)	**MS**	Moist Secretion	**PS**	Potential Saliva	**SW**	Swelling	**WL**	Wood's Lamp +

Locator #	Type	Description	Locator #	Type	Description

RECORD ALL CLOTHING AND SPECIMENS COLLECTED ON PAGE 5

3

G. GENITAL EXAMINATION
Record all findings using diagrams, legend and a consecutive numbering system

1. **Examine the inner thighs, external genitalia, and perineal area. Check the box(es) if there are assault related findings.**
   - ❑ No Findings
   - ❑ Inner thighs ❑ Glans penis ❑ Scrotum
   - ❑ Perineum ❑ Penile shaft ❑ Testes
   - ❑ Foreskin ❑ Urethral meatus
2. **Circumcised.** ❑ No ❑ Yes
3. **Collect dried and moist secretions, stains, and foreign materials. Scan the area with a Wood's Lamp.** ❑ Findings ❑ No Findings
4. **Collect pubic hair combing of brushing.**
5. **Collect pubic hair reference samples according to local policy.**
6. **Collect 2 penile swabs, if indicated by assault history.** ❑ N/A
7. **Collect 2 scrotal swabs, if indicated by assault history.** ❑ N/A
8. **Record other findings per history.** ❑ No ❑ Yes
   If yes, describe:

Patient Identification

Diagram G

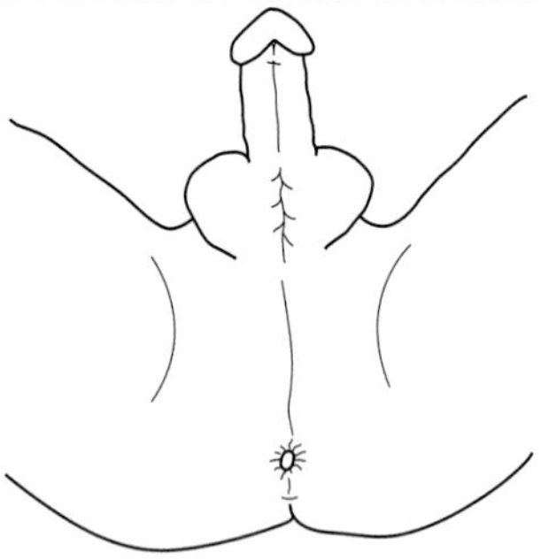

Diagram H

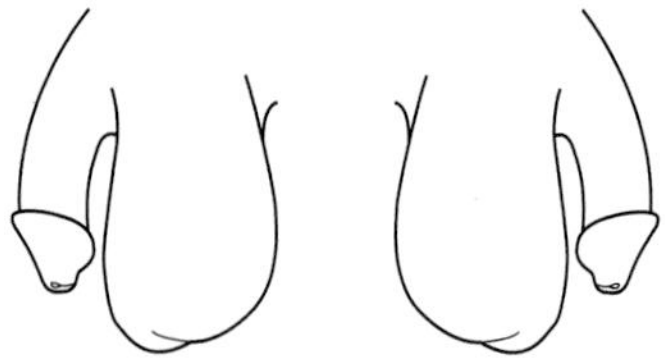

Diagram I

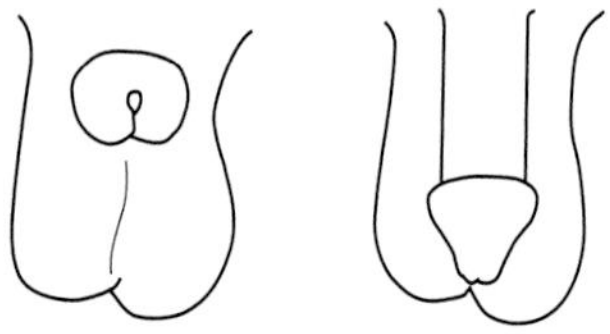

Diagram J

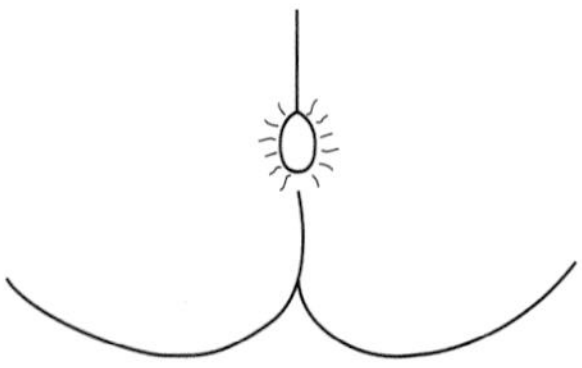

LEGEND: Types of Findings

AB	b	**DE**	eb	**F/H**	be/h	**OF**	OtheeMte I (ecbe)	**SC**	Sc	**TA**	Tt t
BI	Bte	**DF**	ef ty	**IN**	lut			**SHX**	Splepe Hty	**TB**	Tl ueBlue+
BP	ByPec	**DS**	ySec et	**IW**	IceW u	**OI**	Othelju y(ecbe)			**TE**	Te ee
BU	Bu	**EC**	Ecchy(b ue)	**LA**	Lcet	**PE**	Peteche	**SI**	Suctljuy	**V/S**	Ve ett/Sl
CS	CtlSwb	**ER**	Eythe(ee)	**MS**	MtSecet	**PS**	Pt etlSlv	**SW**	Swell	**WL**	W 'Lp+

Locator #	Type	Description	Locator #	Type	Description

RECORD ALL CLOTHING AND SPECIMENS COLLECTED ON PAGE 5

4

H. EVIDENCE COLLECTED AND SUBMITTED TO CRIME LAB

1. Clothing placed in evidence kit	Other clothing placed in bags

2. Foreign materials collected

	No	Yes	Collected by:
Swabs/suspected blood	❑	❑	
Dried Secreations	❑	❑	
Fiber/loose hairs	❑	❑	
Vegetation	❑	❑	
Soil/debris	❑	❑	
Swabs/suspected semen	❑	❑	
Swabs/suspected saliva	❑	❑	
Swabs/Wood's Lamp+ area(s)	❑	❑	
Control swabs	❑	❑	
Fingernail scrapings/cuttings	❑	❑	
Matted hair cuttings	❑	❑	
Pubic hair combings/brushings	❑	❑	
Other types	❑	❑	

If yes, describe:________________

3. Oral/genital samples

	# Swabs	# Slides	Time collected	Collected by:
Oral				
Penile				
Scrotal				

I. TOXICOLOGY SAMPLES

	No	Yes	Time	Collected by:
Blood alcohol/toxicology (gray top tube)				
Urine toxicology				

J. REFERENCE SAMPLES

	No	Yes	Collected by:
Blood (lavender top tube)			
Blood (yellow top tube			
Blood card (optional)			
Buccal swabs (optional)			
Saliva swabs			
Chest hair			
Facial hair			
Pubic hair			
Head hair			

K. PHOTO DOCUMENTATION METHODS

	No	Yes	Colposcope/ 35mm	Macrolens/ 35mm	Colposcope/ Videocamera	Other optics
Body	❑	❑	❑	❑	❑	❑____
Genitals	❑	❑	❑	❑	❑	❑____

Photographed by:

Patient Identification

L. RECORD EXAM METHODS

	No	Yes
Direct visualization only	❑	❑
Colposcopy	❑	❑
Other magnifier	❑	❑
Other	❑	❑

If yes, describe: ________________

M. RECORD EXAM FINDINGS

❑ Physical Findings ❑ No Physical Findings

N. SUMMARIZE FINDINGS

O. PRINT NAMES OF PERSONNEL INVOLVED

	Telephone
History taken by:	
Exam performed by:	
Specimens labeled and sealed by:	
Assissted by: ❑ N/A	
Signature of examiner: License No.	

P. EVIDENCE DISTRIBUTION	GIVEN TO:
Clothing (item(s) not placed in evidence kit)	
Evidence kit	
Reference blood samples	
Toxicology samples	

Q. SIGNATURE OF OFFICER RECEIVING EVIDENCE

Signature: ________________

Print name and ID#: ________________

Agency: ________________

Date:__________ Telephone: __________

5

Appendix 8-2: Suspect Examination Protocols and Procedures

Appendix 8-2. Suspect Examination Protocols/Procedures

Protocols and Procedures

Purpose: To provide consistent and comprehensive evidentiary examinations of suspects evaluated by the Meriter Hospital SANE/Forensic Nursing Program.

1. The suspect will be registered and issued an Emergency Services (ES) Medical Record. A copy of the search warrant, court order, and/or authorizing documentation will be made and kept on file with the ES medical record. See Wisconsin Statute 968.255(2)(d).
2. If the suspect consents to the evidentiary exam, the appropriate consents must be signed.
3. If the suspect consents to the exam, a Medical Records Release of Information should be made out to the law enforcement agency that is requesting the exam.
4. If the suspect does not consent/sign a Medical Records Release of Information, the police officer may obtain a copy of the ES medical record by signing a Medical Records Release of Information and must indicate that the records are needed for an ongoing legal investigation.
   a. There are two exceptions to the release of medical records to law enforcement—HIV results and psychiatric information/history. Law enforcement may call Medical Records at 267-6030 during normal business hours if this information is needed.
5. If the suspect requests STI or HIV testing, refer him/her to their primary health care provider. Instruct the suspect to use condoms until testing is completed. If the police request STI testing and the suspect consents, the SANE nurse may test for STIs/HIV with the appropriate consents signed.
6. The suspect and the victim should not encounter each other in the medical facility.
7. The evidentiary examination of the suspect and victim will not be performed in the same room or by the same nurse. The room in which the exam is performed will be noted on the SANE Evidence Collection Sheet.
8. A law enforcement officer of the same sex as the suspect should be present in the examination room throughout the evidentiary exam. See Wisconsin Statute 968.255(2)(a).
9. Blood for forensic purposes may only be drawn if the suspect consents to having blood drawn, if the search warrant/court order asks that it be drawn, or if drug and/or alcohol exigency exists.
10. The nurse will obtain historical information and necessary data from the law enforcement officer. This exchange of information should not be shared with the suspect and should include:
    a. Date/time/location of assault
    b. Alleged sexual acts
    c. Salient information from the victim exam, if known
11. Cursory medical interview (if suspect willing):
    a. Medications
    b. Allergies
    c. Major medical/surgical conditions

(continued)

Appendix 8-2. *(continued)*

PROTOCOLS AND PROCEDURES

12. Evidence collection should be done using the Wisconsin Crime Lab Sexual Assault Evidence Collection Kit or the Wisconsin Crime Lab Sexual Assault Suspect Evidence Collection Kit. In addition to the standard evidence collection, swabs from around the mouth and/or hands/fingers should be obtained when appropriate. Scan the entire body of the suspect with the Wood's lamp and if fluorescence is noted, obtain a wet to dry swab of the area.
13. Photograph all nongenital trauma. No photographs or video recording may be made of the genitals unless stated in the search warrant. See Wisconsin Statute 968.225(2)(c).
14. General physical examination:
    a. Vital signs
    b. Objective behavior—note right- or left-handedness
    c. Breath, body odor
    d. Tattoos, scars, birthmarks
    e. Other identifying marks or lesions
    f. Colposcope may be used for examination, but no photographs may be made of the genitals unless stated in the search warrant.
    g. Check for signs of injury—measure and document all trauma noted. The SANE should ask how an injury was acquired in order to ascertain if any further medical assessment and intervention is needed.
15. Any injury or unusual finding that requires intervention beyond the scope of practice of the forensic examiner should be referred to the ES physician for assessment and treatment.
16. Urine and blood may be collected for toxicology if the suspect consents. If the suspect does not consent, see #10.
17. Any statements made by the suspect about the crime should be documented as exact quotes. The forensic examiner is NOT responsible for questioning the suspect about the alleged assault and should not do so.
18. Maintain chain of custody throughout the exam—documentation of the chain of custody will be on the SANE Evidence Collection Sheet.
19. The forensic examiner is primarily collecting physical evidence and does not render an opinion as to whether a particular individual is indeed the assailant.

Prepared by Gretchen Hayward, Assistant District Attorney; Marion Morgan, Detective—Madison Police Department; C. Jill Poarch, SANE Program Coordinator; Peter Ouimet, Meriter Risk Management; and Julie Callies, Meriter Medical Records on January 11, 2001. Revised by Jill Poarch, SANE Program Coordinator, and Kim Macaulay, SANE Clinical Educator on July 18, 2003.

References

1. Archambault J; Sexual Assault Training & Investigations. Time limits for conducting a forensic examination: Can biological evidence be recovered 24, 36, 48, 72, 84 or 96 hours following a sexual assault? http://www.mysati.com/enews/May2005/practices_0505.htm. Published May 19, 2005. Accessed September 15, 2009.

2. Poarch CJ. Evidence collection and physical examination of the sexual assault suspect. *On the Edge*. 2007;13(2):5-7. http://www.iafn.org/associations/8556/files/OTESummer2007.pdf. Accessed December 1, 2009.

3. International Association of Chiefs of Police. Investigating sexual assault. http://www.ncdsv.org/images/InvestigatingSexualAssaultsModelPolicy.pdf. Published 2005. Accessed December 1, 2009.

4. US Department of Justice. *National Protocol for Sexual Assault Medical Forensic Examinations: Adult/Adolescent*. http://samfe.dna.gov/. Published September 2004. Accessed September 15, 2009.

5. North Dakota Office of the Attorney General. *North Dakota Sexual Assault Evidence Collection Protocol*. 4th ed. http://www.nsvrc.org/publications/guides/north-dakota-sexual-assault-evidence-collection-protocol. Accessed December 1, 2009.

6. Lonsway K; National Center for Women and Policing. Successfully Investigating Acquaintance Sexual Assault: A National Training Manual for Law Enforcement. http://www.mincava.umn.edu/documents/acquaintsa/acquaintsa.html. Accessed December 1, 2009.

7. Girardin BW. The sexual assault nurse examiner: a win-win solution. *Top Emerg Med*. 2005;27(2):124-131.

8. Archambault J. Forensic examinations of sexual assault suspects. http://www.mysati.com/resources.htm. Accessed September 15, 2009.

9. Keel et al. Physical evidence associated with fingernails. Presented at: Third Joint Meeting of the California Association of Criminalists and the Forensic Science Society; 2000; Sacramento, CA.

10. State of California, Office of Emergency Services. California Sexual Assault Medical/Evidentiary Suspect Exam, Form OES 950. California Emergency Management Agency. http://www.oes.ca.gov/WebPage/oeswebsite.nsf/ClientOESFileLibrary/CJP%20Med%20Forms/$file/SA%20Suspect%202-950.pdf. Accessed September 15, 2009.

11. Caain IT. *The Use of Physical Evidence in the Investigation and Prosecution of Sexual Assault Cases* [master's thesis]. National University; 2002.

12. Blackledge RD; The FBI Law Enforcement Bulletin. Condom trace evidence: a new factor in sexual assault investigations. http://www.findarticles.com/p/articles/mi_m2194/is_n5_v65/ai_18535197/print. Published May 1996. Accessed September 15, 2009.

13. The DOVE Program, Summa Health System. Suspect Examination and Evidence Collection Protocol. Akron, OH.

14. Montana State Hospital. Allegations of Rape or Sexual Assault. http://msh.mt.gov/volumei/emergencyresponse/allegationofrape.pdf. Published August 22, 2008. Accessed September 15, 2009.

15. International Association of Forensic Nurses. SANE Adult/Adolescent Education Guidelines. Arnold, MD: International Association of Forensic Nurses; 2008.

Chapter 9

VICTIM IMPACT AND RECOVERY

Patricia A. Frazier, PhD
Linda E. Ledray, RN, SANE-A, PhD, FAAN

Numerous studies have examined the effects of sexual assault on its victims. The purpose of this chapter is to review the research on the most common short- and long-term aftereffects of rape. Because women are much more likely to be sexually assaulted than men, most research on the effects of sexual assault is on women. Thus, this chapter's review focuses primarily on research on female victims, although research on male victims is also covered. Prior to the review of the research on the effects of rape, some methodological issues and limitations of existing research that can affect the interpretation of study findings will be described. In the last section, clinical implications of this research for the provider who conducts the initial examination will be discussed in addition to effective interventions for reducing immediate and long-term distress.

METHODOLOGICAL ISSUES

One very important methodological issue concerns sample recruitment. Several different methods have been used, and each has its strengths and limitations. One method is to recruit participants from clients seen at rape crisis centers. Investigators who use this method are able to assess immediate and short-term reactions and longitudinally assess symptoms over time. However, because many victims do not seek help at such centers, those who do may not be representative of most victims. To further compound the problem, often a small percentage of the minority who do report participate in the research.[1] Another recruitment method is to advertise for research participants who have been sexually assaulted. The representation of samples is also a concern in studies that rely on this method because research volunteers may differ in various ways from other victims. A third method is to identify rape victims through screening questions in surveys of larger samples. The validity of studies that identify victims in this manner depends in large part on the screening questions used to assess sexual assault. Because many people do not define experiences as "rape," even if those experiences meet the legal definition, many victims will be undetected if that terminology is used.[2] Questions that describe rape in behavioral terms are much more likely to identify victimization experiences.

There are other characteristics of the existing research that can affect conclusions that can be drawn about the effects of sexual assault. One problem is that investigators, particularly those who have recruited victims through rape crisis centers, often do not include the definition of sexual assault used in their studies. Alternatively, studies that identify victims through screening questions often use very broad definitions of sexual assault that range from unwanted kissing to forced intercourse. Although this may not necessarily be considered a problem, it complicates the comparison of findings across studies. Studies that recruit victims through advertisements or surveys do not always specify the time since the rape occurred, which also makes comparisons across studies difficult. Finally, because many victims do not want to participate in research, samples are often small, which reduces the power of statistical analyses.

Review of the Scientific Research on Rape Trauma

The review is organized in the following manner: studies are categorized in terms of whether they assess immediate (within the emergency room [ER]), short-term (within one year postrape), or long-term (more than one year postrape) effects. Within each of the latter 2 sections, studies are organized in terms of whether or not they employed a comparison group of nonvictims because comparative studies provide more information on whether symptoms are more common in victims than in nonvictims. No studies of immediate reactions employ comparison groups of nonvictims. Results obtained using standardized symptom measures are emphasized. With regard to short- and long-term effects, a review is conducted on research on posttraumatic stress disorder (PTSD), depression, fear and anxiety, social adjustment problems, health problems, and substance abuse, which are the most commonly studied aftereffects of rape. Also included are sections on other effects of rape that have been studied less frequently, including risky sexual behaviors, eating disordered behaviors, and positive life change. Additionally, a section is included on the effects of male sexual assault and gender differences in the effects of sexual assault. A discussion of clinical implications and treatment recommendations concludes the chapter.

Relevant research was identified through searches of psychological and medical databases of articles published. Only articles published in peer-reviewed journals were reviewed; unpublished papers, conference presentations, and book chapters were excluded. Even if peer-reviewed, studies were excluded if they were conducted outside of the United States, if they focused exclusively on the effects of childhood sexual victimization, or if they combined victims of sexual assault with victims of other traumas, such as physical assault, unless otherwise noted.

Immediate Reactions

There are very few studies of immediate reactions to rape because of the difficulty of gathering data from victims when they are in an acute state of distress. Nevertheless, early reactions are important to assess because they are strongly related to the development of later distress. For example, in one study, victims who reported more anxiety after the medical exam in the ER reported more PTSD symptoms at 6 weeks postrape.[3]

In a landmark study of the effects of rape, Burgess and Holmstrom interviewed 92 rape victims immediately after the assault in the ER.[4] They reported that victims mainly showed 2 emotional styles: (1) an expressed style in which fear, anger, and anxiety were exhibited through crying, sobbing, and tenseness and (2) a controlled style in which feelings were masked or hidden. They reported that both styles were equally common.

Other qualitative studies involved asking victims to recall their immediate reactions rather than interviewing victims in the ER. In one study, 70 victims were interviewed within 48 hours of the initial ER visit and were asked to describe their immediate reactions.[5] The most common reactions were terror, numbness and disbelief, shame, and anger; however, fewer than 25% mentioned shame or anger, and only 7% mentioned guilt. In another retrospective qualitative study, Bletzer and Koss interviewed 62 Native-American, Mexican-American and Anglo-American victims who had been raped several years previously about the experience.[6] With regard to immediate reactions, the women reported feeling shame, embarrassment, fear, anger, and humiliation. Many felt a sense of helplessness and confusion over what they had experienced, and a feeling of nausea.

Ruch et al have developed 2 measures that can be used in the ER to assess rape trauma more systematically: the Clinical Trauma Assessment (CTA) and the Sexual Assault Symptoms Scale (SASS). The CTA is designed to be completed by clinicians (eg, crisis workers, Sexual Assault Nurse Advocates) in the ER with regard to the immediate impact of the rape on the victim.[7] The CTA consists of 16 items that assess behavioral, emotional, and cognitive trauma. Each item is rated on a 5-point scale. Overall, the emotional trauma items were rated more highly than the behavioral items, followed by the cognitive trauma items. The specific items that had the highest ratings were fear or anxiety, concern about others' reactions, and anger.

The SASS[8] was developed to provide a measure of rape trauma symptoms that can be completed by victims rather than clinicians. It contains 32 items and can be administered as a structured interview or as a self-report measure. Items are rated on 5-point scales. Factor analysis using data from 253 women interviewed in the ER within 72 hours of the assault yielded 4 factors: disclosure shame, safety fears, depression, and self-blame. The specific symptoms reported as most severe were anger at the assailant, depression about the assault, and concern about telling others. Ruch and Wang have recently developed the SASS-II, which assesses issues that may be more relevant later on (not in the ER).[9] It can also be used as an interview or self-report measure and assesses safety fears; self-blame; depression; anger and emotional lability; health fears; and fear and anger directed at the criminal justice system.

The final study that assessed immediate impact focused on reactions to secondary victimization experiences from the police or hospital staff rather than the impact of the rape itself.[10] Interviews with 81 victims immediately after their discharge from the ER revealed that secondary victimization experiences, such as police or hospital staff questioning their choices or behavior, the way they dressed, or about their prior sexual history, were common, especially if an advocate were not present. All behaviors were rated as quite distressing if encountered. Victims were then asked whether they experienced various emotions as a result with their interaction with the police or hospital staff. Negative emotions, including feeling depressed, guilty, violated, distrustful, and reluctant to seek help were very common, especially if an advocate were not present.

Short-Term Reactions

Posttraumatic Stress Disorder

The essential feature of PTSD is the development of characteristic symptoms following a psychologically distressing event. Although the criteria differ somewhat in the various editions of the diagnostic manual (DSM) of the American Psychiatric Association, the basic elements of the PTSD diagnosis include the following:

— Experiencing a traumatic event

— Reexperiencing the trauma (eg, intrusive recollections, nightmares)

— Avoidance and numbing (eg, avoiding thoughts or feelings about the trauma, feelings of detachment from others)

— Increased arousal (eg, difficulty concentrating, hypervigilance, exaggerated startle response)

— Functional impairment (eg, impairment in social or occupational functioning)

Studies with Comparison Groups

No studies were located that compared recent victims to nonvictims in terms of the prevalence of a diagnosis of PTSD or symptoms of PTSD. It is difficult to assess PTSD symptoms in nonvictims because many of the symptoms refer to a specific trauma.

Studies Without Comparison Groups

Several studies have reported data on the prevalence of PTSD diagnoses among rape victims without using a comparison group. In 2 studies by Foa and her colleagues, PTSD symptoms were assessed weekly for 12 weeks among recent victims of rape and attempted rape.[11,12] Across the 2 studies, 90-94% of the victims met the criteria for PTSD at 2 weeks postassault, 60% to 65% met criteria at 1 month postassault, and 47% to 51% met criteria at 3 months postassault. In another longitudinal study, PTSD rates were 78% at 2 weeks, 63% at 2 months, 58% at 6 months, and 48% at 1 year.[13] Other studies assessing PTSD among recent rape victims report prevalence rates between about 50% and 75%.[14]

These and other investigators have also reported levels of PTSD symptoms on self-report measures in recent rape victims, regardless of whether they met the diagnostic criteria for the disorder.[12,14-16] Across these studies, victims scored at least one standard deviation above norm group means. In one interesting longitudinal study, PTSD symptoms were found to peak at 3 to 4 weeks postrape on average.[17] Having a delayed peak reaction was associated with higher levels of subsequent trauma symptoms.

Depression

Symptoms of depression are also commonly studied aftereffects of rape. Typically, they are assessed through self-report measures of depressive symptoms, although some studies assess whether victims meet the criteria for a diagnosis of major depressive disorder (MDD) or major depressive episode (MDE) as outlined in the DSM. Symptoms of depression, which overlap somewhat with the symptoms of PTSD, include depressed mood, diminished interest or pleasure in activities, weight loss or gain, sleep disturbances, feelings of worthlessness, inability to concentrate, and suicidal thoughts.

Studies with Comparison Groups

Several studies have assessed the prevalence of depression among victims and nonvictims within one year of the assault. These studies consistently find higher rates of depressive disorders and symptoms among victims than nonvictims. For example, in 2 studies, 33% to 38% of rape victims met the criteria for a depressive disorder at 6 months postrape in comparison to 11% to 16% of a nonvictim control group.[18,19] Other studies reported higher scores on depression measures among victims recruited from rape crisis centers than among nonvictims,[20] with longitudinal studies suggesting that victims differ from nonvictims until about 2 months postrape.[21-23] Studies of female undergraduate students who experienced unwanted sexual contact within the past year also found that victims scored higher than nonvictims[24] and were more likely to report suicidal ideation,[25] although one study of female undergraduates found no differences between victims and nonvictims on depressive symptoms.[26]

Studies Without Comparison Groups

Several additional studies provide information on levels of depression within rape victims without comparing victims to nonvictims. Specifically, longitudinal studies suggest that victims score, on average, in the moderately depressed range on self-report measures of depression at one month postrape and in the mildly depressed or nondepressed range by one year postrape.[12,27-29]

Fear and Anxiety

Both fear and anxiety are also common symptoms among rape victims. Fears can either relate specifically to the rape, such as fear of men, or involve more general fears. Several symptoms of anxiety overlap with the diagnosis of PTSD, including difficulty concentrating and avoidance of situations due to anxiety, and this overlap is not surprising because PTSD is itself an anxiety disorder. Most studies have assessed anxiety through self-report measures, although some investigators have assessed whether victims meet the criteria for anxiety-related disorders other than PTSD, such as generalized anxiety disorder (GAD), panic disorder, phobic disorder, and obsessive compulsive disorder.

Studies with Comparison Groups

Studies that have assessed short-term reactions to rape have found differences between victims and nonvictims on fear measures for up to one year postrape, particularly on a measure of rape-related fear.[22,23] Another study found that rape victims reported higher levels of fear than victims of 4 other crimes—domestic assault, nondomestic assault, robbery, and burglary—at both 1 and 6 months postcrime.[30]

Longitudinal studies that compared recent victims and nonvictims on self-report measures of anxiety, as opposed to fear, found that victims score higher than nonvictims[23] for up to 12 months postrape. They also score higher than victims of other crimes until one month postrape.[30] In a cross-sectional study, Gidycz et al also reported differences between victims assaulted within the past 9 weeks and nonvictims.[24] One study that assessed the prevalence of diagnosable anxiety disorders other than PTSD among recent victims in comparison to nonvictims found higher rates of GAD in victims (82%) than in nonvictims (32%), although there were no differences in the prevalence of phobic disorder.[18]

Studies Without Comparison Groups

Studies in which anxiety and fear measures have been administered to groups of recent victims without comparing victims' scores either to those of a comparison group or to nonvictim norms indicate that victims score higher than nonvictims in other studies.[12,20,28]

Using a nonstandard measure, Becker et al assessed symptoms among 20 rape victims at one year postassault.[31] Most (80%) reported fear of being alone; 75% reported fear of being indoors, outdoors, or in crowds; and 55% reported fear of people behind them.

Social Adjustment and Interpersonal Functioning

The impact of sexual assault on social adjustment and interpersonal functioning has also received some research attention. The areas of social adjustment assessed include work adjustment, interpersonal relationships, and social and leisure activities. Investigators have assessed social adjustment through self-report measures and structured interviews.

Studies with Comparison Groups

Two studies have examined social adjustment among victim and nonvictim comparison groups within one year postrape. The first study assessed role performance in several major areas of interpersonal functioning (ie, work; economic; social and leisure activities; relationships with extended family members; roles as a spouse, parent, and family member) at 6 points, from 2 weeks to 12 months postrape.[32] Victims reported more adjustment problems (collapsing across role areas) than nonvictims for the first 2 months postrape. At 4 months postrape, victims continued to show more impairment in extended family relationships than did the comparison group. The other study[33] assessed social adjustment among victims and nonvictims using a measure of self-esteem in 8 life domains (self, others, children, authority, work, reality, parents, and hope) at 7 time points, from 2 weeks to 2 years postrape. On the total scale, victims reported lower self-esteem than nonvictims through the 6-month assessment. The only domain in which victims differed from nonvictims at 2 years postrape was family relationship problems, such as the quality of relationships with parents.

Studies Without Comparison Groups

Frank et al assessed social adjustment in 4 specific role areas: work, household, external family, and social/leisure activities as well as overall social functioning among victims recruited from rape crisis centers.[27-29] One interesting finding was that victims who were able to testify in court had lower work adjustment scores at 6 months postrape than those who wanted, but were unable, to have their case prosecuted.[27] In a more recent study, victims' social adjustment scores were similar to those of norm groups at 3 months postrape.[16]

Health Problems

A growing body of research suggests that a history of sexual assault is associated with poorer physical and mental health. Most of these studies have focused on long-term health problems, including perceptions of poor health, various health problems, and medical service utilization.

Studies with Comparison Groups

Few studies have assessed short-term health problems in victims in comparison to nonvictims. In one longitudinal study, victims and nonvictims were compared from 2 weeks to one year postrape in terms of physical symptoms, perceived health, and physician visits.[34] Victims differed from nonvictims on all 3 measures at 4 months postrape. At one year postrape, victims still reported more physician visits than nonvictims. The most common physical symptoms reported by victims were tension headaches, stomachache or nausea, and back pain. Another study examined physical health status among homeless women who had been raped in the past year in comparison to homeless women who had not been raped.[35] Compared to nonvictims, homeless women who had been raped were more likely to report fair or poor health, at least one current physical health limitation, and at least 2 gynecological symptoms and 2 serious physical health symptoms in the past year.

Studies Without Comparison Groups

Norris and Feldman-Summers asked women who had been raped an average of 3 years previously about the symptoms that they had experienced within the 6 months following the rape.[36] With regard to physical symptoms, 18% reported cystitis, 29% reported menstrual irregularity, and 40% reported headaches.

Substance Abuse

Several studies have assessed the prevalence of alcohol and drug abuse among victims, typically in comparison to nonvictims. Some used structured diagnostic interviews to assess whether participants meet the criteria for substance abuse disorders outlined in the

DSM, ie, substance abuse and substance dependence. A key feature of these disorders is a maladaptive pattern of substance abuse leading to clinically significant impairment or distress. Other investigators have used self-report measures of alcohol and drug use.

Studies with Comparison Groups

Several studies have compared victims and nonvictims in terms of substance abuse within one year postassault using very different kinds of samples. In the earliest study, Frank and Anderson[18] recruited victims from a rape crisis center and found no differences between victims and a matched comparison group in terms of previous diagnoses of alcohol or drug abuse or in terms of alcohol abuse after the assault; however, victims were more likely to have met the diagnostic criteria for drug abuse after the assault (28%) than were nonvictims (3%). Similarly, among a sample of homeless women, when several demographic variables were controlled, victims were more likely to report a lifetime diagnosis of drug abuse/dependence and reported more current drug use but did not differ from nonvictims in terms of lifetime alcohol abuse/dependence or current alcohol use.[35] Among a sample of female sorority members on a college campus, those who had unwanted sexual experiences scored higher than nonvictims on measures of alcohol use, alcohol-related negative consequences, and symptoms of alcohol dependence.[26] Whether the alcohol problems came before or after the assault was unclear. Finally, in a large national sample of 16- to 20-year-old females, having experienced attempted or actual forced sex was associated with binge drinking and recent marijuana use.[37]

Kilpatrick et al[38] specifically addressed the issue of the timing of substance abuse relative to an assault (either physical or sexual) using data from the National Women's Study, which involved phone interviews with a national household probability sample of over 4000 women. They found that using drugs or drugs and alcohol was associated with increased risk of assault over a 2-year time span and that having experienced an assault during the 2-year time span increased the risk of alcohol and drug abuse. In other words, abusing drugs appeared to lead to subsequent assaults, and assaults appeared to lead to drug abuse in a reciprocal relationship. Alcohol abuse, on the other hand, appeared to result from having been assaulted sexually or physically.

Studies Without Comparison Groups

No studies were located that assessed substance abuse in recent victims without the use of a comparison group.

Long-Term Effects

Posttraumatic Stress Disorder

Several studies have assessed the prevalence of PTSD diagnoses among nonrecent victims of sexual assault in comparison to victims of other traumas. The current and lifetime PTSD prevalence rates for victims of sexual assault differ widely across these studies as a function of the nature of the samples and the ways in which sexual assault is defined.

Studies with Comparison Groups

At least 2 studies have assessed PTSD among large representative samples of women using behaviorally specific questions to assess completed rape, which is an experience involving nonconsent, force or threat of force, and penetration.[39,40] In these 2 studies the lifetime prevalence of PTSD ranged from 32% to 57%, and the current PTSD prevalence rates ranged from 12% to 17% among rape victims.

Lifetime and current PTSD prevalence rates vary widely across other studies that have not used behaviorally specific questions, have used a broad definition of sexual assault, or have used nonrepresentative samples. Specifically, lifetime PTSD prevalence rates have varied from 4% to 80%,[41-43] and current PTSD prevalence rates have varied from 3% to 76%.[44-48] Several studies suggest that current and lifetime rates of PTSD following rape, or sexual assault defined more broadly, are higher than the PTSD rates associated with other traumatic events.[39-42]

Other investigators have assessed the severity of PTSD symptoms among nonrecent victims in comparison to nonvictims without determining whether all criteria for the diagnosis of PTSD are met. Using a variety of samples, symptom measures, and definitions of sexual assault, these studies have consistently shown that victims of sexual assault report more symptoms of PTSD than do nonvictims.[46,49-52] Other studies have found that sexual assault victims generally report more symptoms of PTSD than do victims of other traumas.[53,54]

Studies Without Comparison Groups

Studies assessing the prevalence of PTSD among nonrecent sexual assault victims without comparison to nonvictim groups have yielded PTSD prevalence rates ranging from 23% to 77%.[55,56] For example, in a large community sample of women who had been sexually assaulted as adults, 70% met criteria for PTSD.[56]

Studies that assess PTSD symptoms among nonrecent victims have also reported higher scores among victims than among nonpatient norm groups.[15,57-59] However, in a longitudinal study in which victims were assessed at 3 months and 2 years postassault, there was a highly significant decrease in PTSD symptoms over time, such that rape victims' scores were similar to those of norm groups at 2 years postassault.[16]

Depression

Studies with Comparison Groups

Studies comparing the prevalence of depressive diagnoses among nonvictims and victims assaulted more than one year previously consistently have shown higher rates of depression among victims than nonvictims. For example, studies that have used structured interviews to assess MDD/MDE according to some versions of the DSM generally show that victims of sexual assault (variously defined) have higher rates of MDD than do nonvictims.[43,44,50,60,61] The rates of MDD for victims in these studies ranged from 12% to 33% (versus 0% to 16% for nonvictims). Studies that have assessed the prevalence of various mood disorders (including major depression, bipolar disorder, and dysthymia) also find higher rates among abused (48%) than among nonabused females (27%).[52] Studies that have assessed depressive symptoms using methods other than structured interviews also reported higher rates of depressive diagnoses among victims than nonvictims.[35,48,62] Rates of depression among these studies ranged from 41% to 70% for rape victims and 29% to 46% for nonvictims. The overall rates of depression were high in these latter studies because they included samples of inpatients, outpatients, and homeless women.

Other studies have compared nonrecent victims to nonvictims using standardized self-report measures of depression. Virtually all of these studies found that victims scored significantly higher than nonvictims on these measures of depressive symptoms.[51,54,63-67]

Several studies have also reported data on suicidal thoughts and attempts, which are symptoms of depression. These studies have consistently shown higher rates of suicidal thoughts and attempts among women who have been assaulted than among those who have not been assaulted.[68] For example, in a large sample of adolescents, 39% of the girls who had been raped had attempted suicide compared to 13% of those who had not been raped.[69] Research that addresses the timing of the attempt relative to the assault suggests that most attempts came after the assault.[70]

Studies Without Comparison Groups

Studies assessing depression among victims more than one year postrape without using comparison groups also reported significant levels of depression among victims. For example, victims score higher than nonpatient norm groups[15,71] and similar to outpatient norm groups.[15,58] Mean depression scores tend to be in the mild to moderate range.[72,73] Rape victims also tend to score higher than victims of other traumas on depression measures.[74] Among studies that use nonstandard measures, 50% to 80% of victims reported having been depressed as a result of the rape,[36,75,76] and 11% reported a suicide attempt.[77]

Fear and Anxiety

Studies with Comparison Groups

Although studies of recent victims yield consistent evidence that victims differ from nonvictims on fear measures for up to one year postrape, studies assessing long-term fear reactions have yielded inconsistent results. For example, Santiago and colleagues[78] found that victims who had been assaulted from 2 to 46 years previously scored higher than nonvictims on a fear measure, but 2 other studies found no differences between victims and nonvictims on fear scores several years postrape.[63,79]

Studies assessing differences between nonrecent victims and nonvictims on anxiety—as opposed to fear—measures have also produced rather varied results. Several studies have found differences between victims and nonvictims on various self-report measures of anxiety, with victims scoring significantly higher than nonvictims[49,51,64,67]; however, several other studies have found no differences between victims and nonvictims on self-report anxiety measures.[54,59,80] Frazier and Schauben also found no differences between victims of rape and other stressors on an anxiety measure.[74]

Studies assessing the prevalence of various diagnosable anxiety disorders among nonrecent victims and nonvictims also have yielded somewhat mixed results. Several studies have found higher rates of anxiety disorders among victims than nonvictims, including having been diagnosed with any anxiety disorder,[42,48,81] panic disorder,[43,60] phobic disorder,[60,61] and obsessive-compulsive disorder.[43,60] Another study only found differences between women victimized as both children and adults and comparison groups in terms of generalized anxiety disorder (GAD) and phobic disorders.[44] A few studies have found no differences between victims and nonvictims in terms of panic disorder[44,50] and GAD.[43]

Studies Without Comparison Groups

Studies that have compared fear scores among nonrecent rape victims to published norms suggest high levels of fear among rape victims. For example, Cohen and Roth[71] reported that victims scored higher than nonvictims on general and rape-related fear and anxiety measure several years postrape. Other studies suggest that fear scores in treatment-seeking samples assessed pretreatment are more than one standard deviation above nonvictim norm group means.[58,82] Finally, studies that have assessed fear and anxiety among victims more than one year postrape using nonstandard measures have also found high levels of fear among victims. For example, in one study, 83% of victims reported that they had experienced fear of being alone since the rape, and 49% reported that they were still fearful several years postrape.[75] Finally, 53% of the victims in another study reported being tense, nervous, or anxious as a result of the assault.[76]

Social Adjustment Problems

Studies with Comparison Groups

Studies that have assessed longer-term impairment in social adjustment among rape victims in comparison to nonvictims generally do not find differences between groups on global measures of social adjustment[42,79] or fear of intimacy.[65] Another study found significant differences between victims and nonvictims only in terms of family problems.[63]

Studies Without Comparison Groups

In studies of the long-term effects of rape on social adjustment without comparison groups, one found that victims scored significantly below standardized norms for women,[71] whereas another found that the rape victim group was within one standard deviation of norm group means.[16] Using nonstandard measures, Burgess and Holmstrom[77] reported that 59% of the victims in their sample, who had been raped an average of 4 to 6 years previously, reported disruptions in their relationships after the rape. Thus, the findings regarding the effects of rape on social adjustment are fairly mixed.

Health Problems

Studies with Comparison Groups

Golding et al have published several papers comparing victims and nonvictims, identified via large-scale population surveys, on various indicators of physical health. In these studies, sexual assault is generally defined as pressured or forced sexual contact as a child or adult. These studies indicate that, in comparison to nonvictims, victims report poorer health, more physical symptoms of various kinds, more physical limitations, more chronic diseases, and more physician visits.[83-86] With regard to particular symptoms, victims report more headaches, reproductive and sexual health problems, pain, premenstrual distress, and gastrointestinal, cardiopulmonary, and neurological problems.[83-85,87] Other investigators have replicated Golding's findings, with victims reporting more health problems in general, more gynecological problems, more sick days, more physician visits, and more health risk behaviors, such as smoking or driving after drinking, than nonvictims.[45,55,88,89]

Other studies have assessed the prevalence of victimization experiences among women who have a specific medical problem in comparison to women who do not have the medical problem (vs. comparing victims and nonvictims in terms of the prevalence of a specific medical problem). For example, there is a higher prevalence of sexual assault among women who are HIV-positive than among women who are HIV-negative[90,91]; among women with gynecological or breast problems (48%) than among women seeking routine care (24%)[92]; and among women referred for laparoscopy for chronic medically unexplained pelvic pain than among women referred for laparoscopy for other reasons, like tubal ligation or infertility evaluation.[93]

Studies Without Comparison Groups

Only one well-known study exists of the long-term health effects of sexual assault that did not have a comparison group.[57] In this study, all the women were seeking treatment for rape-related sleep disturbances. At least 50% of the sample reported 16 of the 54 symptoms assessed, with headaches (86%), upset stomach (75%), and back pain (70%) being most common.

Substance Abuse

Studies with Comparison Groups

Most studies that compare victims to nonvictims in terms of the prevalence of substance abuse or dependence have found that victims are more likely to meet diagnostic criteria for these disorders than are nonvictims.[48,81,94] Rates of substance abuse range from 16% to 33% in the victim groups and 1% to 24% in the nonvictim groups. Studies that assess drinking or drug use without assessing diagnosable substance abuse disorders also find links between victimization and substance use. For example, using data from the National Violence Against Women Survey, Kaukinen and DeMaris[66] examined the relations among both adolescent and adult sexual assault and heavy drinking and illicit drug use. Adolescent sexual assault was associated with illicit drug use but not heavy drinking. Adult sexual assault was related to illicit drug use and heavy drinking but only for minority women. In minority women, the odds of heavy drinking and illicit drug use were 3 to 4 times higher for victims than for nonvictims. Women who have experienced more than one sexual victimization appear to be particularly at risk for substance abuse.[81,95] For example, in the McFarlane et al study, women who had experienced more than one sexual assault were 3.5 times more likely to report beginning or increasing substance use compared to women who reported only one sexual assault. Only women who reported more than one sexual assault reported illicit drug use, which was most often crack or cocaine.

Studies Without Comparison Groups

Studies that report rates of substance abuse disorders among victims without reporting data from comparison groups also indicate that victims of sexual assault have high rates of substance abuse disorders. For example, using data from the large-scale National Comorbidity Survey, Ullman and Brecklin reported that 38% of adult sexual assault victims met criteria for alcohol dependence.[96] This is a higher rate than any of the comparison groups in the previously reviewed studies.

Other Effects

Although PTSD, depression, fear and anxiety, social adjustment problems, health problems, and substance abuse are the most commonly studied effects of rape, there are some additional effects of rape that represent either new or smaller areas of research. Studies assess long-term effects unless otherwise stated.

Risky Sexual Behaviors

Several studies have found that victims of sexual assault reported engaging in more risky sexual behaviors (eg, report more lifetime sexual partners, more current sexual partners) than women who have not experienced sexual assault. This has been found among large national samples of female adolescents[97] and college women,[88] female veterans,[45] and urban American Indian/Alaska Native women.[98] One study of a national sample of 16- to 20-year-old females, most of whom had been assaulted within the past year, also found that those who had experienced attempted or actual forced sex were much more likely to have engaged in sex without birth control in the past 30 days.[37] Thus, sexual assault may have both short- and long-term effects on risky sexual behavior. Finally, in an interesting approach, Campbell, Sefl, and Ahrens[99] identified 3 groups of assault survivors who differed in terms of postrape risky sexual behaviors based on their self-reported sexual behaviors before and after the assault. About one-third (34%) of the sample fell into the high-risk group, in which they reported more sexual activity and partners, less condom use, and more alcohol use after the rape. This group also had more physical and psychological problems. Almost half (48%) of the sample was in a low-risk group who reported less frequent sex after the rape. The rest of the sample was in a moderate risk group who reported more sex but also more condom use and less frequent alcohol use during sex.

Eating Disordered Behavior

A few studies have reported associations between sexual assault and eating disordered behavior. For example, in a large sample of high school girls, having experienced date violence or rape was associated with significantly higher rates of binge eating, fasting or skipping meals, taking diet pills, vomiting, and taking laxatives.[69] Similarly, rates of eating disorders were higher among women who had been sexually assaulted as adults (29%) than among those with no sexual assault history (8%).[81] Those who had been assaulted as children and adults had the highest prevalence rate of eating disorders (52%).

Costs of Rape

Two studies have broadened the assessment of the effects of rape to include what they call resource loss, eg, income loss and relationship loss. The first study involved a nationally representative sample of women who were assessed at baseline and at 2 one-year follow-ups.[100] Women who experienced a physical or sexual assault after the first assessment were more likely to fall into poverty, become divorced, and become unemployed than those not experiencing interpersonal violence. Following up on this study, Monnier, Resnick, Kilpatrick, and Seals[101] examined resource loss among recent rape victims and found that 36% of the survivors had lost a job, 21% had had a relationship breakup, and 7% reported a serious illness between 6 weeks and 3 months postassault. Victims who were more distressed at 6 weeks postrape were more likely to experience resource loss.

While these 2 studies focus on costs to the victim, other studies have tried to calculate the costs of sexual assault to society. For example, Post and colleagues[102] estimated the cost of rape based on lost productivity, medical care/ambulance costs, mental health care services, police/fire services, social/victim services, property loss/damages, and effects on quality of life. Their estimated costs were $94 000 per incident for rapes/sexual assaults in the United States and $108 000 per incident for the state of Michigan in 1996. Total costs for sexual assaults, including rapes, in Michigan in 1996 were estimated to be $6 678 000, which would amount to an almost $700 per year rape tax for every person in Michigan. Focusing on medical costs in female veterans, having a sexual assault history was associated with a significant increase in cost for all medical services as well as psychiatric and ER visits.[48] For example, for all health care services combined, average health care costs for female veterans without a sexual assault history were about $10 061 per year, compared to about $17 689 for female veterans with histories of nonmilitary sexual assault. This is particularly important because only about one-third of the sample did not have a sexual assault history.

Positive Life Change

Although the previously reviewed studies clearly point to the detrimental effects of rape on victims and society, there is also research suggesting that a sexual assault can lead to positive changes in victims' lives. For example, in one study, 57% of female victims reported on an open-ended question that the rape had caused some positive change in their life at 3 days postrape.[103] The most frequent positive change, reported by 22% of the sample, was that they were now more cautious (eg, "It taught me to be more cautious and alert"). Other positive life changes included greater life appreciation, positive changes in relationships, reevaluating life and goals, and becoming more assertive.

Studies that have assessed positive and negative life changes more systematically have found that 91% of sexual assault survivors described at least one positive life change that resulted from the assault at 2 weeks postrape.[13] The most common positive changes at both 2 weeks and 12 weeks postassault were more concern for others in similar situations, better relationships with family, greater appreciation of life, and greater ability to recognize strengths; however, 95% also reported negative life changes 2 weeks following the assault. The most common negative changes were with regard to mental health and beliefs about the safety and fairness of the world. Similar positive and negative life changes were common among nonrecent victims.[104] In this sample of women assaulted an average of 16 years previously, increased empathy for others in similar situations was the most commonly reported positive change (78%), followed by increased assertiveness (60%) and a greater ability to recognize strengths (61%). Finally, a substantial proportion of the sample reported negative changes in beliefs about the fairness and safety of the world (44% to 48%) and in mental health (44%). Other studies report positive changes in self, relationships, life philosophy, and empathy, and increased involvement in social or political action[105] and increased spirituality.[106]

Male Victims and Gender Differences

Although it is generally difficult to accurately identify incidence or prevalence rates for sexual assault, it is especially difficult with male victims because this crime is so often hidden. While estimates vary greatly, it is widely acknowledged that male victims, even more so than female victims, do not seek help or report the crime to law enforcement. In a stratified random sample of the general population, Elliott et al[51] found 3.8% of the men surveyed were sexually assaulted as an adult. The National Violence Against Women Survey reported a 0.8% prevalence rate in 1998[107] and a significantly higher rate of 2.8% in 2006.[108] In a survey of men seeking counseling services, out of 115 male victims of rape, 15% had reported to law enforcement, and 79% sought no help after the assault.[109] At the Sexual Assault Resource Service (SARS) in Minneapolis between June 2006 and June 2007, 27 male victims were seen, which represents 5% of all sexual assault victims seen by SARS. The male victims were injured 53% of the time, compared to 27% of the female victims seen. Unfortunately, data are not available on the percentage of these male victims who came to the hospital because of concerns about injuries but did not initially report the assault (Ledray, unpublished data). Another study reported somewhat higher rates of injury in male (46%) than female (34%) victims of acquaintance rape.[110] In addition, 6% of these men were admitted to the hospital as a result of the rape, while none of the female victims required hospital admission.

Access to research and understanding of the impact of sexual assault on male victims is more limited than with female sexual assault victims. In reviewing the limited literature on the impact of male sexual assault, a number of studies were not included because they did not distinguish among the impact of child sexual abuse, physical abuse, and sexual abuse after 17 years of age. It is also likely that the few studies included are evaluating a somewhat different population of adult male victims because the victims were identified after they went to a hospital for care of physical injuries and, thus, may involve more violent rapes. Studies completed in Canada and Great Britain are included in this section because of the small number of studies overall.

Immediate Reactions

The studies of the immediate reactions of male rape victims were focused on populations seen at hospital sexual assault nurse examiner (SANE) programs. The first compared 74 male victims to 1380 female rape victims seen by a SANE program. The male victims were more depressed and more hostile than the female victims immediately after the rape but did not differ on anxiety.[111]

The second study is included, though it was conducted in Canada. In this study, records were reviewed for 29 male victims, 7% of the total number of rape victims seen at a hospital sexual assault program.[112] Although the authors report that "emotional trauma was evident in the initial presentation of the clients at the crisis unit in the majority of the cases (59%, N=17)," they do not indicate what trauma was evident or how this was determined.[112] They also reported that the emotional trauma following the rapes resulted in 2 of the male victims' being admitted to the hospital. Unfortunately, more details were not provided, and it does not appear that any standardized measures were used.

Long-term Effects

Posttraumatic Stress Disorder

Few studies have examined the prevalence of PTSD in male victims. The studies that do exist suggest that PTSD diagnoses and symptoms are common. In the National Comorbidity Study of 5877 adults,[41] 0.7% of men and 9.2% of women reported having been raped. For both men and women, rape was most likely to be nominated as their worst lifetime event if more than one event had been experienced. For both men and women, rape was also more likely to lead to PTSD than any other event if nominated as the worst event. For example, 65% of the men and 46% of the women who said rape was their worst event met criteria for a diagnosis of PTSD. In a much smaller study, 9 of 22 (41%) male rape victims referred to a British Forensic Psychiatric service were diagnosed with PTSD. The assaults occurred an average of 6 years previously.[113]

Elliott et al[51] compared PTSD symptoms in 469 male victims of adult sexual assault (ASA) to those of 472 female ASA victims and to adults not victimized as adults (non-ASA), identified in a stratified random sample of the general population. The male ASA victims reported more symptoms of intrusion, avoidance, and dissociation than did female ASA victims. Both groups scored higher than nonvictims. Among a sample of 40 male rape victims recruited from advertisements in the United Kingdom,[114] the majority reported symptoms of PTSD. For example, 93% reported flashbacks, 85% reported emotional distancing, and 75% reported intrusive thoughts.

Depression

Symptoms of depression are also common among male victims. For example, depression was the most frequently reported symptom (98%) in the Walker et al study.[114] In the Elliott et al[51] study described above, both the male and female ASA victims reported more depression than the non-ASA victims, and the male ASA victims were more depressed than the female ASA victims. Finally, male veterans who had been sexually assaulted as adults reported more depression and had poorer mental health than nonvictims.[115]

Anxiety and Fear

Elliott et al[51] found that both male and female victims of ASA were more anxious than non-ASA individuals and that male ASA victims were more anxious than female ASA victims. Anxiety (93%) and fear of being alone with men (83%) were reported by nearly all male victims in the Walker et al study.[115]

Hostility

Although the differences were not statistically significant, Elliott et al[51] found that both male and female ASA victims were more angry and irritable than individuals who had not experienced ASA and that male ASA victims reported more anger than female victims. In the Walker et al[115] study, the second most common response, reported by nearly all (95%) male victims, was fantasies about revenge and retaliation. Some reported fantasizing about killing the perpetrator and one reported he actually bought a knife but could not go through with killing the perpetrator. Slightly fewer (80%) reported increased anger and irritability.

Impact on Sexuality

In the Walker et al[115] study, long-term sexual identity crises were reported by 70% of the male victims and damaged masculine identity was reported by 68%. Some of the men reported confusion and disgust about their sexual response during the rape. Several reported getting erections and ejaculating during the rape. These men reported that although sex had been pleasurable for them before the rape, after experiencing an erection or ejaculation during the rape they were disgusted at the thought of sex and by their response. One heterosexual man thought this response must mean that he was actually homosexual and had not been aware of it before the rape. He reported being confused for a long time after the rape. Several men reported changes in their sexual behavior after the assault. Some became promiscuous, while others refused to have sex with men or women for a considerable time after the assault.

With regard to gender differences, Elliott et al[51] found that male ASA victims were more symptomatic than female ASA victims on dysfunctional sexual behaviors, sexual concerns, and impaired self-reference.

Although these 2 studies suggest that impaired sexuality is an important issue for many male victims, another study found that only 12% of male ASA victims reported sexual problems as a result of the assault. Slightly more (16%) of the child sexual assault victims reported sexual problems as adults.[116]

Substance Abuse and Self-Harming Behaviors

Drug abuse and other self-harming behaviors also appear to be common among male victims. In the Walker et al[115] study, abuse of drugs was reported by 53%, alcohol abuse by 63%, and increased use of tobacco by 68%. Self-harming behaviors were reported by 50% and nearly half (48%) reported a suicide attempt.

In another British study, 3% of patients of general practitioners reported having been sexually assaulted compared to 18% of male patients attending a genitourinary medicine.[116] Of these, 23% reported substance abuse and 18% reported self-harming behaviors. They also identified 150 patients who had been victims of sexual abuse as children. Twenty-three percent of the child sexual abuse victims reported self-harming behaviors, and 23% reported substance abuse.[116]

Other Effects

The Walker et al[115] study also identified that male victims often reported a loss of self-respect (90%), increased sense of vulnerability (90%), guilt and self-blame for not being able to prevent the rape (82.5%), and impaired performance (70%).

Summary

On the most general level, there is considerable agreement across studies that victims report more psychological distress than nonvictims, particularly in the first year following the assault. Victims report more symptoms of PTSD, depression, fear, and anxiety; more social adjustment and health problems; more substance abuse than nonvictims; and more symptoms of PTSD than victims of other traumatic events. In terms of prevalence, these symptoms also are common among victims of rape. A meta-analysis of research on psychological distress associated with interpersonal violence reported an effect size of .21 for the effects of rape across 38 studies. This indicates that, on average, there is a 21% increase in the prevalence of psychological distress in rape victims compared to nonvictims.[117]

There are, however, some areas of disagreement in the research literature that also need to be mentioned. First, studies that have assessed the lifetime prevalence of PTSD among rape victims report estimates varying from 4% to 80%. Part of this variability may be due to differences in how rape/sexual assault is defined. As mentioned, studies that use strict definitions of rape tend to produce higher estimates of PTSD while those that use broader definitions produce lower PTSD estimates. Second, although there is agreement across studies that victims report more depressive symptoms, social adjustment problems, and health problems than do nonvictims, cross-sectional and longitudinal studies tend to produce different results in terms of the duration of these differences. For example, although several studies have found that victims report more depressive symptoms several years postrape than nonvictims, longitudinal studies have found that victims do not differ from nonvictims past 2 months postrape. This may be partly because victims in longitudinal studies improve more rapidly than other victims. To address this issue, Atkeson et al[21] compared victims who participated in one assessment with victims who completed repeated assessments and found that those in the repeated assessment group improved more quickly. It may also be the case that individuals who volunteer to participate in a research study several years postrape are those who continue to be distressed; therefore, these studies of long-term effects show significant differences between victims and nonvictims.

With regard to gender differences, female victims are more likely than male victims to seek help and report rape. The few studies on male victims suggest that sexual victimization may be especially trauma-producing for men. As Elliott et al[51] pointed out, our society expects men to be strong and aggressive and to avoid any—even forced—sexual contact with other men. When they are raped, it may be especially traumatic to their sense of self-identity and sexuality.

Clinical Implications

Because victims who experience more distress immediately postrape are at higher risk for distress later on,[3] it is very important for ER staff to do everything possible to ease that distress and to avoid secondary victimization.[10] The clinician treating the sexual assault survivor in the ER or clinic needs to be aware of the significant psychological impact likely to result. Knowing this, the clinician can normalize this response by letting the victim know it is common to experience intrusive thoughts of the rape, nightmares, difficulty concentrating, hypervigilance, and difficulty returning to work or school and socializing with friends, and that symptoms may peak at 3 to 4 weeks postassault.[17]

Suggesting that victims take a few days off from work or school after the rape is often helpful. This suggestion can reduce any potential self-blame or shame for not being able to go on with life as usual immediately, which is an unrealistic but not uncommon expectation among victims or their friends or family. It can also be helpful to recommend that they let someone they trust know what happened at their work or school in case they have trouble performing up to their usual standard. They do not need to know the details; victims can decide to disclose that they were attacked but not raped, or that they needed emergency medical care. Employers and schools can be very helpful in accommodating the needs of the survivor, but they are understandably more likely to be willing to make these accommodations if they are made aware of the issue before problems arise. Schools and universities will sometimes allow survivors to delay exams or even take time off and return when they are more comfortable and capable without suffering serious consequences. Additional trauma and long-lasting work or career consequences should be prevented. Anticipating these very common responses and taking additional steps to minimize the consequences is as important as the initial emergency care.

Because depression and sleep disturbances, such as nightmares, are also common, it can be helpful to provide the sexual assault survivor with sleep aids for the first few days. Although the abuse of drugs and alcohol needs to be assessed and discouraged, it also is important to recognize that sleep aids can be helpful. This is true with providing pain medications for injuries as well.

Most medical records today prevent the clinician who might see the rape victim after the assault from having access to the record of the assault. Although this is done in an attempt to protect the victim's confidentiality, it also can prevent the clinician from having access to information that may be helpful in accurately diagnosing and treating resulting problems. The victim needs to know this information will not be readily available and needs to be strongly encouraged to disclose the assault to clinicians at subsequent visits, especially if there are concerns about sexually transmitted infections, pregnancy, eating problems, sexual issues, abdominal or vaginal pain, general malaise, or any other medical or psychological issue for which the cause is not readily apparent. This could avoid costly, invasive, and unnecessary medical evaluation and treatment.

Asking how the victim has responded during past crises can be helpful for both the provider and the victim to anticipate responses during this trauma. Recalling past effective coping strategies, as well as ineffective ones, may help victims decide to rely on the good and avoid the pitfalls after this assault. It can be helpful to talk these through at the end of the exam and to ask about referral needs. If the victim has seen a counselor in the past for any issue, it can be helpful to recommend that he or she reconnect with that trusted individual at least once before problems arise.

When the victim's current condition is a concern; if he or she is not oriented to person, place, and time; if his or her memory is not intact for recent or past events; or if he or she expresses any suicidal thoughts, it is essential to have a mental health professional perform an evaluation prior to discharge. Although many rape victims do express suicidal thoughts, most do not attempt suicide during the first few days. The immediate postrape period during the first few weeks or months can, however, be a dangerous time for victims.[118]

When the initial contact includes a sexual assault response team (SART), the advocate and the sexual assault nurse examiner (SANE) should both normalize these likely responses by letting victims know that they may experience some or many of them. They should also have information about what to do if that occurs and should know whom to call for help and whenever possible have the first appointment scheduled. If they need an order of protection, the clinician should know how to initiate that process and ensure that they have the information and help to start this process prior to discharge. It is important to know the local resources. Always offering to make the initial appointment when possible is helpful. When the local rape crisis center's or counseling center's number is unavailable, the Rape, Abuse and Incest National Network (RAINN) can be reached at the following number: 1-800-656-HOPE. RAINN's information can be accessed at www.rainn.org.

Getting victims' permission to have the follow-up counselor call them for the initial appointment is always preferable to waiting for victims to reach out for support. As the caregiver, it is important to remember that reaching out to an unknown resource is always more difficult than accepting help that is being offered.

Although rape is never a good thing, by becoming more cautious in the future, more assertive, more selective in relationships, and developing stronger, more effective boundaries, the ultimate result can be positive changes for the survivor. Rape brings about the realization that a profound change must be made. These changes may result in improved personal safety and empowerment.

Beyond following these guidelines, an additional way to decrease distress is to implement more structured interventions in the ER. Specifically, Resnick et al[3] have developed a 17-minute video that can be used in the ER to reduce distress regarding the forensic exam as well as later symptoms. In comparison to those who did not watch the video, victims who watched the video reported less distress and anxiety after the exam. More interventions like this need to be developed that can be delivered in the ER because many victims do not return for follow-up counseling.

If victims do seek treatment later, there are several effective interventions for reducing PTSD and other forms of distress. Bisson and Andrew[119] reviewed 33 studies of psychological treatments for PTSD, 12 of which involved primarily sexual female assault survivors. All studies were randomized controlled trials that compared one or more defined psychological treatments to a placebo or other control (eg, usual care or waiting list control) condition. They concluded that individual trauma-focused cognitive behavioral therapy (TFCBT), eye movement desensitization and reprocessing (EMDR), stress management, and group TFCBT are all effective in treating PTSD. Other non-trauma-focused psychological treatments (eg, supportive therapy, psychodynamic therapy) did not reduce PTSD symptoms as significantly. Individual TFCBT and EMDR were recommended as the treatments of choice.

Another review focused on pharmacological treatments for PTSD.[120] This review included 35 short-term randomized controlled trials in which medication treatments were compared to a placebo (active or nonactive) or other medication. Results indicated that a significantly larger proportion of patients responded to medication (59%) than to placebos (39%). They concluded that medications can be effective in reducing the core symptoms of PTSD. Although there is also no clear evidence that any particular class of medication is more effective or better tolerated than any other, the greatest number of trials showing efficacy to date, as well as the largest, have been with the selective serotonin reuptake inhibitors (SSRIs).

There are numerous resources available for clinicians wanting further information on responding to sexual assault survivors. One of the best resources is a book by Foa and Rothbaum[121] entitled *Treating the Trauma of Rape*. Their step-by-step guidelines for conducting various forms of cognitive-behavioral treatment for rape survivors are very helpful. Resick and Schnicke's[122] treatment manual is a step-by-step guide for cognitive processing therapy. The guidelines on the treatment of PTSD from the expert consensus guideline series are also very useful, especially for selecting treatment strategies,[123] which are also available on the World Wide Web at www.psychguides.com. The guidelines also contain a list of additional resources, such as the International Society for Traumatic Stress Studies, which has a comprehensive web site (www.istss.org). More condensed expert consensus guidelines on PTSD are also available.[124]

References

1. Roy-Byrne PP, Russo J, Michelson E, Zatzick D, Pitman RK, Berliner L. Risk factors and outcome in ambulatory assault victims presenting to the acute emergency department setting: implications for secondary prevention studies in PTSD. *Depression Anxiety*. 2004;19:77-84.

2. Koss MP. The underdetection of rape: methodological choices influence incidence estimates. *J Soc Issues*. 1992;48:61-75.
3. Resnick H, Acierno R, Holmes M, Kilpatrick DG, Jager N. Prevention of post-rape psychopathology: Preliminary findings of a controlled acute rape treatment study. *J Anxiety Disord*. 1999;13:359-370.
4. Burgess A, Holmstrom L. Rape trauma syndrome. *Am J Psychiatry*. 1974;131:981-986.
5. McCombie SL. Characteristics of rape victims seen in crisis intervention. *Smith Coll Stud Soc Work*. 1976;46:137-158.
6. Bletzer KV, Koss MP. After-rape among three populations in the southwest: a time of mourning, a time for recovery. *Violence Against Women*. 2006;12:5-29.
7. Ruch LO, Gartrell JW, Amedeo SR, Coyne BJ. The clinical trauma assessment: Evaluating sexual assault victims in the emergency room. *Psychol Assess*. 1991;3:405-411.
8. Ruch LO, Gartrell JW, Amedeo SR, Coyne BJ. The sexual assault symptom scale: Measuring self-reported sexual assault trauma in the emergency room. *Psychol Assess*. 1991;3:3-8.
9. Ruch L, Wang C. Validation of the Sexual Assault Symptom Scale II (SASS II) using a panel research design. *J Interpersonal Violence*. 2006;21:1440-1461.
10. Campbell R. Rape survivors' experiences with the legal and medical systems: Do rape victim advocates make a difference? *Violence Against Women*. 2006;12:30-45.
11. Foa E, Riggs D. Posttraumatic stress disorder following assault: theoretical considerations and empirical findings. *Curr Dir Psychol Sci*. 1995;4(2):61-65.
12. Rothbaum BO, Foa EB, Riggs DS. A prospective examination of post-traumatic stress disorder in rape victims. *J Trauma Stress*. 1992;5:449-456.
13. Frazier P, Conlon A, Glaser T. Positive and negative life changes following sexual assault. *J Consult Clin Psychol*. 2001;69:1048-1055.
14. Kramer T, Green B. Post-traumatic stress disorder as an early response to sexual assault. *J Interpersonal Violence*. 1991;6(2):160-173.
15. Burge S. Post-traumatic stress disorder in victims of rape. *J Trauma Stress*. 1988;1(2):193-210.
16. Koss M, Figueredo A. Change in cognitive mediators or rape's impact on psychosocoial health across 2 years of recover. *J Consult Clin Psychol*. 2004; 72(6):1063-1072.
17. Gilboa-Schechtman E, Foa E. Patterns of recovery from trauma: the use of intraindividual analysis. *J Abnorm Psychol*. 2001;110:392-400.
18. Frank E, Anderson B. Psychiatric disorders in rape victims: past history and current symptomatology. *Compr Psychiatry*. 1987;28(1):77-82.
19. Sorenson S, Golding J. Depressive sequelae of recent criminal victimization. *J Trauma Stress*. 1990;3(3):337-350.
20. Moss M, Frank E, Anderson B. The effects of marital status and partner support on rape trauma. *Am J Orthopsychiatry*. 1990;60:379-391.

21. Atkeson BM, Calhoun KS, Resick PA, Ellis EM. Victims of rape: repeated assessment of depressive symptoms. *J Consult Clin Psychol.* 1982;50:96-102.

22. Kilpatrick D, Resick P, Veronen L. Effects of a rape experience: a longitudinal study. *J Soc Issues.* 1981;37:105-122.

23. Kilpatrick D, Veronen L, Resick P. The aftermath of rape: recent empirical findings. *Am J Orthopsychiatry.* 1979;49:658-669.

24. Gidycz C, Coble C, Latham L, Layman M. Sexual assault experience in adulthood and prior victimization experiences: a prospective analysis. *Psychol Women Q.* 1993;17(2):151-168.

25. Stephenson H, Pena-Shaff J, Quirk P. Predictors of college student suicidal ideation: gender differences. *Coll Student J.* 2006;40(1):109-117.

26. Larimer M, Lydum A, Anderson B, Turner A. Male and female recipients of unwanted sexual contact in a college student sample: prevalence rates, alcohol use, and depression symptoms. *Sex Roles.* 1999;40(3-4):295-308.

27. Cluss P, Boughton J, Frank E, Stewart B, West B. The rape victim: psychological correlates of participation in the legal process. *Criminal Justice Behav.* 1983;10(3): 342-357.

28. Frank E, Turner S, Duffy B. Depressive symptoms in rape victims. *J Affective Disord.* 1979;1(4):269-277.

29. Stewart BD, Hughes C, Frank E, Anderson B. The aftermath of rape: profiles of immediate and delayed treatment seekers. *J Nervous Ment Dis.* 1987;175(2):90-94.

30. Wirtz P, Harrell A. Victim and crime characteristics, coping responses, and short and long term recovery from victimization. *J Consult Clin Psychol.* 1987;55(6):866-871.

31. Becker J, Skinner L, Abel G, Howell J, Bruce K. The effects of sexual assault on rape and attempted rape victims. *Victimology: An Int J.* 1982;7(1–4):106.

32. Resick P, Calhoun K, Atkeson B, Ellis E. Social adjustment in victims of sexual assault. *J Consult Clin Psychol.* 1981;49(5):705-712.

33. Murphy SM, Amick-McMullan AE, Kilpatrick DG, Haskett ME, Veronen LJ, Best CL, Saunders BE. Rape victims' self-esteem: a longitudinal analysis. *J Interpersonal Violence.*1988;3:355-370.

34. Kimerling R, Calhoun K. Somatic symptoms, social support, and treatment seeking among sexual assault victims. *J Consult Clin Psychol.* 1994;62(2):333-40.

35. Wenzel S, Leake B, Gelberg L. Health of homeless women with recent experience of rape. *J General Intern Med.* 2000;15(4):265-268.

36. Norris J, Feldman-Summers S. Factors related to the psychological impact of rape on the victim. *J Abnorm Psychol.* 1981;90(6):562-567.

37. Champion H, Foley K, DuRant R, Hensberry R, Altman D, Wolfson M. Adolescent sexual victimization, use of alcohol and other substances, and other health risk behaviors. *J Adolesc Health.* 2004;35:321-328.

38. Kilpatrick D, Acierno R, Resnick H, Saunders B, Best C. A 2-year longitudinal analysis of the relationships between violent assault and substance use in women. *J Consult Clin Psychol.* 1997;65(5):834-847.

39. Kilpatrick D, Saunders B, Veronen L, Best C, Von J. Criminal victimization: lifetime prevalence, reporting to police, and psychological impact. *Crime Delinquency.* 1987;33:479-489.

40. Resnick HS, Kilpatrick DG, Dansky BS, Saunders BE, Best CL. Prevalence of civilian trauma and posttraumatic stress disorder in a representative national sample of women. *J Consult Clin Psychol.* 1993;61:984-991.

41. Kessler R, Sonnega A, Bromet E, Hughes M, Nelson C. Posttraumatic stress disorder in the national comorbidity survey. *Arch Gen Psychiatry.* 1995;52(12): 1048-1060.

42. Krupnick JL, Green BL, Stockton P, Goodman L, Corcoran C, Petty R. Mental health effects of adolescent trauma exposure in a female college sample: exploring differenctial outcomes based on experiences of unique trauma types and dimensions. *Psychiatry.* 2004;67(3):264-279.

43. Winfield I, George LK, Swartz M, Blazer DG. Sexual assault and psychiatric disorders among a community sample of women. *Am J Psychiatry.* 1990;147:335-341.

44. Cloitre M, Scarvalone P, Difede J. Posttraumatic stress disorder, self- and interpersonal dysfunction among sexually retraumatized women. *J Trauma Stress.* 1997;10:437-452.

45. Lang AJ, Rodgers CS, Loffaye C, Satz LE, Dresselhaus TR, Stein MB. Sexual trauma, posttraumatic stress disorder, and health behavior. *Behav Med.* 2003;28: 150-158.

46. Layman MJ, Gidycz CA, Lynn SJ. Unacknowledged versus acknowledged rape victims: situational factors and posttraumatic stress. *J Abnorm Psychol.* 1997;105: 124-131.

47. Norris FH. Epidemiology of trauma: Frequency and impact of different potentially traumatic events on different demographic groups. *J Consult Clin Psychol.* 1992;60: 409-418.

48. Suris A, Linda L, Kashner M, Borman P, Petty F. Sexual assault in women veterans: an examination of PTSD risk, health care uilization, and cost of care. *Psychosomatic Med.* 2004;66:749-756.

49. Briere J, Elliott DM, Harris K, Cotman A. Trauma Symptom Inventory: psychometrics and association with childhood and adult victimization in clinical samples. *J Interpersonal Violence.* 1995;10(4):387-401.

50. Davidson JRT, Hughes DC, George LK, Blazer DG. The association of sexual assault and attempted suicide within the community. *Arch Gen Psychiatry.* 1996;53:550-555.

51. Elliott D, Mok D, Briere J. Adult sexual assault: prevalence, symptomatology, and sex differences in the general population. *J Trauma Stress.* 2004;17:203-211.

52. Hutchings P, Dutton M. Symptom severity and diagnoses related to sexual assault history. *J Anxiety Disord.* 1997;11(6):607-618.

53. Kaltman S, Krupnick J, Stockton P, Hooper L, Green B. Psychological impact of types of sexual trauma among college women. *J Trauma Stress.* 2005;18(5):547-555.

54. Vrana S, Lauterbach D. Prevalence of traumatic events and post-traumatic psychological symptoms in a nonclinical sample of college students. *J Trauma Stress*. 1994;7:289-302.

55. Conoscenti L, McNally R. Health complaints in acknowledged and unacknowledged rape victims. *J Anxiety Disord.* 2006;20(3):372-379.

56. Ullman S, Filipas H, Townsend S, Starzynski L. Trauma exposure, posttraumatic stress disorder and problem drinking in sexual assault survivors. *J Stud Alcohol.* 2005;66(5):610-619.

57. Clum GA, Nishith P, Resick PA. Trauma-related sleep distrubance and self-reported physical health symptoms in treatment-seeking female rape victims. *J Nerv Meantla Dis*. 2002;189:618-622.

58. Resick P, Clifford G, Jordan C, Girelli S, Hutter C, Marhoefer–Dvorak C. A comparative outcome study of behavioral group therapy for sexual assault victims. *Behav Ther*. 1988;19:385.

59. Riggs D, Kilpatrick D, Resnick H. Long-term psychological distress associated with marital rape and aggravated assault: a comparison to other crime victims. *J Fam Violence*. 1992;7:283-296.

60. Burnam MA, Stein JA, Golding JM, Siegel JM, Sorenson SB, Forsythe AB, Telles CA. Sexual assault and mental disorders in a community population. *J Consult Clin Psychol.* 1988;56:843-850.

61. Kilpatrick DG, Best CL, Saunders BE, Veronen LJ. Rape in marriage and in dating relationships: how bad is it for mental health? *Ann N Y Acad Sci.* 1988;528:335-344.

62. Briere J, Woo R, McRae B, Foltz J, Sitzman R. Lifetime victimization history, demographics, and clinical status in female psychiatric emergency room patients. *J Nerv Ment Dis*. 1997;185:95-101.

63. Ellis E, Atkeson B, Calhoun K. An assessment of long-term reaction to rape. *J Abnorm Psychol.* 1981;90:263-266.

64. Gidycz CA, Koss MP. Predictors of long-term sexual assault trauma among a national sample of victimized college women. *Violence Victims*. 1991;6:175-190.

65. Harris HN, Valentiner DP. World assumptions, sexual assault, depression, and fearful attitudes toward relationships. *J Trauma Stress*. 2002;19:837-846.

66. Kaukinen C, DeMaris A. Age at first sexual assault and current substance use and depression. *J Interpersonal Violence*. 2005;20:1244-1270.

67. Shapiro B, Schwarz JC. Date rape: its relationship to trauma symptoms and sexual self-esteem. *J Interpersonal Violence*. 1997;12(3):407-419.

68. Ullman SE. Sexual assault victimization and sucidal behavior in women: a review of the literature. *Agression Violent Behav*. 2004;9(4):331-351.

69. Ackard D, Neumark-Sztainer D. Date violence and date rape among adolescents: associations with disordered eating behaviors among adolescent females and males with type 1 diabetes: associations with sociodemographics, weight concerns, familial factors, and metabolic outcomes. *Diabetes Care*. 2002;25(8):1289-1296.

70. Ullman SE, Brecklin LR. Sexual assault history and suicidal behavior in a national sample of women. *Suicide Life-Threatening Behav*. 2002;32:117-130.

71. Cohen L, Roth S. The psychological aftermath of rape: long-term effects and individual differences in recovery. *J Soc Clin Psychol.* 1987;5(4):525-534.

72. Foa E, Hearst-Ikeda D, Perry K. Evaluation of a brief cognitive-behavioral program for the prevention of chronic PTSD in recent assault victims. *J Consult Clin Psychol.* 1995;63(6):948-955.

73. Mackey T, Sereika SM, Weissfeld LA, Hacker SS. Factors associated with long-term depressive symptoms of sexual assault victims. *Arch Psychiatr Nurs.* 1992;6: 10-25.

74. Frazier P, Schauben L. Causal attributions and recovery from rape and other stressful life events. *J Soc Clin Psychol.* 1994;13:1-14.

75. Nadelson C, Notman M, Zackson H, Gornick J. A follow-up study of rape victims. *Am J Psychiatry.* 1982;139:1266-1270.

76. Siegel J, Golding J, Stein J, Burnam M, Sorenson S. Reactions to sexual assault: a community study. *J Interpersonal Violence.* 1990;5(2):229-246.

77. Burgess AW, Holmstrom LL. Adaptive strategies and recovery from rape. *Am J Psychiatry.* 1979;136:1278-1282.

78. Santiago J, McCall-Perez F, Gorcey M, Beigel A. Long-term psychological effects of rape in 35 rape victims. *Am J Psychiatry.* 1985;142:1338-1340.

79. Roth S, Wayland K, Woolsey M. Victimization history and victim-assailant relationship as factors in recovery from sexual assault. *J Trauma Stress.* 1990;3(1): 169-180.

80. Surrey J, Swett C, Michaels A, Levin S. Reported history of physical and sexual abuse and severity of symptomatology in women psychiatric outpatients. *Am J Orthopsychiatry.* 1990;60:412-417.

81. Thompson KM, Crosby RD, Wonderlich SA, Mitchell JE, Redlin J, Demuth G, Smyth J, Haseltine B. Psychopathology and sexual trauma in childhood and adulthood. *J Trauma Stress.* 2003;16:35-38.

82. Becker J, Skinner L, Abel G, Axelrod R, Treacy E. Depressive symptoms associated with sexual assault. *J Sex Marital Ther.* 1984;10:185-192.

83. Golding JM. Sexual assault history and physical health in randomly selected Los Angeles women. *Health Psychol.* 1994;13:130-138.

84. Golding JM. Sexual assault history and women's reproductive and sexual health. *Psychol Women Q.* 1996;20:101-121.

85. Golding J. Sexual assault history and headaches: five general population studies. *J Nerv Ment Dis.* 1999;187(10):624-629.

86. Golding JM, Cooper ML, George LK. Sexual assault history and health perceptions: seven general population studies. *Health Psychol.* 1997;16:417-425.

87. Golding J, Taylor D. Sexual assault history and premenstrual distress in two general population samples. *J Women's Health.* 1996;5(2):143-152.

88. Brener ND, McMahon PM, Warren CW, Douglas KA. Forced sexual intercourse and associated health-risk behaviors among female college students. *J Consult Clin Psychol.* 1999;67(2):252–259.

89. Campbell J, Soeken K. Forced sex and intimate partner violence: effects on women's risk and women's health. *Violence Against Women*. 1999;5(9):1017-1035.

90. Kimerling R, Armistead L, Forehand R. Victimization experiences and HIV infection in women: associations with serostatus, psychological symptoms, and health status. *J Trauma Stress*. 1999;12:41-58.

91. Wyatt GE, Myers HF, Williams JK, Kitchen CR, Loeb T, Carmona JV, Wyatt LE, Chin D, Presley N. Does a history of trauma contribute to HIV risk for women of color? Implications for prevention and policy. *Am J Public Health*. 2002;92:660-665.

92. Read J, Stern A, Wolfe J, Ouimette P. Use of a screening instrument in women's health care: detecting relationships among victimization history, psychological distress, and medical complaints. *Women Health*. 1997;25(3):1-17.

93. Walker E, Katon W, Hansom J, Harrop-Griffiths J, Holm L, Jones M, Hickok L, Russo J. Psychiatric diagnoses and sexual victimization in women with chronic pelvic pain. *Psychosomatics*. 1995;36(6):531-540.

94. Kilpatrick DG, Acierno R, Schnurr PP, Saunders B, Resnick HS, Best CL. Risk factors for adolescent substance abuse and dependence: data from a national sample. *J Consult Clin Psychol*. 2000;68:19-30.

95. McFarlane J, Malecha A, Gist J, Watson K, Batten E, Hall I, Smith S. Intimate partner sexual assault against women and associated victim substance use, suicidality, and risk factors for femicide. *Issues Ment Health Nurs*. 2005;26:953-967.

96. Ullman SE, Brecklin LR. Sexual assault history, PTSD, and mental health service seeking in a national sample of women. *J Community Psychol*. 2002;30:261-279.

97. Upchurch D, Kusunoki Y. Associations between forced sex, sexual and protective practices, and sexually transmitted diseases among a national sample of adolescent girls. *Womens Health Issues*. 2004;14(3):75-84.

98. Evans-Campbell T, Lindhorst T, Huang B, Walters K. Interpersonal violence in the lives of urban American Indian and Alaska Native women: implications for health, mental health, and help-seeking. *Am J Public Health*. 2006;96(8):1416-1422.

99. Campbell R, Sefl T, Ahrens C. The impact of rape on women's sexual health risk behaviors. *Health Psychol*. 2004;23:67-74.

100. Byrne C, Resnick H, Kilpatrick D, Best C, Saunders B. The socioeconomic impact of interpersonal violence on women. *J Consult Clin Psychol*. 1999;67(3):362-366.

101. Monnier J, Resnick H, Kilpatrick D, Seals B. The relationship between distress and resource loss following rape. *Violence Victims*. 2002;17(1):85-91.

102. Post LA, Mezey NJ, Maxwell C, Wibert WN. The rape tax: tangible and intangible costs of sexual violence. *J Interpersonal Violence*. 2002;17:733-782.

103. Frazier P, Burnett J. Immediate coping strategies among rape victims. *J Counseling Dev*. 1994;72:633-639.

104. Frazier P, Conlon A, Steger M, Tashiro T, Glaser T. Positive life changes following sexual assault: a replication and extension. In: Columbo F, ed. *Post-traumatic Stress: New Research*. Hauppauge, NY: Nova Science Publishers; 2006:1-22.

105. Burt M, Katz B. Dimensions of recovery from rape: focus on growth outcomes. *J Interpersonal Violence*. 1987;2(1):57-81.

106. Kennedy JE, Davis RC, Taylor BG. Changes in spirituality and well-being among victims of sexual assault. *J Sci Study Religion*. 1998;27:322-328.

107. Tjaden P, Thoennes N. Full report of the prevalence, incidence, and consequences of violence against women: findings from the national violence against women survey. Washington, DC: National Institute of Justice; 1998.

108. Tjaden P, Thoennes N. Extent, nature, and consequences of rape victimization: findings from the national violence against women survey. Washington, DC: National Institute of Justice; 2006. http://www.ncjrs.gov/pdffiles1/nij/210346.pdf. Accessed October 14, 2009.

109. King M, Woollett E. Sexually assaulted males: 115 men consulting a counseling service. *Arch Sex Behav*. 1997;26:579-588.

110. Stermac L, Del Bove G, Addison M. Stranger and acquaintance sexual assault of males. *J Interpersonal Violence*. 2004;11:52-64.

111. Frazier P. A comparative study of male and female rape victims seen at a hospital-based rape crisis program. *J Interpersonal Violence*. 1993; 8:64-76.

112. Stermac L, Sheridan P, Davidson A, Dunn S. Sexual assault of adult males. *J Interpersonal Violence*. 1996;11:52-64.

113. Huckle P. Male rape victims referred to a forensic psychiatric service. *Med Sci Law*. 1995;35:187-192.

114. Walker J, Archer J, Davies M. Effects of rape on male survivors: A descriptive analysis. *Arch Sex Behav*. 2005;34:69-80.

115. Chang B, Skinner K, Zhou C, Kazis L. The relationship between sexual assault, religiosity, and mental health among male veterans. *Int J Psychiatry Med*. 2003;33(3):223-239.

116. King M, Coxell A, Mezey G. Sexual molestation of males: associations with psychological disturbance. *Br J Psychiatry*. 2002;181(2):153-157.

117. Weaver TL, Clum GA. Psychological distress associated with interpersonal violence: a meta-analysis. *Clin Psychol Rev*. 1995;15:115-140.

118. Little K. *Sexual Assault Nurse Examiner Programs: Improving the Community Response to Sexual Assault Victims*. Office for Victims of Crime Bulletin. 2001;4:1-19.

119. Bisson J, Andrew M. Psychological treatment of post-traumatic stress disorder (PTSD). *Cochrane Database Syst Rev*. 2005;(2):CD003388.

120. Stein DJ, Ipser JC, Seedat S. Pharmacotherapy for post traumatic stress disorder (PTSD). *Cochrane Database Syst Rev*. 2006;(1):CD002795.

121. Foa E, Rothbaum B. *Treating the Trauma of Rape: Cognitive-Behavioral Therapy for PTSD*. New York, NY: Guilford; 1998.

122. Resick P, Schnicke M. *Cognitive Processing Therapy for Rape Victims: A Treatment Manual*. Newbury Park, CA: Sage Publications; 1993.

123. Foa E, Davidson J, Frances A, Culpepper L, Ross R, Ross D. The expert consensus guideline series: treatment of posttraumatic stress disorder. *J Clin Psychiatry.* 1999;60(suppl 16):4-76.

124. Ballenger J, Davidson J, Lecrubier Y, Nutt D, Foa E, Kessler R, McFarlane A, Shalev A. Consensus statement on posttraumatic stress disorder from the International Consensus Group on Depression and Anxiety. *J Clin Psychiatry.* 2000;61(suppl 5):60-66.

Chapter 10

The Psychobiology of Traumatic Stress Responses After Sexual Assault

Donna A. Gaffney, DNSc, PMHCNS-BC, FAAN

Sexual assault is a trauma of unparalleled depth and potentially long-lasting impact, and is the most common cause of posttraumatic stress disorder (PTSD) among women.[1-3] Its often shattering emotional repercussions raise an important question: How does a human being psychologically cope with such a searing and traumatic experience? Clinicians and researchers attempting to answer this question have begun to recognize that a complex set of psychological and biological mechanisms are responsible for the physiological response to trauma. These practitioners and scientists acknowledge the need to integrate the psychological and biological aspects of trauma response into a unified field of psychobiology, which combines an understanding of the structure and function of the brain with an understanding of affective and somatic processes. This chapter will describe how human beings respond to traumatic events, particularly the trauma of sexual violence. After an overview of brain function, memory, and trauma, specific assessment skills and interpersonal communication strategies will be discussed in an effort to assist clinicians working with survivors of sexual assault.

Trauma, Stress, and Crisis

The terms *traumatized*, *in crisis*, and *stressed out* are often used interchangeably in everyday language. However, trauma, stress, and crisis, although related, have vastly different effects on the human experience. Researcher Rachel Yehuda describes how trauma and stress differ from each other. She points out that the effects of stress are alleviated once the stressor is removed. Traumatic events are more extreme versions of stressful events and their effects continue well after the events have passed. Finally, the memory of the traumatic event lingers on, with continued arousal.[4]

Crisis is described by Caplan as a threat to homeostasis, a temporary disruption of coping and problem-solving skills, which does not necessarily present as a life-threatening experience.[5] Crises very often represent a turning point, and can be developmental or situational in nature. Crises may also offer opportunities for learning and growth.

Considering these characteristics, one can understand that sexual assault clearly falls into the category of a traumatic event rather than that of a crisis or stressful event. However, stress and crisis are also present. The assault itself presents as a life-threatening traumatic event. The consequences of that assault—going to the hospital, starting therapy, or going to court—suggest a cumulative effect of these ongoing stressful events and crises. The emotions that are evoked by the trauma of sexual assault last long after the event is over. The fear of death and the terror and helplessness experienced during the assault persist even when one is out of harm's way. The stress of going to the hospital for a nonassault patient may leave one frustrated, anxious, or angry, but those emotions tend to subside once the patient leaves the hospital. As Yehuda points out, once a stressor is eliminated, all physical and psychological reactions disappear along with it.[4] Emotions and memories of traumatic events, by contrast, continue on. The sound of the perpetrator's voice, breaking glass, or other sights and sounds accompanying the traumatic assault may intrude into daytime consciousness or nightmares, unbidden, but present just the same. Patients reporting sexual assault often continue to experience a sense of hyperalertness similar to what was felt in those first moments after the traumatic event. Trauma encompasses every aspect of one's being. The physical responses persist, and, as with PTSD, individuals may never fully recover.

Sexual assault can also disrupt and challenge coping and problem-solving strategies, resulting in a crisis. Skills that may have worked for the survivor in the past no longer seem effective. Resolving a crisis eliminates the state of emotional turmoil and disequilibrium; the crisis event passes and normal functioning returns. While a crisis can be an opportunity for learning and raising one's functioning to a higher level, a traumatic event may have the opposite effect, leaving one in a position of instability and vulnerability.

Human responses to stressful events or traumatic events can vary depending on a number of factors, including age, the specific situation, and the individual's prior coping skills. It is important to make a distinction between normal coping responses and pathological responses. There is a constellation of body and brain reactions that are normal responses to traumatic events. These are often called peritraumatic or posttraumatic responses. However, in some situations the traumatic event and the individual's response to it cause long-term dysfunction in cognition and affect. This is when PTSD may be identified.

The mental health community did not address the study of trauma, stress, and the condition ultimately called posttraumatic stress disorder until the latter half of the 20th century. The next section will briefly explore the historical evolution of the current understanding of sexual assault as a trauma.

Historical Perspectives

The study of trauma, until recently, was not undertaken systematically or sustained consistently. Although trauma symptoms have been noted as early as the sixth century BCE, those first writings characteristically related to the reactions of soldiers in combat.[6] Centuries later, Samuel Pepys wrote about traumatic responses to the Great Fire of London in 1666.[7] Charles Dickens also experienced traumatic symptoms after witnessing a tragic rail accident outside of London.[8] However, interest in trauma has waxed and waned. At the end of the 19th century, a number of European physicians began to grapple with a mysterious constellation of symptoms in some of their patients—most notably their female patients. These included uncontrollable behavior, extreme emotions, and odd physical events such as numbing of various body parts. Freud, Janet, and Charcot, in particular, were fascinated by what was regarded as "hysteria" in some of their female patients. Today, these symptoms could be identified as the manifestations of posttraumatic stress reactions. However, in Freud's era, these behaviors were regarded as strange and inexplicable. Moreover, since they seemed to be present in women only, the term originally used by Plato was ***hysteria***—a word that comes from the root *hyster*, meaning "uterus." It was presumed that the symptoms originated in the woman's uterus, which wandered throughout the woman's body causing distress.[9] Freud addressed the cause of this dysfunction in his paper, "The Etiology of Hysteria." He believed that a "premature" sexual experience was the core of the "hysterical" woman's mental state. This was Freud's "Seduction Hypothesis," in which an environmental event (the sexual assault) served as the cause of psychic motivation. Freud believed it was this psychic motivation that caused the toxic symptoms of hysteria.[10]

Herman notes that the social and political climate of late 19th-century Europe was such that even Freud's followers did not support Freud's theory on hysteria. He was urged to redefine his work or at least not to present it to public or professional audiences.[11]

However, Reisner suggests that Freud did not completely abandon this environmental theory of psychic motivation but modified it to imply that it was not the event itself (the assault) but how the individual reacted to such an experience that caused the symptoms.[10] Pierre Janet, a colleague of Freud, also studied trauma in his patients. He believed that traumatic memories were stored in a different manner in the brain than other types of experiences and was the first to suggest the concept of dissociation. The study of trauma was abandoned until 2 decades later, when World War I forced the medical community to confront trauma again. Certain soldiers seemed to have a hysterical or numbed response to combat. They were unable to function on the battlefield. The soldiers were diagnosed with shell shock. After World War I, research on trauma was limited until World War II, when the medical and psychiatric communities were forced once more to come to grips with the symptoms of traumatized soldiers. Battle fatigue was the new name for this mysterious condition.[12] After World War II and into the 1950s, a number of studies addressed the psychological consequences of concentration camps and natural and human-inflicted disasters. Vietnam veterans spoke about their difficulties when returning to the United States. In the midst of the American public's antiwar sentiment and confused by their symptoms, veterans met informally to talk about the difficult adjustment they faced upon their return from combat. Their newly formed group, the Vietnam Veterans Against the War, consulted 2 psychiatrists, Chaim Shatan and Robert J. Lifton, about their situation. They organized a number of smaller "rap" groups designed to provide one another with support and raise consciousness. Ultimately, they helped to organize the first systematic psychiatric research on PTSD.[13]

During the next 5 years, the feminist movement brought attention to the harrowing experiences of women who were sexually assaulted. Two researchers in Boston, Ann Burgess and Linda Holmstrom, followed over 100 women who were admitted to a city hospital emergency department for sexual assault. In clinical interviews, they observed that the women experienced symptoms quite similar to those of combat veterans. The researchers identified and described "Rape Trauma Syndrome" based on their observations of this sample. The groundwork laid by combat veterans paved the way for an understanding of the psychological syndrome seen in survivors of rape, domestic assault, and incest. It became clear that these women were suffering from the same syndrome seen in survivors of war.[11]

The diagnostic criteria for what would be called posttraumatic stress disorder went through a series of definitions and revisions. The first *Diagnostic and Statistical Manual of Mental Disorders* (DSM),[14] published in 1952, classified stress responses as "transient situational personality disturbance, gross stress reaction, or adjustment reaction." However, the second edition, published in 1968,[15] omitted the concept of a stress reaction, including only "adjustment reactions" (of infancy, childhood, adolescence, adult, or late life). The DSM-III, published in 1980, reincorporated the concept of a stress response by adding the first description of PTSD.[16,17] In 1994, acute stress disorder (ASD) was added to the DSM-IV. The criteria for both PTSD and ASD are listed at the end of this chapter and appear in the most current version of the DSM.[18]

Kira points out that the DSM IV-TR defines a traumatic event as one in which there are actual or potential physical consequences.[19] In an effort to consider other nonphysical traumatic events, the American Psychological Association Trauma Group defined a ***traumatic stressor*** as one that causes a process culminating in disorganization of a person's core sense of self and world.[18] In addition, it changes one's worldview with long-lasting results that can include mental health disorders. Such traumatic events are not limited to physical outcomes (eg, combat, rape, life-threatening accidents, death of a significant or loved one, domestic violence, community collective trauma).

There is, however, a lack of clarification in the literature on taxonomy of trauma events or clear definitions of trauma types. Previously, Terr theorized that there were 2 types of trauma: a Type I traumatic event, in which there is a singular incident, and Type II trauma, in which there are multiple occurrences over time.[20] Kira and associates propose that there are more than 2 types of trauma.[19] They hypothesize that there are multiple types of trauma determined by 2 dimensions: a developmental basis and the objective characteristics of the trauma itself.[19] The objective characteristics are cumulative stress trauma, internal trauma, and nature-made or person-made trauma. Types of trauma in this system include Type I, a single event that is person-made; Type II, repeated person-made trauma that no longer occurs; Type III, repeated person-made trauma that is ongoing; and Type IV, cumulative trauma.[19] Sexual assault can be either a singular event or, as in the case of sexual abuse, ongoing traumatic events.

It appears that the issues surrounding trauma and its effects on human beings are finally being addressed. Certainly the terrorist attacks of September 2001, the devastating Gulf Coast hurricanes in 2005, and the wars in Afghanistan and Iraq underscore the need to revisit this important mental health diagnosis. It remains to be seen how the current understanding of the traumatic nature and impact of sexual assault will influence the next DSM, and how the mental health community will continue to evolve in its treatment and conception of rape.

One of the most important areas of ongoing research and understanding concerns the impact of trauma in general and sexual trauma in particular on brain structure and function. The next section will examine the neurophysiology of the posttraumatic response.

The Impact of Traumatic Events on the Structure and Function of the Human Brain

Structure, Function, and Memory

The seat of intellectual functioning that distinguishes human beings from all other species is the cerebral cortex. It is the largest part of the brain and possesses higher cognitive functioning, where information is processed with accuracy and complexity. However, there are several crucial structures located deep in the brain that are most important when responding to threat or danger. Among these structures are the thalamus, the hippocampus, and the amygdala.

The ***thalamus*** is the central processor for visual and auditory stimuli. It sorts sensory cues by their characteristics (ie, size, shape, color, volume, etc) and then sends them to the appropriate areas of the cortex. The ***amygdala***, which is comprised of 2 almond-shaped structures located in the left and right hemispheres of the brain, prompts the fear response. The amygdala is the structure most involved with the emotional interpretation of incoming stimuli.[21]

The ***hippocampus*** is located near the amygdala and is concerned with the initial consolidation and subsequent storage of memory. It processes an event and places it in time and place. In other words, it provides the context for the event. The hippocampus is especially vital to short-term memory, holding an event in place until it is either filed into long-term memory (where it lasts for a lifetime) or lost. The hippocampus allows the individual to remember the actual, "real-life" context of a memory—the *who, what, when*, and *where* of a given event. The amygdala indicates the emotional context of the event and initiates physiological changes in response to the trauma.[21-23] The hippocampal and amygdalate memory systems work in concert with and parallel to each other. ***Conscious memory*** (also known as declarative or explicit memory) is mediated by the hippocampus. By contrast, ***implicit memory***—memory that is stored but not readily accessible to conscious awareness—is mediated by other memory systems, one of which involves the amygdala.

Since a defining characteristic of trauma is that the event continues to live on in the psyche of the survivor, it should be clear what role each of these structures plays in the processing of a traumatic event. The amygdala processes and then facilitates the storage of emotions and sensory reactions to events that are defined by intense feelings, especially fear, threat, and anger. The hippocampus holds the event in short-term memory. Although still in their infancy, neuroimaging studies have demonstrated significant neurobiological changes related to PTSD. Recent findings of studies using magnetic resonance imaging (MRI) and positron emission tomography (PET) techniques have shown that the volume of the hippocampus is reduced in adults who suffer from chronic PTSD.[24-27] This hippocampal volume reduction may affect the survivor on several levels. Clear and integrated recall of the trauma may not be readily accessible to the survivor. Even the survivor's ordinary memory functions, such as short-term memory and reasoning abilities, may be impaired. However, Stein et al, who conducted some of this pioneering research, warns, "It is far from proven that these defects are caused by trauma. It is equally possible that the findings represent a preexisting structural anomaly which might serve as a risk factor for the development of PTSD following trauma exposure."[24]

Kolassa et al demonstrated other changes in the brain following repeated trauma.[28] The ***insula*** is a structure deep in the brain that is believed to process convergent information and provide the sensory context of an event. Kolassa et al measured slow waves in the brain and found these changes, specific to the insula, could play a key role in understanding how a person may have difficulty in identifying, expressing, and regulating emotional responses to reminders of traumatic events.[28] Rausch et al studied the effects of dysfunction in the prefrontal cortex.[29] They proposed that such dysfunction might contribute to diminished extinction of conditioned fear and reduced inhibition of the amygdala. Broca's area, the part of the brain necessary for labeling emotions, was found to be deactivated. As in earlier studies, Rausch and associates found Broca's area changes during symptom provocation in PTSD. These studies may indicate that Broca's area symptom provocation may be related to insular dysfunction.

Finally, the ***neocortex*** is unique to higher mammals and accounts for nearly 85 percent of human brain mass. It consists of many structures, each with several functions. The ***cerebrum***, which is covered by the cerebral cortex, is responsible for thought and language acquisition and expression, while the ***frontal lobes*** handle language processing and complex thinking. The parietal lobes are responsible for perceptual processing, the occipital lobes deal with vision, and the temporal lobes are responsible for hearing, expression, and short-term memory.

Trauma and Neurotransmitters

Each of the structures within the brain contains millions of connecting neurons. These neurons do not actually touch one another, but they do communicate via chemically transmitted electrical impulses. The impulses jump from neuron to neuron across the ***synapse***, the gap between the ends, or ***dendrites***, of the neurons. The chemicals used in the transmission process—neurotransmitters—are stored in the nerve cell's nucleus, or ***axon***. When an electrical impulse traveling along the nerve reaches the axon, the neurotransmitter is released and travels across the synapse, either facilitating or inhibiting the passage of electrical impulses along the nerve.

More than 300 neurotransmitters have been identified in human beings; the most common are acetylcholine, dopamine, norepinephrine, serotonin, and the endorphins. Research in the past few decades has further illustrated the roles of these chemicals produced by neurons.[30] Certain drugs increase the availability of neurotransmitters in the brain, while other drugs can inhibit neurotransmitter activity. These can have a profound impact on memory, because the formation of new memories involves permanent alterations in the synapses between neurons. Benzodiazepines, alcohol, marijuana, and certain amnesiacs (eg, ketamine, gamma-hydroxybutyrate) may affect the formation of new memories by disrupting or blocking the neurotransmitters involved in the storage of an event into a memory.[30]

The body responds to trauma or a threatening stimulus with a chain of events that involves 2 aspects of the autonomic nervous system. The first is the ***sympathetic nervous system*** (SNS), which regulates the smooth muscles of body organs. When the body is in a state of physical effort or stress, the SNS is in operation. The second is the ***parasympathetic nervous system*** (PNS), which is activated when the body is relaxed or in a state of rest.

When the senses receive information that signals danger, there are 2 pathways of response. The "high" road is described as the passage of sensory information from the sensory thalamus up into the cortex, where the stimuli are thoroughly analyzed. This is a very important step, but it has one significant disadvantage. It is relatively slow and can take a few seconds to analyze a new sensory stimulus. However, at times of threat another pathway is also used, the "low road," which involves the transmission of sensory information from the sensory thalamus *directly* to the amygdala. This pathway provides no opportunity for the slower analysis of the stimulus, but it does one very important thing: within milliseconds, it fires off neurons in the amygdala that in turn trigger the body's emergency response systems. With this triggering, there is a chain of neurobiological events that protects one from danger.[22]

With the first indication of threat, the amygdala is activated. It then stimulates the hypothalamus, which calls on the pituitary gland to stimulate the adrenal cortex. These are the elements of the hypothalamic-pituitary-adrenal axis (HPA axis), which is a major part of the neuroendocrine system that manages the body's response to stress. The adrenal glands release 2 steroid hormones, ***epinephrine*** and ***cortisol***, into the bloodstream. ***Norepinephrine***, another hormone, is released from other parts of the body. Epinephrine and norepinephrine prepare the body for survival of threatening situations by stimulating the rapid release of energy from stored glucose and by assisting immune functions.

The steroid hormones also circulate back to the brain. When cortisol reaches the hippocampus, it inhibits further activation. The body is now primed for relaxation and a return to the base state. However, as long as the threat remains, the body will remain in a state of arousal. Only when the stressful event is over does cortisol act upon the hippocampus, returning the body to its nonalert state.

During extreme episodes of traumatic stress, excessive neurotransmitters may be released, damaging the brain and inhibiting memory functions. Ongoing or intense trauma may cause the threat response system to function abnormally.[31] Yehuda found that in patients with PTSD the adrenal glands do not produce enough cortisol to return the body to a nonstressed state.[32] In another study, Yehuda found significantly attenuated cortisol responses in female sexual assault survivors compared to women who did not have a history of sexual assault.[33] Other researchers have confirmed the finding that individuals suffering from PTSD have lower cortisol levels than those without PTSD.

The expression "fight or flight" has become so commonly used that it requires no further discussion in order to be understood. Most people are not aware, however, that there is a preliminary response to threat that precedes fight or flight. When there is a fear stimulus, an animal or human initially responds by stopping all movement.[34] This state of tonic immobility or freezing allows the organism to assess the environment for escape or defensive aggressive behaviors in the event that escape is not a viable option. There is some indication that when mammals are unable to fight or flee, they continue "freezing" as a final measure when confronting a life-threatening stressor; thus, the rabbit "freezes" as it waits for the hunter to pass, or the mouse hangs lifeless while trapped in the cat's mouth.[35] When the hunter passes or the cat drops the mouse, the animals run away. When faced with the perception of imminent death, unavoidable escape, and a perpetrator so threatening as to preclude rational thought, the human being may respond as an animal does—by remaining in a frozen, death-like state, unable to move. For a sexual assault survivor, this may translate into lying passive and motionless during an assault or being unable to escape or scream for help.[36,37] In 2000, Taylor et al hypothesized that women may have a different response to threats as compared to males. In a review of the large body of research on threat responses, the researchers raised the possibility that women may respond to threat in a "tend or befriend" manner.[38] Women tend to protect others who might be in danger, especially children, or to attempt to negotiate with the perpetrator in an attempt to save their own life or the lives of others. These behaviors may serve to protect the self and future offspring. A pituitary hormone called oxytocin, in conjunction with female reproductive hormones, is thought to have a role in the tend or befriend survival strategy. While this is a new and untested theory, there may be relevance for women. A female may respond with a tend or befriend reaction at times of sexual assault. Women may negotiate, acquiesce, or bargain with perpetrators in an effort to stay alive and protect family members.

Memory and Trauma

An understanding of the complex interplay of trauma and memory lies at the root of the treatment of sexual assault survivors in the acute aftermath as well as in the months and years to come. The survivor may appear detached, be unable to speak, or, when communication is possible, the narrative may seem fragmented or inconsistent. Traumatic experiences are recalled and presented differently than ordinary experiences. The clinician working with the survivor of sexual assault must recognize the symptoms of trauma in the hours and months following the assault and the role that memory plays in the presentation of those symptoms.

Memory involves the recording, storage, and retrieval of information taken in from the senses, thoughts, emotions, and behaviors. ***Implicit memory*** includes aspects of an individual's experience that influence performance, thoughts, and perceptions, even though the individual may be unaware of this impact. ***Explicit memory*** is typically known as remembering, and involves the conscious, deliberate recall or recognition of information.

Memory storage is achieved in 2 ways. ***Short-term memory***, also called working memory, lasts for only a short period, perhaps just seconds. Then, through a process called ***memory***

consolidation, information is moved to long-term storage. The way information is encoded (stored) is the way a person will remember it. In fact, memory is more likely to be retrieved if the individual's mood state matches that experienced at the time of the experience. In other words, experiencing fear even years after an assault and for a reason unrelated to the assault can trigger the emotions of fear experienced during the assault. This concept is especially important in understanding PTSD.[39]

The mechanisms that consolidate everyday memories are different from those responsible for handling traumatic memories.[39] Brown and Kulik refer to the remembering of a new event or experience as a "now print."[40] It is also called a "snapshot" or flashbulb memory. The image of the event is preserved or "frozen" at one precise moment in time. The details of the event are clearly and consistently recalled. Current research suggests that the personal significance of the "now print" will determine its durability and persistence over time. Whether it is retained in the brain on a long-term basis depends on the role it plays in the individual's life and conceptual structure. People experience hundreds of events daily and when asked can probably recall many of them, but most are forgotten unless they hold some sustained importance to one's practical or psychological life. Moreover, the accuracy of one's memory varies. Individuals might believe that they recall an event accurately, but details can be distorted or blurred.

In contrast, memories of personal trauma are particularly durable and accurate. Terr referred to these memories as "burned-in visual representations."[41] They are burned into the memory of the individual and appear to remain there permanently. These memories can leap into the individual's consciousness, unbidden, thrusting the experience before the survivor and causing significant disruption of day-to-day experiences. Although these recurrent memories tend to become less frequent over time, they do not disappear entirely. Moreover, their content is often more vivid, detailed, and accurate than that of ordinary, day-to-day memories. A number of factors can distort or influence memory, including developmental age, current emotional needs, time from event to recall of information, and the emotional climate of the event itself. The neurotransmitters themselves may also have an effect on memory.[25] As Schacter points out, "The release of stress-related hormones, signaled by the amygdala, probably accounts for some of the extraordinary power and persistence that characterize many highly emotional traumatic experiences."[39]

The processing of traumatic events is very different from the processing of ordinary or even novel events. Trauma is first organized in memory on a perceptual level. There may be fragments of sensory components, depending on the manner in which the trauma is first experienced: visual images, olfactory and auditory input, kinesthetic sensations, taste, and even an intense wave of feelings may be recorded as they are experienced. In fact, for many people there are no words to describe the traumatic event, and the narrative emerges over time as the individual tries to explain what has happened.[39] While the construction of the narrative also occurs in day-to-day situations, the sensory elements are not registered separately in consciousness, but are immediately integrated into the personal narrative. Piaget theorized that when memories cannot be integrated on a linguistic level they tend to be organized on a more primitive level of information processing.[42]

Thus, the survivor of a profound trauma such as sexual assault may have recorded the experience as a series of terrifying sensations unaccompanied by verbal interpretation. The stream of sensations—for example, tactile (the texture of the assailant's hand or sleeve) or olfactory (the odor of the assailant's cologne)—form a set of "sensory snapshots" of the event within the survivor's memory before the event can be translated into a verbal narrative.

Individuals who interview or work with survivors of sexual assault should not, therefore, expect a neat, organized, sequential account of the events. While some survivors may be able to verbalize and recount what happened, many experience difficulties with concentration, difficulty with sequencing of events, and memory disturbances. These are common characteristic symptoms of peritraumatic stress.[43] The brain's ability to process, retain, and recall information has been compromised by the trauma.[44] Thus, the retelling of the experience may contain internal inconsistencies. Moreover, the survivor may present slightly or even dramatically different accounts during the numerous interviews that she must undergo in the medicolegal aftermath of the assault. The survivor may not even be able to recall experiencing any pain or the location of the pain felt due to stress-induced analgesia, which is a consequence of the activation of the brain's opiate system following a trauma.[45]

When traumatic memories are stored in the implicit form, as feelings and sensations, the assault experience is remembered in fragments but infused with intense emotion and recollections of sensory cues such as tastes, smells, and sounds. This has implications not only for the survivor's ability to present a coherent chronicle of the events, but also for the survivor's ability to identify sensations and feelings of traumatic origin. Thus, some survivors become haunted by feelings and senses they know are related to the trauma, but have difficulty accurately identifying the source of the feeling or sensation. Being bombarded by a series of sensations, feelings, or memory snapshots extends the terror long beyond the existence of the actual threat.

The phenomenon of ***dissociation*** frequently accompanies a traumatic event. Because trauma severs the links between memory systems within the brain, the past experiences become detached from consciousness. Dissociation compartmentalizes experiences. According to Schachter, "Dissociation causes the mind to be split into streams. Thoughts, feelings, and memories splinter into separate worlds of their own: memory systems and subsystems that ordinarily communicate with each other closely, passing information back and forth, lose touch with each other."[39] Dissociative symptoms include a sense of numbing, detachment, absence of emotional responsiveness, reduction of awareness of one's surroundings, derealization, depersonalization, and dissociative amnesia or the inability to recall an important aspect of the trauma.[18]

Posttraumatic Stress Disorder and Mental Health Consequences Following Sexual Assault

Kilpatrick et al reported that one-third of female survivors developed PTSD at some point after they were assaulted.[46] Other common mental health consequences of rape are major depression and alcohol or drug abuse.[47,48] Ullman and Brecklin studied the relationships between past-year chronic medical conditions and lifetime contact with health care professionals for mental health and substance abuse problems in women with differing histories of sexual victimization. They found that victimization at varying points across the lifespan resulted in different health outcomes. Alcohol dependence symptoms and PTSD were each associated with greater odds of lifetime health care professional contact among women victimized in early and later life.[49] Depression was related to greater odds of help-seeking for women victimized at only one point in their lives.

Determining the factors that may put a survivor at risk for PTSD or any negative mental health outcome is challenging and has been the focus of a number of studies. Rape is one of the most emotionally and physically intrusive traumatic events. The boundaries of the human body are violated in the most intimate way imaginable. The crime itself is fraught with the burden of historical myths and misconceptions, permeating every aspect of society and culture. The stigma resulting from sexual violence prevents many from seeking and receiving social support at a time when it is needed the most. In addition, rape and sexual assault are crimes that are often blamed on their victims. In a review of the literature, Classen et al found that the occurrence and magnitude of childhood sexual abuse are the most recognized predictors of sexual revictimization and PTSD during adulthood.[50] Layering of multiple traumatic events, particularly physical abuse during childhood, also contributes to a greater risk for PTSD later in life. Cultural and familial issues may be significant factors as well.

Frazier and colleagues reported that sexual assault is more likely to result in PTSD than other kinds of traumatic experiences.[51] Some authors suggest that it is a combination of factors that make this event far more significant than other types of trauma: the physically intrusive nature of the assault, the perception that one's life is threatened, and the realization that the perpetrator is another human being (one who may have been trusted and loved by the survivor) increase the risk to the survivor for PTSD. Other researchers have found that the presence of physical injury is a predictor of PTSD.[24] Campbell et al found that survivors who received few services and significant secondary victimization experienced more symptoms of PTSD even when the rape characteristics were controlled.[52] Acierno et al surveyed over 3000 women and identified a history of depression as a risk factor for PTSD in both physical and sexual assault.[53] However, the risk of developing PTSD was 3 times greater for those sexually assaulted women with a history of alcohol abuse or physical injury sustained during the rape than for women without those characteristics.

Prior interpersonal trauma may also contribute to PTSD symptoms in survivors of sexual assault. Nishith et al determined that a higher rate of childhood sexual abuse (not physical abuse) was related to higher rates of subsequent adult sexual and physical assault, which then contributed to a higher rate of PTSD symptoms.[54] In their study of 117 adult rape victims, histories of child sexual abuse, child physical abuse, other adult sexual and physical victimization, and current PTSD symptoms were assessed within 1 month of a recent rape.[54] Results from path analyses revealed that a child sexual abuse history seems to increase vulnerability for adult sexual and physical victimization.[54] The authors hypothesized that these data may be attributed to perceptions of trust or symptoms of unresolved traumatic stressors interfering with cognitive appraisals of risk situations.

While there are few studies that examine the recovery environment, several studies explored negative social reactions and their impact on the survivor. It appears that negative social reactions (eg, silencing of the victim, victim blame, alienating or isolating the victim, controlling responses) correlate with more psychological symptoms and poorer self-assessment of recovery.[51,55-57] Ullman and Fillipas examined the correlating factors of PTSD severity and both negative and positive social reactions among survivors who disclosed their assaults to social support providers (informal and formal). They found a relationship between a range of negative social reactions and PTSD symptom severity.[58] In fact, stigmatizing social responses were the strongest predictor of PTSD symptoms. The same study also identified race and education as predictors of PTSD symptoms; the authors suggested that women of color might be at greater risk for social reactions that stigmatize and isolate them than women of other ethnic and racial backgrounds.

Psychological Assessment of the Sexual Assault Survivor

The focus of care for the sexual assault survivor should include both physical and psychological elements in both the immediate and long-term timeframes. The clinician must attend to a series of survivor needs and demands in the immediate aftermath of an assault. Interacting with someone who has just been assaulted requires an understanding and anticipation of common physical and psychological reactions to traumatic events. Familiarity with these reactions is important for the assessment process. It also has therapeutic value. The strategies employed by the sexual assault nurse examiner (SANE) can facilitate immediate care and treatment while beginning the process of integrating the event into the survivor's life.

The clinician must have a working knowledge of the symptoms related to trauma and must understand the difference between the immediate aftereffects of an assault and the long-term consequences. The long-term goal of treatment is to place the assault in the broader context of a person's life. The survivor should recognize that the assault will never be forgotten, but that the associated pain and memories will lessen and the rape will no longer be the central focus of her life. In other words, the eventual goal is for the survivor to integrate the rape into her other life experiences. While the role of the medical or nursing forensic examiner is quite different from that of a therapist who is seeking to help survivors reach these long-term goals, the work done with survivors in the early hours and days postassault is crucial to establishing the foundation for psychological healing.

The following constitute the various reactions a survivor may have to the trauma of sexual assault (**Table 10-1**).

Remember that the clinician primarily interacts with the survivor in the immediate aftermath of the sexual assault—the early hours, first days, or weeks following an assault. Although some of the reactions listed above overlap with the symptoms of PTSD, it is important to recognize the clinician's role and goals of treatment. The immediate post-assault period may not be the time to diagnose PTSD or ASD. Both PTSD and ASD are diagnosed using a set of criteria that includes a time referent and should not be confused with common peritraumatic responses immediately following a sexual assault. The criteria for diagnosing PTSD and ASD appear at the end of this chapter.

Table 10-1. Common Reactions to Traumatic Events

PHYSICAL REACTIONS	
Gastrointestinal:	— Nausea, indigestion, upset stomach
Cardiovascular:	— Flushing, palpitation or tachycardia, sweating palms, dry mouth, profuse sweating, chills and feeling cold
Respiratory:	— Shortness of breath, pressure or tightness across the chest
Neuromuscular:	— Numbness and tingling of extremities, muscular tension, aches (eg, throat, jaw), vision disturbances, exhaustion or fatigue
EMOTIONAL/AFFECTIVE RESPONSES	
General:	— Fear of separation and abandonment and for personal safety — Anger or outrage — Helplessness, hopelessness, or powerlessness — Sadness or grief — Denial, disbelief, or numbness — Guilt — Distrust

(continued)

Table 10-1. Common Reactions to Traumatic Events *(continued)*

COGNITIVE REACTIONS	
Cognitive Processing Attention:	— Decreased attention span, poor concentration, calculation difficulties
Orientation:	— Time distortion and inability to sequence events, confusion, disorientation
Memory:	— Distortions or inability to remember crucial details or remembering details that don't necessarily have to do with the traumatic events, flashbulb memories of event, flashbacks (intrusive images), nightmares
Thoughts and Statements:	— "How could someone do this?" — "It feels so unreal; it's just like a bad dream."
Denial and Disbelief:	— "I can't talk about it."
Orientation:	— "Time stood still." — "I felt so confused. I'm not sure what happened."
Guilt:	— "I wanted to get help." — "I should have done more."
Separation:	— "I'm all alone." — "No one in my family understands this."
BEHAVIORAL RESPONSES	
Immediate and Long-term:	— Biting lip, clenching fists, tapping fingers, biting nails — Withdrawal or excessive silence — Exaggerated startle response to neutral cues — Episodes of panic or anxiety or crying (episodic or precipitated by a reminder of the event) — Hypervigilance, suspiciousness, excessive humor, joking, laughing — Irritability
Long-term:	— Sleep disturbances — Alteration in risk taking (taking more risks or avoiding any risks) — Initiation or return to drug or alcohol use — Impulsive actions — Increased or decreased eating or smoking
INTERPERSONAL REACTIONS	
General:	— Difficulty with intimacy, affection, or sexual relationships — Conflict and confrontation (fighting and arguing) — Withdrawal, isolation, or being distant from others — Being judgmental (especially about coping and grieving styles) — Overly controlling or overly cautious to the point of limiting another's choices.

The Healing Process: First Steps

As already mentioned, the primary goal of treatment is to integrate the sexual assault into the survivor's life so that it is no longer considered the central focus or defining event. Over time, some survivors come to view the assault as the signature event in their lives; it becomes the line of demarcation between the pre-rape self and the postrape, injured self. The course of healing is often initiated in the emergency department when the survivor first appears for treatment, and care must be taken to begin treatment of both the physical and emotional damage as early as possible. Since sexual assault is an assault not only on the victim's physical self but also on her sense of autonomy and control, the victim feels helpless. Things are being done to her without her consent. Therefore, an important first step in healing is for the victim to regain a sense of control over her body and over events in which she is involved. Again, this process begins in the emergency room. The clinician takes the initial step by returning control to the survivor in the earliest moments of the assessment process. The act of obtaining consent, which involves preparing and educating the survivor about assessment and evidence collection, enables the survivor to make decisions about health care—and, by extension, about her own body. The importance of establishing trust and providing a sense of safety is crucial. There should be no surprises during the time the survivor is being treated.[11] This reverses the experience of victimization, during which the assailant might have acted unpredictably, without concern for the survivor's lack of preparedness and acquiescence. **Table 10-2** details clinician actions that may facilitate the assessment process.

Table 10-2. Clinician Actions During the Assessment Process

Introductions

Purpose: To establish a *trusting relationship*, and provide *safety*.

Give your name. Indicate how you would like to be addressed. Ask how she would like to be addressed.

Carefully consider how you will introduce yourself. Using the title "Sexual Assault Examiner" may be disconcerting especially if the survivor has not used the words *sexual assault* or *rape*. (This is akin to being introduced to one's oncologist before the biopsy results confirm the presence of cancer.) Rather, state your role, ie, "I am a registered nurse and have been especially trained to work with people who have been through situations similar to yours."

Identify your responsibilities at the hospital and your commitment to staying with her for "as long as it takes." Do not indicate that you will remain with the survivor unless you are certain it will be possible for you to do so.

Use language that is clear and nonthreatening. Avoid technical (legal or medical) terminology.

Preparation and Explanation

Purpose: To reinforce *safety* and *security*, ensuring there are no surprises.

Begin by saying what you already know (from the chart, from the triage person, etc). "I understand from your chart that you are here because you were assaulted, hurt..." (use the patient's own words).

(continued)

Table 10-2. Clinician Actions During the Assessment Process *(continued)*

PREPARATION AND EXPLANATION

Tell the survivor that you will be informing her what will happen before it happens. Indicate clearly and repeatedly that if there is anything that occurs during the course of the examination that is painful or uncomfortable, you will stop. Let the survivor know that she can decline any part of the examination or evidence collection steps. If the survivor is fearful of being left alone, indicate that you (and the advocate) will remain with her throughout the process.

OFFERING SUPPORT

Purpose: To reduce the survivor's anxiety and increase the sense of trust.

Avoid emergency department jargon, medical terminology, and the "landmines" of these words that may increase anxiety.

Do not rush to fill silence with words. Some survivors need to sit quietly and process the event. After a few moments, acknowledge the silence. You might say something like: "I can see this is not easy to put into words." "Sometimes it feels easier not to talk." "Sometimes it may feel better to be silent."

Acknowledge that you are a *stranger*, a new person in her life. "I know we have just met, it may be uncomfortable for you to tell me about what happened to you, but I am here for you, to listen to you and make sure you are okay."

Reassure the survivor that you will be *patient* and that she does not need to hurry through her account on your account. You might say: "We can take as long as you need." "I'll wait." "That's okay, take your time."

Use simple support statements when needed. "I'm glad you called." "I'm glad you came here." "It's good you are telling me these things." "I'm sorry this happened to you." "You are safe here." "What would it take for you to feel safe here?" "It's okay to feel..." "Your feelings are not any different than other women (girls, men) your age who are in the very same situation." "You are not to blame." "It's not your fault." "You aren't responsible for what happened." "What you are feeling is very common for someone who has been through what you have." "If you want to stop at any time, we can—just tell me." "If you remember anything else we will stop what we're doing and talk." "You're here—you have survived." "You did all the right things—you've survived."

Provide a safe space for emotional expression. If the interview comes to a halt with shouting or expressions of rage, for example, point out the behavior and ask how you can help the survivor feel more comfortable.

Do not ever say you "know" or "understand" how she feels. Even if you yourself are a survivor of sexual assault, it is impossible to "know" the life experience of someone else either before or after her assault.

You can provide empathy and support by reflecting to the person what she is doing (crying, expressing anger) and asking how you can help. "I see you are angry. You have a right to be angry. Please tell me what I can do to help you feel better." "I see you are crying, we can wait until you are ready to talk. Is there anything that I can do to help you?"

Strategies for Effective Therapeutic Communication

The final section of this chapter is a review of suggestions for facilitating effective communication with sexual assault survivors (**Table 10-3**).

Table 10-3. Strategies for Effective Therapeutic Communication.[59]

Techniques	Examples
Active Listening	— Demonstrating attentive, careful interest in the survivor's statements by reacting verbally or nonverbally. This skill will help the clinician remember details of his/her account, facilitate the creation of trust, and be useful in the problem-solving process.
Using Silence	— Allowing the survivor to take as much time as needed is comforting and assists in the establishment of trust.
Using Open-Ended Questions	— Who? What? When? Where? How? (Avoid "Yes" or "No")
Providing Instructions, Directions, and Information Using Clear, Concrete Words and Terminology	— Avoid using words such as *left* or *right*, as the survivor may be disoriented and unable to comprehend even the simplest of directions. Instead use specific locations in the room. ("Turn and face the window" or "Look towards the door while I examine your neck.")
Accepting	— "Yes." — "I follow what you said." — "I hear what you are saying." — Nodding
Giving Recognition	— Good morning Mrs./Ms./Mr.
Offering Self	— "I'm going to take care of you while you are here." — "I'll stay here with you." — "I'm interested in your comfort."
Giving Broad Openings	— "Tell me what happened." — "What are you thinking about?" — "Where would you like to begin?"
Offering General Leads	— "Go on." — "And then?" — "Tell me about it…"
Placing the Event in Time or in Sequence	— "What happened right before…?" — "Was this before or after…?" — "When did this happen?"
Making Observations	— "Your muscles appear tight." — "I see your fist is clenched." — "I notice you are shifting in your chair." — "I see that you're biting your lips."

(continued)

Table 10-3. Strategies for Effective Therapeutic Communication.[59] *(continued)*

TECHNIQUES	EXAMPLES
Encouraging Description of Perceptions	— Encouraging the conversation and clearer and deeper disclosure by asking questions that allow the victim to elaborate and clarify her needs, options, and desires. — "Tell me when you feel anxious." — "What is happening?" — V: "Do you know what I mean?" C: "No, I don't know exactly. Tell me more about what you are thinking?" — V: "No one will believe me anyway." C: "Help me understand the reason you feel that no one will believe you?" — V: "I try to think why this happened but…" C: "We can try to help you get the answers to your questions, but the most important thing is that you are here."
Encouraging Comparison	— "Was this something like…?" — "Have you had similar experiences?" — "Has anything like this ever happened to you in the past?"
Restating	— Restating (in the clinician's own words) the content and emotion that has been communicated by the survivor. Restating helps assess the accuracy of understanding the survivor's statements as well as offering an opportunity to hear. — "You mentioned feeling frustrated about this assault." — "It sounds to me that you are feeling helpless right now." — "The worry about being pregnant is your first concern, right? It also sounds like you are in a great deal of pain."
Reframing	— Offering an interpretation of alternative ways of looking at or thinking about situations. This may involve providing additional information or raising concerns, ideas, or possibilities the survivor did not think of herself. Remember, the survivor's account and sensibilities are the accurate ones. — V: "I should have been able to figure out what he was doing." C: "It's hard to know what another person will do, even if you know him very well. You couldn't have predicted his behavior." — V: "I shouldn't have taken that street home after work." C: "You have probably taken that street home many times before, and nothing happened. If you knew ahead of time that you would be hurt, you wouldn't have made that choice. We make the best decisions we can with the best information we have at the time."
Focusing	— "Let's go back to this point for a moment..."
Exploring	— "Tell me more about that." — "Would you describe it more fully?"

(continued)

Table 10-3. *(continued)*

TECHNIQUES	EXAMPLES
Offering Information	— Given common misconceptions about sexual assault, the traumatic nature of sexual assault, and the various health, legal, and personal decisions that survivors need to make, some part of the time should be devoted to providing information. It will be helpful to have printed information, but the clinician should not assume that a survivor can read; information should always be presented verbally as well. — "My name is…" — "My purpose in being here is…" — "I'm taking you to the…" — "These are the services we can offer you…" — "Here is a list of the medications you have received…"
Seeking Clarification	— "I'm not sure that I follow." — "You are in the emergency room of Metro hospital."
Presenting Reality	— "Tell me whether my understanding of it agrees with yours."
Seeking Consensual Validation	— "You didn't answer what you want to do, is there something else you'd like to ask me?"
Verbalizing the Implied	— "Let me know what is working for you."
Encouraging Evaluation	— "Perhaps you and I can discuss…"
Suggesting Collaboration	— "You've said that…" — "During the interview you and I have discussed…"
Summarizing	— Drawing on the various elements of your discussion with the survivor, present a series of concise statements that briefly describes what happened, how the survivor feels, what she needs, and what the follow-up plans are. — "Let's review the plan and see if the order feels right for you. I want to be sure that you've had a chance to tell me anything you want me to know, and that I understand what you want now."
Encouraging Formulation of a Plan of Action	— Identifying those aspects of the survivor's situation over which she has decision-making power. This is to illustrate possibilities and options as she begins to reestablish a sense of control. Working as a problem-solving team, the clinician and the survivor will identify problems, make an action plan, and set some goals for resolving the crisis. — "You have some decisions to make about how you are going to respond to the situation. Shall we talk about some of them?" — "Let's make a plan to deal with each of your concerns in the order that you want to. The pregnancy test we can do first, if you like, and then we'll have more information to go on."

Adapted by the author from the work of H. Peplau. Peplau, H. Interpersonal Relations in Nursing: A Conceptual Frame of Reference for Psychodynamic Nursing. *New York, NY: Springer Publishing; 1952.*

DSM IV-TR Criteria for Acute Stress Disorder and Posttraumatic Stress Disorder

The concept of a stress response following trauma went through a series of stages and alterations in the development of the formal diagnostic criteria in the mental health community. The first DSM published in 1952 classified stress responses as "transient situational personality disturbance, gross stress reaction or adjustment reaction."[14] However, the second edition, published in 1968, omitted the concept of a stress reaction, including only "adjustment reactions" (of infancy, childhood, adolescence, adult, or late life).[15] The DSM-III, published in 1980, reincorporated the concept of a stress response by adding the first description of PTSD.[16,17] In 1994, acute stress disorder was added to the DSM-IV. The criteria for both PTSD and ASD are listed here as they appear in the newest version of the DSM.[18]

Acute Stress Disorder

The disorder develops within one month of exposure to the traumatic stressor. The person has been exposed to a traumatic event in which both of the following were present: (1) experienced, witnessed, or was confronted with an event(s) that involved actual or threatened death or serious injury, or threat to physical integrity of self or others and (2) the person's response involves intense fear, helplessness, or horror.

While experiencing or after experiencing the event, the individual has 3 or more of the following dissociative symptoms: a subjective sense of numbing, detachment, or an absence of emotional responsiveness, reduction of awareness of her surroundings (being "in a daze"), derealization (things don't seem "real"), depersonalization, or the inability to recall an important aspect of the trauma.

The traumatic event is persistently reexperienced in at least one or more of the following ways: recurrent images, thoughts, dreams, illusions, flashback episodes, or a sense of reliving the experience, or distress on exposure to reminders of the traumatic event. There is marked avoidance of stimuli that arouse recollections of the trauma. These can be thoughts, feelings or conversations, activities, people, or places. There are also clear symptoms of anxiety or increased arousal such as difficulty falling or staying asleep, irritability or outbursts of anger, poor concentration, hypervigilance, exaggerated startle response, or restlessness.

All of these symptoms cause clinically significant distress or impairment in social, occupational, or other important areas of functioning or impair the individual's ability to pursue some necessary task, such as obtaining assistance or mobilizing personal resources by telling family members about the traumatic experience. The duration of the symptoms lasts for a minimum of 2 days and a maximum of 4 weeks and occurs within 4 weeks of the event. The disturbance is not due to a physiological effect of a substance or general medical condition.

Posttraumatic Stress Disorder

This disorder can be classified as *acute* if symptoms last less than 3 months, *chronic* if symptoms continue for 3 or more months, or *delayed onset* if symptoms begin at least 6 months after the stressor. Like ASD, PTSD occurs when a person has been exposed to a traumatic event in which both of the following were present: (1) a person experienced, witnessed, or was confronted with an event that involved actual or threatened death or serious injury, or threat to physical integrity of self or others and (2) the person's response involves intense fear, helplessness, or horror. For children, fear and helplessness may be expressed as disorganized or agitated behavior.

Symptoms fall within 3 categories that seem to be contradictory in nature: the trauma is unwittingly reexperienced, persistent avoidance of thoughts, feelings and behaviors, and a state of hyperarousal.

The traumatic event is persistently reexperienced in one or more of the following ways. It is essentially relived through recurrent and intrusive distressing recollections of the event as images, thoughts, or perceptions. There are also recurrent distressing dreams of the traumatic situation. In younger children, these dreams may be frightening but without recognizable content. The individual acts or feels as if the traumatic event were recurring; young children may reenact the event in specific detail. There is also the possibility of intense psychological distress at exposure to internal or external cues or reminders that symbolize or resemble some aspect of the event. Finally, there may be physiological reactivity on exposure to internal/external reminders of some aspect of the trauma.

The presence of 3 or more symptoms of persistent avoidance of stimuli associated with the trauma or numbing of general responsiveness is indicative of a diagnosis of PTSD. These behaviors include purposeful efforts to avoid thoughts, feelings, or conversations associated with trauma; avoiding activities, persons, or places that arouse recollections of trauma; or the inability to recall important aspects of the trauma. The individual may have significant diminished interest/participation in important activities or a feeling of detachment or estrangement from others. The person may also have a restricted range of affect and be unable to experience joy or loving feelings. Finally, there may be a sense of a foreshortened future in which the person does not expect to have a career or significant commitment or live to see her children or siblings grow up.

Feelings of persistent increased arousal, which were not present before the trauma, are indicative of PTSD if there are 2 (or more) of the following: difficulty falling or staying asleep, irritability or outbursts of anger/rage, difficulty concentrating or focusing on a task, hypervigilance, or an exaggerated startle response.

The duration of the intrusive, avoidance, or arousal symptoms is more than one month and causes clinically significant distress or impairment in social, occupational, or other important areas of functioning.

Rape Trauma Syndrome

Burgess and Holmstrom described the psychological experiences of the sexual assault survivor in the first year after the assault. The authors observed 2 psychological stages in the first year following the sexual assault: the acute stage and the long-term process of reorganization.[60] The acute stage, primarily characterized by disorganization, consists of the *impact* reaction occurring immediately after the assault. The survivor's emotional reactions may be either *expressive,* which includes agitation, crying, and anxiety, or very *controlled.* Survivors may have difficulty concentrating, making decisions, and doing simple, everyday tasks, or they may act numb or stunned and have poor recall of the rape or other memories.

Somatic and emotional reactions in the weeks that follow the sexual assault often remain hidden behind the survivor's facade of what appears to be normal from the outside. Physical complaints may include gastrointestinal or genitourinary symptoms, muscle tension, soreness, sexual problems, and gastrointestinal disturbances (eg, nausea, vomiting, and compulsive eating related to nature of assault). There is also a disruption of normal everyday routines (eg, high absenteeism at work suddenly or, conversely, working longer than usual hours; dropping out of school; traveling different routes; going out only at certain times). The second stage, the long-term process of reorganization, is comprised of lifestyle changes (residence, job, and phone) and an attempt to reestablish family support systems. The intrusive symptoms noted in the acute stage are often present during the later months following the assault.

Although Rape Trauma Syndrome (RTS) is not included in the DSM-IV-TR, it is recognized as a nursing diagnosis and was revised and clarified by NANDA in 1999 (**Table 10-4**). While RTS has been used in courts to explain a survivor's behavior and actions following an assault, other jurisdictions do not allow it into testimony as it would be improper to use the term *Rape Trauma Syndrome*, when the legal conclusion of rape has not yet been reached. For clinical purposes, RTS is useful in gauging the survivor's reactions during the first months. At the present time, most researchers and clinicians suggest that the behaviors associated with RTS are best characterized as Posttraumatic Stress Disorder–Rape Related Trauma.[61]

Table 10-4. Nursing Diagnosis of Rape Trauma Syndrome

DEFINITION OF RAPE TRAUMA SYNDROME

Rape Trauma Syndrome is defined as sustained maladaptive response to a forced, violent sexual penetration against the survivor's will and consent. This syndrome includes the following 3 subcomponents: (A) rape trauma, (B) compound reaction, and (C) silent reaction.[62] *Note: Although attacks are most often directed toward women, men also may be survivors.*

DEFINING CHARACTERISTICS

A: Rape Trauma

Subjective:	— Shock, fear, anxiety, and anger — Embarrassment — Shame — Guilt — Humiliation — Revenge — Self-blame — Loss of self-esteem — Helplessness — Powerlessness — Nightmare and sleep disturbances — Change in relationships — Sexual dysfunction — Changes in lifestyle (change in residence; seeking family support; seeking social network support)
Objective:	— Physical trauma (eg, bruising, tissue irritation) — Muscle tension and/or spasms — Hyperalertness — Confusion — Disorganization — Inability to make decisions — Mood swings — Vulnerability

(continued)

Table 10-4. *(continued)*

Objective: *(continued)*	— Depression — Dependence — Agitation — Aggression — Denial — Phobias — Paranoia — Substance abuse — Suicide attempts — Dissociative disorders
B: Compound Reaction (All defining characteristics listed under rape trauma and compound reaction.)	
Acute Phase:	— Reactivated symptoms of such previous conditions (ie, physical/psychiatric illness) — Reliance on alcohol and/or drugs
C: Silent Reaction	
Subjective:	— Abrupt changes in relationships with men — Increase in nightmares — Increasing anxiety during interview, that is, blocking of associations, long periods of silence, minor stuttering, physical distress — Pronounced changes in sexual behavior — No verbalization of the occurrence of rape — Sudden onset of phobic reactions

References

1. Kessler R, Sonnega A, Bromet E, Nelson CB. Posttraumatic stress disorder in the National Comorbidity Survey. *Arch Gen Psychiatry.* 1995;52:1048-1060.
2. Frans Ö, Rimmö PA, Åberg L, Fredrikson M. Trauma exposure and post-traumatic stress disorder in the general population. *Acta Psychiatrica Scandinavica.* 2005; 111(4):291-299.
3. McFarlane J, Malecha A, Watson K, Gist J, Batten E, Hall I, Smith S. Intimate partner sexual assault against women: frequency, health consequences, and treatment outcomes. *Obstet Gynecol.* 2005;105:99-108.
4. Yehuda R. Discrepancy Between Theory, Research and Practice. Conference presentation at: Mt. Sinai Medical Center; September 1999; New York, NY.
5. Caplan G. *Principles of Preventative Psychiatry.* New York, NY: Basic Books; 1964.
6. Holmes R. *Acts of War.* New York, NY: Free Press; 1985.
7. Daly RJ. Samuel Pepys and posttraumatic stress disorder. *Br J Psychiatry.* 1983; 143:64-68.
8. Trimble MD. Post-traumatic stress disorder: history of a concept. In: Figley CR, ed. *Trauma and Its Wake: The Study and Treatment of Post-Traumatic Stress Disorder.* New York, NY: Brunner/Mazel; 1985:5-14.

9. Adair M. Plato's view of the 'wandering uterus.' *Classical J.* 1996;91(2):153-163.

10. Reisner S. Reclaiming the metapsychology: classical revisionism, seduction and the self in Freudian psychoanalysis. *Psychoanalytic Rev.* 1991;8(4):439-462.

11. Herman J. *Trauma and Recovery.* New York, NY: Basic Books; 1997.

12. Saigh P, Bremner J. The history of posttraumatic stress disorder. In: Saigh P, Bremner J, eds. *Posttraumatic Stress Disorder: A Comprehensive Text.* Needham Heights, MA: Allyn & Bacon; 1999:1-17.

13. van der Kolk B, McFarlane A, Weisaeth L. *Traumatic Stress: The Effects of Overwhelming Experience on Mind, Body and Society.* New York, NY: Guilford; 1996.

14. American Psychiatric Association. *The Diagnostic and Statistical Manual of Mental Disorders-I.* Washington, DC: Author; 1952.

15. American Psychiatric Association. *The Diagnostic and Statistical Manual of Mental Disorders-II.* 2nd ed. Washington, DC: Author; 1968.

16. American Psychiatric Association. *The Diagnostic and Statistical Manual of Mental Disorders-III.* 3rd ed. Washington, DC: Author; 1980.

17. American Psychiatric Association. *The Diagnostic and Statistical Manual of Mental Disorders-III-R.* 3rd rev ed. Washington, DC: Author; 1987.

18. American Psychiatric Association. *The Diagnostic and Statistical Manual of Mental Disorders-IV-TR.* 4th rev ed. Washington, DC: Author; 2000.

19. Kira IA, Lewandowski L, Templin T, Ramaswamy V, Ozkan B, Mohanesh. J. Measuring cumulative trauma dose, types, and profiles using a development-based taxonomy of traumas. *Traumatology.* 2008;14(2):62-87.

20. Terr L. Childhood traumas: an outline and overview. *Amer J Psychiatry.* 1991;148: 10-20.

21. Pribram KH, Melges FT. Psychophysiological basis of emotion. In: Vinken PJ, Bruyn GW, eds. *Handbook of Clinical Neurology.* Amsterdam, Neth: North-Holland Publication; 1969:316-342.

22. LeDoux J. *Mind and Brain: Dialogues in Cognitive Neuroscience.* New York, NY: Cambridge University Press; 1986.

23. Tulving E, Markowitsch HJ. Episodic and declarative memory: role of the hippocampus. *Hippocampus.* 1998;8(3):198-204.

24. Stein M, Walker J, Forde D. Gender differences in susceptibility to posttraumatic stress disorder. *Behav Res Ther.* 2000;38:619-628.

25. Bremner J, Southwick S, Charney D. The neurobiology of posttraumatic stress disorder: an integration of animal and human research. In: Saigh P, Bremner J, eds. *Posttraumatic Stress Disorder: A Comprehensive Text.* Needham Heights, MA: Allyn & Bacon; 1999.

26. Nutt D, Malizia A. Structural and functional brain changes in posttraumatic stress disorder. *J Clin Psychiatry.* 2004;65(suppl 1):11-17.

27. Smith ME. Bilateral hippocampal volume reduction in adults with post-traumatic stress disorder: a meta-analysis of structural MRI studies. *Hippocampus.* 2005; 15(6):798-807.

28. Kolassa I, Wienbruch C, Neuner F, Schauer M, Ruf M, Odenwald,M, Elbert T. Altered oscillatory brain dynamics after repeated traumatic stress. *BMC Psychiatry.*

2007;7:56. http://www.biomedcentral.com/1471-244X/7/56. Published October 27, 2007. Accessed May 21, 2008

29. Rauch SL, van der Kolk BA, Fisler RE, Alpert NM, Orr SP, Savage CR, Fischman AJ, Jenike MA, Pitman RK. A symptom provocation study of posttraumatic stress disorder using positron emission tomography and script-driven imagery. *Arch Gen Psychiatry*. 1996;53(5):380-387

30. Glannon W. Psychopharmacology and memory. *J Med Ethics*. 2006;32:74-78.

31. de Kloet CS, Palesh OG, Aggarwal R, Vermetten E, Geuze E, Kavelaars A, Heijnen CJ, Westenberg HG. Assessment of HPA-axis function in posttraumatic stress disorder: pharmacological and non-pharmacological challenge tests, a review. *J Psychiatr Res*. 2006;40(6):550-567.

32. Yehuda R, Southwick SM, Nussbaum G, Wahby V, Giller EL Jr, Mason, JW. Low urinary cortisol excretion in patients with posttraumatic stress disorder. *J Nerv Ment Dis*. 1990;178:366-369.

33. Yehuda R, Resnick H, Schmeidler J, Yang R, Pitman R. Predicators of cortisol and 3-methoxy-4-hydroxy-phenylglycol responses in acute aftermath of rape. *Biol Psychiatry*. 1998;43:855-859.

34. Archer J. Behavioral aspects of fear. In: Sluckin W, ed. *Fear in Animals and Man*. New York, NY: Van Nostrand Reinhold; 1979: 56-85.

35. Gallup GG, Maser JD. Tonic immobility: evolutionary underpinnings of human catalepsy and catatonia. In: Seligman MEP, Maser JD, eds. *Psychopathology: Experimental Models*. San Francisco, CA: W.H. Freeman; 1977:334-357.

36. Suarez SD, Gallup GG. Tonic immobility as a response to rape in humans: a theoretical note. *Psychol Record*. 1979;29:315-320.

37. Galliano G, Noble LM, Travis LA, Puechl C. Victim reactions during rape/sexual assault. A preliminary study of the immobility response and its correlates. *J Interpersonal Violence*. 1993;8:109-114.

38. Taylor SE, Klein LC, Lewis BP, Gruenewald TL, Gurung RAR, Updegraff JA. Female responses to stress: tend-and-befriend, not fight-or-flight. *Psychol Review*. 2000;107(3):411-429.

39. Schacter D. *Searching for Memory*. New York, NY: Basic Books; 1996.

40. Brown R, Kulik J. Flashbulb memories. *Cognition*. 1977;5:73-99.

41. Terr L. What happens to early memories of trauma? *J Amer Acad Child Adolesc Psychiatry*. 1988;27:96-104.

42. Piaget JP. *The Origins of Intelligence in Children*. New York, NY: International Universities Press; 1952.

43. Seigel D. Memory, trauma and psychotherapy: a cognitive science view. *J Psychother Pract Res*. 1995;4(2):93-122.

44. Jacobs W, Nadel L. Stress-induced recovery of fears and phobias. *Psychol Rev*. 1985;100:68-90.

45. Bolles R, Fanselow M. A perceptual-defense-recuperative model of fear and pain. *Behav Brain Sci*. 1980;3:291-323.

46. Kilpatrick D, Edmunds C, Seymour A. *Rape in America: A Report to the Nation.* Arlington, VA: National Victim Center; 1992.

47. Kilpatrick DG, Acierno R, Resnick HS, et al. A 2-year longitudinal analysis of the relationship between violent assault and substance abuse in women. *J Consult Clin Psychol.* 1997;65:834-847.

48. Resnick HS, Kilpatrick DG, Dansky BS, et al. Prevalence of civilian trauma and posttraumatic stress disorder in a representative national sample of women. *J Consult Clin Psychol.* 1993;61:984-991.

49. Ullman S, Brecklin L. Sexual assault history and health-related outcomes in a national sample of women. *Psychol Women Q.* 2003;27 (1):46-57.

50. Classen C, Palesh O, Aggarwal R. Sexual revictimization: a review of the empirical literature. *Trauma Violence Abuse.* 2005;6(2):103-129.

51. Frazier P, Byrne C, Glaser T, Iwan A, Seales L. Multiple Traumas and PTSD Among Sexual Assault Survivors. Paper presented at: Annual of the American Psychological Association Meeting; 1997; Chicago, IL.

52. Campbell R, Sefl T, Barnes H, Ahrens C, Wasco S, Zaragoza-Diesfeld Y. Community services for rape survivors: enhancing psychological well-being or increasing trauma? *J Consult Clin Psychol.* 1999;67:847-858.

53. Acierno RE, Resnick HS, Kilpatrick DG, Saunders BE, Best CL. Risk factors for rape, physical assault, and PTSD in women: examination of differential multivariate relationships. *J Anxiety Disord.* 1999;13(6):541-563.

54. Nishith P, Mechanic M, Resnick P. Prior interpersonal trauma: the contribution to current PTSD symptoms in female rape victims. *J Abnorm Psychol.* 2000;109(1): 20-25.

55. Davis R, Brickman E, Baker T. Supportive and unsupportive responses of others to rape victims: effects of concurrent victim adjustment. *Amer J Community Psychol.* 1991;19:443-451.

56. McAuslan P, Abbey A. Do disclosure and the reactions of others affect mental health, physical health and alcohol use following sexual assault? Paper presented at: International Society for the Study of Personal Relationships; 1998; Saratoga Springs, NY.

57. Ullman S. Correlates and consequences of adult sexual assault disclosure. *J Interpersonal Violence.* 1996;11:554-571.

58. Ullman S, Fillipas H. Predictors of PTSD symptom severity and social reactions in sexual assault victims. *J Trauma Stress.* 2001;14(2):369-389.

59. Peplau H. *Interpersonal Relations in Nursing: A Conceptual Frame of Reference for Psychodynamic Nursing.* New York, NY: Springer Publishing; 1952.

60. Burgess A, Holmstrom L. The rape trauma syndrome. *Am J Psychiatry.* 1974;131: 981-986.

61. Foa E, Rothbaum B. *Treating the Trauma of Rape.* New York, NY: Guilford Press; 1998.

62. North American Nursing Diagnosis International. *Nursing Diagnoses: Definitions and Classification 2007-2008.* Philadelphia, PA: NANDA International; 2007.

Chapter 11

Education and Qualifications of the Forensic Nurse in Sexual Assault Evaluation

Patricia M. Speck, DNSc, APN, FNP-BC, DF-IAFN, FAAFS, FAAN
Susan B. Patton, DNSc, PNP-BC, SANE-A, SANE-P*

Violence was unrecognized as a major health care concern until the middle of the 1980s, but an understanding of the connection between health and violence was taking root in the late 1960s.[1] There was a growing realization that the existing health care system was burdened by patients needing emergency and long-term psychological care following sexual violence. While the numbers of nurses[†] responding to rape victims were growing in the 1970s and 1980s, nursing and medical literature had little knowledge of or information about the impact of sexual violence on health.[2] It was not until the 1990s that the "forensic nurse[‡]" appeared in the national media.[3] However, it is well established that nurses have been assisting physicians who were uneducated in the treatment of and evidence collection from rape victims for decades. Unfortunately, it is a practice that persists today, and in many communities, neither licensed health care provider (physician or registered nurse [RN]) has been educated about rape, its evaluation and treatment, or the psychological aftermath and physical injury that follow sexual assault and abuse.

History of the Education of Sexual Assault Nurse Examiners

Prior to the development of sexual assault nurse examiner practice, a complaint of rape from patients would require inordinate amounts of time for care and evaluation—especially for the nonurgent patient who waited 6 to 12 hours to see a physician in the busy emergency department.[4-7] Physicians did not have adequate time to complete evidence collection before being called away to care for a "real" physical emergency. Oftentimes, the evidence was compromised. Consequently, entry-level resident or intern physicians were relegated and often punished with the assignment of a rape victim (D. Muram, MD, personal communication, July 1984). They invested considerable time

* *The authors would like to recognize Ms. Gail Spake, Technical Writer in the Office of Research and Grant Support at UTHSC College of Nursing for providing EndNote support.*

† *The term* nurse *is used in this instance and throughout the text to mean "registered nurse with practice experience and education in the care of patients who have been sexually assaulted."*

‡ *For the purposes of this text, the term* forensic nurse *is used to represent the nurse engaged in the practice of nursing in the specialty of forensic nursing as defined in the* Forensic Nursing Scope and Standards of Practice, *published jointly by the American Nurses Association and the International Association of Forensic Nurses.*

evaluating the patient and collecting evidence for a Vitullo kit by reading instructions printed on the inside of the box.[8] In those days, the prevailing wisdom was that raped patients were not really physically injured and that the patient somehow contributed to her own victimization through her choices or activities because "good girls" didn't get raped. In the social upheavals of the 1960s, these beliefs were challenged. The civil rights movement provided a foundation for a renewal of the women's liberation movement. It was in this climate of change that an RN and social worker evaluated and studied rape victims in an emergency department in Boston. Ann Burgess's landmark article, "Rape trauma syndrome," provided the foundation for understanding the psychological impact of rape.[9]

The subject matter of rape, also confused with "just sex" in the 1960s, was socially taboo. International coverage of the modern conceptualization of rape, now called *Rape Trauma Syndrome* (RTS), resulted in a growth in awareness about the psychological trauma following rape (A.W. Burgess, DNSc, RN, FAAN, personal communication, March 1983). Beverly H. Bounds, a nurse practitioner and University of Tennessee Health Science Center College of Nursing educator, had championed the development of the nurse practitioner role in Tennessee in the early 1970s. After the article about rape victims in the emergency department appeared in the *American Journal of Nursing*, she turned her public health nursing skills to changing the response to problems encountered by rape victims in the local county hospital in Memphis, Tennessee.[5] In 1973, she partnered with emergency room physicians from the local county hospital, law enforcement professionals from the Memphis Police Department, and prosecutors from the Office of the Memphis/Shelby District Attorney General to introduce a new model of care: nurses providing care for and collecting evidence from rape victims. A federal educational grant provided the seed money necessary to educate RNs and to implement the Memphis Rape Crisis Program.[10] The new role's job title was "nurse clinician," which was a reflection of the conceptualization of the nursing role at the time—a role that emanated from nurse specialty areas such as acute care, psychiatry, pediatrics, women's health, and public health during that decade.

Registered nurses are historically educated about the scientific fundamentals that help them to care for patients collaboratively with other professions, and the first nurse clinicians were no exception. Knowledge, skills, abilities, and attitudes evident in the registered nursing practice included relationships between person, environment, health, nurse, and included biopsychosocial and spiritual foundations in health across the life span; this was the theoretical basis for nursing care of the rape victim in the earliest days of the role. While unrecognized at the time, the program infrastructure development, including formative and summative evaluations used to establish the sexual assault programmatic response, are now considered public health nursing competencies.[11] At the time, the legislated independence of the public health nurse working with women in individual states following the passage of Title X: Public Health Service Act in 1970 was timely and contributed to acceptance of the sexual assault nurse clinicians' testimony by state courts.[12,13] Many of the nurses who were hired in the first program, soon to be known as sexual assault nurse examiners (SANEs), had "nurse practitioner certificates," some from early nurse practitioner educational programs.[14] The graduates of the early nurse practitioner programs practiced in community settings such as women's health clinics, making them a natural choice for nursing care of rape victims. The model for sexual assault response by nurses that was proposed in Memphis initially included only nurse practitioners.[10] This is because the evaluations were and continue to be performed in a community-based clinic where RNs could not practice without direct physician oversight under Tennessee law at the time. However, because there were very few nurse practitioners at the time and the numbers of women reporting rape in Memphis doubled from 157 to over 350 in the first year of operation,* experienced OB-GYN nurses were subsequently hired and educated about the "rape nurse" role.[2] The local medical director of the health department considered the nonpractitioner nurse clinicians to be equivalent to the public health nurse role (J. Kirkley, MD, personal communication, August 1984)—an interpretation that would change under another medical director in the 1980s. The additional education necessary for the nonpractitioner rape nurse clinicians included additional psychomotor nursing skills (eg, speculum insertion for examination and to sample for evidence of rape, STI screening, PAP smear).[15] All would be educated in specialty techniques (eg, evidence collection, packaging, secure storage) heretofore considered the purview of law enforcement.[8] These skills were taught by representatives from the collaborating health care and criminal justice agencies, from the local emergency department, forensic laboratory, the Memphis Police Department, and the local district attorney's office.

The focus of the education in the first program was to cover why the nurse clinician would use a particular technical skill in a procedure, use a particular test, give a particular medication, or record a particular type of physical or psychological response to rape trauma. The nurse clinicians needed the information to provide comprehensive nursing and medical care, and the courts needed identical information to adjudicate their cases. These early relationships between law enforcement and nursing eventually created misunderstandings and legal inquiry about whether the nurse witness is a clinical expert or simply an extension of the prosecution as a testimonial witness in a criminal justice process.[16,17] In the 1970s and early 1980s—unaware of the challenges to comprehensive nursing practice that would occur in the clinical and courtroom arenas—nurses in the earliest SANE practices would teach each other using the old adage "see one, do one, teach one."

Further north in another Mississippi River city, Minneapolis, Linda Ledray read the article entitled "Rape trauma syndrome"[9] (L. Ledray, PhD, RN, FAAN, personal communication, May 2007), and, in 1975, she received a research demonstration treatment grant from the National Institute of Mental Health to establish a model of care for rape victims in Minneapolis. She had been asked by clinic nurses to help them address the needs, both medical and psychological, of rape victims and to improve the follow-up rates after evaluation in the local emergency department. During her systematic review of the response to rape victims in the emergency department, Ledray was appalled by the treatment of victims and, in 1977, she established the Sexual Assault Resource Center (SARC) to respond to rape victims using RNs as counselors initially (L. Ledray, PhD, RN, FAAN, personal communication, May 2007). Like the nurses in Memphis, the nurses in Minneapolis brought to the table nursing education, ethical standards, and licensure obligation to the patient. These pioneers added another very important dimension to the rape nurse role: mental health nursing. Their initial work as counselors in the Minneapolis program included repeated contact with the reporting rape victims, during which they received feedback about the adjudication course of their cases. Very quickly, they could see that "it made no sense to counsel or empower the victim when [barriers to] recovery included attitudes of apathy and anger among hospital staff, physicians, and nurses" (L. Ledray, PhD, RN, FAAN, personal communication, November 2007). In addition, there were other barriers to efficient care

* *Reported rapes double in many communities after the establishment of a SANE program, and this phenomenon was seen in early communities that established SANE programs nationally. This increased reporting is felt to be due to public awareness rather than an increase in rapes. Today, new SANE/SART programs should plan for the increased reporting from community populations that become aware of the new services.*

and ultimate recovery, such as distractions in the emergency department (eg, urgent care of patients), compromised evidence due to inordinate amounts of time for the rape victim to wait in the emergency department for care, and poor court outcomes. The mental health nursing education was solid, but the initial education and training in forensic care of rape victims, described as "flying by the seat of our pants," was of little help (L. Ledray, PhD, RN, FAAN, personal communication, November 2007). In the early years of the sexual assault forensic nursing role in Minneapolis, nursing education about the care of victims of sexual assault did not prepare the nurse clinician staff for the frustrating experiences and poor outcomes inherent in the adjudication process. By 1977, the Minneapolis program had partnered with the hospitals, a forensic laboratory, and county attorneys to begin to collect evidence in addition to providing counseling and, more importantly, began to receive feedback about what worked and what did not work in evidence collection and testimony by registered nurses. These initial efforts to impact public health through stakeholder participation and process analysis demonstrated an interprofessional and collaborative fact-finding and evidence-based approach to sexual assault response information that would eventually be formalized and published in the Office for Victims of Crime's *SANE Development and Operations Guide.*[16] When there, the nurse clinician would not only provide therapeutic nursing care utilizing techniques including physical evaluation, crisis intervention, and anticipatory guidance, but, with the patient's permission, they would also collect evidence.[4,6,7,18] Ledray predicted that they could impact the outcome of the adjudication process (L. Ledray, PhD, RN, FAAN, personal communication, March 1984), a prediction that was supported in several communities following evaluation and implementation of evidence-based practice models in the new millennium.[2,19-21]

As in Memphis, the number of registered nurses working in and studying aspects of sexual assault care and the amount of information shared between professions in Minneapolis increased rapidly. While SANEs practiced in isolation in the 1970s, the comprehensive education to prepare them for their new role was strikingly similar. Developing independently, forensic nurses in sexual assault care were able to respond to their specific hospital or community agency with law enforce-ment when there was a rape complaint. The nurse practitioner, rape crisis counselor or activist, and law enforcement officer quickly became part of the sexual assault response team (SART). There were rape crisis programs and activists in many communities in the early 1970s, but in Memphis these early activists were certified counselors or social workers who performed dual roles of counselor and advocate.[22] After a decade of being on call for crisis counseling 24/7, providing long-term mental health counseling, and making court appearances to support the victims, in 1985, grant dollars were secured in Memphis for a funded (but not new) model of rape support: the rape advocate. The program chose to separate the roles of advocate and counselor, and those who wanted to continue as the mental health counselor did so, while others chose the court advocate role to support the rape victim throughout the process of reporting and adjudication. The 24/7 on-call crisis intervention through a telephone hotline was contracted to a community agency hotline that responded to other crises (ie, suicide). This new advocate role would not only provide support to the victim throughout the adjudication process, it would also link the prosecution in the criminal justice system to the existing resource team of counselor, advocate, nurse, and law enforcement (M. Snyder, MSSW and B. Cassinello, CMSW, personal communication, August 1986).

Both Memphis and Minneapolis demonstrated rudimentary permutations of a team approach in the 1970s that would eventually be known as SART. When the team response occurred in a community agency outside hospital emergency departments (eg,

Memphis Rape Crisis Center), it was referred to as "one-stop shopping." Rape victims could receive a planned, comprehensive response from a model in which nurses, rape activist counselors (the future advocates), and law enforcement officers came together in SARTs for education and development of collaborative policies and procedures to serve and care for the reporting victim.[2,16,19,20] The supportive piece of the rape crisis counselor's after-hours role in the 1970s, became the rape crisis advocate services in the mid-to-late 1980s. In Memphis, the counselor's role remained a stable and long-term therapeutic link to recovery, but the practice moved away from the court process and focused on the mental health of the client. Splitting the role of counselor and activist or advocate was a new conceptualization of the 2 roles. While advocates remained the immediate emotional support following the rape and remained a bridge to the criminal justice system, the counselor addressed the morbidities associated with the mental health outcomes through short- and long-term treatment plans. The comprehensive community response model of one-stop shopping demonstrated at the Memphis Rape Crisis Center in the 1970s and 1980s was a precursor to the child advocacy center model of the late 1980s and early 1990s. Today, the family justice and safety center models are one recent permutation of the early SARTs and advocacy center models providing expanded wrap-around services to victims of intimate partner and sexual violence and their children (D.P. Connor, PhD, personal communication, October 2007).[23] Today, with federal mandates to develop interprofessional teams representing all community stakeholders, the evolution of response teams to all types of victims of violence continue. The teams are planned through collaborative and formative processes with all stakeholder interprofessional team members through community partnerships. The newest language to describe this process is called a coordinated community response (CCR), and many communities divide teams to respond to specific populations, eg, older and vulnerable persons in cases of abuse, neglect, and exploitation (OVPANE). These teams have hammered out the roles and responsibilities of the unique disciplines and have included decision tree algorithms for timing the immediate and ongoing wrap-around responses necessary to respond to individuals subjected to violence. In the past, many agencies operated in silo systems, uncoordinated and duplicative; they failed to coordinate care of victims and consequently increased costs to their communities. The CCR resembles the first SART and usually includes law enforcement, health care, and advocacy. Today there is a realization that many services are needed for vulnerable raped individuals at the time of the report of the criminal act. These may include things like 24-hour hotlines or legislated institutional investigation and emergency specialized housing for a vulnerable person with intellectual or physical disabilities or dementia. The immediate evaluation is just the beginning of a collaborative effort to help the victim. The larger stakeholder community members are considered partners with the CCR who also respond to the victim, her immediate needs, and the safety needs of the community. Removing barriers that prohibit sharing of vital information in confidential venues is one hurdle faced by all CCR teams and stakeholders; however, a shared vision of a "victim-centered" approach to services and mutual respect for the need to know specific information is central to all stakeholder agencies, including the CCR.[24]

All programs that respond to sexual assault victims represent a strong public health approach designed to improve care and speed recovery of patients who are sexually victimized. Today, centers that promote prevention of sexual violence are working hand in hand with response and resource teams and their agencies to implement permanent changes for the at-risk person in the community, whether a youth or an elder, male or female. Each evolutionary phase has been integrated in the educational and clinical education of the SANE and sexual assault forensic examiner (SAFE). ("SANE" will be used throughout this chapter for expediency with the realization that there are other licensed health care providers operating in the role of the SAFE, including physicians and physician assistants [PAs].)

A third program in Amarillo, Texas, began using RNs in the emergency room to collect evidence as early as 1979.[18] Nurses initially assisted physicians in evidence collection, but eventually demonstrated comprehensive care to victims of sexual assault. Sexual assault nurse examiner education at Amarillo was remarkably like the other 2 programs, a phenomenon that would repeat itself in many communities as programs developed throughout the 1980s.

As individuals within SART programs developed early publications[4-7,15,18,25-27] and described the early forensic nurse response to sexual assault in not-for-profit and government programs, the need for consistent and collaborative educational content was realized as necessary for the new SANE practice. Although there was no communication between the programs prior to the early 1980s, it is anecdotally reported that the early education was similar. Specifically, there was a heavy reliance on a solid scientific foundation in nursing and practice expertise at the generalist and advanced nursing practice level of care (Memphis and Minneapolis), physician supervision in hospital-based practices (Amarillo) that employed primarily generalist nurses, and informal education that was taught by personnel from the local health department, forensic laboratory, law enforcement, and the Office of the District Attorney General. It is important to point out that early education for all 3 types of programs included instructions about why and how to collect evidence, its implication in the criminal justice system, and information about rules of evidence and attorney strategies in courtroom testimony. It was presumed that the licensed health care professionals, specifically RNs, knew how to assess the patient, collect the medical history of the event, evaluate and document the physical injuries, and make medical referrals. Lacking was the rationale and standardized procedure for evidence collection. The literature was sparse and the rationale for specific forensic techniques was generally opinionated conjecture or tradition (eg, pulling hair); therefore, there was a general lack of evidence base for SANE practice. On the other hand, there was a considerable evidence base for nursing practice with patients who had been sexually assaulted. Consequently, non-nurses taught borrowed forensic science and anecdotal experience to new SANEs during this early period.

For the first decade, nursing education about sexual assault was provided to new nurse clinicians by those practicing in the forensic science specialty, such as the medical examiner (ME) and the ME's staff in Memphis. As education about content associated with rape was integrated into continuing education in nursing programs, more formalized education began to develop. The earliest educational offerings were taught in hospitals and community organizations as part of employee orientation and in-services (eg, grand rounds). By the early 1980s, these educational programs provided continuing education units for the nurses by partnering with their local universities and professional organizations. In 1986, the University of Tennessee Department of Continuing Medical Education, in collaboration with the Memphis Sexual Assault Resource Center (formerly the Memphis Rape Crisis Program), formalized presentations taught by SANEs in the 1970s and 1980s and embedded them in a curriculum for OB-GYN resident practical education.[2,13] Evidence over the next 3 years confirmed that hospital nurses, medical students, and residents changed their behavior, retained the information provided by the forensic nurse educators, and found the education about rape and victim responses useful in their daily medical practices.[28] This educational program continued under a contract until 2003, when it was discontinued.

Who Should Be Conducting SANE Education, and Why?

As with most new nursing specialties, pieces that are missing in nursing education are taught by professionals with expertise and experience in specific areas. Clinicians and other professionals involved in forensic care, including physicians, nurse practitioners, forensic laboratory personnel, both prosecutors and defense attorneys, and law enforcement officers, were the teachers of the first registered nurses and nurse practitioners caring for sexual assault victims in the 1970s. Historical precedence for these educational methods and processes impacting the nursing process has been set by a number of emerging specialties. Physicians trained midwives in the 1930s and nurse practitioners in the 1960s. In fact, "many nurses have had to go outside of nursing to learn forensic skills."[29] This was not lost on forensic nurses with a decade or more of experience in the subspecialty of sexual assault care. Others predicted that, as nurses entered the new specialty of forensic nursing, experience and content expertise would grow, providing the forensic nurse educators of sexual assault care content in the future.[30]

Today, a handful of nurses have 25 or more years of experience in SANE practice with adult and pediatric patients. With hundreds of forensic nurses approaching 10 to 15 years of experience in the care of adult, adolescent, and child sexual assault and abuse patients, it is rare for nurses to need to look outside the experts in forensic nursing circles to learn emerging scientific information about patient evaluation and treatment. In this context, the expert forensic nurse develops education that incorporates this new information into curricula.[31] Forensic nurses have been leaders in collaboration, and they share scientific discoveries and experiences with physicians, attorneys, law enforcement, advocacy, and expert nurses in other areas of nursing. The camaraderie demonstrated by forensic nurses is also found among SART members and can be seen in the documents that have been produced by professional consensus.[32,33] These important documents help establish the evidence base and guidelines as standards for care as well as maintain consistency between and among responders to the targeted event, specifically the rape or abuse victim. However, for the most part, nursing certification bodies require nursing experts to teach nurses in a program certified by the American Nurses Credentialing Center (ANCC); the same applies for maintenance of certifications.[34] Borrowed science has historically played a large part in nursing specialties. Science developed by non-nurse specialties is foundational to the application of nursing process in the care of rape and sexual assault victims. The registered nurse educator is highly qualified to understand the relationships between the borrowed science and theoretical underpinnings of nursing and nursing practice; in addition, registered nurses teach the nursing process, which is absent in education provided by non-nurses. Accordingly, this method has improved as the SANE has gained experience and developed an understanding of health and human responses to disease and injury following rape and abuse. The nursing profession takes methods of scientific evidence collection from forensic science, legal, psychological, sexual assault, and public health literature and applies it to the nursing process, creating a unique patient-focused relationship with the victims of sexual assault, rape, and abuse and with the victims' communities. However, nurses who choose this role and respond to rape and sexual assault or abuse patients primarily bring their nursing education and experience in providing holistic care. They then incorporate information unique to forensic nursing of sexual assault patients (ie, wounding and healing, ethical dilemmas, evidence collection and other legal nuisances [WHEEL]), or public health and prevention.[2,11,31] Education and psychomotor skills for care of all persons experiencing injury are taught in undergraduate nursing education. Subsequently, continuing education courses provide the foundation for practice in specific practice areas and with specific groups of patients, such as sexual assault victims in an emergency department or community setting.

Graduate forensic nurse specialists with an expertise in the sexual assault content area will be sought out for direct care and leadership functions (eg, administration, education, consultation), particularly if the program curriculum completed by the nurse meets or exceeds the national standards for graduate curriculum.[31,35] Early sexual assault nurses were trained in technical procedures to improve psychomotor skills (eg, kit collection, PAP smears, microscopy, other technical skills). Through a modern lens, the knowledge of yesterday now appears primitive and even risky (although it was felt at the time to be cutting edge). Registered nurses have always been taught how to approach the patient; to evaluate the patient for injury, physical and mental healing, and the community response to the event; and to counsel or anticipate health care needs or apply systems change to populations in nursing education.[2,31,36] Along with the additional knowledge and experience in the content areas of evidence and law, the sexual assault forensic nursing role will continue to produce the subject matter experts and educators of the future.[2,36]

What Is Included in SANE Educational Programs?

Historically, the *Sexual Assault Nurse Examiner: Scope and Standards of Practice* provided structure to the practice role of the SANE and the first *IAFN Sexual Assault Nurse Examiner Educational Guidelines* provided a comprehensive nursing foundation for the development of basic SANE coursework along with an outline of content topics to address.[34,37] Today, the curriculum designer of SANE education programs has a number of documents that frame the scope, domains, and levels of nursing for use in the creation of education and training for the SANE. The documents identified below represent a small selection of the resources to be considered:

— *Forensic Nursing: Scope and Standards of Practice:* a consensus document that reflects forensic nursing content while maintaining alignment with all other specialties in nursing, and which includes guidelines and protection for every level of nursing practice.[38]

— The Forensic Nurse's Code of Ethics[39]

— *Code of Ethics for Nurses with Interpretative Statements*[40]

— *Nursing's Social Policy Statement:* a consensus document that describes nursing's accountability to the public and the mechanisms necessary to maintain public trust.[41]

— *A National Protocol for Sexual Assault Medical Forensic Examinations: Adults/Adolescents:* a consensus document that was created as a supplement to state and local protocols and as a guide for criminal justice and health care professionals in response to the need for standardization of response by health care providers.[32]

— *National Training Standards for Sexual Assault Medical Forensic Examiners:* a consensus document created in response to a federal statutory mandate to develop guidelines for the minimum preparation of sexual assault care providers who are expected to work in coordination with other team members.[42]

An understanding of these and other national and international consensus documents provides a framework to guide and uniformity between the trainer and educator. These frameworks are the basis for the forensic nursing specialty, of which SANE is a subspecialty. The educational guidelines are particularly useful, as they define content areas for educational and clinical goals. The SANE educator should also use the International Association of Forensic Nurses (IAFN) documents to guide the content of the material. The IAFN has developed consensus documents for forensic nursing care of both young (pediatric or adolescent) and more mature (older adolescent and adult) victims of sexual assault and abuse. These resources identify topical areas for educational content. Both documents are proprietary and remain available from the IAFN at http://www.iafn.org.[43]

The *Forensic Nursing Scope and Standards of Practice* were revised to reflect the current thinking of international nursing experts in both practical and research positions using the template designed by the American Nurses Association (ANA).[31,38] Care is influenced by the varying levels of educational preparation and certification (ie, generalist versus specialist) within the group of nurses desiring to practice as SANEs. Since the majority of SANEs are prepared to practice nursing at the undergraduate level and many RNs are directly supervised by advanced practice nurses with graduate degrees or physicians, SANE programs should also look to local and state or province literature and legislation to improve quality by guiding practice through policies and procedures. For example, *Advanced Nursing Practice: A National Framework* defines the minimum education of the advanced nursing practice as a graduate education and the *Nursing: Scope and Standards of Practice* presents expectations for all registered nurses in the United States.[44,45] Importantly, both of these documents differentiate between the undergraduate general and graduate advanced nursing practice. To that end, the IAFN, through its leadership, has created documents consistent with professional nursing organizations' positions on appropriate practice.[31,32,46] In addition, the documents align with federal publications detailing the expected qualifications of trainers and training materials.[42] For the most part, training and education for SANEs is divided into either the SANE-A (adult and adolescent) or SANE-P (pediatric) category. As seen in the list below, topic areas and evidence base in SANE education are overlapping, albeit distinct within and influenced by the developmental stage of the patient. In both SANE-A and SANE-P, the educational content guide for forensic nursing education includes the following topic areas[42,43]:

— Interprofessional teams and their roles

— Forensic nursing role with targeted population (pediatric, adolescent, or adult) in specific settings and systems

— Forensic nursing role in sexual assault/abuse care

— Dynamics of sexual assault/abuse

— Medical history/forensic interview

— Physical evaluation and findings

— Evidence collection and evaluation

— Documentation of findings, diagnosis, treatment, and patient management

— Ethics

— Criminal justice system

There is content that is of necessity duplicated between the SANE-A and SANE-P courses. This content includes core knowledge, skills, abilities, and attitudes of both the SANE-A and SANE-P. When the SANE-A and SANE-P courses are taken separately, the content should be, and normally is, offered in both. When a course combines both SANE-A and SANE-P educational and clinical materials, not only does the coursework mimic nursing education across the life span, but the length of the course is shortened and the student saves time and expense because there is a lack of duplication.

While no demonstration of clinical skills is required by any standard of education for the SANE, whether caring for adult, adolescent, or pediatric patient populations, there is a growing movement toward requiring demonstrations of clinical skills to be included in the courses through simulation and standardized patients. These clinical skills include, but are not limited to, basic nursing skills of creating a clean environment where contamination is reduced or eliminated, advanced therapeutic nursing assessment (including a focused history and complete physical evaluation), sample collection and handling of laboratory specimens (forensic or medical), objective documentation of findings and conclusions, reporting of findings in different venues (eg, after the evaluation, in court), and improvement of psychomotor skill sets (eg, sample collection, microscopy, photography, speculum use). The following list includes the different skill areas that make up the clinical content guide for forensic nursing education for both SANE-A and SANE-P[42,43]:

— Initial wellness and developmental assessment

— Injury recognition and description

— Sample collection, handling, and security

— Interview and history taking

— Photography

— Microscopy

— Instruments of magnification

— Physical assessment, including anogenital evaluation

— Tools for documentation and classification of findings

— Formulation of diagnosis and treatment

— Systems response (notification, referral, and follow-up)

— Courtroom proceedings

In at least 5 states (Kentucky, Maryland, New Jersey, Nevada, Texas), the SANE must adhere to a specific rule, regulation, or legislation regarding preparation or practice. The varied state regulations (eg, specified education, state certification or approval, mandated national certification process, mandated certification process through state agency) were created in an attempt to ensure quality care before formal education and professional certification were available nationally. However, national certification is now available and demonstrates competence in sexual assault forensic nursing. As the SANE model of care within SARTs is accepted and spreads, states should continue to remove institutional barriers and to provide resources (including financial backing) that will promote patient access to qualified SANEs, particularly in geographically large rural areas. In summary, clinical competence is determined by the certification process and validated by an experienced clinician—whether an employer, a contractor, or a peer. By determining distinct levels of knowledge, possession or lack of certain skills and abilities, and understanding provider attitudes, expert educators are able to teach to the level of the provider's practice, whether that be general care or a more advanced specialization. In order to address the large number of clinicians in remote areas who will require education and the more general movement toward providing online access to educational content, as well as the growing numbers of SANE students and the expanding base of evidence and research, educators will need to continue to develop their technological skills. Further, future clinical demonstrations will occur through simulation in an effort to protect the patient until competence is demonstrated.[22,47-49] Decisions regarding who is capable of doing this work in remote areas will require a common goal of access for all victims, maintenance of the highest standards of care, development of emotional intelligence in communication, and equality in interprofessional collaboration.

Continuing Education: CEU, Undergraduate, or Graduate Education?

One way to promote increasing knowledge about sexual assault care is to encourage participation in accredited continuing education activities related to sexual assault care. ***Continuing education*** is an inclusive term that includes a spectrum of postsecondary education learning activities and programs. Broadly defined, it is postsecondary education that does not lead to a degree or diploma. Recognized forms of postsecondary learning activities include degree credit courses by nontraditional students, nondegree career training, workforce training, formal personal enrichment courses (both on campus and distance online), self-directed learning (such as through Internet interest groups, clubs, or personal research activities), and experiential learning. In the 1990s, nurse educators moved toward ANCC-approved accreditation because renewal of specialty certification requires at least 50% of contact hours be derived from ANCC-approved providers and taught by a registered nurse educator.[50] Accreditation of educational courses is a voluntary process that grants recognition to an organization or institution that "meets established standards based on predetermined criteria."[51] ANCC will accredit organizations as either an approver or a provider of continuing education units (CEUs) in nursing.[51] Many state nursing boards now require that a certain percentage of CEU credit be ANCC approved.[51]

Through learning activities focused on subject topics like sexual assault, nursing and health care provided to victims and offenders, evidence, and the criminal justice system, the SANE today has acquired a knowledge base regarding the subject matter before learning the SANE role. Additional subject matter must be addressed in a continuing education format for each geographic community; it is often unaccredited but may meet additional certification needs for SANEs. For example, specific policies and procedures for the agency (ie, government, commercial, or not-for-profit), local customs and collaborative relationships (ie, MOUs, SARTs, CACs, or Family Violence or Safety Centers), and information about applicable legislation and rulings are all necessary to meet the standards set in *Forensic Nursing: Scope and Standards of Practice*.[31] Documents guiding SANE practice are revised periodically to reflect current research findings. The SANE will use the guidelines to provide validation for the content in local SANE education programs that may be the only accredited providers of continuing education for SANE.

Continuing education is also valuable to the nurse seeking professional certification. Forensic nurses, like those from other nursing roles and specialties, have developed certification methods to demonstrate to the public that they are competent not only as nurses, but as practitioners of forensic skills. Professionals earn certifications to assure that they are qualified to perform a role, job, or task. For the most part, certification is granted for demonstration of a complex combination of knowledge, skills, abilities, and attitudes at the level of competence set by the organization bestowing certification. Competency is not to be equated with expertise. According to Benner, expertise is developed beyond the level of competence through the acquisition of knowledge and experience over time.[52,53] In some communities, clinical ladders for SANEs are based on Benner's framework for advancement.[54]

The Forensic Nurse Certification Board is the certifying arm of the IAFN. Utilizing publications on promising and best practice methods, standards of practice, and the judgment of expert clinicians, the certification board has developed certification exams for SANEs caring for injured adolescents and adults (SANE-A) and those caring for pediatric patients (SANE-P). Registered nurses who pass a standardized course on sexual assault and whose clinical evaluation by an independent SANE is considered competent are eligible to take the exam(s). Upon successful completion of all requirements, the certification affords the nurse a distinction among her peers as one qualified to make assessments, offer treatments, and make recommendations to the courts regarding individuals with injuries related to sexual assault. In some states, certification through the Forensic Nurse Certification Board is required for practice with this population. In addition, credibility in the courtroom can be enhanced by methods of credentialing that demonstrate the competence of successful candidates to make critical judgments in forensic venues.

The IAFN criteria for certification by examination includes the following[34]:

— Educational coursework focused on forensic nursing care of sexual assault patients

— Demonstrated competency in this subspecialty area

— Holding an RN license for at least 2 years

The content outline includes the dynamics of sexual assault, the evaluation and clinical management of sexual assault patients, and interaction throughout the judicial process. The content also includes the roles and responsibilities of the SART and includes professional practice trends and issues. In addition, knowledge and skills inherent in general RN practice are needed to perform the SANE role.[43] Those seeking recertification from the IAFN Forensic Nursing Certification Board in 2009 will require 45 hours of educational activities over a 3-year period, at least 60% of which must be earned through continuing education offerings. Further, 20% of those continuing education hours must be from accredited nursing organizations, and all of the educational activities must be related to the SANE content outline.

The effectiveness of continuing education in demonstrating ongoing or current competence remains controversial, although it is now well-known that knowledge in isolation of appropriate clinical experience is not well correlated to the development of a clinical skill set.[55] In that vein, the development of a portfolio method of assessing competence in advanced practice forensic nursing that incorporates additional evidence of mastery (eg, peer review, scholarship, continuing education with posttesting, self-evaluation, case studies) will most likely begin to influence recertification methods for SANEs and other professional roles in the near future.

Formal forensic-specific continuing education courses generally result in a certificate of completion or a CEU and can prepare health care providers to respond correctly to victims of sexual violence and to collect and preserve evidence. However, graduate education is now necessary for those who wish to assume leadership positions in the broader field of forensic nursing rather than focus on the subspecialty of sexual assault care. Preparation leading to a degree provides comprehensive and, in most institutions, accredited credentials necessary for a variety of leadership roles overseeing nursing care of patients with specialized forensic needs.

The first postprofessional certificate in forensic nursing from an accredited institution was offered by Mount Royale College in Canada in 1996. Other institutions were slow to follow, because there was no documentation of need at that time. To assist institutions in developing curricula for forensic nursing practice, an IAFN Education Committee resolution in support of the development of graduate education for forensic nurses was presented to and adopted by the Board of Directors of IAFN in 2002. Under the guidance of the IAFN President, this was followed by the appointment of an IAFN Ad Hoc Committee Chair who was charged with creating a consensus document through a series of regional meetings that defined the forensic nursing domains, content areas, and performance measures. The participants and developers of these documents were primarily educators with experience in curriculum development and content mapping. When completed, these 2 documents provided the necessary foundation for justification of a framework for programs in forensic nursing to be developed at many schools of nursing, including the first Doctor of Nursing Practice (DNP) in forensic nursing at the University of Tennessee Health Science Center College of Nursing. Most nongraduate SANE programs offer a certificate of completion or CEUs. Most graduate programs include the SANE content in the larger curriculum of forensic nursing, and these institutions offer a wide range of academic credentials—from graduate diplomas (ie, MSN, DNP) to postgraduate or postdoctoral certificates. Today the type of credential awarded often reflects where advanced practice nurses are educated (ie, in a specific country, state, province) and the level of education each has achieved.

Program Evaluation, Safety, and Educational Outcomes

Program evaluation is one way to critically examine the foundational education and clinical experience of nurses beginning their SANE education. There are 2 stages of program evaluation: formative and summative.[56] Formative evaluation answers questions regarding the quality and improvement of the program in its developmental stages. Summative evaluation examines outcomes identified as benchmark indicators of the effectiveness of the program. This holds true not only for sexual assault programs, but also for all levels of education that prepare sexual assault forensic nurses.[2]

For example, it is expected that an advanced practice forensic nurse with a certification in women's health care will demonstrate pelvic evaluation technique during her graduate educational preparation, because integration of forensic principles into specialized nursing education forms the basis and rationale for advanced forensic nursing practice. All education and experience meant to meet the ANA mandate that nurses should continue to seek knowledge builds from the concept of attaining competence through proficiency expertise.[11,45] During the formative evaluation of SANE programs, plans that address educational foundations and coursework should be assessed for evidence of the most current research and scholarship.[2] Examples of some questions to ask in the formative stages of an educational program evaluation include, but are not limited to, the following:

— Does the educational program meet the stated guidelines and newest evidence in publication?

— Do the teachers meet the standards set forth for content expertise and education?

— What is the profile of the students enrolled?

— What steps are in place to assist the nursing student in the transition from knowledge to competence?

— Will there be clinical simulations, and, if so, what elements will be highlighted?

— What measures are in place to establish that educational information has been understood and integrated into the student's nursing process?

— For how long will a nurse completing this program require clinical supervision?

— How many simulated clinical experiences are available to each student?

— How many students are assigned to each simulated clinical experience?

— Should the formative processes involve an outside evaluator?

When developing summative evaluation benchmarks, use validated tools for assessment of SANE programs.[2] Some questions to ask in the summative evaluation of the educational program include the following:

— How many students were enrolled in the educational activities?

— What were the demographics of the class?

— Are the former students employed in SANE programs? If not, why?

— Did the cohort meet the benchmarks for competency with each skill?

— After this course, are the nurses in the course competent to see patients without direct supervision? How many required remedial attention? In what areas did they require attention?

— Are students who complete the educational experience adequately prepared in the foundations of sexual assault nursing to perform at their level of education (basic or advanced)?

As the matrix for the formation of the program progresses using the published evidence to support the educational activities, summative outcomes can be developed concurrently as demonstrated in **Table 11-1**.

Table 11-1. Example of Formative and Summative Outcome Matrix Using An Activity

Activity	Formative Questions/Inputs	Summative Questions/Outputs
Simulation activity – Speculum insertion	What are the criteria for competency with speculum insertion?	Did the evaluator and student report quality improvement and demonstrate competency with the speculum?
	How much time is needed with each student?	Was the time adequate to develop competence with the psychomotor technical skill?
	What location and equipment is necessary to facilitate learning?	Were the equipment and location adequate to facilitate learning?

With all activities associated with SANE education, including the example above, the supervisor or coordinator of the nursing program is responsible for regularly documenting demonstrated activities to ensure continuous quality improvement and staff competency within the program.[2] This is made particularly important by the spread of the SANE model to rural and remote locations nationwide as programs use technology to meet the quality assurance and improvement activities necessary for competent practice for SANE.

Educational Preparation for Program Development and Administration

As RNs gain experience or show an interest in the care of rape or child abuse victims, some are asked to take the lead in their communities by developing SANE programs. However, most are not educationally prepared to administer SANE programs, and many do not have program management or supervisory experience outside hospital department supervision as a charge nurse or department manager.[2] Consequently, there are a number of basic development discussions at meetings and through the IAFN-SANE list server about formative and summative program development and sustainability. Initially, the *SANE Development and Operations Guide*[16] provided a graduate public health nursing approach to SANE program development that included competencies such as needs assessment, community assessment, stakeholder involvement, and financing activities. Many undergraduate nurses became a driving force in the development of SANE programs, and they utilized the *SANE Development and Operations Guide* to justify and establish the foundation for sexual assault response in their communities. Today, the graduate public health competencies continue to be used to establish new programs.[2,11] Those educated at the graduate level will utilize formative and summative methods of evaluation to examine additional public health nursing skills and will choose validated tools to use in the development of programs (eg, SANE Program Evaluation Questionnaire [SPEQ]).[2] Growth as a SANE includes both acquisition of new technical skills (ie, training) and, more importantly, continuing education on providing care to victims of sexual violence. This parallels the evolution of nursing scholarship and practice as the profession continues to develop skills, knowledge, and attitudes at each level of training and education.

In 1999, a survey of 35 SART programs reported that 89% of staff held diplomas, associate degrees, or bachelor of science in nursing (BSN) degrees and that graduate nursing staff accounted for 11% of all staff working in the responding programs.[16] The initial training programs for SANE focused on imparting the technical skills of evidence collection and providing factual testimony. Most educational activities for SANEs provide CEUs, and training events have proliferated nationally and internationally; 17 were listed in the first quarter of 2008 on the IAFN Web site.[57] Equal numbers of degree and certificate programs are listed, but different educational programs should not be assumed to be equal. The consumer should be aware that graduate diplomas (eg, MSN, DNP) and certificates are not the same as CEUs or certificates of completion; the consumer should examine the qualifications of the educator and how the training or educational program fits their personal needs and career goals and choose accordingly.

In 2008, 18 graduate programs in forensic nursing were listed on the IAFN Web site, and they have begun to accumulate the forensic nursing knowledge base, including that of the SANE subspecialty, in order to meet new accreditation guidelines.[58,59] The accreditation process evaluates the effectiveness of the institution at meeting its stated mission, goals, and expected outcomes and in complying with regulatory standards pertaining to the key program elements.[60] These elements include the development of the forensic nursing framework, developing clinical judgment, and encouraging leadership as they are relevant to the individual interests and talents of forensic nurses. As a subspecialty in forensic nursing, the SANE role is a platform for forensic nurses to enter clinical practice and is leading the development of the evidence base for sexual assault clinicians. SANE skills, knowledge, and education embedded in college and university coursework promise to produce the forensic nurse leaders who will continue the development of a firm foundation for future educational offerings and practice advances.

General Topics of Interest Related to SANE Education

Scholarship

Leaders in forensic nursing and other content experts in sexual assault are driving the improvement of SANE education. Representing a variety of educational backgrounds, these professionals have been early pioneers in initiating programs throughout the world. Increasingly, evaluation of program outcomes is conducted by nurses holding graduate degrees in public health or forensic nursing to demonstrate the quality and effectiveness of these educational models.[2,11] Additionally, the publication of these and other measures of quality establishes the knowledge base for practice and further program development.[2] Dissemination of scholarship in peer-reviewed presentations and publications discourages practice based on anecdotal experience, exchange of forms, or inaccurate information, which is often encouraged by other sources (eg, list servers, blogs). Also, there is a mechanism inherent in peer-reviewed journals that discourage plagiarism—a continual problem on list servers. Therefore, all SANEs need to develop a habit of validating information through scientific publications where proper credit is given to the seminal author.

Guidelines for Practice

At one time, inconsistency in educational offerings existed among SART programs. In recognition of this problem, the IAFN Board of Directors charged the SANE Council to develop educational guidelines for SANEs.[60] The first published guidelines outlined the primary topics and time in the classroom that should be included in basic SANE training. Introduction to these content topic areas, terminology, and the basic technical skills was essential before the SANE certification examination was developed. Today, however, other published documents and training guidelines recognize that meeting a quota of hours in class does not necessarily meet the needs of some individuals.[32,42] Also, these documents were collaborative efforts involving recognized experts, including SANEs, who were members of SART teams that presented basic training courses nationally. The consensus documents glossed over the number of classroom and experiential hours needed; they focused instead on establishing competency among health care professionals caring for sexually assaulted patients and recommended that community standards prevail.[2,32,42] The value of these consensus documents has been demonstrated, and, at this point, they should be incorporated into graduate programs in forensic nursing and SANE education in order to ensure consistency between national and international standards set forth in these and other documents. For all SANEs, continued training to maintain and improve skills or introduce new technical devices (ie, cameras or light sources) can be provided through simulation activities overseen by those deemed proficient in the role.[47,61-63] As local expertise develops, many SANE programs begin to provide the initial education and training for their staff, either by using their local experts or by bringing in an expert from another program.[30] Then SANE care, including technical skills, must be evaluated and determined to be satisfactory before employees can be considered competent in the care of sexually assaulted patients.

The Future of SANE/SAFE Education

Foundation for SANE Education

Future education for forensic nurses and SANEs will incorporate the nursing specialty statements and essential documents for nurses at all levels internationally. For SANEs, this education should include the foundational documents that form the core domains of nursing. The second edition of *Nursing's Social Policy Statement* describes nursing's accountability to the public and the mechanisms necessary to maintain trust.[42] *Nursing: Scope and Standards of Practice* presents detailed guidelines for all RNs and advanced practice nurses.[45] In addition, essential care documents define the provider levels and delineate the scope of practice for each.[38,45] These documents and the related frameworks are the basis for specialty practice (ie, forensic nursing) and are the foundation for the current revisions of the *Forensic Nursing: Scope and Standards of Practice*.[45] The subspecialty of SANE adheres to the scope and standards of forensic nursing as they are used internationally to design educational programs for SANEs.[45,64,65]

Learning Styles

Learning theories will also guide the development of educational programs for the forensic nurses. There are multiple types of intelligence and styles of learning, and each nurse brings prior experience and skills to the educational process. In addition, individuals learn in different ways. Historically, all SANEs in a classroom have received a lecture using slide presentations, videotapes, and audio clips. But face-to-face courses require up to 40 hours in the classroom, meaning 5 to 6 days away from jobs, family, and home. Today, an increasing number of SANE programs exist online. Literature about online education validates that learner satisfaction and retention are equivalent to that found in traditional classroom work.[66] In the new millennium, online distance learning has the distinct advantage of being asynchronous and, therefore, available at a location and time more convenient to the student. Synchronous online sessions can also be scheduled to enhance learning for those who desire a live chat or face-to-face contact through webcam activities. Modules are currently being developed for online programs to present the students with educational material following published guidelines for SANE education.[43] Modular material is then released at regular intervals. Online learning provides a variety of educational opportunities that possess a clear advantage over traditional classroom lectures. Specifically, this material addresses multiple learning styles through a format that includes slide presentations, video clips, essays, articles, live chats, interactive DVDs, and discussion boards for key issues by design. Students in these programs with access to hospital or university libraries are also encouraged to research key topics and bring additional material to the discussion, ensuring that it is retained.

Distance Learning

While current technology is necessary to participate in online SANE programs, the advantages for distance learners are considerable. Those living in rural communities, who are at a significant distance from SANE courses, or who have limited staff to cover their absence from their agencies, are able to participate in distance learning. Online distance learning that provides CEUs and online graduate course offerings will proliferate as resources are maximized both for the provider of education and the student who needs flexibility in scheduling educational activities. Future SANEs will minimize lost productivity and gather to demonstrate competency, reducing the expense to the SANEs as well as to their employers. These savings will result in more time in the clinical setting for SANEs and more time for them to work with community stakeholders. SANE education is now available in every region of the United States and Canada and increasingly throughout the rest of the world. Modalities include online SANE programs accredited within institutions; virtual interactive DVD programs[67] for the maintenance of skills in the SANE role; vignettes of sample cases and appropriate interventions; and live Web presentations with expert SANEs and simulation laboratories that include mock courts, evidence collection, photography, and other technical skills acquisition activities. The future of SANE education is bright.

Accredited nursing institutions are ensuring that future SANEs will benefit from the evolution of SANE education and practice, including scholarly research.

Simulation Labs

One major drawback in SANE education is that it is difficult to evaluate clinical competence when many SANE students find it hard to develop and maintain skills. Historically, students have looked to their communities to find opportunities to master the skills needed to complete a sexual assault evaluation with evidence collection. These experiences included conducting pelvic examinations in family planning clinics, visiting laboratories, riding with law enforcement, and witnessing trials. Few classroom programs offered clinical skills laboratories to the students, but this is changing. The School of Nursing at Rutgers University in New Jersey is a pioneer in offering clinical skills practice and demonstration since the SANE education inception in the late 1990s (E. Allen, MSN, RN, personal communication, September 2008). Today, simulation laboratories have demonstrated utility in many venues and promise to do so in SANE education as well. Clinical skills amenable to simulation training include injury detection and treatment, forensic pelvic inspection and evaluation, phlebotomy, colposcope and digital camera use, photography and videography, evidence collection (including sampling from the sexually assaulted patient and clothing management), interviewing, and documentation of findings. Simulation activities in basic training programs should become standard as the SANE emerges as the preferred role for care of sexual assault victims.

Quality Improvement

Use of technology will improve SANEs' knowledge and clinical skills by providing immediate feedback through electronic transmission (ie, telemedicine), thereby creating an electronic consultation through the use of electronic communication and information technology. In 1995, Alaska used an early version of software to enable electronic transfer of information called *Second Opinion* to communicate with experts about findings in sexual assault cases when the patient was located in remote areas accessible only by plane or during blizzard conditions when any travel was unsafe; the equipment was also used to provide distance education and quality assurance (C. James, RN, personal communication, January 2008). Utah used the same equipment and pioneered telemedicine for the care of child abuse patients on reservations.[68] All programs that use similar technology to communicate with content experts at regional centers from remote locations find the access valuable and cost saving (C. James, RN, personal communication, January 2008).[68] While digital photographs were crude a decade ago, the technology today has clarity not heretofore seen in electronic applications (A. Ward, SDFI President, personal communication, September 2008). This emerging technology is beginning to be incorporated into SANE education and promises to improve clinical skills in the safe environment of a simulation laboratory by providing immediate feedback through telemedicine. These simulated clinical laboratories allow the SANE to make mistakes in technique or decision making without the risk of compromising the health of a real patient.[49,62,63,69]

This technology is now spreading to rural communities in states with large geographical areas, where it is being used for quality improvement and to expand access to SANE expertise and education. Telemedicine has already created a connectedness and uniformity of care in the hierarchy of regional health care delivery in both remote rural areas and military outposts. Future sexual assault evaluation and care in remote areas may be completed by laypersons in the community under the supervision of an experienced SANE with a graduate-level education via electronic models of health care delivery. Today, telemedicine provides an opportunity for SANEs with little experience to speak with regional experts about forensic cases. Additionally, international programs in large metropolitan or regional centers are also using the technology to consult with nursing experts in the United States and Canada. This technology has become a preferred mode of communication for many SANE programs due to its versatility and the robust security measures involved in the transfer of sensitive materials, setting the stage for future educational applications.

Conclusion

Education for the SANE has evolved since the 1970s. While many SANEs entered the field through classroom presentations, future SANE education will combine online educational experiences with simulation laboratory training as an alternative to the very expensive 40 to 80 hours of classroom lectures. Historically, the 40-hour training was followed by myriad inconsistent clinical experiences for the SANE. In the future, the number of continuing education hours will vary because the educational level of the nurse will direct the development of customized basic coursework and competency. Those from certain advanced practice backgrounds or who hold certification need only demonstrate the psychomotor skill of speculum insertion for forensic purposes. Simulation laboratories will be useful to programs as they initially train and retrain SANEs in the basic psychomotor skills necessary to clinical practice, particularly in programs where the volume of patients is sparse and there is a serious risk of skill atrophy without maintenance activities. In addition, telemedicine consults with clinicians in remote areas will continue to enhance communication between the RN responding to sexual assault and the supervising graduate forensic nurse expert or the supervising physician. This technology can be adopted by rural communities in need of expert graduate clinicians for validation of competency, supervisory, or quality improvement activities. Telemedicine also promises to provide synchronous expert consultation through other Internet applications, such as Adobe Connect Professional. As the evidence from research molds the future practice activities of the SANE, there will remain a need for rapid dissemination of this important information through educational venues. Through institutions of higher education, technology can provide that infrastructure for rapid dissemination of SANE education curricula and materials.

In the last 4 decades, SANE education has come far from its origins from the addition of technical skills for collecting evidence and testifying about it. Today's SANE enjoys a basic introductory education with skills training that is comprehensive in its approach, guided by current research, and grounded in nursing theory and practice. In the past, introduction to SANE practice occurred in a local continuing education venue and was taught by a content expert in SANE nursing and additional community team members. For many, it was also their introduction to forensic nursing and to the first professional organization for forensic nurses, the International Association of Forensic Nurses. As in other nursing specialties, collaboration with the multidisciplinary team members will always be part of the SANE approach to education, training, and quality improvement. However, in the future, the evolving complexity of SANE practice requires nursing educators with graduate preparation to provide the foundations in nursing theory and clinical practice, awareness of issues within the field, and education that will satisfy accreditation requirements in institutions and meet the evolving credentialing standards for forensic nurses practicing as SANEs.

References

1. The C. Everett Koop Papers: Reproduction and Family Health. National Libraries in Science. Web site. http://profiles.nlm.nih.gov/QQ/Views/Exhibit/narrative/abortion.html. Accessed January 20, 2008.

2. Speck PM. *Program evaluation of current SANE services to victim populations in three cities* [unpublished dissertation]. Memphis, TN: University of Tennessee Health Science Center; 2005.

3. Gaffney DA. The power of the press: how one media spark ignited interest in forensic nursing. *J Forensic Nurs.* 2005;1(2):82-83.

4. Arndt S. Nurses help Santa Cruz sexual assault survivors. *California Nurse.* 1988; 84(8):4-5.

5. Burgess AW, Holmstrom LL. The rape victim in the emergency ward. *Am J Nurs.* 1973;73(10):1740-1745.

6. Solola A, Scott C, Severs H, Howell J. Rape: management in a noninstitutional setting. *Obstet Gynecol.* 1983;61(3):373-378.

7. Speck PM. *Anxiety in the acute phase of the rape trauma syndrome* [unpublished thesis]. Memphis, TN: University of Tennessee Health Science Center; 1985.

8. The Last Link on the Left. Final credits—Louis R. Vitullo. http://lastlinkontheleft.com/fc0601vitullo.html. Published 2006. Accessed October 20, 2008.

9. Burgess AW, Holmstrom LL. Rape trauma syndrome. *Am J Psychiatry.* 1974; 131(9):981-986.

10. Mills B, Stegbauer C. *History of the Memphis Rape Crisis Center.* Memphis, TN: University of Tennessee Health Science Center College of Nursing; 2004.

11. QUAD Council Public Health Nursing Competencies. QUAD Council Web site. http://www.achne.org/i4a/pages/index.cfm?pageid=3292. Accessed January 18, 2008.

12. Gold RB. Title X: three decades of accomplishment. *Guttmacher Rep Public Policy.* 2001;4(1):5-8.

13. History, Landscape, and Future Directions for SARTs. National Sexual Violence Resource Center. http://www.nsvrc.org/projects/154/sart-history. Accessed January 18, 2008.

14. FSMFN: School History. Frontier School of Midwifery and Family Nursing. http://www.midwives.org/about.asp?id=7&pid=29. Accessed January 18, 2008.

15. Memphis Rape Crisis Center. Memphis RCC nurse's protocol [unpublished protocol]. Updated 1978.

16. Ledray LE. *SANE Development and Operations Guide.* Washington, DC: Office for Victims of Crime, Department of Justice; 1999.

17. The Oyez Project. *Crawford v Washington.* 541 U.S. 36 (2004). http://oyez.org/cases/2000-2009/2003/2003_02_9410. Accessed December 7, 2009.

18. Antognoli-Toland P. Comprehensive program for examination of sexual assault victims by nurses: a hospital-based project in Texas. *J Emerg Nurs.* 1985;11: 132-135.

19. Campbell R. The effectiveness of sexual assault nurse examiner (SANE) programs. *VAWnet.* 2004;1:1-8

20. Littel K. Sexual assault nurse examiner programs: improving the community response to sexual assault victims. *Office for Victims of Crime Bulletin.* 2001;4:1-19.

21. McLaughlin SA, Monahan C, Doezema D, Crandall C. Implementation and evaluation of a training program for the management of sexual assault in the emergency department. *Ann Emerg Med.* 2007;49(4):489-494.

22. Kilpatrick DG, Whalley A, Edmunds C. Chapter 10: sexual assault. In: Seymour A, Murray M, Sigmon J, Hook M, Edmunds C, Gaboury M, Coleman G, eds. *National Victim Assistance Academy Textbook* (NCJ 197109); 2002. URL: http://www.ojp.usdoj.gov/ovc/assist/nvaa2002/chapter10.html. Accessed September 24, 2009.

23. About the President's Family Justice Center Initiative. Office on Violence Against Women. http://www.ovw.usdoj.gov/pfjci.htm. Accessed January 19, 2008.

24. Wisconsin Coalition Against Domestic Violence, modified by the Wisconsin Coalition Against Sexual Assault, Inc. Domestic Violence and Sexual Assault CCR Toolkit. http://www.ncdsv.org/images/WCADV_DV-SA_CCR_Toolkit_2009.pdf. Published in 2009. Accessed February 15, 2010.

25. Ledray LE. Services to sexual assault victims in Hennepin County. *Special Issue Eval Change.* 1980;131-134.

26. Ledray LE. *Recovering from Rape.* New York, NY: Henry Holtz and Company, Inc; 1986.

27. Moynihan B, Coughlin P. Sexual assault: a comprehensive response to a complex problem. *J Emerg Nurs.* 1978;4:22-26.

28. Muram D, Speck PM, Cassinello B. Teaching Forensic Evaluation of Sexual Abuse Victims to Medical Residents. Memphis, TN: Tennessee Dept of Human Services; 1989:1-5.

29. Sheridan DJ. The role of the battered woman specialist. *J Psychosoc Nurs Ment Health Serv.* 1993;31(11):31-37.

30. Speck PM, Aiken MM. Education, Scope and Standards of Practice for Sexual Assault Nurse Clinicians. Paper presented at: 1st International Association of Forensic Nurses; 1992; Sacramento, CA.

31. American Nurses Association. *Forensic Nursing: Scope and Standards of Practice.* Silver Springs, MD: American Nurses Association; 2009.

32. *A National Protocol for Sexual Assault Medical Forensic Examinations: Adults/Adolescents.* Office on Violence Against Women Web site. www.ncjrs.gov/pdffiles1/ovw/206554.pdf. Published September 2004. Accessed January 18, 2008.

33. Evaluation and Management of the Sexually Assaulted or Sexually Abused Patient. American College of Emergency Physicians Web site. http://www.acep.org/practres.aspx?id=29562. Accessed September 24, 2009.

34. Certification renewal. International Association of Forensic Nurses. http://www.iafn.org/certification/certRecert.cfm. Accessed January 18, 2008.

35. The Essentials of Doctoral Education for Advanced Nursing Practice. American Association of Colleges of Nursing. http://www.aacn.nche.edu/DNP/pdf/Essentials.pdf. Accessed October 30, 2008.

36. Speck PM. Things you didn't learn in nursing school: forensic nursing principles—WHEEL. Paper presented at: Emergency Nurses Association; 2000; Chicago, IL.

37. International Association of Forensic Nurses. *SANE: Scope and Standards of Practice*. Arnold, MD: International Association of Forensic Nurses; 1997.

38. American Nurses Association. Recognition of a nursing specialty, approval of a specialty nursing scope of practice statement, and acknowledgment of specialty nursing standards of practice. Paper presented at: the Congress on Nursing Practice and Economics; September 2005; Washington, DC.

39. The forensic nurse's code of ethics. International Association of Forensic Nurses Web site. http://www.iafn.org/displaycommon.cfm?an=1&subarticlenbr=56. Published in 2006. Updated November 2008. Accessed June 11, 2008.

40. American Nurses Association. *Code of Ethics for Nurses with Interpretative Statements*. Washington, DC: American Nurses Association; 2005.

41. American Nurses Association. *Nursing's Social Policy Statement*. Washington, DC: American Nurses Publishing; 2003.

42. Office on Violence Against Women. *National Training Standards for Sexual Assault Medical Forensic Examiners*. http://www.safeta.org/displaycommon.cfm?an=4. Accessed January 18, 2008.

43. International Association of Forensic Nurses. *Sexual Assault Nurse Examiner Adult/Adolescent and Pediatric Education Guidelines*. Arnold, MD: International Association of Forensic Nurses; 2008.

44. Canadian Nurses Association. *Advanced Nursing Practice: A National Framework*. Ottawa, ON: Canadian Nurses Association; 2008.

45. American Nurses Association. *Nursing: Scope and Standards of Practice*. Washington, DC: American Nurses Association; 2004.

46. International Association of Forensic Nurses. Core Competencies for Advanced Practice Forensic Nursing. IAFN Web site. http://www.forensicnurse.org/associations/8556/files/APN%20Core%20Curriculum%20Document.pdf. Published in 2004. Accessed June 11, 2008.

47. Goolsby MJ. The role of computer-assisted simulation in nurse practitioner education. *J Am Acad Nurse Pract*. 2001;13(2):90-97.

48. Letterie GS. How virtual reality may enhance training in obstetrics and gynecology. *Am J Obstet Gynecol*. 2002;187(suppl 3):S37-40.

49. Wood RY. Use of the nursing simulation laboratory in reentry programs: an innovative setting for updating clinical skills. *J Continuing Educ Nurs*. 1994;25(1): 28-31.

50. American Nurses Credentialing Center. Category 1: Continuing Education Hours. http://www.nursecredentialing.org/Certification/CertificationRenewal/UniqueRequirements/ContinuingEducationHours.aspx. Published in 2006. Accessed December 7, 2009.

51. American Nurses Credentialing Center. Accreditation Process. http://www.nursecredentialing.org/ContinuingEducation/Accreditation/AccreditationProcess.aspx. Published 2006. Accessed December 7, 2009.

52. Benner P. *From Novice to Expert: Excellence and Power in Clinical Nursing Practice.* Menlo Park: Addison-Wesley; 1984.

53. Nolan TF. N312: Introduction to professional nursing: Benner's stages of clinical competence. http://www.sonoma.edu/users/n/nolan/n312/benner.htm. Accessed July 15, 2008.

54. Sievers V, Stinson S. Excellence in forensic practice: a clinical ladder model for recruiting and retaining sexual assault nurse examiners (SANEs). *J Emerg Nurs.* 2001;28(2):172-175.

55. Gragnola CM, Stone E. *Considering the Future of Health Care Work Force Regulation: Policy Considerations for the 21st Century.* San Francisco, CA: University of California, Center for Health Professions; 1997.

56. Weiss CH. *Evaluation.* 2nd ed. Upper Saddle River, NJ: Prentice Hall, 1998.

57. International Association of Forensic Nurses. Local training and events. https://m360.iafn.org/ViewCalendar.aspx. Published in 2008. Accessed February 28, 2008.

58. Graduate & Certificate Programs. International Association of Forensic Nurses Web site. http://www.iafn.org/displaycommon.cfm?an=1&subarticlenbr=50. Accessed February 28, 2008.

59. Commission on Collegiate Nursing Education. *CCNE Standards for Accreditation of Baccalaureate and Graduate Degree Nursing Programs.* Washington, DC: CCNE; 2008.

60. International Association of Forensic Nurses. *Sexual Assault Nurse Examiner Educational Guidelines.* Pittman, NJ: Author, 1998.

61. Haskvitz LM, Koop EC. Students struggling in clinical? A new role for the patient simulator. *J Nurs Educ.* 2004;43(4):181-184.

62. Lasater K. Clinical judgment development: using simulation to create an assessment rubric. *J Nurs Educ.* 2007;46(11):496-503.

63. Metcalfe SE, Hall VP, Carpenter A. Promoting collaboration in nursing education: the development of a regional simulation laboratory. *J Professional Nurs.* 2007;23(3):180-183.

64. American Nurses Association, International Association of Forensic Nurses. *Forensic Nursing Scope and Standards of Practice.* Washington, DC: American Nurses Association; 1997.

65. International Association of Forensic Nurses. *Sexual Assault Nurse Examiner Standards of Practice.* Pittman, NJ: Author; 1996.

66. Coma del Corral JJ, Guevara JC, Luquin PA, Pena H, Mateos Otero JJ. Usefulness of an Internet-based thematic learning network: comparison of effectiveness with traditional teaching. *Med Inform Internet Med.* 2006;31(1):59-66.

67. Speck PM. Sexual assault: forensic and clinical management DVD practicum: virtual SANE is on the horizon. *IAFN: On the Edge.* 2008;14(1).

68. Powers J. Assessment of victims of child sexual abuse in a rural setting: a successful new program at the Ft. Duchesne Indian health center. *IHS Clin Support Center.* 1998;23(4):37-39.

69. Theroux R, Pearce C. Graduate students' experiences with standardized patients as adjuncts for teaching pelvic examinations. *J Am Acad Nurse Pract.* 2006;18(9):429-435.

Chapter 12

Sexual Assault Response Team Operation

Linda E. Ledray, RN, SANE-A, PhD, FAAN
Colleen O'Brien, RN, MS, SANE-A, SANE-P
Susan Chasson, JD, MSN, SANE-A

Until the late 1970s, advocates, medical personnel, law enforcement officers, and prosecutors worked independently on sexual assault cases. During these early years, roles were based on what those in the field "thought" worked best, as there was little evidence-based research to define best practice. Advocates often found themselves in an adversarial role working against both medical personnel providing forensic examinations and law enforcement officers investigating the crime as the advocates attempted to help the victims.

In the mid-1970s, a handful of communities began to create multidisciplinary teams designed to respond to sexual assault and to care for victims. Fortunately, all of the invested disciplines soon recognized that their individual goals could be more easily and effectively accomplished and that the needs of victims could be more fully met through a team-based approach. In addition, it was hoped that a team-based approach would increase reporting and prosecution rates by developing collaborative relationships between the various actors. The initial cooperative relationships that were formed were as varied as the individuals and organizations forming them. As the potential practices and approaches to collaborative sexual assault responses have been explored, however, the multidisciplinary approach has begun to coalesce. This chapter will review options for sexual assault response team (SART) operations and the findings available to date on their impact and efficacy. While the goal of the team is to assist the *victim* of the sexual assault to move towards *survivor* status, this takes time. Since many victims do not feel like they are survivors during the first few days after the assault, these terms will be used interchangeably when taking about this early period.

What Is a Sexual Assault Response Team?

While some communities may use other terminology, such as *coordinated community response team* or *sexual assault resource team*, for the sake of consistency we will use SART to refer to all sexual assault response teams following the example of the National Protocol for Sexual Assault Medical Forensic Examinations. According to the National Protocol, a SART is a "multidisciplinary team that provides specialized immediate response to recent victims of sexual assault."[1] This team is most often comprised of sexual assault nurse examiners (SANEs) or sexual assault forensic examiners (SAFEs), rape crisis advocates, law enforcement officers, prosecutors, and forensic laboratory specialists. Team members work collaboratively to better meet the needs of the sexual assault survivor, as well as to maximize reporting and prosecution of the crime. Their goal is to reconcile patient care with medicolegal investigation; a balancing act that has led Dr. Michael Weaver (personal communication, March 2008) to develop what he refers to as the 5 Cs of SART operation (**Table 12-1**).

Often individuals from other agencies, such as social services, domestic violence programs, chaplaincy, or mental health services, may also be involved in the SART process. These additional professionals primarily provide the victim with support services to facilitate her recovery. Using the word *team* may be somewhat confusing, because it implies that the same stable group of individuals will function as a unit in each response. This is usually not the case, as individual team members may only become involved if his or her skills are needed to respond to elements of a given assault.

Table 12-1. The 5 Cs of SART Operation

Compassionate	SART team members must be compassionate and nonjudgmental or the victim will not agree to begin the sexual assault forensic exam process. Trust is critical for follow-up counseling and maintaining victim cooperation if the case goes to trial.
Victim Centered	SART members must always remember that each victim brings with her a unique sociocultural identity and an array of individual life experiences. Race and ethnicity, religion, age, health, gender and sexuality, social economic status, educational level, and geographic location are all important considerations. The exam provider must always consider these individual aspects to ensure culturally respectful care.
Coordinated	Everyone on the multidisciplinary SART team should know his or her role and its boundaries. A victim may be willing to go forward because of a compassionate initial response, but procedural issues such as interviewer priority should be clearly explained to the survivor.
Collaborative	During the SAFE process, *appropriate* information should be shared between law enforcement, health care, and advocacy in a timely and professional manner.
Competent	Regardless of discipline, anyone conducting a sexual assault forensic exam should carefully follow the appropriate policies and, when possible, evidence-based procedures. This competency is the essential foundation for the multidisciplinary SART process and ultimate successful outcomes.

Some of the team members (usually the SANE, advocate, and law enforcement officer) may actually respond to the medical facility together when the victim comes in for an evidentiary exam. While in some communities they may even do a single joint interview, more often they work independently but collaborate closely to see that all of the victim's needs are adequately addressed.

Sexual Assault Response Team Operations and Roles

It is important to recognize that SART members have distinct and specified roles. SART activities are, however, comprehensive and often include the following:

— Providing the victim and her friends or family with initial support, information, advocacy, and crisis intervention

— Performing a medical evaluation and providing care for injuries

— Making referrals or providing follow-up care for the victim

— Collecting and interpreting forensic evidence

— Investigating the crime

— Prosecuting the offender

— Developing policies and procedures for SART operation

— Providing continued education for SART members

— Evaluating SART operation

— Providing community education

The individual roles of SART members include advocates, law enforcement officers, and SANEs and SAFEs.

Advocate

The role of the advocate is to provide victims with support, crisis intervention, information about the medicolegal or judicial process and their options, and information about the impact of choices they may make. Ultimately, the advocate will support and facilitate these choices. While services differ depending upon community resources and policies, the advocate may accompany victims to the emergency department (ED) for the initial medical exam, to law enforcement appointments, and when they meet with the prosecutor. While follow-up services also vary greatly depending on resources, the advocate will see that victims have information about where to get additional support and care and will keep victims informed about the progress of the criminal case. Advocates typically keep minimal, if any, records, and are not involved in evidence collection or investigation.

Advocate programs may be independent, community-based, or system-based (ie, based within a law enforcement or prosecutor's office). System-based advocates often do not have the same ability to maintain a confidential relationship with the victim, since they may be required to disclose information to other members of the agency for which they work. It is important that the victim be made aware of the limits of confidentiality the advocate can provide, so that the victim understands which conversations will be kept confidential and which may be shared. Advocate programs also typically take the lead in providing community education, often in conjunction with other SART members.

Law Enforcement Officer

In addition to providing for victims' initial personal safety, a law enforcement officer will transport victims to the medical facility for the evidentiary exam. An officer will interview the victim, make an initial report, and investigate the crime. It is also the role of the law enforcement officer to apprehend the suspect(s), interview any possible witnesses, and collect all relevant evidence for the prosecutor. Depending on the situation, more than one law enforcement officer or jurisdiction may be involved (eg, tribal police, military police, Federal Bureau of Investigation, sheriff, state patrol, or campus police). One officer may work the case from the initial report to resolution, or a number of officers may be involved in the different stages of investigation.

The SANE and SAFE

The SANE is a registered nurse who has special training in clinical and forensic issues relating to victims of sexual assault. SAFE is a more generic term used to refer to all specially trained health care providers including the nurse, physician, or physician's assistant who can also complete the initial medicolegal exam. The most common term, SANE, will be used throughout the remainder of this chapter, however, the information applies to all health care providers as well.

The initial exam performed by a SANE will include an in-depth interview to guide the medicolegal exam, including care and treatment of injuries, evaluation of risk and prevention of sexually transmitted infections (STIs) and pregnancy, collection of evidence, documentation, and providing the patient with information, crisis intervention, and support (see Chapter 4).

Nurse or Advocate?

There is currently much discussion amongst SANEs about their role in providing crisis intervention, support, and patient advocacy to sexual assault victims in the ED. The discussion centers around both what their role should include and how it should be described: *patient advocacy* or *support and crisis intervention*. This discussion has become important because in an attempt to discredit SANE testimony in court, defense attorneys have tried to paint the SANE as biased by referring to them as "advocates."

The SANEs' initial response was to combat this by emphasizing that, while they do provide crisis intervention and support for their patients, they are not advocates. The supportive role they play for their patients is different from that of the advocate on the team, who is biased. They emphasized that the SANE provides support and crisis intervention, not advocacy. It was thought that by using different terminology the concept would be less confusing, especially to jurors in cases that go to trial, and this approach has been effective.[2] While the American Nurses Association (ANA) code of ethics describes the nurse as "an advocate for the patient,"[3] there was no concern about confusion in the use of the term *advocate* in that context as there was no need to distinguish the role of the nurse from that of another team member.

Some SANEs went further and actually became forensic technicians focusing solely on the evidence collection portion of their role. They no longer provided support and crisis intervention, but abdicated that role entirely to the advocate.[2] This solution was supported by some advocates who felt that the SANE was infringing on their role.[4] These advocates were concerned that if the SANE provided support, information, and advocacy, which they saw as the role of the advocate, they would be forced out of the exam room. In some isolated areas this did, unfortunately, occur[5]; however, since the National Protocol recognizes the dual role of the SANE to "address the needs of the individual" victim of rape, as well as to "address justice system needs,"[1] many SANEs would argue this is an unfortunate and limiting solution that does not fully meet the role expectations of the SANE. Most SANEs support the importance of working collaboratively with the advocate to maximize role overlap in this area to facilitate victim recovery.[4]

Downing and Mackin conducted a study looking at role conflict in SANE practice. They found that most SANEs did not experience role conflict and clearly stated that SANEs are not advocates.[6] Unfortunately, they also found that many of these same SANEs interpreted not being an advocate as not providing support and empathy to their patients. Their response to their role in providing support and empathy is concerning. She distinguished 2 definitions of advocacy: the dictionary definition of *advocate* and the nursing definition of *patient advocate.*

Some nurses do not want to give up the term *patient advocate* since the ANA Code of Ethics states that the nurse is "an advocate for the patient."[3] They therefore see this as an integral part of their nursing role. The dictionary definition of *advocate*, however, is "one that pleas the case of another, specifically: one that pleas the case of another before a tribunal or judicial court. One that defends or maintains a cause or proposal. One that supports or promotes the interests of another."[7] This definition is clearly a biased description and one that is distinct from the nursing definition.

The advocate (in health care) is a practitioner, usually a nurse, who utilizes this role to promote and safeguard the well-being and interests of his or her patients or clients by ensuring they are aware of their rights and have access to information to make informed decisions. Advocacy in health care is an integral part of professional practice.[8] The *Forensic Nursing: Scope and Standards of Practice* states, "the forensic nurse serves as a patient advocate assisting patients in developing skills for self-advocacy and empowerment."[9]

Since most SANEs recognize how important this supportive part of their role is for their patients, the primary controversy centers around what this role should be called and how it should be described when they testify in court to prevent confusion with the role of the victim advocate on the SART, which, unlike the SANE role, is biased. Should they describe this supportive function as "patient advocacy" or "support and crisis intervention"?

SANE and Law Enforcement Role Distinction

As a part of the medicolegal exam, SANEs collect evidence from the victim's body that can assist the prosecutor in the decision to charge or not to charge the suspect or suspects. Unlike the law enforcement officer, however, the SANE does not get a description of the assailant and does not ask about details of the assault other than those that will guide his or her exam to identify injuries and areas where he or she may collect evidence on the patient's body. The SANE will document any additional information the patient volunteers that may be pertinent to the assault, but that is not the focus of the SANE's interview. If the law enforcement officer is available after the exam, the SANE will likely discuss the exam findings with the officer.

When the case goes to trial, the SANE may also be called upon to testify in court as a factual witness to present what was collected and how it was collected, or as an expert witness to provide an opinion about the physical or emotional injury that was or was not seen and the evidence collected.

Prosecutor

Unlike the previously mentioned SART members, the prosecutor is not a first responder; this professional typically becomes involved later in the investigation process. Based on the history of events as reported and the evidence collected, the prosecutor will decide whether or not to charge a suspect with the assault. The prosecutor will use all available evidence to make the charging decision, including evidence collected by the SANE and the law enforcement officer as well as the final laboratory test results returned by the crime lab.

When a suspect has been identified, apprehended, and charged, the prosecutor will either negotiate a plea agreement or take the case to trial. While it is important and helpful to keep the victim informed about this process and to solicit her input into the progress of the case, it is ultimately the prosecutor's place to determine whether the case will be charged, plead, or taken to trial.

Forensic Laboratory Specialist

The laboratory specialist is also not a first responder, but is an equally important team member. This professional is responsible for analyzing the evidence collected by both the SANE and law enforcement officers and is often called to testify in court as a factual or expert witness. In many communities, the forensic laboratory specialist will also perform another important role. The specialist works closely with the SART to provide feedback on the evidentiary collection process and its results.

Sexual Assault Response Team Operation Models

The SART begins its work with the victim at the initial report, typically within 72 hours of the assault. With advances in DNA recovery techniques, many communities have chosen to increase this initial evidence recovery period to 96 to 120 hours or more. Others are considering making this change of policy. It is important to note that it is not necessary for the team members to respond as a unit when the sexual assault victim comes in for a medical evidentiary exam in order to be considered a SART. There are 2 primary models of SART operation: the single-interview model and the multiple-interview model.

Single-Interview Model

In the single-interview model, when a sexual assault survivor reports to a medical facility following a sexual assault, she will be asked to wait until the SANE, advocate, and law enforcement officer have all arrived so that a single initial interview can include all of these SART members. While the rape victim will be made comfortable and urgent medical care provided, no interview, additional non-urgent medical care, or evidence collection is begun until all team members are present. The team then does one joint interview with the victim.

One rationale for this model is the belief that it is traumatic for victims to repeat their account of the assault multiple times. Sexual assault response teams who use this model feel very strongly that it is important to ask the victim for the specifics of the assault, and, in this model, a patient will only have to recall and relive the details of the assault once. Another rationale is that since all team members hear the same assault history, there is less chance that conflicting information will be recorded, as this could later be used by a defense attorney to suggest inconsistencies in the victim's recall, which can confuse the jury and make prosecution more difficult. While this rationale may seem reasonable, research is not available to support either of these conclusions. The state of California has mandated a single-interview model in their state sexual assault protocol for many years. Since they are viewed as leaders in the field, many other developing SARTs have chosen to follow their model without benefit of evidence-based findings that this model either serves victims better or produces more prosecution of suspects.

A recent US Supreme Court decision, *Crawford v. Washington*, is causing many SARTs to reconsider the single-interview protocol. The Crawford decision has placed significant restrictions on hearsay testimony that is considered to be "testimonial," or that the victim could reasonably believe would be used for courtroom testimony.[10]

Health care providers can testify to statements made by victims because of hearsay exceptions for statements made for the purpose of medical diagnosis and treatment. Under *Crawford*, that exception may be invalidated if the patient is questioned by a SANE in the presence of law enforcement. The health care provider hearsay exception may be the only way to enter statements about who committed an assault in a pediatric or geriatric case where the patient is unable to testify due to deteriorating health, memory issues, or other problems at the time of the trial.

Clearly, this model will require at least an initial report to law enforcement before the SART can be mobilized. This makes the single-interview model less accommodating for victims who do not want to report or who are uncertain about reporting. Since one study found 38% of rape victims who report to the hospital ED after a sexual assault are uncertain if they want to report, this model may not meet the needs of 1 in 3 rape victims.[11]

This model may be even more problematic now that the reauthorized 2005 Violence Against Women Act (VAWA) clearly mandates states that receive VAWA STOP funds are obligated to certify that the state does not require victims to participate in the criminal justice system or cooperate with law enforcement to have a medical forensic exam completed.[12] The National Sexual Assault Protocol also recommends that reporting not be required for exam payment.[1]

Multiple-Interview Model

A continuum of interview practices exists in communities that employ the multiple-interview model. In this model, the victim may enter the system through a variety of avenues. The victim may come to the medical facility first and, in this case, the SANE and advocate will be paged to the hospital. If the victim knows she wants to report, an evidentiary exam will be completed and law enforcement called to take the initial report. If she is uncertain about reporting, but willing to have an evidentiary exam, medicolegal evidence will be collected and held at either the medical facility or police department as determined by local policy, for a specified period of time while the victim decides if she wants to move forward with the criminal case. In Ledray's study, it was found that, after talking with the SANE or advocate, an additional 17% to 20% of victims made the decision to report to law enforcement, even though they were initially uncertain.[11] While the single-interview model may work well for the 2 out of 3 victims who have made the decision to report to law enforcement, the multiple-interview model that allows intervention as well as options for holding the evidentiary kit may increase reporting for the undecided group.

If the victim calls law enforcement first, the police will likely take an initial statement immediately and then bring the victim to the hospital for an evidentiary exam. Once the victim arrives at the hospital, the SANE and advocate will be paged. With the victim's consent, the advocate will be present during the medicolegal interview and evidentiary examination of the victim. Law enforcement will not be present during the evidentiary exam but may be called back to the hospital when the examination is completed to pick up the evidence, discuss the findings with the SANE, and transport the victim home or to additional interviews. If another investigative interview is conducted that day, or later, the advocate will likely be available to provide support to the victim during these follow-up interviews.

In the initial multiple-interview model, a law enforcement officer, advocate, and SANE may each conduct independent interviews. The rationale for this model is based on the belief that it may shorten the overall time victims are in the medical facility because they do not need to wait until the entire team is present to be interviewed. Victims may also find it easier to tell one or two people at a time rather than the entire team. SANEs often report the victim will disclose more intimate or embarrassing details of the assault to them that they did not disclose to a male law enforcement officer. This is information that may otherwise have been lost.

Finally, exposure therapy, the repeated recounting and processing of the traumatic event, is the treatment of choice for posttraumatic stress disorder (PTSD) and may make the multiple-interview model advantageous to the victim's recovery.[13] Currently, there is considerable debate about which of these models is the most appropriate and effective. Research on these 2 SART models remains limited and inconclusive.[14]

Additional SART Collaboration

The SART members may meet regularly, once a month, or quarterly for continued education, case discussion, and policy and procedure development. The team may communicate informally about specific cases or procedures as well. The more formal the SART, the more likely they will be to have a designated, paid coordinator (often called a sexual assault response coordinator [SARC]), and regularly scheduled SART meetings. Location of meetings may rotate through disciplines or be at one fixed site.

SART collaboration means ensuring that each discipline knows the roles and responsibilities of all other team members and the limitations and boundaries of each role. For example, the advocate who understands that her handling the evidence may limit its admissibility in court will ensure that the victim gives the evidence to the SANE or law enforcement officer rather than taking custody of it herself. She will also encourage the victim to tell the SANE or law enforcement officer important information concerning the case, even if it may be embarrassing or have unknown consequences.

In addition to looking at the team members' immediate responses to victims of sexual assault, some SARTs attempt to deal with issues of sexual violence within their community. For example, they may become involved in primary prevention programs or work with local media to discuss ways to report sexual assault while minimizing trauma to the victim. SARTs may also play an important role in developing services designed to meet the unique needs of special populations such as homeless, incarcerated, elderly, disabled, or GLBT victims.

SANE Operation Options

As indicated by a survey of 110 SANE programs, providing high-quality medical care to patients who present following a sexual assault is the primary goal of these professionals.[15] In fact, 90% of the survey's respondents rated providing high-quality care as their highest priority. Additional goals included collecting evidence for identification and prosecution of the assailant and providing timely and comprehensive medical, legal, and support services to survivors to prevent further victimization.

Just as there are a variety of SART options, there are a variety of SANE program models. While it is certainly important to have a goal that every rape victim who requests an exam at a health care facility be seen by a specially trained SANE, not every hospital needs to have its own SANE program. Hospitals do, however, have a responsibility to ensure that a specially trained medical professional is available to perform an evidentiary exam for every rape victim who needs or requests one. It is no longer acceptable to have insufficiently trained staff reading directions for the procedure as they complete the evidence collection kit. This would be an unacceptable standard of care with any other patient, and it is unacceptable for rape victims as well.

Medical facilities that see few victims may, however, choose to contract or collaborate with other facilities that have SANEs for this service. It is not financially or clinically feasible for every medical facility to have its own independent SANE program. Facilities that do not see sufficient numbers of victims will not be able to develop or maintain medicolegal and clinical expertise. In many communities today, a single SANE program may provide services to multiple hospitals in multiple counties over a large geographic area. The SANE on call will go to any medical facility with a service agreement in order to complete the requested medicolegal exam. As a result, these SANEs may work collaboratively with a number of law enforcement agencies and prosecutors. Today, this is an effective model both in large metropolitan areas and rural communities.[11,16] Plichta, Clements, and Housman completed an evaluation of SANE models that supports the conclusion that more effective care is provided by calling in SANEs from another site, rather than referring the victim to another facility.[17] Ledray also found that even when victims were put into a cab with a voucher and referred to another hospital for services, only 1 out of 3 arrived at the other facility.[18] This indicates that, on average, far more victims will receive needed services and medicolegal examinations when the SANE comes to them than when the victim is asked to report for treatment at a second hospital.

Creating a Sexual Assault Response Team

While the initial teams that evolved during the 1970s and 1980s struggled to develop the first protocols for a multidisciplinary response, communities today have many resources to help them with this process. In September 2004, the US Department of Justice published *A National Protocol for Sexual Assault Medical Forensic Examination: Adult/Adolescent*. The Protocol emphasizes the role of each team member in a victim-centered approach and outlines the issues that must be addressed by SARTs.[1] The Kansas Sexual Assault Network has written a "Community Development Manual" for establishing a community response to sexual assault. Their manual includes checklists and tools for performing a community assessment, organizing a multidisciplinary team, and creating a community protocol.

In addition to creating the National Protocol, the Department of Justice, in collaboration with the International Association of Forensic Nurses (IAFN) and other professional organizations, has created the Sexual Assault Forensic Examiner Technical Assistance Project (SAFE TA). The SAFE TA Project disseminates the National Protocol, the interactive virtual practicum, provides a national toll-free help line for questions about SANE and SART response, and provides limited on-site assistance to communities that want to develop or improve their response to victims of sexual assault (www.SAFEta.org). The SAFE TA Web site also contains numerous resources for the development of SARTs. In addition to these resources, many communities with existing programs are often willing to share their protocols to help other teams get started.

SANE-SART PROGRAM IMPACT

Although the number of SART programs is expanding rapidly, evidence-based data that can provide information to improve the program design and the outcome of these programs continues to be limited. Because the SART model has 2 distinct goals (to better meet the needs of sexual assault victims and to meet the needs of the legal system), evaluation of the SART model needs to focus on its effectiveness in dealing with both issues. Still, there is little scientific data available today from victims or SART members regarding their satisfaction with the SART process; there are also no definitive answers to questions about what makes a SART helpful (or unhelpful) to the individual or the legal system. Anecdotal data seem to indicate that victims are satisfied with the care they receive from the SANE, appreciate the care, and respond well to the SANE as a caregiver.[19-21] Victims treated by SANEs also report feeling safe, personally respected, in control, and reassured by the knowledge and expertise of the SANE.[22] Regarding members of SART teams, again there is only anecdotal data suggesting that SARTs and SANEs are well-received and that advocates believe that having more SART programs would improve the treatment of rape victims.[20,21,23] Evidence regarding the effectiveness of SANE-SART programs is beginning to accumulate. Derhammer and colleagues compared the treatment of sexual assault victims in the ED prior to and after the implementation of a SANE program and found that victims spent less time waiting in the ED after the SANE program was implemented.[24] Evidence collection also improved.[19] Campbell found that victims received better treatment if their community had more coordinated services.[21] Other authors report evidence that SANE programs result in better evidence collection, significantly better maintenance of the chain of custody of evidence once it has been collected, reduced waiting times, and increased reporting rates.[11,19,20,25-27]

Victims who were seen in SANE programs have been found to report to law enforcement more often.[16,28] This is significant to a person's overall emotional and physical health as victims who report to law enforcement were found to seek medical care 9 times more often than those who did not report.[29] The American Prosecutors Research Institute and Boston College examined the difference between the single-interview model with the SANE, law enforcement officer, and advocate performing a joint initial hospital interview, and the multiple-interview model, in which the SANE and law enforcement officer conduct independent initial interviews.[30] They also compared these 2 models to a model in which the victim refused to see a SANE or SART, never sought their assistance, or for unspecified reasons did not get a SANE exam. In the multiple-interview model, the SANE, law enforcement officer, and prosecutor may collaborate on the case, but they work independently.[30] It is important to note that in the SANE-only cases an average of 3.4 days lapsed between the incident and the report, an average of 5.6 days lapsed in the SANE-SART cases, and an average of 33 days lapsed in the cases in which there was no SANE or SART intervention. Taking this time factor into consideration, it is not surprising that DNA evidence was most often found in the SANE-only exam (97% of the time) and less often in the SANE-SART cases (37% of the time). DNA evidence was recovered in only 10% of the non–SANE/SART exams. Unfortunately, the authors of this study did not report when the exams that yielded evidence in non–SANE/SART cases were performed so it is not possible to clearly determine if time or SANE/SART involvement was the most important variable. However, it is very likely that this data could be better explained by the time frame in which the evidence was collected rather than by the identity of the examiner at the time of collection. The researchers also found that using a single SART initial intervention model is a factor in the identification and arrest of a suspect, which is the strongest predictor that charges will be filed and a conviction will follow. They found the single-interview SART approach was 3.3 times more likely to result in the filing of charges than other approaches. While only 39% of all cases resulted in an arrest and 12% of these were not charged, the majority of the cases charged resulted in convictions (68%). Nearly half of these cases (47.7%) were settled with a pretrial guilty agreement, and 23% were convicted at trial.

A study completed in Minnesota found results that were similar but that featured some interesting disparities. This study compared 155 cases in which sexual assault victims were seen at the hospital for the initial exam using the single-interview model to 198 cases in which the SANE and law enforcement officer did independent interviews.[14] An advocate was present for the SANE exam in 93% of the single-interview model cases and only 10% of the time for the multiple-interview model cases. A friend was present with the victim in the hospital in nearly half of all cases. It is interesting to note that the hospital whose policy it was to use the single-interview model was only able to do so 21% of the time for a variety of reasons, the primary reason being a desire not to delay victim care. In 53 cases, law enforcement went ahead and did their interview without waiting for the SANE to arrive, and in an additional 30 cases, the SANE decided to complete the exam instead of waiting for law enforcement to arrive. In 10 additional cases, the victim did not want to report, but agreed to have the SANE complete an exam in case she changed her mind later. There was no difference noted in overall victim satisfaction with the care received and, initially, there was no difference expressed by the victims in preference of either the single-interview or multiple-interview model. However, at the time of the third follow-up interview, which occurred 6 months after the initial hospital visit, 67% of the victims reported that they would have preferred a single interview because they would only have had to tell the story once; they wanted to forget about the assault, and they believed the exam would not have taken as long. Unlike the previous study, this study found that cases with the single-interview model resulted in charges filed 33% of the time, slightly less than the 36% in the instances in which multiple initial interviews occurred.[14] In other studies, SANE programs have also been found to increase the rate of guilty pleas and community prosecution rates[16,31]; this is likely the result of a number of factors. Health care professionals who are educated in medical forensics do a more thorough job of collecting evidence,[32] and, as a result of their extensive experience and training, also make excellent expert witnesses when the case goes to trial. Unlike medical personnel who lack specific knowledge and training on forensic issues and practice, SANEs understand the necessity and process of testifying in court. They may be more available to the prosecutor, are more knowledgeable on medicolegal issues and protocols and, consequently, are more comfortable answering tough questions.[16,33,34] Campbell et al found that SANEs were more likely to report a positive experience testifying in court when they had more clinical forensic experience; these professionals were often also in administrative positions within their programs, affiliated with SANE programs that had a higher census, and possessed of strong, collaborative relationships with their prosecutors.[34]

SANE programs are also more likely to meet the victims' medical needs, including evaluating risk of pregnancy and STIs and offering medications to prevent both. According to a national study, only 20% of rape survivors nationally receive emergency contraception (EC) to prevent a pregnancy caused by the assault.[35] This is troubling, as Holmes estimated that 32 000 pregnancies each year result from sexual assault.[36] The situation is much improved when SANE programs are evaluated separately. One Canadian study found that 45% of rape victims seen initially by a SANE program received EC.[37] While this is still surprisingly low, the percentage of patients who were initially offered EC was not indicated. Ciancone et al found that 97% of sexual assault victims seen in the 61 SANE programs they surveyed were offered both pregnancy testing and EC.[38] The number who chose to take the EC was not reported. In this same survey of 61 SANE programs, 90% were offered STI prophylactic care.[38] This compares favorably to a national study of SANE and non-SANE programs, in which only 58% of sexual assault victims were screened and given prophylactic treatment for STIs.[35]

It is also important to determine whether specific procedures in the ED increase or decrease patient distress, as early distress is highly predictive of later distress including PTSD. For example, Rothbaum and colleagues found that PTSD symptoms detected soon after a sexual assault predicted PTSD at 3 months postassault.[13] Several recent studies also suggest that acute stress disorder (ASD) soon after a trauma is predictive of later PTSD (eg, Brewin, Andrews, Rose, & Kirk, 1999).[39] Therefore, implementing procedures during the interview and exam process that will reduce stress may help prevent chronic PTSD.

Unfortunately, most sexual assault victims do not return for follow-up counseling, and, consequently, the ED may be the only opportunity health care professionals have to implement interventions to reduce victim stress.[40] One recent study suggests that ED interventions are feasible and effective. Specifically, Resnick and colleagues assigned rape victims to 1 of 2 groups in order to determine the feasibility of dealing with victim stress during the initial ED visit: (1) standard treatment in the ED or (2) standard treatment following a 17-minute video that provided information designed to explain the examination procedures and to prevent future PTSD symptoms.[41] Those in the video study group had lower anxiety scores in the ED, which in turn were strongly related to lower PTSD scores at 6 weeks postassault, suggesting that ED protocols can affect later stress responses. Thus, implementing procedures in the ED that reduce stress and prevent chronic PTSD is critical to victim recovery.

It is important to document whether victim and assault variables are related to the quality of care received, even in SART programs. In a series of studies, Campbell has documented the "secondary victimization" experienced by victims who seek help from the medical, legal, and mental health systems.[42] Interviews with advocates, mental health professionals, and victims all suggest that many victims do not receive the services they need and that negative experiences with these systems are not uncommon.[43-45] Victims who are most at risk for receiving substandard care and treatment are women of color, victims of acquaintance rape, and those who do not fit the profile of "good victim behavior."[42,43]

Conclusion

Initial studies suggest that the more than 600 SANE-SART programs in the United States today have improved the quality of medical and psychological services to sexual assault victims, as well as having improved the collection of evidence and increased the rate and success of prosecution of this violent, interpersonal crime.[46,47] It is encouraging to note that, by working together as a team, SART members, the SANE, advocate, law enforcement officer, prosecutor, and crime laboratory specialists have better met the needs of both the victim and the system. While there have been only a few controlled studies, and most of the evidence available is anecdotal case studies or evidence from a few programs that were developed in the 1970s, the evidence that exists is overwhelmingly positive in its support of the SANE-SART response. Evidence-based research on all aspects of SART operation is still clearly needed to improve the feasibility and sustainability of these programs. Future research should include replicating existing studies, expanding knowledge of diverse SART practices, improving policies and procedures for delivery of care, and examining the impact these SART models have on the treatment of the victims of interpersonal violence.

References

1. US Department of Justice, Office on Violence Against Women. *A National Protocol for Sexual Assault Medical Forensic Examinations: Adults/Adolescents.* Washington, DC: Office on Violence Against Women, US Dept of Justice; 2004.

2. Ledray LE, Faugno D, Speck P. SANE: advocate, forensic technician, nurse? *J Emerg Nurs.* 2001;27(1):91-93.

3. American Nurses Association. Code of Ethics for Nurses with Interpretive Statements—Provision 3.5. http://nursingworld.org/ethics/code/protected_nwcoe813.htm. Accessed March 22, 2010.

4. Gaffney D, Ledray L. Sexual assault examiners and rape crisis advocates: rising to the challenge together. *Sex Assault Rep.* 1999;3(2):17-32.

5. Sloan L. Sexual assault nurse examiners: the new challenge. *Sex Assault Rep.* 1999;2(6):81-96.

6. Downing N, Mackin ML. The Perception of Role Conflict in Sexual Assault Nursing and its Effect on Care Delivery. Paper presented at the International Association of Forensic Nurses Conference; October 2009; Atlanta, GA.

7. Advocate. Merriam-Webster. http://www.merriam-webster.com/dictionary/advocate. Accessed February 8, 2010.

8. Martin, E, ed. *A Dictionary of Nursing.* 5th ed. New York, NY: Oxford University Press; 2008.

9. American Nurses Association. *Scope and Standards of Forensic Nursing Practice.* Washington, DC: American Nurses Association and the International Association of Forensic Nurses; 1997.

10. *Crawford v. Washington,* 124 S. Ct. 1354, 2004.

11. Ledray L. *SANE Development & Operation Guide.* Washington, DC: US Dept of Justice, Office of Victims of Crime; 1999.

12. Violence Against Women Act of 2005, Pub L No. 109-162, 119 Stat 2964-3077.

13. Rothbaum B, Foa E. Exposure treatment of PTSD concomitant with conversion mutism: a case study. *Behav Ther.* 1992;22:449-456.

14. Ledray L, Frazier P, Peters J. Final Report, Grant # 2002-VF-GX-0007, Sexual Assault Response Team Operation Evaluation. Published in 2007.

15. Campbell R, Townsend SM, Long SM, Kinnison KE, Pulley EM, Adames SB, Wascon SM. Responding to sexual assault victims' medical and emotional needs: a national study of the services provided by SANE programs. *Res Nurs Health.* 2006;29:384-398.

16. Littel K. *Sexual Assault Nurse Examiner (SANE) Programs: Improving the Community Response to Sexual Assault Victims.* Washington, DC: US Dept of Justice, Office for Victims of Crime, Office of Justice Programs; 2001.

17. Plichta SB, Clements PT, and Housman C. Why SANEs matter: models of care for sexual violence victims in the emergency department. *J Forensic Nurs.* 2007;3(1):15-23.

18. Ledray L, Arndt S. Examining the sexual assault victim: A new model for nursing care I. *J Psychosoc Nurs.* 1994;32(2):7-12.

19. Ledray LE, Simmelink K. Sexual assault: clinical issues. Efficacy of SANE evidence collection: a Minnesota study. *J Emerg Nurs.* 1997;23(2):182-186.

20. Thomas M, Zachritz H. Tulsa sexual assault nurse examiners (SANE) program. *J Okla State Med Assoc.* 1993;86:284-286.

21. Campbell R, Ahrens C. Innovative community services for rape victims: an application of multiple case study methodology. *Am J Community Psychol.* 1998;26(4):537-571.

22. Ericksen J, Dudley C, McIntosh G, Ritch L, Shumay S, Simpson M. Clients' experiences with a specialized sexual assault service. *J Emerg Nurs.* 2002;28(1):86-90.

23. Smith K, Holmseth J, Macgregor M, et al. Sexual assault response team: overcoming obstacles to program development. *J Emerg Nurs.* 1998;24(4):365-367.

24. Derhammer F, Lucent V, Reed JF, Young MJ. Using a SANE interdisciplinary approach to care of sexual assault victims. *Joint Commission J Quality Improvement.* 2000;26(8):488-496.

25. Hohenhaus S. SANE legislation and lessons learned. *J Emerg Nurs.* 1998;24:463-464.

26. Sievers V, Murphy S, Miller J. Sexual assault evidence collection more accurate when completed by sexual assault nurse examiners: Colorado's experience. *J Emerg Nurs.* 2003;29:511-514.

27. Selig C. Sexual Assault Nurse Examiner and Sexual Assault Response Team (SANE/SART) program. *Nurs Clin North Am.* 2000;35(2):311-319.

28. Ledray L. The sexual assault nurse clinician: a fifteen-year experience in Minneapolis. *J Emerg Nurs.* 1992;18:217-222.

29. Resnick H, Holmes M, Kilpatrick D, Clum G, Acierno R, Best C, Saunders B. Predictors of post rape medical care in a national sample of women. *Am J Preventative Med.* 2000;19(4):214-219.

30. Nugent-Borakove E, Fanflik P, Troutman D, Johnson N, Burgess AW, O'Connor AL. *Testing the Efficacy of SANE/SART Programs: Do They Make a Difference in Sexual Assault Arrest & Prosecution Outcomes?* (Final Report). National Institute of

Justice. http://www.ncjrs.gov/pdffiles1/nij/grants/214252.pdf. Accessed February 4, 2010.

31. Crandall C, Helitzer D. *An Impact Evaluation of a Sexual Assault Nurse Examiner (SANE) Program*. Washington, DC: National Institute of Justice; 2003. http://www.ncjrs.org/pdffiles1/nij/grants/203276.pdf. Accessed September 28, 2009.

32. Ledray LE. Do all emergency physicians have an obligation to provide care for victims of sexual assault or is there a more effective alternative? *Ann Emerg Med.* 2002;39:61-64.

33. Ledray L, Barry L. Sexual assault: clinical issues: SANE expert and factual testimony. *J Emerg Nurs.* 1998;24(3):284-287.

34. Campbell R, Long S, Townsend K, Kinnison E, Pulley S, Bibiana Adamees, Wascon S. Sexual Assault Nurse Examiners' experiences providing expert witness court testimony. *J Forensic Nurs.* 2007;3(1):7-14.

35. Amey A, Bishai D. Measuring the quality of medical care for women who experience sexual assault with data from the national hospital ambulatory medical care survey. *Ann Emerg Med.* 2002;39:631-638.

36. Holmes M, Resnick H, Kilpatrick D, Best C. Rape-related pregnancy: estimates and descriptive characteristics from a national sample of women. *Am J Obstet Gynecol.* 1996;175(2):320-324.

37. Stermac L, Dunlap H, Bainbridge D. Sexual assault services delivered by SANE practitioners. *J Forensic Nurs.* 2005;1:124-128.

38. Ciancone AC, Wilson C, Collette R, Gerson LW. Sexual assault nurse examiners in the United States. *Ann Emerg Med.* 2000;35(4):353-357.

39. Bryant RA, Moulds ML, Gutherie RM. Acute stress disorder scale: a self-report measure of acute stress disorder scale. *Psychol Assess.* 2000;12:61-68.

40. Frazier P, Rosenberger S, Moore N. Correlates of service utilization among sexual assault survivors. Poster presented at: The annual meeting of the American Psychological Association; August 2000; Washington, DC.

41. Resnick H, Acierno R, Holmes M, Kilpatrick DB, Jager BA. Prevention of post-rape psychopathology: preliminary findings of a controlled acute rape treatment study. *J Anxiety Disord.* 1999;13:359-370.

42. Campbell R. The community response to rape: victims' experiences with the legal, medical and mental health systems. *Am J Community Psychol.* 1998;26:355-379.

43. Campbell R, Bybee D. Emergency medical services for rape victims: detecting the cracks in service delivery. *Women's Health.* 1997;3:75-101.

44. Campbell R, Raja S. The secondary victimization of rape victims: insights from mental health professionals who treat survivors of violence. *Violence Victims.* 1999;14:261-275.

45. Campbell R, Sefl T, Barnes HE, Ahrens CE, Wasco SM, Zaragonza-Diesfeld Y. Community services for rape survivors: enhancing psychological well-being or increasing trauma? *J Consult Clin Psychol.* 1999;67:847-858.

46. Sexual Assault Nurse Examiner, Sexual Assault Response Team. Sexual Assault Resource Service Web site. http://sane-sart.com. Accessed January 22, 2010.

47. International Association of Forensic Nurses. IAFN Web site. http://www.iafn.org. Accessed March 23, 2010.

Chapter 13

Sexual Assault Response in the Military

CDR Barbara Mullen (FNP), NC, USN*
Tawnne O'Connor, RN, BSN

Women have volunteered to serve side-by-side in the US military—functioning as nurses, cooks, and laundresses to name a few—since the founding of the United States.[1] It was not until the turn of the 20th century, however, that women began to serve in an official capacity in the US military forces. In 1901, the US Army established the Army Nurse Corps, and, in 1908, the US Navy followed suit with the Navy Nurse Corps. As of September 2009, women accounted for 15% of active duty forces.[2]

An Overview of the United States Military

The US military is a culture within itself. There are policies, procedures, languages, and legal systems unlike those found in civilian life. To understand sexual assault and official military policy, one must understand the overall organization of the US military. The military falls under the Department of Defense (DoD) and is directed by the Secretary of Defense. The Secretary of Defense is a Cabinet member and reports to the president of the United States.

The Branches of the Department of Defense

The 3 main branches of the DoD are (1) the Army, (2) the Navy (which includes the Marine Corps), and (3) the Air Force. Each branch of the DoD has unique missions and unique guiding principles, referred to as "core values." Also, each branch is comprised of an active component and a reserve component: individuals on active duty serve full-time in the military and individuals on reserve duty serve part-time in the military. These individuals can be changed to an active or full-time status based on state or federal government needs.

The United States Army

The US Army, founded on June 4, 1775, protects the interests of the country through the use of ground force. It consists of the active duty component, the Army Reserves, and the National Guard. There are 7 core values of the US Army[3]:

— *Loyalty:* Bear true faith and allegiance to the US Constitution, the Army, and all soldiers

— *Duty:* To fulfill one's obligations

* *This contributor would like to note the following disclaimer:*
"The views expressed in this article are those of the author and do not necessarily reflect the official policy or position of the Department of the Navy, Department of Defense, nor the U.S. Government."
"I am a military service member. This work was prepared as part of my official duties. Title 17, USC, §105 provides that 'Copyright protection under this title is not available for any work of the United States Government.' Title 17, USC, §101 defines a U.S. Government work as a work prepared by a military service member or employee of the U.S. Government as part of that person's official duties."

— *Respect:* Treating people as they should be treated

— *Selfless service:* Put the needs of others, including the nation and the Army, first

— *Honor:* Living up to all the Army values

— *Integrity:* Do what is right, legally and morally

— *Personal courage:* Face fear, danger, or adversity

The United States Navy

The US Navy, which achieves sea-based military strategy via amphibious operations with the US Marine Corps, was founded on October 13, 1775. The US Marine Corps, which falls under the Department of the Navy, was founded on November 10, 1775, and functions as the United States' amphibious expeditionary force. Both the Navy and Marine Corps have an active duty and reserve component, and they share the same set of core values[4]:

— *Honor:* Maintain professionalism at all times

— *Courage:* The strength, both mentally and morally, to do what is right

— *Commitment:* Work as a team to achieve the mission

The United States Air Force

As the youngest of the services, the US Air Force was officially chartered on September 17, 1947, though it began as part of the US Army on August 1, 1907. The Air Force is composed of the active duty components, reserve components, and the Air National Guard. The mission of the Air Force is to protect US interests through air support. There are 3 core values of the US Air Force[5]:

— *Integrity first:* Do what is right

— *Service before self:* Professional duty comes before personal desires

— *Excellence in all we do:* Continuously improve performance

The Legal System

Though each branch of the military has its own set of core values, all service members are subject to the Uniform Code of Military Justice (UCMJ), a codified statute enacted to ensure good order and discipline and deal with service members who violate the law. Established in 1950 and updated on an almost annual basis, the UCMJ is comprised of 146 articles. The UCMJ ultimately falls under Title 10, Subtitle A, Part II, Chapter 47 of the US Code.[6,7] The UCMJ defines criminal acts ranging from relatively minor violations and military specific offenses, such as unauthorized absence, to serious common law offenses, such as murder. Balancing good order and discipline with the pursuit of justice, the Code sets forth the methods through which commanding officers can legally manage such violations. The outline for the UCMJ is listed in **Table 13-1**.

Courts-Martial and Other Military Discipline

When an individual violates the UCMJ, options range from hearing the case before the command officer to a courts-martial. A courts-martial is a military trial, heard in a military courtroom setting. There are 3 types of courts-martial. Each one varies with respect to who can convene the court-martial.

General Court-Martial

The first type of court-martial is known as a General Court-Martial (Article 22). This can only be convened by flag officers, general officers, or commanding officers at an

Table 13-1. Outline of Uniform Code of Military Justice (from 2008 Courts-martial Manual).[7]

PART*	CHAPTER	TITLE
I		Preamble
II		Rules for Courts-martial
	I	General Provisions
	II	Jurisdiction
	III	Initiation of Charges; Apprehension; Pretrial Restraint; Related Matters
	IV	Forwarding and Disposition of Charges
	V	Courts-martial Composition and Personnel; Convening Courts-martial
	VI	Referral, Service, Amendment, and Withdrawal of Charges
	VII	Pretrial Matters
	VIII	Trial Procedure Generally
	IX	Trial Procedures Through Findings
	X	Sentencing
	XI	Post-Trial Procedure
	XII	Appeals and Review
	XIII	Summary Courts-martial
III		Military Rules of Evidence
IV		Punitive Articles

** There are 57 articles under which an individual can be charged.*

overseas command. Similar to a civilian felony court, it is reserved for the most serious offenses, similar to a civilian felony court. Both officers and enlisted service members may be tried at a General Court-Martial. In this type of court-martial, the accused may choose whether it is a judge alone or a judge and panel comprised of at least 5 military members who hear the case. The maximum punishments vary by offense but include the death penalty; dishonorable discharge or bad-conduct discharge for enlisted members; a dismissal for officers (generally viewed as the equivalent to a dishonorable discharge); confinement of up to life in a military prison; loss of all rank for enlisted members, loss of all pay and allowances; and fines.[8,9]

Special Court-Martial

A Special Court-Martial (Article 23) can be convened by an individual authorized to convene a General Court-Martial or by any commanding officer, regardless of command location. This type of court-martial is used for lesser offenses similar to a civilian misdemeanor court. Like the General Court-Martial, both officers and enlisted members can be tried. In this type of court-martial, the accused decides if a judge or a judge and at least 3 military members will hear the case. The maximum punishments include hard-labor confinement for one year, "forfeiture of two-thirds of one month's pay for one year," loss of all rank for enlisted members, and a bad-conduct discharge.[8]

Summary Court-Martial

A Summary Court-Martial (Article 24) can be convened by any individual authorized to convene a Special Court-Martial, an Officer-In-Charge of a unit, and all other active duty commanding officers. A Summary Court-Martial is reserved for enlisted members charged with minor offenses. One commissioned officer presides over the proceeding, and maximum punishments include reduction in grade, hard labor confinement for one month, "forfeiture of two-thirds of one month's pay for one month, hard labor without confinement for 45 days, or restriction for two months."[8]

Other Military Discipline

Nonjudicial punishment is another method of military discipline. It is authorized under Article 15 and permits the commanding officer to hear a case and determine punishment, which may include restriction, pay or grade reductions, or extra duty.

Finally, commanders may use administrative action as a form of punishment. An administrative action holds the military member accountable for his or her actions, when deemed problematic. Punishments may include administrative separation, reassignment, and career field reclassification, to name a few.

Definitions of Rape and Sexual Assault in the Military

Offenses Chargeable Under Article 120

Article 120 of the UCMJ covers rape and sexual assault. Effective October 1, 2007, a total of 14 offenses fall under this article. The following are offenses chargeable under Article 120[10]:

— Rape

— Rape of a child

— Aggravated sexual assault

— Aggravated sexual assault of a child

— Aggravated sexual contact

— Aggravated sexual abuse of a child

— Aggravated sexual contact with a child

— Abusive sexual contact

— Abusive sexual contact with a child

— Indecent liberty with a child

— Indecent act

— Forcible pandering

— Wrongful sexual contact

— Indecent exposure

Definitions of Rape and Sexual Assault

— ***Rape***, if the victim is an adult, occurs when there is sexual penetration (penis, finger, hand, or object forced, no matter how deep, into the vaginal opening) with grievous bodily harm resulting from the force used.

— ***Grievous bodily harm*** is defined as force that results in serious bodily injury including fractures or dislocation, deep lacerations, torn members of the body, severe internal damage, or other severe bodily injuries. Rape also occurs when a perpetrator threatens grievous bodily harm; when a perpetrator uses force in such a way that prevents the victim from avoiding the sexual contact including the display of a deadly weapon; when a perpetrator renders the victim unconscious; or when the perpetrator, without the victim's knowledge, administers an intoxicant leaving the victim unable to consent to the sexual act.

— ***Sexual assault*** occurs when there is sexual penetration with bodily harm that is not grievous or when the perpetrator makes threats against the victim that do not amount to threats of bodily harm. An example of sexual assault would be a threat by a supervisor to ruin a victim's military career whether or not the sexual act occurs. Another example would be when the victim is unable to appraise the nature of the sexual conduct or unable to voluntarily consent to the act. This would involve a victim who is asleep or intoxicated, for instance.

— ***Aggravated sexual contact*** occurs when there is no sexual penetration, but, had there been penetration, the surrounding circumstances would have met one of the theories of rape.

— ***Abusive sexual contact*** occurs when there is no sexual penetration, and the surrounding circumstances would have met one of the theories of aggravated sexual assault.

— ***Wrongful sexual contact*** is any sexual contact done without consent.

These are just a few of the possible charges under Article 120. From the definitions above, it becomes clear, according to Article 120 of the UCMJ, that sexual assault and rape occur only when there is contact involving the vagina. In the event that the victim is a woman or a man who is sexually assaulted orally or anally, the charge would be made under Article 125, sodomy.

— ***Sodomy*** is defined as "unnatural copulation with another person of the same or opposite sex or with an animal....[P]enetration, however slight, is sufficient to complete the offense."[10] If this occurs without consent and by use of force, it is considered an aggravated event.

When a child is the victim, age becomes one of the differentiating factors. If the victim is under 12 years of age and any sexual act occurs, then *rape* is the offense; if the victim is 12 years old, the criteria for *rape* of an adult must be met for the offense to be charged as *rape of a child*. In the event of sexual intercourse with a child between 12 and 15 years of age, *aggravated sexual assault of a child* is charged, absent one of the adult rape theories. As with the adult, there are a multitude of other charges that may be brought against the accused when dealing with sexual conduct with a child.

Whether the victim is an adult or a child, sexual assault is taken very seriously in the military. The UCMJ should be referenced for full definitions of each section of Articles 120 and 125. **Table 13-2** reflects the maximum punishments that may be rendered to the accused during a court-martial under Article 120.

Table 13-2. Article 120 and Maximum Punishments as of 2008.[10]

USMC Violation (Article 120)	Maximum Punishment
Rape and Rape of Child	Death/Life
Aggravated Sexual Assault	30 yrs
Aggravated Sexual Assault of a Child	20 yrs
Aggravated Sexual Abuse of a Child	20 yrs
Aggravated Sexual Contact (Adult or Child)	20 yrs
Abusive Sexual Contact with Child	15 yrs
Indecent Liberty with a Child	15 yrs
Abusive Sex Contact	7 yrs
Indecent Act/Forcible Pandering	5 yrs
Wrongful Sex Contact	1 yr
Indecent Exposure	1 yr

The Evolution of Sexual Assault Policy

The views and management of sexual misconduct in the military have evolved over the years. Concerns initially focused on the integration of women into the armed services and sexual discrimination. In 1988, the first DoD-wide survey regarding sexual issues focused on sexual harassment in the military. Three years later, a scandal named Tailhook in which 90 men and women came forward with allegations of sexual assault at the annual naval aviation conference in 1991 in Las Vegas rocked the US Navy.[11] In 1996, the US Army confronted harassment and sexual assault issues at Aberdeen Proving Grounds. When a hotline was established, 200 investigations were launched in response to more than 1000 phone calls,[12] and, in 2003, more than 50 cases of sexual assault were identified as having occurred at the US Air Force Academy between January 1993 and December 2002.[13]

In early 2004, then Secretary of Defense Donald Rumsfeld expressed his concern regarding the number of sexual assault cases in the military, particularly in the combat theaters of Afghanistan, Iraq, and Kuwait[14]; there were more than 100 reported sexual assaults in these combat areas over 18 months.[15] He authorized the formation of a task force to investigate current reporting and prevention policies and to provide recommendations for improvement.[8] Ellen Embrey, then deputy assistant secretary for defense for health, protection, and readiness, spearheaded the Care for Victims of Sexual Assault Task Force. This task force had 90 days to investigate current practices within the DoD and report back to Donald Chu, then the undersecretary for personnel and readiness.[16,17]

Three months following the authorization of this task force, the report was delivered to the undersecretary for personnel and readiness. This report reviewed current barriers to effective reporting and management of sexual assault cases. It summarized 35 factors influencing and affecting the reporting of sexual assault and proposed 9 corrective actions.[8]

The Care for Victims of Sexual Assault Task Force report divided the 35 influencing factors, which were categorized into 7 categories and are summarized in **Table 13-3**.

Table 13-3. Categorization and Description of the Findings from the Task Force

Sexual Assault Data and Definition*	
Prevention	Training programs aimed at preventing sexual assault were limited in content and audience. Not all officers and enlisted service members received introductory and refresher training. Commanders were concerned that this lack of introductory training complicated training requirements once troops were there as there were time constraints due to operational requirements.
Reporting	Individuals were often unsure of how to report sexual assaults, and many believed they had to go through their chain-of-command. This presented several barriers as individuals were often reluctant to report sexual assault due to fear of reprisal, fear of impact on reputation, and fear of impact on unit cohesiveness. Also, there was often confusion about what legally constituted sexual assault due to varying definitions within the services and lack of training.
Response–Safety and Protection	There were several challenges within this category. First, there was the need to segregate the victim and offender in a timely manner without adversely impacting either party's career or the unit mission. Second, jurisdiction was often problematic when the offender was a foreign national or member of a coalition force.
Response–Care for Victims	There was no uniform response system for sexual assault, often leading to a delay in care and improper tracking of the victims. Additionally, victims were often without support services and were not updated on the investigation or the legal status of the case.
Response–Investigation and Prosecution	Investigating and prosecuting sexual assault cases are challenging, and delays in processing DNA evidence and the combat environment further complicated this issue.
System Accountability for Sexual Assault	There was no DoD-appointed individual, committee, or office tasked with dealing with sexual assault and setting forth policies or a data collection system. This resulted in difficulty with managing and resolving sexual assault cases.

** Each military service utilized independent reporting methods and definitions of sexual assault.*

The 9 items proposed for corrective action were categorized as immediate, short-term, and long-term and are listed in **Table 13-4**; however, no timeline was referenced in the task force report regarding implementing the corrective actions.[8]

As a result of these findings, the Joint Task Force for Sexual Assault Response and Prevention was established in October 2004, and Air Force Brigadier General K.C. McClain was assigned as the commander.[15] This task force would lay the groundwork for the development of a permanent program, which would be established in October of 2005, known as the Sexual Assault Prevention and Response Office.[16,17]

The New Mandate

An October 2005 directive from DoD (DODD 6495.01) established the Sexual Assault Prevention and Response (SAPR) program, with the objective of establishing a standardized system for training, prevention, and responding to and reporting sexual assault.[18]

With this directive, the DoD established the definition for sexual assault. ***Sexual assault*** is defined as "intentional sexual contact, characterized by the use of force, threats, intimidation, abuse of authority, or when the victim does not or cannot consent." Rape, forced sodomy—oral or anal sex and "other unwanted sexual contact that is aggravated, abusive, or wrongful (to include unwanted and inappropriate sexual contact), or attempts to commit these acts"—fall under this definition.[18]

Table 13-4. Summary of Recommendations by Task Force

Recommendations for Immediate Action

1. Establish a single point of accountability for all sexual assault policy matters within DoD.
2. During the upcoming Combatant Commanders Conference, allocate time on the agenda to discern how the findings and recommendations of this report should apply to their areas of responsibility.
3. Ensure broad dissemination of relevant sexual assault information through DoD-wide communication outlets.
4. [By July 2004], convene a summit of DoD leaders (military and civilian) and recognized experts on sexual assault, to develop strategic courses of action on critical, unresolved issues.

Recommendation for Near-Term Action

5. Establish an Armed Forces Sexual Assault Advisory Council.
6. Develop policies, guidelines, and standards for sexual assault prevention, reporting, response, and accountability.
7. Assure manpower and fiscal resources are authorized and allocated, especially in the near years, to implement required policies and standards.
8. Develop an integrated strategy for sexual assault data collection to aid commanders, service providers, legal staff, and law enforcement entities in evaluating response effectiveness and system accountability.

Recommendation for Longer-Term Action

9. Establish institutional sexual assault program evaluation, quality improvement, and oversight mechanisms.

This directive also led to the development of the sexual assault response coordinator (SARC). The function of the SARC is to serve as the installation or regional coordinator, manage the sexual assault response team (SART), coordinate care for victims, and oversee training regarding sexual assault in the region.

Responsibilities of the Sexual Assault Response Coordinator

The SARC ensures appropriate care is coordinated and provided to victims of sexual assault from the initial report through final disposition and resolution.[18] As in the nonmilitary setting, victim safety is a top priority. Medical care is readily available to the victim. This care occurs either within a military treatment facility or at a civilian facility that has a memorandum of understanding (MOU) with the local military base to provide care for assault victims.

The SARC also oversees awareness training in the community and specialized training for first responders. Awareness training is offered to both military and nonmilitary personnel. For the military members, this training is provided upon entry into the military and on an annual basis. Training focuses on sexual assault awareness, prevention, and what to do if an assault occurs. First responder training for victim advocates, health care providers, chaplains, and those involved in the legal and investigative processes is extensive and correlates to the role the individuals play in the process of caring for the sexual assault victim.[19]

The SARC is also responsible for the victim advocate (VA) program. The VA is a volunteer specially trained in sexual assault victim advocacy. The VA stays with the victim from the time of medical treatment until the case is resolved and provides support and education on reporting options as applicable.

The Sexual Assault Victim Intervention Program

The US Navy established the Sexual Assault Victim Intervention (SAVI) program in 1994 under the Office of the Chief of Naval Operations Instruction (OPNAVINST) 1752.1.[20] This instruction mandates that all Department of the Navy commands provide training and advocacy for victims of sexual assault. Updated most recently in 2006, the current instruction mandates that annual sexual assault awareness training be conducted for active duty members, that there is a 24-hour on-call victim advocate, that the victim is afforded protection from the assailant, and that the victim has full access to counseling.[21]

Restricted versus Unrestricted Reporting

To encourage active duty members to report when these events occur, the DoD established 2 types of reporting under DoD Directive (DODD) 6495.01: unrestricted and restricted reporting. Both options allow the victim to receive medical care (for any trauma, prevention of sexually transmitted infections, and emergency contraception), evidence collection (if desired), follow-up care, and counseling services.

If a victim chooses unrestricted reporting, a full investigation is initiated involving legal, security, and investigative services. The individual's commander is also notified of the event and provided with the name of the victim. A case management team reviews each case of unrestricted reporting on a monthly basis. This team includes the SARC, the VA, a military criminal investigator, a member of military law enforcement, a health care provider, the chaplain, a command legal representative, the clinic counselor, and possibly the victim's commander.[19]

In a restricted report, there is no legal, security, or investigative service notification. The commander is notified only that there was a sexual assault against a member of that command, and no identifying information is provided (ie, name of individual, age, sex, rank, job, location of assault). Restricted reporting allows a victim to "confidentially disclose the details of his or her assault to specific individuals and receive medical treatment and counseling, without triggering the official investigative process."[18] This type of reporting ensures the victim has access to an advocate, counseling services, and follow-up care, while maintaining confidentiality. Both the SARC and the VA remain in close contact with the victim to ensure all services are available. The victim has up to one year to change the report to unrestricted and allow an investigation to be launched.[18]

Initially, if the victim disclosed a sexual assault to anyone aside from a health care provider, victim advocate, or chaplain, then an unrestricted report had to be filed.[18] However, the directive was modified to allow victims to confide in friends or family members without the assault being mandated to an unrestricted report. The stipulation with this modification is that if a friend or family member notifies the chain-of-command or law enforcement, then the report becomes unrestricted, and an investigation is initiated. In the event the victim is believed to be in serious or imminent danger, then the assault must be reported to law enforcement, and it becomes an unrestricted report (T. Joyner, SARC, oral communication, January 2009).

At the time of the writing of this chapter, only active duty service members and victims of domestic violence involving sexual assault may choose unrestricted or restricted reporting (though state mandatory reporting laws may affect the ability of the assault victim to select a restricted report) (T. Joyner, SARC, oral communication, January 2009).[20,22] All other individuals such as family members, retirees, or DoD contractors must file an unrestricted report.

Improving the Sexual Assault Prevention and Response Program

In 2006, the Department of Defense Instruction (DODI) 6495.02, Sexual Assault Prevention and Response Program Procedures, was developed to provide direction and guidance regarding care for victims of sexual assault. Based on this directive, the majority of the military treatment facilities (MTFs) within the continental United States have developed an MOU with civilian facilities to conduct forensic exams. An MTF overseas is required to train health care providers in performing these forensic exams. The directive dictates that licensed physicians, advanced practice nurses, physician assistants, and registered nurses with specialized training and practice in sexual assault exams are utilized.[19] Both DODD 6495.01 and DODI 6495.02 provide guidelines, instructions, and requirements for prevention and response to sexual assault.

One Region's Experience: Training in Naval Facilities in the Pacific Region

In the Pacific, specifically US Naval Hospitals (USNH) Guam, USNH Okinawa, and USNH Yokosuka, registered nurses (RNs) and nurse practitioners (NPs) are employed as sexual assault nurse examiners (SANEs). As early as 2000, RNs have been trained to perform forensic exams for sexual assault victims at USNH Yokosuka (L. Robinson, RN, verbal communication, December 2009). Until 2007, only a few nurses had received training, limiting the number of individuals qualified to conduct the forensic exams. Additionally, the training received by the few individuals was sponsored by a variety of agencies, leading to program inconsistencies.

Since 2007, however, the Navy Far East Pacific commands have streamlined training by hosting an annual training conference for all area SANEs ensuring all staff receive uniform training. One subject matter expert, Linda Ledray of the Sexual Assault Resource Services, has provided the formal training. Her program is enhanced by presentation from the SARC, Naval Criminal Investigative Services, and a member of Judge Advocate General Corps, and it provides the most current information from these fields.

Upon completion of training, each SANE has the opportunity to work with providers in the Family Practice Clinic, and perform cervical exams to ensure competency and ease with speculum exams. When each newly trained SANE is on call, he or she is accompanied by an experienced SANE to assist with the first forensic exam.

As this program has expanded and evolved over the past 2 years, Ledray has provided vital guidance for program development. The current forensic exam form and standard operating procedures enhance evidence collection and protocols, which help to deliver the best services possible to victims.

Raising Sexual Assault Awareness in Yokosuka, Japan

While many advances have been made to the SANE program at the Naval Far East Pacific Commands, changes are constantly being addressed to better serve victims of sexual assault. Within the team of SANEs, quarterly telephone conferences are held with USNH Yokosuka and its branch clinics located throughout mainland Japan, USNH Okinawa, and USNH Guam to maintain a rapport, ensure consistency within the programs, and address any issues that may arise. Annual training is offered to ensure adequate staffing and competency. Future training will also involve the independent duty corpsmen who are often stationed aboard small ships to ensure that the exams they conduct for sexual assaults are completed appropriately.

Training has also focused on educating the community on sexual assault. Upon arrival to the region, individuals assigned to Command Fleet Activities Yokosuka (CFAY) attend an Area Orientation Brief (AOB) to become familiar with the services available through the base. The brief includes a concise introduction to the SANE program and its services to increase awareness about sexual assault reporting. During Sexual Assault Awareness Month (SAAM) held in April, members of the SART (including the SARC, SAVI, and SANE representatives) participate in an annual awareness performance that highlights the importance of sexual assault awareness. In 2008, approximately 1000 civilians and active duty members assigned to CFAY attended, with an increase in attendance by 200 individuals in 2009 for this annual performance. This community awareness program is offered at no charge.

Sexual Assault Statistics

The DoD has maintained statistics on sexual assault in the military prior to the revision of its current policy offering service members the option of restricted or unrestricted reporting. Unfortunately, upon review in 2005, it was acknowledged that the data had been incomplete in the past because of the lack of uniform reporting requirements within the DoD. The report for calendar year (CY) 2004 (signed May 6, 2005) serves as the baseline for sexual assault reporting.[22]

One must be cognizant when reviewing these statistics collected over the past several years as several factors have impacted the results. First, until 2007, the annual reports regarding sexual assault were based on the CY. This changed in 2007 when the report began in the fiscal year (FY). The military FY begins October 1st and ends September 31st of the following year; consequently, the data for October through December 2006 is reflected in the reports for both CY 2006 and FY 2007. Second, restricted reporting did not become an option to victims until June 2005. Therefore, it was not until CY 2006 that individuals had the choice of restricted or unrestricted reporting.[22-26] **Table 13-5** reflects the total number of sexual assaults in the military per year from 2004 through 2008.

Table 13-5. Reporting Summary of Sexual Assaults in the Military

Type*	CY 2004	CY 2005	CY 2006	FY 2007	FY 2008	FY 2009
Restricted Reporting	N/A	327	670	603	643	714
Unrestricted Reporting	1700	2047	2277	2085	2265	2516
Total	**1700**	**2374**	**2947**	**2688**	**2908**	**3230**

* *CY: calendar year–January 1st through December 31st; FY: fiscal year–October 1st through September 31st.*

Conclusion

The DoD, with its major branches being the US Army, US Navy, and the US Air Force, has worked aggressively to attack the issue of sexual assault in the military since 2004. This began with the creation of a task force and has since led to several policy revisions over the past several years.

Current policies regarding sexual assault in the military allow service members on active duty to choose reporting options. If an unrestricted report is filed, a full investigation is launched. If a restricted report is filed, no investigation is launched, unless the victim changes his or her mind within one year of the report. Regardless of the type of report filed (restricted versus unrestricted), the service member is afforded medical care, forensic evidence collection, and counseling services. The DoD has been very clear in these policies that there is no tolerance for sexual assault in the military and that victims will be cared for with the highest level of respect and compassion.

References

1. Highlights in the History of Military Women. Women in Military Service for America Memorial Foundation Web site. http://www.womensmemorial.org/Education/timeline.html. Accessed November 21, 2008.

2. Military Personnel Statistics. Department of Defense's Web site. http://siadapp.dmdc.osd.mil/personnel/MILITARY/Miltop.htm. Accessed December 3, 2009.

3. Department of the Army. US Army Web site. http://www.goarmy.com. Accessed December 3, 2008.

4. Department of the Navy. US Navy Web site. http://www.navy.mil. Accessed December 3, 2008.

5. Department of the Air Force. US Air Force Web site. http://www.airforce.com. Accessed December 3, 2008.

6. Uniform Code of Military Justice. Delaware Consulting Group. http://www.ucmj.us. Accessed December 23, 2008.

7. Joint Service Committee on Military Justice. Manual for Courts-martial US (2008 Edition). Washington DC: US Dept of Defense; 2008.

8. Task Force on Care for Victims of Sexual Assault. DoD Care for Victims of Sexual Assault Task Force Report. http://www.defenselink.mil/news/May2004/d20040513SATFReport.pdf. Published April 2004. Accessed November 30, 2009.

9. Naval Justice School. *Note Taking Guide for Legal Officers*. San Diego, CA: Naval Justice School—Detachment San Diego; 2006.

10. Dewey E. Sexual Assault Nurse Examiners and the Courtroom. Presented at: The Sexual Assault Nurse Examiner Training Course; October 28, 2008; Yokosuka, Japan.

11. PBS. Tailhook `91. PBS Frontline Web site. http://www.pbs.org/wgbh/pages/frontline/shows/navy/tailhook. Accessed December 30, 2008.

12. CNN. Army's highest ranking enlisted soldier accused of assault, harassment. CNN Interactive Web site. http://www.cnn.com/US/9702/03/pentagon.miseries/index.html. Accessed January 2, 2009.

13. Robert J. Air Force Rape Scandal Grows. CBS News Web site. http://www.cbsnews.com/stories/2003/03/11/national/main543490.shtml. Accessed January 2, 2009.

14. Rumsfeld D. Memorandum for the Under Secretary of Defense 05 FEB04. http://www.sapr.mil/contents/references/d20040213satf.pdf. Published February 5, 2004. Accessed November 15, 2008.

15. ABC News. Soldiers Raping Soldiers. ABC News Nightline. ABC television. May 14, 2004.

16. Chu D, McClain KC. Joint Task Force Sexual Assault Prevention and Response. DoD News Briefing. http://www.defenselink.mil/transcripts/transcript.aspx?transcriptid=1628. Published January 4, 2005. Accessed November 15, 2008.

17. Sexual Assault Prevention and Response. Sexual Assault Prevention and Response Offices Web site. http://www.sapr.mil. Accessed December 18, 2008.

18. Department of Defense. Sexual Assault Prevention and Response (SAPR) Program. October, 6, 2005. DODD 6495.01.

19. Department of Defense. Sexual Assault Prevention and Response (SAPR) Program Procedures. June 23, 2006. DODI 6495.02.

20. Department of the Navy. Sexual Assault Victim Intervention Program. March 23, 1990. OPNAVINST 1752.1A.

21. Department of the Navy. Sexual Assault Victim Intervention Program. December 29, 2006. OPNAVINST 1752.1B.

22. Department of Defense. Reported Sexual Assaults in the Military for Calendar Year 2004. http://www.sapr.mil/contents/references/Signed%20DOD%20report%20of%20sexual%20assaults%20in%20CY2004.pdf. Published May 6, 2005. Accessed December 18, 2008.

23. Department of Defense. Reported Sexual Assaults in the Military for Calendar Year 2005. http://www.sapr.mil/contents/references/2005%20RTC%20Sexual%20Assaults.pdf. Published March 14, 2006. Accessed December 18, 2008.

24. Department of Defense. Reported Sexual Assaults in the Military for Calendar Year 2006. http://www.sapr.mil/contents/references/2006%20Annual%20Report.pdf. Published March 14, 2007. Accessed December 18, 2008.

25. Department of Defense. FY07 Report on Sexual Assault in the Military. http://www.sapr.mil/contents/references/2007%20Annual%20Report.pdf. Published March 13, 2008. Accessed December 18, 2008.

26. Department of Defense. FY08 Report on Sexual Assault in the Military. http://www.sapr.mil/contents/ResourcesReports/AnnualReports/DoD_FY08_Annual_Report.pdf. Published March 12, 2009. Accessed December 1, 2009.

Chapter 14

Campus Sexual Assault

Donna M. Barry, RN, MSN, APN-C, FN-CSA

According to a US Department of Education survey, there were 16 million students enrolled in 4200 colleges and universities across the United States in 2002.[1] The average age range for undergraduate students is 18 to 24 years, with enrollment at coeducational institutions being somewhere between 55% and 62% female.[1] National surveys reveal that women in the United States between the ages of 17 and 24 are at the greatest risk for sexual assault.[2] Specifically, a college-focused survey showed that the incidence of rape and attempted rape of female college students within a 9-month period (the academic year) was 5.8%.[3] The National Institute of Justice Study in 2000 found that 35 of every 1000 (2.8%) female college students had experienced rape or attempted rape while at school.[2] The National Violence Against Women Survey in 2006 showed that 29.4% of female victims were 18 to 24 years old when they were raped.[4] One can easily conclude from this data that female students at colleges and universities are at a significantly higher risk for sexual assault and that a large number of incidents of sexual violence occur each year.

Most of these incidents go unreported. Prior studies demonstrate that less than 5% of completed or attempted rapes committed against students were reported to campus or community law enforcement.[2] Victims are more likely to turn to a peer or mentor for support.[2] These support systems traditionally lack the training and specialized knowledge needed to assist a sexual assault victim, resulting in a high number of campus sexual assault victims being underserved and unable to begin the process of healing and recovery. Lack of reporting also results in a large number of offenders not being held accountable for their actions, with no opportunity for justice to be served for the victim or the community.

The vast majority of incidents are nonstranger assaults. Ninety percent of college women who are victims of rape or attempted rape know their assailant, and 13% of college women indicate that they have been forced to have sex in a dating relationship.[2,5] Since the offender is most often someone the victim knows and possibly even trusts, many have difficulty defining their experience as rape.[2] The inability to identify the incident as an assault and the struggle to label an acquaintance as a rapist have a powerful effect on the desire to report an assault or obtain assistance from trained individuals. This is compounded by the fear of being rejected by peers and the community.

Relationship violence is also prevalent within the campus setting. The most recent American College Health Association-National College Health Assessment (ACHA-NCHA) report indicates that 12.7% of the respondents reported emotionally abusive relationships, 2% experienced physical abuse, and 15% stated they have been sexually abused by a current or former partner.[3]

In a high number of incidents, alcohol or drugs are involved. A recent nationwide alcohol survey of college student alcohol use indicated that 72% of women who reported being raped were intoxicated at the time of the assault.[6] A report on college drinking by the National Institute on Alcohol Abuse and Alcoholism in 2002 indicates that over 70 000 traditionally college-age students experience alcohol-related sexual assault each year across the country.[7] In many cases of alcohol-related sexual assault, the victim is unable to consent to or remember details of the incident, often focusing on her own alcohol use as the cause of the assault. The uncertainty and fear of potential disciplinary or legal action against one's own behaviors is common as well.

Although alcohol is by far the substance most highly abused by college students, the use of prescription and street drugs continues to occur. In the fall 2006 report of the ACHA-NCHA, 5.2% of the respondents indicated marijuana use 1 to 2 times in the past 30 days. Cocaine and amphetamines were used 1 to 2 times by 0.7% of the participants during the same time frame.[3] None of the respondents indicated intentional use of Rohypnol or GHB, traditionally categorized as "date rape drugs."

The impact of the illegal use of other drugs on victim reporting is significant. Many fear charges for drug use will occur if an assault is reported to law enforcement or campus officials. When combined with alcohol use, the amnesic or incapacitating effect of many of these drugs results in minimal if any recollection of events. Law enforcement and campus officials are gravely hindered in the investigative process for those victims who choose to seek criminal or disciplinary charges.

The frequency of use of date rape drugs such as Rohypnol and GHB by offenders to incapacitate a victim has not been accurately measured. Both substances are illegal in the United States but commonly available in other countries and through the black market. Although less frequently used than alcohol and other drugs, some victims report intentional self-use prior to an assault. Others delay reporting. Since both substances become undetectable in blood and urine in a short period of time, conclusive evidence of a suspected drug-facilitated sexual assault is lost, and only an anecdotal report remains.

Alcohol continues to be the drug of choice for acquaintance rapists and campuses can provide an opportunistic setting for assault due to the inherent nature of the environment. Social events often involve the use of alcohol, with student housing on and off campus serving as the most frequent location for socialization and parties. This creates a high-risk environment and frequent opportunity for sexual assault. The survey conducted by Fisher et al revealed that 91% of the reported assaults took place in student residences and that more than 10% occurred in fraternity housing.[2] Research by Thompson reveals behavioral patterns indicative of acquaintance rapists who use these scenarios to offend.[8] An acquaintance rapist "plans to score" and selects a target who is younger, naïve, trusting, submissive, and flattered by the attention, typically an upper-classman male that singles out a freshman anxious to be a part of the college experience. Alcohol is most often used to reduce a victim's ability to resist and increase the rapist's chance to control the victim. The upperclassman invites the younger woman to a party and then repeatedly gives her drinks to the point of intoxication. The victim is then isolated in another room and the assault occurs.[8] Lisak has developed a similar profile of offenders he terms "the Undetected Rapist." His research identified similar attributes of premeditation and the use of alcohol and drugs to increase victim vulnerability. These studies also demonstrated that the majority of these individuals are serial offenders who are never prosecuted for their crimes.[9]

A Population at Risk

The inherent risk of sexual assault to the college-age population is exacerbated by a culture in which commitment and loyalty to the institution and its members is a priority and in which the primary means of socialization is an ideal opportunity for offenders.

College students who are victims of sexual violence have unique needs, options, and rights just as other groups or communities for whom culturally competent care is necessary do. Recognition and understanding of these victims as a special population is crucial to an effective response. It requires a sound understanding of the campus culture, its impact on victims, and adaptive protocols that offer an inclusive response.

The *National Training Standards for Sexual Assault Medical Forensic Examiners* refers to culture by defining diversity using Blue's definition from "The Provision of Culturally Competent Care": "Any group that has 'learned beliefs, traditions, and guides for behaving and interpreting behavior that are shared among members.'"[10,11]

Thus, a college environment can be recognized as a diverse population and a unique culture—a city within a city of sorts, regardless of its size or structure. Each institution has it own mission statement, governing body, internal policies, and regulations that define behavioral expectations and form a culture specific to its campus. The mission of most traditional institutions of higher education is to provide opportunities for strong academic achievement; further develop skills and talents that enhance future success; and encourage behaviors that will have a positive impact on society as a whole. Institutions achieve the objectives of their mission through a wide range of academic, athletic, and social activities and provide an extensive array of events for the purpose of learning, socialization, and community development.

Culture and Dynamics

Traditional campuses encourage a communal relationship by creating an environment where students live, share meals, learn, work, and socialize within close proximity to one another. Student housing serves as a common place to sleep, eat, study, and socialize. Dining facilities promote socialization during meals and strengthen a sense of community. Formal campus groups (ie, athletic teams, Greek organizations, and other clubs) further support this concept through activities in which commitment and loyalty to each member and the institution occurs and bonds of friendship form that last throughout a lifetime.

All campuses maintain a unique, internal set of policies and regulations by which students, staff, and faculty are obligated to abide. Often called a code of conduct, these regulations state the behavioral expectations of a campus community and potential sanctions if individuals violate these regulations. Each institution's administrative structure is ultimately responsible for the development of all policies and regulations, approval and oversight of activities, and upholding the behavioral standards of the community developed through these regulations.

Academic programs are usually the primary consideration for young adults determining which college or university to attend. The culture of an institution also plays a significant role. Applicants seek a school that will offer them opportunities to take part in activities of personal interest, to develop new friendships, to engage with the campus community, and to transition smoothly into collegiate life. Once enrolled, students participate in activities in an effort to become accepted members of the community and eventually become ingrained into its culture. Throughout the college experience, beliefs, traditions, and behaviors of the community are learned, furthering the mission of the institution and the desires of the student.

As a result, college students who are victims of sexual assault will react in a variety of ways based on this culture, which will impact victim response, frequency of reporting, access to care, and effective prosecution. The fear of being ostracized by peers or rejected by the community is common after an assault and is compounded by the strong bond that has developed among group members in organizations like athletics, Greek life, and clubs. In some cases, such relationships can even exist within small groups, such as among roommates.

Each institution's policies will determine how it responds to a sexual assault incident. The code of conduct and sanctions may or may not reflect the seriousness of sexual offenses. Campus services range from a comprehensive, accessible, and victim-friendly response to a response featuring minimal resources and little or no support for victims. Administrative reactions can also vary considerably, from attempts to avoid negative publicity to a victim-centered approach. Institutional leaders are often torn between the responsibility to protect the institution and the need to uphold the rights of victims and to report offenders as mandated by law.

External Regulations that Govern Institutions

Institutions of higher education must abide by numerous federal regulations. Those that are most pertinent to sexual assault include the Campus Sexual Assault Victim's Bill of Rights of the Higher Education Act Amendment of 1992, the Clery Act, and Title IX of the Education Amendments of 1972 Federal Gender Equity Requirements. Individual states may also have statutes specific to colleges and universities. An example is the New Jersey Campus Sexual Assault Victim's Bill of Rights (**Appendix 14-1**). These laws serve to protect victim rights, provide adequate victim services, mandate institutions of higher education to address sexual assault issues, and provide accurate crime reports for their respective campuses.

The Campus Sexual Assault Victim's Bill of Rights

The Campus Sexual Assault Victim's Bill of Rights was developed as part of the Higher Education Act Amendments of 1992.[12] (**Appendix 14-2**). This federal statute states that each institution of higher education must develop and distribute a policy for sexual assault that includes the following:

— Procedures students should follow if a sex offense occurs, including who should be contacted, the importance of preserving evidence, and to whom the alleged offense should be reported.

— Procedures for on-campus disciplinary action in cases of alleged sexual assault.

— Possible sanctions to be imposed following the final determination of an on-campus disciplinary procedure regarding rape, acquaintance rape, or other sex offenses, forcible or nonforcible.

— The option to notify proper law enforcement authorities, including on-campus and local police, and the option to be assisted by campus officials in notifying such authorities, if the student so chooses.

— Notification to students of options for, and available assistance in, changing academic and living situations after an alleged sexual assault incident, if so requested by the victim and if such changes are reasonably available.

— Entitlement of both accuser and accused to the same opportunities to have others present during a campus disciplinary proceeding.

— Entitlement of both accuser and accused to be informed of the outcome of any campus disciplinary proceeding brought alleging a sexual assault.

— Educational programming that aims at sexual assault prevention.

This statute delineates specific rights of campus victims that are in addition to community victim rights. It considers the dynamics and culture of a campus environment and offers options for victims to assist in the recovery process.

Filing a disciplinary action against the accused is a viable option for campus victims if one considers that often the accused is a fellow student, known to the victim, and frequently someone the victim trusts. Victims tend to view their experience as something that the individual should not have done, struggle with using the label "rapist," and decline the option of filing criminal charges. Typically, campus victims will respond to offers to file criminal charges by indicating that the assailant should not have committed the assault but does not deserve lifelong consequences. A disciplinary action allows the victim to seek justice through a charge of violation of institutional regulations that can be filed in addition to or instead of criminal charges, based on the victim's preference.

Academic accommodations are an important aspect of the healing process for college victims. Many times they share classes with the offender and revictimization can occur each time the victim must face the assailant in the classroom, regardless of whether there is any interaction. Without this accommodation, the victim is forced to choose between academic performance and revictimization. The trauma of the incident tends to overshadow the desire for academic achievement, and the victim no longer participates in the classroom experience. This right offers the option to have class schedules changed to avoid further contact with the offender and possible revictimization so that academic progress may continue.

As stated previously, inherent in the campus community is a communal living environment for many students. Victims may live in the same residence hall and often on the same floor as the offender. The fear of returning to housing and being revictimized or having to see the offender again can have a negative impact on victim recovery. If reasonably available, housing reassignments must be provided when requested by a victim. This can be in the form of offender relocation or the victim may choose to move to another room.

THE CLERY ACT

The Clery Act (**Appendix 14-3**), formally known as the Jeanne Clery Disclosure of Campus Security Policy and Campus Crime Statistics Act, is named in memory of college freshman Jeanne Clery, who was raped and murdered while asleep in her residence hall at Lehigh University in 1986. The law was enacted as a mechanism to increase the awareness of campus communities to crime incidents and therefore reduce the risk of a student or employee becoming a victim.

This statute reiterates the mandates required by the Campus Sexual Assault Victim's Bill of Rights, such as policy content requirements and educational programming, and adds the following additional regulations for all colleges and universities receiving federal student aid:

- Notification to students of existing on- and off-campus counseling, mental health, or other student services for victims of sex offenses.
- Reporting of sexual offenses to campus security officials by all individuals who hold a position of "security authority" on campus.
- Publication of an annual security report of all crimes including sexual offenses that have occurred at the institution.

The additional component of counseling services is a critical piece in supporting postassault campus victims. Advocacy services may be utilized during the initial sexual assault response team (SART) intervention, although victims sometimes decline this option or hesitate to contact crisis centers or hot lines in the days that follow an assault. The option to access mental health services is a viable one and many campuses have comprehensive counseling departments that can provide consistent and ongoing mental health interventions to victims.

The Clery Act is enforced by the US Department of Education, which may impose financial penalties against schools that fail to comply. Compliance is the responsibility of individuals recognized as security authorities on campus. This is most often the security or law enforcement department of the institution. However, anyone who is responsible for monitoring or maintaining security within the institution must report crimes that have been identified to them; this may include less obvious members, such as student employees who monitor the security of residence halls or athletic coaches responsible for the safety of their teams.

Clery Act regulations officially define the position of security authority as the following:

(a) Any individual or individuals who have responsibility for campus security but who do not constitute a campus police department or a campus security department, such as individuals responsible for monitoring entrances into institutional property.

(b) Any individual or organization specified in an institution's statement of campus security policy as an individual or organization to which students and employees should report criminal offenses.

(c) An official of an institution who has significant responsibility for student and campus activities, such as student housing, student discipline, or campus judicial proceedings. If such an official is a pastoral or professional counselor, the official is not considered a campus security authority when acting as a pastoral or professional counselor.[13,14]

Title IX of the Education Amendments of 1972

Title IX of the Education Amendments of 1972 prohibits discrimination on the basis of sex in any education program or activity at an institution receiving federal aid, and includes sexual harassment as a form of discrimination.[15] Sexual assault is currently viewed as an extreme form of sexual harassment. In *A Guide to Understanding What Is Expected of Colleges & Universities Under Federal Gender Equity Requirements When A Sexual Assault Occurs*, it states:

Sexual assault, a term which includes rape and other forms of sexual abuse like forcible fondling, is an extreme form of sexual harassment. It is "unwelcome conduct of a sexual nature," and, more specifically, "unwelcome sexual advances" and "unwelcome physical conduct of a sexual nature."[16,17]

Therefore, institutions must take the following actions related to incidents of sexual assault:

— Develop a policy and grievance procedure for sexual harassment that involves timely and impartial resolution.

— Address both informal and formal complaints with advisement on the grievance procedure for the school.

— Take steps to resolve the harassment.[17]

Students have the right to file a Title IX grievance with the Office of Civil Rights after an incident of sexual assault if they feel the institution violated their right to address the complaint or failed to take appropriate steps to resolve the harassment.

Internal Regulations: Judicial Affairs

Most institutions develop a code of conduct that parallels federal, state, and local statutes. Administrative leadership may, however, impose additional regulations. For example, a campus may have a policy that prohibits the possession or consumption of alcohol anywhere on school premises. All community members must abide by this regulation, regardless of the legal age for consumption established by state statutes. These policies and regulations set the tone for a campus' culture by providing behavioral expectations of all members and the accepted type and nature of events that are sponsored by the institution.

Enforcement is accomplished through a judicial or disciplinary board hearing that determines if a violation has occurred and imposes a sanction based on the severity of the action. The board composition and hearing process will vary from institution to institution, but all schools must publish the regulations, disciplinary process, and potential sanctions and provide due process to both the victim and the accused.

A review of potential institutional violations is a completely separate process from criminal or civil action. It is an internal procedure of the institution that determines only if a member of the community has violated campus regulations, not the law. Campus sexual assault victims may request disciplinary action against an individual who is also a student at the same institution. Using this option, a victim can seek justice and hold an individual accountable for an offense without going through the legal court system.

It is imperative for SART members to be aware of the additional rights and options of college students who seek services in the community and for team members to have a heightened awareness of the unique obstacles faced during the recovery process.

Impact on Health Care Providers

Primary Prevention Strategies

Primary prevention is a key intervention to reduce sexual violence. Individuals who provide health care to college students on campus or within the community can utilize this approach by integrating strategies as a standard of care for all routine and problem-focused patient visits. Recommendations for prevention and screening adolescents and young adults have traditionally included screenings for potential high-risk behaviors such as the use of alcohol, recreational drugs, or tobacco products; unsafe sex practices; eating disorders; and mental health concerns. These are vital issues that need to be addressed and an assessment of these areas should be included for any college student in order to gain a comprehensive patient history. The integration of screening for sexual violence risk, past history, and recent incidence is critical when caring for all individuals, especially with the high-risk college population.

In order to effectively use primary prevention against sexual assault when working with college students, the following areas need to be considered.

Development of Culturally Competent Skills to Work Effectively with College Students

The provision of culturally competent care is based on certain fundamental principles, including the beliefs that a clinician should understand and respect a given group or culture; should recognize its needs and how they impact patient care and response; should utilize this knowledge to make effective, culturally sensitive clinical decisions; and should provide care in a nonjudgmental, compassionate, patient-centered manner. The application of these principles to the care of campus sexual assault victims can be accomplished by employing certain core competencies.

Recognition of College Students as a Population at High Risk for Sexual Assault

Highly publicized cases of sexual assault on campuses represent a minute percentage of the incidents that occur. Invariably when students attend outreach programs or trainings on the subject of sexual violence, most can identify with situations where an attempted or completed assault occurred. The unfortunate outcome of these discussions is that many do not see themselves at risk. The belief that these crimes only happen to others is prevalent until an incident actually occurs, similar to the attitudes many young adults maintain regarding arrest for underage drinking or driving while intoxicated. Recognition of this population as inherently vulnerable and addressing these issues during care is a necessary intervention in the primary prevention of sexual assault on campus.

Understanding of the Dynamics and Culture of Campus Communities

Despite fundamental similarities in structure and regulations, the unique dynamics of an individual campus create different cultural environments. A basic understanding of the campus culture within the relevant geographic area will heighten professionals' awareness of the specific social risk behaviors for that campus. Small, private, or faith-based schools may differ significantly from large public institutions in the type of social events that occur as well as in the prevalence of student alcohol use. This is not to imply that some schools are entirely devoid of sexual assault incidents; as stated earlier, certain forms of socialization, especially involving the use of alcohol, increase risk factors and vulnerability—causing sexual assault to be potentially more prevalent.

Self-Assessment of Individual Bias and Assumptions Regarding College Student Behaviors

All health care providers bring to their practice personal values, beliefs, and attitudes developed over time, each of which influences clinician behaviors. Differences in age can also affect the health care provider's ability to appreciate a victim or patient's perspective of certain behaviors. Viewing a situation through the more mature frame of an adult can provide a vastly different understanding of a given situation than to do so through the frame of a 19-year-old college student. Self-reflection is important to determine whether biases and assumptions are present and whether nonjudgmental care can be offered. Assumptions and beliefs on the part of a provider concerning the impact of a victim's attire, alcohol use, prior sexual activities, or behaviors prior to the assault can be expressed through the format of questions posed, facial expressions as the incident is related, and body language during the interview process. In essence, the provider creates an interaction that supports a victim's feelings of self-blame for the assault. In 2006, the media response to the alleged rape of a college female is an example. The alleged victim was hired as an exotic dancer by the lacrosse team at Duke University for entertainment at a party. Numerous editorials and commentaries questioning the morals and behavior of the victim were written, and it was assumed that because she was employed as an exotic dancer she was also promiscuous and, therefore, had consented to sexual intercourse that evening. A true understanding of campus culture would contradict this assumption. Frequently, female college students work as exotic dancers to support themselves and to provide for their education. It is seen as a lucrative source of income that normally does not involve sexual contact and has hours that do not conflict with academic schedules. A provider's opinion may differ dramatically regarding the appropriateness of this type of employment, and it may be a struggle to maintain a nonjudgmental, noncritical approach during care.

The provision of culturally competent care to campus victims requires an examination of a provider's view of college student behaviors and resolution of areas that may undermine the provision of sensitive care to campus victims.

Integration of a Methodology for Sexual Violence Screening into All Patient Histories, Especially Those of College Students

Health care providers routinely screen populations at high risk for specific chronic diseases, cancers, and substance abuse. In the same manner, clinicians in community practice and college health providers can develop an approach to working with the college population regarding sexual assault and rape. Seasoned clinicians have always relied on thorough patient histories as the foundation for clinical decisions. Implementation of primary prevention techniques can be accomplished through the integration of questions into patient history forms, use of health assessment tools, and inclusive verbal histories taken at each visit. It is advisable to recognize that college students often share only the information asked of them, as do other consumers of health care. Questions about social and sexual behaviors are an uncomfortable and personal topic that even clinicians have difficulty discussing with patients. The importance of increasing a clinician's level of comfort in broaching these topics is as important as asking necessary questions about these topics. Questions should be phrased in a nonthreatening and nonjudgmental manner and often can be prefaced with an explanation of the reasoning behind the questions. General questions regarding seatbelt use and exercise habits should be included to emphasize the objective of determining safety and lifestyle habits and not just information on private or assumptive behaviors.

Many college students tend to seek assistance for sexual violence issues through what has been called the "back door approach" to services. College victims often enter the health care system after an assault by requesting screening for sexually transmitted infections (STIs) or emergency contraception (EC). This is a common and accepted reason to seek health care in the college setting. If clinicians do not ask questions about the possibility of unwanted sexual activity during these encounters, victims tend to withhold the underlying reason for the visit. Shame and self-blame experienced secondary to the sexual assault is reflected in the use of a more acceptable reason for the patient visit. A recent interaction with a patient demonstrates an all-too-familiar patient encounter with a college victim.

Case Study 14-1

The patient's chart indicated that the reason for her visit was to obtain emergency contraception. I asked routine questions about menstrual and contraceptive history and the time of the unprotected sexual activity. I then asked a simple but direct question: "Did something happen to you that you did not want to happen?" She began to weep and asked me, "Why would you believe me? No one ever did when it's happened before." I explained to her that I was there to help her in any way I could. She shared with me the following story:

"When I was 16, I was going with a guy in my school for about 3 months when he began pressuring me to have sex. We had been doing some stuff but not real 'sex.' I wasn't ready for going that far with anyone. It felt wrong somehow, so I kept telling him, 'No.' One night, we were alone, and he started trying to convince me again. He said everyone was doing it and if I really loved him I would want to. He made me feel like some kind of a freak, but I kept saying, 'No.' He started touching me and just kept going. I tried to stop him and was crying but it didn't matter so I just gave up resisting him. When it was over I asked him why he did it and he said he just couldn't stop. He went home right after that, and I was still crying when he left. The next day in school my best friend said she heard we had hooked up last night. I told her what happened and she just laughed at me. She said, 'Get over it. It wasn't rape. He was just being a guy.' I never told anyone else about it and the guy broke up with me afterward anyway. The next year, I started dating a guy from another school who seemed so different to me. There was never any pressure to have sex so I felt safe with him. His friends were that way, too—protective and nice to me and my friends all the time. He graduated the year before me and went to college, but we stayed together. So, when my senior prom came around and he couldn't come home, he offered to have his best friend take me to the prom. The night of the prom, I drank but not a lot, and we had a great time. On the way home he 'claimed' to get lost, and we ended up on a deserted road somewhere. He pulled over and raped me twice. I told my parents and they blamed me for all of it. They said it was my fault because I was drinking. So I didn't tell my boyfriend. I was sure he wouldn't believe me and would blame me, too. That was four months ago. My boyfriend and I stayed together and I went to visit him this weekend at his school. Everything seemed to be great between us until Saturday night when we came back from a party. We had both been drinking, but I wasn't drunk. I fell asleep right away and woke up to find him on top of me trying to have sex. We had never done it before, and I told him, 'No.' He got really angry and wouldn't stop. After it was over, he fell asleep like he hadn't done anything wrong. I got up and left and drove back to school last night."

When she left my office with resources and referrals for services, she turned and said to me, "If you hadn't asked me that question, I never would have told you what really happened to me. Thank you." I asked myself at the time how many victims we had missed because we did not ask the right questions.

This victim's experience emphasizes the importance of integrating queries about sexual assault into all aspects of patient histories. Primary prevention in this form seeks to prevent sexual assault from ever happening, assists victims with a history of sexual assault to access care, and can prevent revictimization.

Patient Education Methodology that Addresses Vulnerability and Risk Reduction

Educating patients has always been a critical aspect of overall care. Clinicians of all professions strive to inform patients of their health care status and to pass on methods to assist in health management. Identification of behaviors through patient history that increase individual vulnerability and the provision of educational information to avoid risk situations is an effective method to implement risk reduction. This can easily be applied to college students by identifying individual behaviors that increase vulnerability to sexual assault. **Table 14-1** provides educational guidance that can be used for all patients.

Information sheets and brochures that are readily available in provider waiting rooms can assist in heightening awareness of risk factors among family members and college students seeking routine care. General information of this type can be used to open lines of communication between students and their immediate support system about risk behaviors that can increase their vulnerability to sexual assault.

Table 14-1. Identifying Individual Behaviors that Increase Vulnerability to Sexual Assault

In General

— Be wary of behavior that makes you feel uncomfortable.

— Trust your instincts: If an individual makes you feel uncomfortable, find a safe place to remove yourself from the situation.

— You always have the right to set sexual limits in any relationship.

— Avoid excessive use of alcohol and other drugs.

— Be aware of what's going on around you.

— Educate yourself, your friends, and family members about sexual assault.

— Communicate your boundaries/limits clearly. If someone makes you feel uncomfortable, tell him or her early and firmly. ***Say "No" when you mean "No."***

— Take a look at the people around you and be wary of anyone who puts you down or tries to control how you dress or your choice of friends.

(continued)

Table 14-1. *(continued)*

ON THE STREETS

- — Try not to walk alone at night. If you must do so, walk in lighted areas and at a steady pace, looking confident. If you're on campus, call university police for an escort.
- — Be aware of your surroundings at all time; even in areas that you consider "safe."
- — It is not necessary to stop and be polite when a stranger or slight acquaintance asks a question in a public place.
- — Keep one hand free when carrying packages.
- — Avoid dark, empty places.
- — Listen for footsteps. Turn around if you think you are being followed and check. If you think you are, cross the street and go quickly to the nearest area where there are other people.
- — Have door and car keys ready before you need them.
- — Avoid walking alone if you are distracted, upset, or under the influence of any substance that may impair your action.

BEVERAGE SAFETY

- — Never accept beverages, including nonalcoholic ones, from someone not known or trusted well.
- — Keep track of your drink wherever you might be at the time.
- — Never leave your drink unattended; get a new one if you do.
- — Never drink from open beverage containers, including punch bowls at parties.
- — In a bar or restaurant, accept drinks only from the bartender or wait-staff.
- — Watch out for your friends. If someone appears disproportionately drunk for the amount of alcohol consumed, be concerned and closely monitor the person's behavior.[18]

Patient Education Methodology that Includes Healthy Relationships

Utilization of health histories to identify college students that are in abusive relationships is another important aspect of working with the campus community. Relationship violence is prevalent among college students, with sexual assault being part of the cycle of violence that occurs. Data from an ongoing NCHA survey demonstrated that 12.7% of college women experienced emotional abuse, 2% physical abuse, and 15% sexual abuse in the year prior to the study.[1] Assessing a patient's relationship with a partner is important in order to determine whether it is a healthy interaction or abusive in nature. Characteristic behaviors that serve as warning signs for abusive relationships are delineated in **Table 14-2**.

Simple conversations with a college student can reveal a wealth of information regarding relationships. Demonstrating an interest in their life along with the other, traditional health concerns offers a holistic approach to care and assists the health care professional in gathering information regarding risks and areas for patient education. Observing behaviors is another means of identifying patient needs. A brief encounter with a college student seeking care for the common cold demonstrates the importance of this.

Table 14-2. Characteristic Behaviors of Abusive Relationships

Abuse	Action
Emotional Abuse	— Threatening to harm individual or loved ones — Intimidation, ridicule, belittling, name-calling, humiliation, degradation — Extreme jealousy — False accusations — Physical or social isolation — Deprivation of basic needs or money
Sexual Abuse	— Making the victim perform sexual acts against his or her will — Forcing sex when victim cannot consent or is afraid to refuse — Intentional physical harm through sexual activity — Coercion to have sex without protection against disease or pregnancy
Physical Abuse	— Pushing, shoving, slapping, punching, kicking, biting, restraining victim — Strangling victim, pulling hair — Inflicting bruises, burns — Inflicting injuries to pets, children

Case Study 14-2

As I took a basic medical history from a student, her cell phone rang. She apologized, ignored the call, and we continued. The phone rang 3 more times within about 5 minutes. I commented that someone was anxious to speak with her and that perhaps she should answer it. She informed me it was her boyfriend and that he called like that all the time. The phone rang again, and this time it was a text message that read, "Bitch-answer your phone!"

The choice between ignoring the warning signs in her partner's behavior or addressing this area of concern and educating this student was obvious. A discussion of the dynamics of healthy relationships and further questions to determine safety concerns may protect a patient from further abuse, including sexual assault.

Awareness of Options and Rights of College Students

As stated earlier, college students have additional rights and options as victims of sexual assault. Most students are unaware of the existence of the Campus Sexual Assault Victim's Bill of Rights and need to be provided with this information at the time of an incident. Providers who are aware of its contents and have quick access to the document can easily assist a college victim with this information. A printed copy can be downloaded from the Security on Campus Web site (http://www.securityoncampus.org) and kept with other patient education materials and in provider waiting rooms. Students can also be directed to their institution's Web site to access the Student Handbook. This document covers all regulations, rights, and processes related to sexual assault that can assist in the adjudication procedure and access to campus resources.

Awareness of Available Campus and Community Resources for Referral

Clinicians whose practices are located in proximity to college or university campuses can access information about campus services with relative ease via the Web sites of local academic institutions or by contacting the campus offices of health services. The regulations, policies, and campus resources are available to the public in written and electronic form via the Internet. This can be a valuable tool for community providers caring for college victims when utilized as a patient education resource or referral guide.

College health professionals need to be cognizant of community resources for victim services as well. These services should be evaluated to determine the convenience, quality, and comprehensiveness of care and whether the care is compassionate and victim-centered. In an ideal response, a collaborative relationship is formed between community and campus resources, with one individual assigned to assure a comprehensive, coordinated response and continued care for the victim post assault.

Responding to Campus Victims

A campus victim's response to sexual assault will impact all members of the SART and the role they may play in the provision of services. Whether the response is from within the institution, from the community, or from both groups, communication, coordination, and evaluation of ongoing services is essential in offering a comprehensive and effective response.

In general, women who are attacked by a partner or acquaintance are more likely to present for treatment 2 or more days after the attack.[19] Campus victims normally present in a similar time frame. However, since campus victims commonly do not identify their experience as rape, it is more likely that they will seek medical care for EC or STI treatment than to access services through advocacy or law enforcement. Self-blame and a significant hesitancy to report the incident are commonly seen, as are similar behaviors. As the victim's first contact, the campus or community clinician should perform appropriate interventions:

1. Pose pertinent, victim-sensitive questions to screen for the possibility of sexual assault.
2. Assess victim safety.
3. Instill trust in victim through supportive statements (eg, "This was not your fault," "I believe you").
4. Explain the traditional services available to victims (eg, advocacy, forensic medical examination, law enforcement involvement) as well as the purpose of each role.
5. Explain campus options for disciplinary action, housing and academic accommodations, and follow-up counseling.
6. Explain confidentiality issues related to each option available to the victim.
7. Assist the victim in accessing care through available community and campus services.
8. Educate other response team members regarding considerations and needs unique to campus victims.
9. Inform response members of victim choices that are specific to campus victims in writing to ensure victim rights are upheld.
10. Provide a copy of the Campus Sexual Assault Victim's Bill of Rights to the victim.
11. Use anticipatory guidance to discuss potential peer and social group responses the victim may encounter when returning to campus and provide campus resources for assistance.
12. Determine a point of contact for the victim for coordination of initial care and follow-up.

Conclusion

Addressing the needs of campus victims in a comprehensive and victim-centered manner requires that all SART members recognize this special population as one with unique needs and options. This is especially important for health care providers who may be members of SARTs, community clinicians, or those who specialize in college health within the campus environment. Campus victims frequently access care directly through these providers rather than through the traditional routes of law enforcement and advocacy services.

Key concepts have been identified as necessary components to provide culturally competent, comprehensive care for campus victims:

— Recognition of campus victims as a group at high risk for sexual assault and other forms of sexual violence

— Understanding and sensitivity to the dynamics and culture of campus communities

— Comprehension of internal and external regulations that govern institutions of higher education

— Self-assessment of individual bias and assumptions regarding college student behaviors

— Utilization of primary prevention strategies to screen for sexual violence

— Implementation of a patient education methodology that addresses vulnerability and risk reduction

— Implementation of a patient education methodology that includes healthy relationships

— Thorough knowledge of options and rights of campus victims for access to care, reporting, and discharge planning

— Coordination of services between campus and community providers with an identified leadership role

Implementation of these concepts by clinicians as a standard of care will assure that the needs of campus victims are addressed, improve access to care, and potentially reduce the rate of sexual violence among college students.

Appendix 14-1: Campus Sexual Assault Victim's Bill of Rights

State of New Jersey
(UPDATED THROUGH P.L. 2007, ch. 41 and J.R. 4)
TITLE 18A EDUCATION
18A:61E-2. "Campus Sexual Assault Victim's Bill of Rights"; development; content

(2) The Commission on Higher Education shall appoint an advisory committee of experts which shall develop a "Campus Sexual Assault Victim's Bill of Rights" which affirms support for campus organizations which assist sexual assault victims and provides that the following rights shall be accorded to victims of sexual assaults that occur on the campus of any public or independent institution of higher education in the State and where the victim or alleged perpetrator is a student at the institution or when the victim is a student involved in an off-campus sexual assault.

(a) The right to have any allegation of sexual assault treated seriously; the right to be treated with dignity; and the right to be notified of existing medical, counseling, mental health or student services for victims of sexual assault, both on campus and in the community whether or not the crime is reported to campus or civil authorities.

"Campus authorities" as used in this act shall mean any individuals or organizations specified in an institution's statement of campus security policy as the individuals or organizations to whom students and employees should report criminal offenses.

(b) The right to have any allegation of sexual assault investigated and adjudicated by the appropriate criminal and civil authorities of the jurisdiction in which the crime occurred, and the right to the full and prompt cooperation and assistance of campus personnel in notifying the proper authorities. The provisions of this subsection shall be in addition to any campus disciplinary proceedings which may take place.

(c) The right to be free from pressure from campus personnel to refrain from reporting crimes, or to report crimes as lesser offenses than the victims perceive the crimes to be, or to report crimes if the victim does not wish to do so.

(d) The right to be free from any suggestion that victims are responsible for the commission of crimes against them; to be free from any suggestion that victims were contributorily negligent or assumed the risk of being assaulted; to be free from any suggestion that victims must report the crimes to be assured of any other right guaranteed under this policy; and to be free from any suggestion that victims should refrain from reporting crimes in order to avoid unwanted personal publicity.

(e) The same right to legal assistance, and the right to have others present, in any campus disciplinary proceeding, that the institution permits to the accused; and the right to be notified of the outcome of any disciplinary proceeding against the accused.

(f) The right to full, prompt, and victim-sensitive cooperation of campus personnel in obtaining, securing, and maintaining evidence, including a medical examination if it is necessary to preserve evidence of the assault.

(g) The right to be informed of, and assisted in exercising, any rights to be confidentially or anonymously tested for sexually transmitted diseases or human immunodeficiency virus; the right to be informed of, and assisted in exercising, any rights that may be provided by law to compel and disclose the results of testing of sexual assault suspects for communicable diseases.

(h) The right to have access to counseling under the same terms and conditions as apply to other students seeking such counseling from appropriate campus counseling services.

(i) The right to require campus personnel to take reasonable and necessary action to prevent further unwanted contact of victims with their alleged assailants, including but not limited to, notifying the victim of options for and available assistance in changing academic and living situations after an alleged sexual assault incident if so requested by the victim and if such changes are reasonably available.

L.1994,c.160,s.2.

18A:61E-3. Implementation of Bill of Rights

(3) In developing the "Campus Sexual Assault Victim's Bill of Rights," established by P.L.1994, c.160 (C.18A:61E-1 et seq.), the committee created pursuant to section 2 of P.L.1994, c.160 (C.18A:61E-2) shall review existing policies and procedures of public and independent institutions of higher education within the State and shall, as

appropriate, incorporate those policies into a proposed bill of rights. The committee shall make a recommendation to the commission which incorporates a proposed "Campus Sexual Assault Victim's Bill of Rights." The commission following consultation with the New Jersey Presidents' Council, established pursuant to section 7 of P.L.1994, c.48 (C.18A:3B-7), shall adopt a "Campus Sexual Assault Victim's Bill of Rights." The commission shall make the "Campus Sexual Assault Victim's Bill of Rights" available to each institution of higher education within the State. The governing boards of the institutions shall examine the resources dedicated to services required on each campus to guarantee that this bill of rights is implemented, and shall make appropriate requests to increase or reallocate resources where necessary to ensure implementation.

L.1994,c.160,s.3.

18A:61E-4. Distribution to Students

(4) Every public and independent institution of higher education within the State shall make every reasonable effort to ensure that every student at that institution receives a copy of the "Campus Sexual Assault Victim's Bill of Rights."

Appendix 14-2: Campus Sexual Assault Victim's Bill of Rights

Statute Text-20 USC § 1092 (f)(8)

(A) Each institution of higher education participating in any program under this subchapter and part C of subchapter I of chapter 34 of Title 42 shall develop and distribute as part of the report described in paragraph (1) a statement of policy regarding—

(i) such institution's campus sexual assault programs, which shall be aimed at prevention of sex offenses; and

(ii) the procedures followed once a sex offense has occurred.

(B) The policy described in subparagraph (A) shall address the following areas:

(i) Education programs to promote the awareness of rape, acquaintance rape, and other sex offenses.

(ii) Possible sanctions to be imposed following the final determination of an on-campus disciplinary procedure regarding rape, acquaintance rape, or other sex offenses, forcible or nonforcible.

(iii) Procedures students should follow if a sex offense occurs, including who should be contacted, the importance of preserving evidence as may be necessary to the proof of criminal sexual assault, and to whom the alleged offense should be reported.

(iv) Procedures for on-campus disciplinary action in cases of alleged sexual assault, which shall include a clear statement that—

(I) the accuser and the accused are entitled to the same opportunities to have others present during a campus disciplinary proceeding; and

(II) both the accuser and the accused shall be informed of the outcome of any campus disciplinary proceeding brought alleging a sexual assault.

(v) Informing students of their options to notify proper law enforcement authorities, including on-campus and local police, and the option to be assisted by campus authorities in notifying such authorities, if the student so chooses.

(vii) Notification of students of options for, and available assistance in, changing academic and living situations after an alleged sexual assault incident, if so requested by the victim and if such changes are reasonably available.

(C) Nothing in this paragraph shall be construed to confer a private right of action upon any person to enforce the provisions of this paragraph.

Implementing Regulations-34 CFR § 668.46 (b)(11)

(b) Annual security report. An institution must prepare an annual security report that contains, at a minimum, the following information:

(11) A statement of policy regarding the institution's campus sexual assault programs to prevent sex offenses, and procedures to follow when a sex offense occurs. The statement must include—

(i) A description of educational programs to promote the awareness of rape, acquaintance rape, and other forcible and nonforcible sex offenses;

(ii) Procedures students should follow if a sex offense occurs, including procedures concerning who should be contacted, the importance of preserving evidence for the proof of a criminal offense, and to whom the alleged offense should be reported;

(iii) Information on a student's option to notify appropriate law enforcement authorities, including on-campus and local police, and a statement that institutional personnel will assist the student in notifying these authorities, if the student requests the assistance of these personnel;

(iv) Notification to students of existing on- and off-campus counseling, mental health, or other student services for victims of sex offenses;

(v) Notification to students that the institution will change a victim's academic and living situations after an alleged sex offense and of the options for those changes, if those changes are requested by the victim and are reasonably available;

(vi) Procedures for campus disciplinary action in cases of an alleged sex offense, including a clear statement that—

(A) The accuser and the accused are entitled to the same opportunities to have others present during a disciplinary proceeding; and

(B) Both the accuser and the accused must be informed of the outcome of any institutional disciplinary proceeding brought alleging a sex offense. Compliance with this paragraph does not constitute a violation of the Family Educational Rights and Privacy Act (20 U.S.C. 1232g). For the purpose of this paragraph, the outcome of a disciplinary proceeding means only the institution's final determination with respect to the alleged sex offense and any sanction that is imposed against the accused; and

(vii) Sanctions the institution may impose following a final determination of an institutional disciplinary proceeding regarding rape, acquaintance rape, or other forcible or nonforcible sex offenses.

Appendix 14-3: "The Clery Disclosure of Campus Security Policy and Campus Crime Statistics Act."

20 USC § 1092(f) Disclosure of campus security policy and campus crime statistics

(1) Each eligible institution participating in any program under this subchapter and part C of subchapter I of chapter 34 of Title 42 shall on August 1, 1991, begin to

collect the following information with respect to campus crime statistics and campus security policies of that institution, and beginning September 1, 1992, and each year thereafter, prepare, publish, and distribute, through appropriate publications or mailings, to all current students and employees, and to any applicant for enrollment or employment upon request, an annual security report containing at least the following information with respect to the campus security policies and campus crime statistics of that institution:

(A) A statement of current campus policies regarding procedures and facilities for students and others to report criminal actions or other emergencies occurring on campus and policies concerning the institution's response to such reports.

(B) A statement of current policies concerning security and access to campus facilities, including campus residences, and security considerations used in the maintenance of campus facilities.

(C) A statement of current policies concerning campus law enforcement, including—

(i) the enforcement authority of security personnel, including their working relationship with State and local police agencies; and

(ii) policies which encourage accurate and prompt reporting of all crimes to the campus police and the appropriate police agencies.

(D) A description of the type and frequency of programs designed to inform students and employees about campus security procedures and practices and to encourage students and employees to be responsible for their own security and the security of others.

(E) A description of programs designed to inform students and employees about the prevention of crimes.

(F) Statistics concerning the occurrence on campus, in or on noncampus buildings or property, and on public property during the most recent calendar year, and during the 2 preceding calendar years for which data are available—

(i) of the following criminal offenses reported to campus security authorities or local police agencies:

(I) murder;

(II) sex offenses, forcible or nonforcible;

(III) robbery;

(IV) aggravated assault;

(V) burglary;

(VI) motor vehicle theft;

(VII) manslaughter;

(VIII) arson; and

(IX) arrests or persons referred for campus disciplinary action for liquor law violations, drug-related violations, and weapons possession; and

(ii) of the crimes described in subclauses (I) through (VIII) of clause (i), and other crimes involving bodily injury to any person in which the victim is intentionally selected because of the actual or perceived race, gender, religion, sexual orientation, ethnicity, or disability of the victim that are reported to campus security authorities or local police agencies, which data shall be collected and reported according to category of prejudice.

(G) A statement of policy concerning the monitoring and recording through local police agencies of criminal activity at off-campus student organizations which are recognized by the institution and that are engaged in by students attending the institution, including those student organizations with off-campus housing facilities.

(H) A statement of policy regarding the possession, use, and sale of alcoholic beverages and enforcement of State underage drinking laws and a statement of policy regarding the possession, use, and sale of illegal drugs and enforcement of Federal and State drug laws and a description of any drug or alcohol abuse education programs as required under section 1011i of this title.

(I) A statement advising the campus community where law enforcement agency information provided by a State under section 14071(j) of Title 42, concerning registered sex offenders may be obtained, such as the law enforcement office of the institution, a local law enforcement agency with jurisdiction for the campus, or a computer network address.

(2) Nothing in this subsection shall be construed to authorize the Secretary to require particular policies, procedures, or practices by institutions of higher education with respect to campus crimes or campus security.

(3) Each institution participating in any program under this subchapter and part C of subchapter I of chapter 34 of Title 42 shall make timely reports to the campus community on crimes considered to be a threat to other students and employees described in paragraph (1)(F) that are reported to campus security or local law police agencies. Such reports shall be provided to students and employees in a manner that is timely and that will aid in the prevention of similar occurrences.

(4)(A) Each institution participating in any program under this subchapter [20 U.S.C. § 1070 et seq.] and part C of subchapter I of chapter 34 of Title 42 [42 U.S.C. § 2751 et seq.] that maintains a police or security department of any kind shall make, keep, and maintain a daily log, written in a form that can be easily understood, recording all crimes reported to such police or security department, including—

(i) the nature, date, time, and general location of each crime; and

(ii) the disposition of the complaint, if known.

(B)(i) All entries that are required pursuant to this paragraph shall, except where disclosure of such information is prohibited by law or such disclosure would jeopardize the confidentiality of the victim, be open to public inspection within two business days of the initial report being made to the department or a campus security authority.

(ii) If new information about an entry into a log becomes available to a police or security department, then the new information shall be recorded in the log not later than two business days after the information becomes available to the police or security department.

(iii) If there is clear and convincing evidence that the release of such information would jeopardize an ongoing criminal investigation or the safety of an individual, cause a suspect to flee or evade detection, or result in the destruction of evidence, such information may be withheld until that damage is no longer likely to occur from the release of such information.

(5) On an annual basis, each institution participating in any program under this subchapter and part C of subchapter I of chapter 34 of Title 42 [42 U.S.C. § 2751 et seq.] shall submit to the Secretary a copy of the statistics required to be made available under paragraph (1)(F). The Secretary shall—

(A) review such statistics and report to the Committee on Education and the Workforce of the House of Representatives and the Committee on Labor and Human Resources of the Senate on campus crime statistics by September 1, 2000;

(B) make copies of the statistics submitted to the Secretary available to the public; and

(C) in coordination with representatives of institutions of higher education, identify exemplary campus security policies, procedures, and practices and disseminate information concerning those policies, procedures, and practices that have proven effective in the reduction of campus crime.

(6)(A) In this subsection:

(i) The term "campus" means—

(I) any building or property owned or controlled by an institution of higher education within the same reasonably contiguous geographic area of the institution and used by the institution in direct support of, or in a manner related to, the institution's educational purposes, including residence halls; and

(II) property within the same reasonably contiguous geographic area of the institution that is owned by the institution but controlled by another person, is used by students, and supports institutional purposes (such as a food or other retail vendor).

(ii) The term "noncampus building or property" means—

(I) any building or property owned or controlled by a student organization recognized by the institution; and

(II) any building or property (other than a branch campus) owned or controlled by an institution of higher education that is used in direct support of, or in relation to, the institution's educational purposes, is used by students, and is not within the same reasonably contiguous geographic area of the institution.

(iii) The term "public property" means all public property that is within the same reasonably contiguous geographic area of the institution, such as a sidewalk, a street, other thoroughfare, or parking facility, and is adjacent to a facility owned or controlled by the institution if the facility is used by the institution in direct support of, or in a manner related to the institution's educational purposes.

(B) In cases where branch campuses of an institution of higher education, schools within an institution of higher education, or administrative divisions within an institution are not within a reasonably contiguous geographic area, such entities shall be considered separate campuses for purposes of the reporting requirements of this section.

(7) The statistics described in paragraph (1)(F) shall be compiled in accordance with the definitions used in the uniform crime reporting system of the Department of Justice, Federal Bureau of Investigation, and the modifications in such definitions as implemented pursuant to the Hate Crime Statistics Act. Such statistics shall not identify victims of crimes or persons accused of crimes.

(8)(A) Each institution of higher education participating in any program under this subchapter and part C of subchapter I of chapter 34 of Title 42 shall develop and distribute as part of the report described in paragraph (1) a statement of policy regarding—

(i) such institution's campus sexual assault programs, which shall be aimed at prevention of sex offenses; and

(ii) the procedures followed once a sex offense has occurred.

(B) The policy described in subparagraph (A) shall address the following areas:

(i) Education programs to promote the awareness of rape, acquaintance rape, and other sex offenses.

(ii) Possible sanctions to be imposed following the final determination of an on-campus disciplinary procedure regarding rape, acquaintance rape, or other sex offenses, forcible or nonforcible.

(iii) Procedures students should follow if a sex offense occurs, including who should be contacted, the importance of preserving evidence as may be necessary to the proof of criminal sexual assault, and to whom the alleged offense should be reported.

(iv) Procedures for on-campus disciplinary action in cases of alleged sexual assault, which shall include a clear statement that—

(I) the accuser and the accused are entitled to the same opportunities to have others present during a campus disciplinary proceeding; and

(II) both the accuser and the accused shall be informed of the outcome of any campus disciplinary proceeding brought alleging a sexual assault.

(v) Informing students of their options to notify proper law enforcement authorities, including on-campus and local police, and the option to be assisted by campus authorities in notifying such authorities, if the student so chooses.

(vi) Notification of students of existing counseling, mental health or student services for victims of sexual assault, both on campus and in the community.

(vii) Notification of students of options for, and available assistance in, changing academic and living situations after an alleged sexual assault incident, if so requested by the victim and if such changes are reasonably available.

(C) Nothing in this paragraph shall be construed to confer a private right of action upon any person to enforce the provisions of this paragraph.

(9) The Secretary shall provide technical assistance in complying with the provisions of this section to an institution of higher education who requests such assistance.

(10) Nothing in this section shall be construed to require the reporting or disclosure of privileged information.

(11) The Secretary shall report to the appropriate committees of Congress each institution of higher education that the Secretary determines is not in compliance with the reporting requirements of this subsection.

(12) For purposes of reporting the statistics with respect to crimes described in paragraph (1)(F), an institution of higher education shall distinguish, by means of separate categories, any criminal offenses that occur—

(A) on campus;

(B) in or on a noncampus building or property;

(C) on public property; and

(D) in dormitories or other residential facilities for students on campus.

(13) Upon a determination pursuant to section 1094(c)(3)(B) of this title that an institution of higher education has substantially misrepresented the number, location, or nature of the crimes required to be reported under this subsection, the Secretary shall impose a civil penalty upon the institution in the same amount and pursuant to the same procedures as a civil penalty is imposed under section 1094(c)(3)(B) of this title.

(14)(A) Nothing in this subsection may be construed to—

(i) create a cause of action against any institution of higher education or any employee of such an institution for any civil liability; or

(ii) establish any standard of care.

(B) Notwithstanding any other provision of law, evidence regarding compliance or noncompliance with this subsection shall not be admissible as evidence in any proceeding of any court, agency, board, or other entity, except with respect to an action to enforce this subsection.

(15) This subsection may be cited as the "Jeanne Clery Disclosure of Campus Security Policy and Campus Crime Statistics Act."

References

1. US Department of Education, National Center for Educational Statistics (2002). Digest of Educational Statistics (NCES 2001-22). http://nces.ed.gov. Accessed December 2006.
2. Fisher B, Cullen F, Turner M. *The Sexual Victimization of College Women.* Washington DC: US Dept of Justice; 2000.
3. American College Health Association. Fall 2006 National College Health Assessment. http://www.acha-ncha.org. Accessed December 2006.
4. Tjaden P, Thoennes N; National Institute of Justice. *Extent, Nature and Consequences of Rape Victimization: Findings from the National Violence Against Women Survey.* Washington DC: US Dept of Justice, Office of Justice Programs; 2006.
5. Johnson I, Sigler R. Forced sexual intercourse among intimates. *J Interpers Violence.* 2000;15(1):95-108.
6. Mohler-Kuo M, Dowdall G, Koss M, Wechsler H. Correlates of rape while intoxicated in a national sample. *J Alcohol Stud.* 2004;65(1):37-45.
7. National Institute of Alcoholism and Alcohol Abuse. Alcohol Alert: Changing the Culture of Campus Drinking. http://pubs.niaaa.nih.gov/publications/aa58.htm. Published October 2002. Accessed December 14, 2009.
8. Thompson S. Date/Acquaintance rape: the crime and criminal. *Campus Law Enforcement J.* 1995;25(3):21-22, 36.
9. Lisak D. *The Undetected Rapist.* Boston, MA: University of Massachusetts; 2002.
10. Blue AV. The Provision of Culturally Competent Care. Medical University of South Carolina Web site. http://www.musc.edu/fm_ruralclerkship/culture.html. Accessed December 14, 2009.

11. US Department of Justice Office on Violence Against Women. National Standards for Sexual Assault Medical Forensic Examiners. June 2006. NCJ213827.

12. Higher Education Amendment of 1992. Campus Sexual Assault Victims' Bill of Rights. PL 102-325 section 486 (c).

13. The Jeanne Clery Disclosure of Campus Security Policy and Campus Crime Statistics Act (Clery Act). Higher Education Act Amendment of 1992. 20 USC § 1092 (f).

14. The Jeanne Clery Disclosure of Campus Security Policy and Campus Crime Statistics Act (Clery Act). Higher Education Act Amendment of 1992 Revision July 2003. 34FR668.46.

15. Title IX, Education Amendments of 1972. 20 USC § 1681-1688.

16. Lowery JW. Revised Sexual Harassment Guidance: Harassment of Students by School Employees, Other Students, or Third Parties. Washington, DC: US Dept of Education, Office of Civil Rights: 2001. URL: http://www.ed.gov/about/offices/list/ocr/docs/shguide.pdf. Accessed December 14, 2009.

17. Hogan H. Title IX Requires Colleges & Universities to Eliminate the Hostile Environment Caused by Campus Sexual Assault: A Guide to Understanding What Is Expected of Colleges & Universities Under Federal Gender Equity Requirements When a Sexual Assault Is Reported. Security On Campus, Inc. http://www.securityoncampus.org/pages/titleixsummary.html. Published in 2005. Accessed December 2006.

18. Kirkland C. Sexual Assault Services 2007. George Mason University Web site. www.gmu.edu/sas. Accessed January 5, 2007.

19. Miller G, Stermac L, Addison M. Immediate and delayed treatment seeking among adult sexual assault victims. *Women Health*. 2002;35(1):53-63.

Chapter 15

Drug-Facilitated Sexual Assault

Marc A. LeBeau, PhD

Drug-facilitated sexual assault (DFSA) is a term that describes a situation in which a person is subjected to a sexual act due to the incapacitating effects of alcohol and/or drugs.[1] The pharmacological effects of the drugs prevent the victim from being able to legally consent to the sexual act or fight off the attacker.[2]

While it is generally thought that the drug must be secretly administered to a person through food or drink for it to be considered a DFSA, many of these crimes most likely occur after voluntary consumption of recreational drugs with strong central nervous system (CNS) depressant effects.[1] In some cases, prescription and over-the-counter medications have been coingested with small amounts of alcohol, causing incapacitation and leading to DFSA. The key element is that the pharmacological effects of the drugs assist the crime.

The true prevalence of DFSAs is unlikely to ever be fully recognized.[3] Nonetheless, studies have tried to quantify the problem. The first such study was supported by Roche Pharmaceuticals,[4] the manufacturer of the benzodiazepine Rohypnol. In this study, free toxicological analyses for drugs in urine specimens collected in suspected DFSA cases were performed by an independent, forensic toxicology laboratory. A total of 3303 samples were analyzed, with 73% of the urine specimens having been collected within the first 24 hours after the alleged drugging. Over 61% of the samples were positive for one or more drugs, including ethanol. Critics of the study have noted that while the urine specimens were screened for Rohypnol at a very low concentration, other benzodiazepines were not screened for at such low levels. Additionally, the study reported that 3% of the urine samples were positive for gamma hydroxybutyrate (GHB); however, it is now recognized that the cutoff value used to differentiate between endogenous and exogenous GHB was too low, so GHB's prevalence was likely overestimated.[5,6]

More recent studies in the United Kingdom have found that nearly 50% of 1014 cases of alleged DFSA analyzed by the Forensic Science Service in London over a 2-year period were positive for ethanol and/or other incapacitating drugs.[7] Operation Mattise examined 120 cases of suspected DFSA over a 1-year period and agreed that ethanol is still the most common agent associated with DFSA.[8] More importantly, the report highlights the difficulties in investigating DFSA cases. Other studies have been conducted in Australia,[9] Canada,[10] France,[11] and Poland.[12]

Most cases of sexual assault are prosecuted at the state level, but there are 2 federal statutes available to charge offenses of DFSA: the Drug-Induced Rape Prevention and Punishment Act of 1996 and the Hillary J. Farias and Samantha Reid Date-Rape Drug Prohibition Act of 1999.

Challenges of DFSA Investigations

Drugs

The most important challenge facing investigators of DFSA allegations centers on the drugs used to commit this crime.[1] The mainstream media has led the general public, including investigators and prosecutors, to believe that there are only 3 or 4 drugs used to commit DFSA. In reality, over 50 drugs are known or suspected to have been used to commit DFSA.[13] Many are well-known recreational drugs of abuse, prescription medications, or over-the-counter pharmaceuticals. In many cases the drugs are self-administered by the eventual victim. One study found that fewer than 5% of sexual assault cases involved a drug surreptitiously administered to the victim. Further, when voluntary drug use is considered, over one-third of sexual assault cases could be classified as having been facilitated by drugs.[3]

Since most drugs exist in a solid, tablet formulation, surreptitious administration requires preparation on the part of the criminal, particularly if the drug is to be given in the drink of the victim. The pill or tablet may not immediately disappear if it is simply dropped into a drink. It may fizz as it slowly dissipates into the beverage. Additionally, most tablets contain insoluble, cellulose-based fillers that do not completely dissolve into the drink and leave a grainy residue. For these reasons, perpetrators commonly pre-dissolve the pill in small amounts of alcohol, filter the alcohol to remove insoluble materials, and then transfer the drug/alcohol mixture into a small eyedropper bottle. Additionally, some drugs, such as GHB, drugs found in gelatin capsules, and injectable drugs, are already in a liquid form, minimizing the preparation required.

Many drugs used in DFSAs are fast-acting, strong CNS depressants that mimic ethanol intoxication.[14] They can cause myriad pharmacological effects, including relaxation, euphoria, decreased inhibitions, amnesia, impaired perceptions, difficulty maintaining balance, impaired speech, drowsiness, complete loss of motor functions, vomiting, incontinence, unconsciousness, and possible death. Nearly all of these drugs can produce symptoms of general anesthetic agents, a common description used by victims of DFSAs. Because the CNS depressant effects imitate one another, it is highly unlikely one can determine the drug used by symptoms alone.

To further complicate DFSA investigations, the pharmacokinetics (ie, absorption, distribution, biotransformation, and elimination) of these drugs vary significantly.[1] There is a variable window of time after ingestion that drugs can be detected. For example, some drugs are detectable only for a few hours after ingestion.[15] In other instances, a drug may be detectable weeks after ingestion.[16] Without the knowledge of which drug may have been ingested, it is difficult to interpret a negative toxicological finding.

Reporting the Crime

Sexual assaults are significantly underreported, but common sense suggests that the percentage of DFSA cases reported must be considerably lower than reporting of forcible sexual assaults. In many cases, the victim suffers from amnesia. In other instances, the victims may be unclear as to the sequence of events, so they may delay reporting the crime while they try to piece together their memories.[17]

Delays in reporting usually mean specimens are not collected in a timely fashion, making it much more difficult for the toxicology laboratory to identify the agents used.[18] Additionally, it is vital that the victim is forthright about any prescription, over-the-counter, or recreational drugs that were voluntarily ingested.[1]

Evidence Collection

Another challenge facing investigators of DFSA is ensuring that the proper amount of specimens is collected as quickly as possible and properly preserved.[18] Urine is the most useful specimen in typical DFSA investigations because drugs and their metabolites become concentrated in urine specimens before elimination from the body, making them more readily detectable.[6] This becomes most important when attempting to determine if the victim had any drug exposure in the 1 to 4 days prior to the specimen collection. Current recommendations by the Society of Forensic Toxicologists (SOFT) DFSA Committee are that urine specimens be collected as soon as possible after a DFSA, not to exceed 120 hours after the suspected exposure.[19] If possible, 100 mL of urine should be collected to ensure the laboratory can adequately perform a sensitive and thorough analysis.[1]

After ingestion, most drugs are below detectable levels in the blood within 24 hours, thereby limiting the usefulness of a blood specimen. When blood can be collected a short time after drug ingestion, the combination of blood and urine specimens may assist in narrowing the window in which the drug exposure most likely occurred.

Blood specimens should be placed into collection tubes containing sodium fluoride. In addition to urine, at least 7 to 10 mL of blood should be collected when it can be provided within 24 hours of the suspected drug exposure.[1]

In many cases, a DFSA victim delays a report of the crime to medical and/or law enforcement personnel for days or weeks after the alleged crime.[16] At this point, it is no longer possible to find meaningful evidence of a drug in blood or urine specimens, but hair specimens have shown some promise.[20-23] Typically, head hair is used, although other body hair may also prove of some value. It is advised to wait at least 1 month after the suspected drug exposure before collecting the hair sample. This allows the portion of hair exposed to the drug via the bloodstream to grow above the scalp or skin. Using a hair clip, twist tie, string, aluminum foil, or rubber band, a twist of hair (about the diameter of a pencil) from the crown of the head should be tightly secured and then cut as close to the scalp as possible. The cut hair should be clearly labeled to differentiate the cut end from the distal end. The cut hair should then be properly sealed in a paper envelope and labeled.

Hair does present additional challenges compared to blood and urine specimens. Studies are lacking to fully evaluate if all drugs that may potentially be used in DFSA will incorporate into the hair matrix. Without this information, a negative hair result may be misleading. Furthermore, a positive hair result can also be challenging. Head hair grows at a rate of about 1 cm per month. Segmental analysis of hair is necessary to pinpoint the portion of hair that corresponds to the growth period during the alleged drug exposure and to demonstrate that the drug was not ingested outside of that growth period. For example, if, a month before an alleged DFSA, the victim took a strong sedative, the hair test must not confuse that previous ingestion with any drugs ingested the night of the DFSA. Only laboratory personnel skilled with handling hair specimens should be relied on to attempt segmental hair analyses.

In some cases, a vomit specimen may be useful.[18] If a drug is not fully absorbed before vomiting occurs, it may be detected in relatively high amounts in a vomit stain.

Laboratory Analysis of DFSA Specimens

Many of the drugs used to facilitate sexual assault are potent CNS depressants. Because of their high potency, only small amounts are required to achieve the desired pharmacological effect. Unfortunately, in many cases, the DFSA specimens were completely consumed or prematurely discarded because they were sent to laboratories that did not have appropriate methods or instrumentation to carry out the toxicological analyses. In general, clinical laboratories cannot detect subtherapeutic concentrations of the primary DFSA drugs, so they should not be relied on to determine if an individual was exposed when specimens are collected more than a few hours after the drug was likely ingested. Forensic toxicology laboratories may be unable to provide much better service, unless they have adequate sensitivities in their methods.

To improve consistency in laboratory results, the SOFT DFSA Committee developed a chart of the most prevalent drugs associated with DFSAs and their recommended maximum detection limits[13] when analyzing urine specimens (**Table 15-1**). These recommended detection limits are based on published analytical methods that use standard laboratory instrumentation. The committee's goal was to encourage laboratories to evaluate their current capabilities and make improvements as necessary. Furthermore, this tool provides a means of simplifying communication between analytical toxicologists and their customers, usually law enforcement personnel.

Table 15-1. Drug-Facilitated Sexual Assault Recommended Maximum Detection Limits for Urine Specimens

Target Drug/Metabolite	Recommended Max Detection*
Ethanol 10 mg/dL	
GHB and Analogs	10 mg/L
Benzodiazepines:	
Alprazolam	10 μg/L
Chlordiazepoxide	
Diazepam	
Hydroxyalprazolam	
Lorazepam	
Nordiazepam	
Oxazepam	
Temazepam	
7-amino-clonazepam	5 μg/L
7-amino-flunitrazepam	
Clonazepam	
Flunitrazepam	
THCCOOH	10 μg/L
Barbiturates:	
Amobarbital	25 μg/L
Butalbital	
Pentobarbital	
Phenobarbital	
Secobarbital	20 μg/L

(continued)

Table 15-1. *(continued)*

Target Drug/Metabolite	Recommended Max Detection*
Antidepressants:	
Amitriptyline	10 µg/L
Citalopram	
Desipramine	
Desmethylcitalopram	
Desmethyldoxepin	
Doxepin	
Fluoxetine	
Imipramine	
Norfluoxetine	
Norsertraline	
Paroxetine	
Sertraline	
Over-the-Counter Medications:	
Brompheniramine	10 µg/L
Chlorpheniramine	
Desmethylbrompheniramine	
Desmethylchlorpheniramine	
Desmethyldoxylamine	
Dextromethorphan	
Diphenhydramine	
Doxylamine	
Opiates and Nonnarcotic Analgesics:	
Codeine	10 µg/L
Hydrocodone	
Hydromorphone	
Meperidine	
Methadone	
Methadone Metab (EDDP)	
Morphine	
Normeperidine	
Norpropoxyphene	
Oxycodone	
Propoxyphene	
Miscellaneous Drugs:	
Carisoprodol	50 µg/L
Meprobamate	
Valproic Acid	

(continued)

Table 15-1. Drug-Facilitated Sexual Assault Recommended Maximum Detection Limits for Urine Specimens *(continued)*

Target Drug/Metabolite	Recommended Max Detection*
Miscellaneous Drugs: ***(continued)***	
Cyclobenzaprine	10 µg/L
MDA	
MDMA	
PCP	
Scopolamine	
Zolpidem	
Clonidine	1 µg/L
Ketamine	
Norketamine	

* *mg/dL = miligram/deciliter; mg/L = miligram/liter; µg/L = microgram/liter.*
Reprinted with permission from the Society of Forensic Toxicologists (SOFT).

Drugs Used to Commit DFSA

Ethanol

Although ethanol (alcohol) is the most common "drug" used to facilitate sexual assault, it is rarely recognized as such. This is in part due to its acceptance as a social drug by most of the world. When ethanol has a role in facilitating a crime, the alcohol is usually voluntarily ingested. However, in some cases, especially those involving children, ethanol was surreptitiously administered to the victim.

Numerous factors affect the level of intoxication reached from drinking ethanol.[24-29] Some variables are easily controlled, such as type of alcoholic beverage consumed (beer, wine, or mixed drinks), size of the beverages, whether ethanol is consumed with or after eating a meal (as opposed to an empty stomach), if the alcohol is mixed with a carbonated or a fatty beverage, and where the beverage is consumed (eg, at high altitude or in a hot tub). All of these variables affect ethanol's absorption into the bloodstream. The faster ethanol is absorbed and distributed to the brain, the more intoxicated the user generally becomes. Additionally, as with all CNS drugs, the more alcohol consumed, the more severe the intoxication.[30,31]

Ethanol impairment has been extensively studied in relation to operating motor vehicles, therefore, much is known about its effects on behavior. Users generally pass through different phases of intoxication, beginning with a subclinical stage where there are no appreciable symptoms of intoxication. The next phase is euphoria, in which the user becomes more talkative and social with diminished inhibitions. This is followed by a stage of excitement where the user may begin to feel drowsy, have indications of emotional instability, and demonstrate impaired perceptions, memory, and comprehension. The next stages are more serious, with symptoms of confusion, stupor, coma, and death. Throughout these stages, the user may experience severe disorientation, lack of coordination, slurred speech, vomiting, blackouts, unconsciousness, anesthesia, and respiratory depression.

Ethanol is generally eliminated following zero-order kinetics.[32] This allows for the average elimination rates for both men (0.015 g/dL/hour) and women (0.018 g/dL/hour) to be used to predict the blood ethanol concentration of an individual based on the number, type, and size of the drinks that they consumed in a given evening, as well as their body weight. Commercially available software programs allow toxicologists to estimate the blood alcohol concentration range a person likely reached based on the history of alcohol consumption. This helps evaluate the role ethanol may have played in contributing to the symptoms the DFSA victim described, particularly when the blood alcohol concentration range is compared to research, as presented in **Table 15-2**. However, factors such as chronic alcoholism, genetic factors, and liver disease must also be considered.

Table 15-2. Concentration, Stages, and Clinical Signs and Symptoms of Alcoholic Influence

Blood Alcohol Concentration	Stages of Alcoholic Influence	Clinical Signs/Symptoms
0.01-0.05 (g/dL)	Subclinical	— Influence/effects no apparent or obvious — Behavior nearly normal by ordinary observation — Impairment detectable by special tests
0.03-0.12 (g/dL)	Euphoria	— Mild euphoria, sociability, talkativeness — Increased self-confidence; decreased inhibitions — Diminution of attention, judgment, and control — Some sensory motor impairment — Slowed information processing — Loss of efficiency in critical performance tests
0.09-0.25 (g/dL)	Excitement	— Emotional instability — Loss of critical judgment — Impairment of perception, memory, and comprehension — Decreased sensitory response; increased reaction time — Reduced visual acuity, peripheral vision, and glare recovery — Sensory motor incoordination; impaired balance — Drowsiness
0.18-0.30 (g/dL)	Confusion	— Disorientation; mental confusion — Dizziness — Exaggerated emotional states (fear, sorrow, rage, etc) — Disturbances of vision and perception of color, form, motion, dimensions — Increased pain threshold — Increased muscular incoordination; staggering gait — Slurred speech — Apathy — Lethargy

(continued)

Table 15-2. Concentration, Stages, and Clinical Signs and Symptoms of Alcoholic Influence *(continued)*

Blood Alcohol Concentration	Stages of Alcoholic Influence	Clinical Signs/Symptoms
0.25-0.40 (g/dL)	Stupor	— General inertia — Approaching loss of motor functions — Markedly decreased response to stimuli — Marked muscular incoordination — Inability to stand or walk — Vomiting — Incontinence of urine and feces — Impaired consciousness — Sleep or stupor
0.35-0.50 (g/dL)	Coma	— Complete unconsciousness; coma — Anesthesia; depressed or abolished reflexes — Subnormal temperature — Incontinence of urine and feces — Impairment of circulation and respiration — Possible death
0.45+ (g/dL)	Death	— Death from respiratory arrest

Reprinted with permission from K.M. Dubowski, University of Oklahoma College of Medicine, Oklahoma City, Oklahoma, 1997.

GHB and Analogs

Of all the drugs used to facilitate sexual assault and other crimes, GHB and its metabolic precursors—gamma butyrolactone (GBL) and 1,4-butanediol (1,4-BD)—are probably among the most favored. Unfortunately, solid proof of their use in many cases is difficult to obtain because GHB, GBL, and 1,4-BD have strong sedative, amnesiac effects and are very rapidly eliminated after ingestion. To further complicate the matter, GHB is a metabolite of GABA, a natural neurotransmitter in humans.[33] Therefore, measurable amounts of endogenous GHB are found in blood (< 2 mg/L) and urine specimens (< 10 mg/L) from most humans.[6,34] After ingestion, exogenous GHB is not likely to be differentiated from endogenous concentrations of GHB in as little as 2 to 8 hours in blood specimens or 3 to 12 hours in urine samples.[15]

Another factor that makes GHB, GBL, and 1,4-BD popular with some rapists is their availability. GHB is very simple to synthesize, requiring only GBL (found in many cleaning or degreasing solutions in home improvement stores), a strong alkaline solution (ie, lye or drain cleaners), vinegar (to neutralize the mixture), and water (to dilute the final product). GHB, GBL, and 1,4-BD are also relatively easy to illegally purchase.

The French physician Henri Laborit first developed GHB in the 1960s while he was studying GABA.[35] Later that decade, GHB was introduced as an intravenous general anesthetic agent, but its use was limited by side effects such as grand mal seizures and coma. Nonetheless, today GHB is still employed as a general anesthetic in France (Gamma-OH) and Germany (Somsanti). It has also been studied for its ability to suppress the symptoms of alcohol dependence, opiate-withdrawal, treatment of fibromyalgia, and the management of narcoleptic patients.[36-45] In 2002, the US Food and Drug Administration (FDA) approved sodium oxybate (Xyrem)–a medically formulated form of GHB–for the treatment of cataplexy.[43,46] When used as medically prescribed, Xyrem is a Schedule III controlled substance, but its illicit use continues to carry the penalties of Schedule I substances in the United States.

GHB and its analogs belong to a group of drugs often referred to as "club drugs." These recreational drugs are often encountered at nightclubs and all-night dance parties called raves. Club drug users tend to be teenagers and young adults who abuse GHB for its strong CNS depression, which leads to euphoria, reduced inhibitions, and sedation. As with other CNS depressants, the effects largely depend on the amount consumed and degree of tolerance to the drug. Thus an individual consuming GHB may experience a variety of symptoms, from wakefulness and euphoria to deep sleep or coma.[47]

GHB, GBL, and 1,4-BD are nearly always administered as an oral solution. They may be disguised as bottled water, sport drinks, juices, hairsprays, eye drops, breath drops, or mouthwashes. Consumption is usually by the capful or teaspoon; however, GHB has also been abused in a powder form or as a gummy ball.[48] After ingestion, GHB and its analogs are rapidly absorbed. Peak plasma concentrations occur within 30 to 60 minutes[47,49,50]; however, GHB's absorption is likely to be capacity-limited and may be enhanced when it is absorbed on an empty stomach.[51-53]

GBL and 1,4-BD are rapidly metabolized into GHB (**Figure 15-1**), so their pharmacological effects mimic those of GHB. In most DFSA cases, findings of GBL or 1,4-BD would be unexpected, as there should be complete conversion to GHB by the time the victim provides specimens. The same enzymes used to metabolize ethanol metabolize 1,4-BD,[54] so if there is coingestion of 1,4-BD and alcohol, the effects of 1,4-BD may be more severe and the detection times of GHB may be longer than expected. Because GHB is also rapidly and extensively metabolized, less than 5% of an oral dose is excreted unchanged in the urine.[49,51]

Individuals exposed to GHB or one of its analogs may pass from complete alertness into deep unconsciousness within 10 to 15 minutes after ingestion.[55] Because of GHB's rapid clearance, the GHB-assisted sleep generally only lasts 3 to 4 hours.[56] Contrary to many other drugs used in DFSA, people exposed to GHB usually wake up without a so-called "hangover" effect.

Figure 15-1. *GBL and 1,4-BD rapidly metabolize into GHB.*

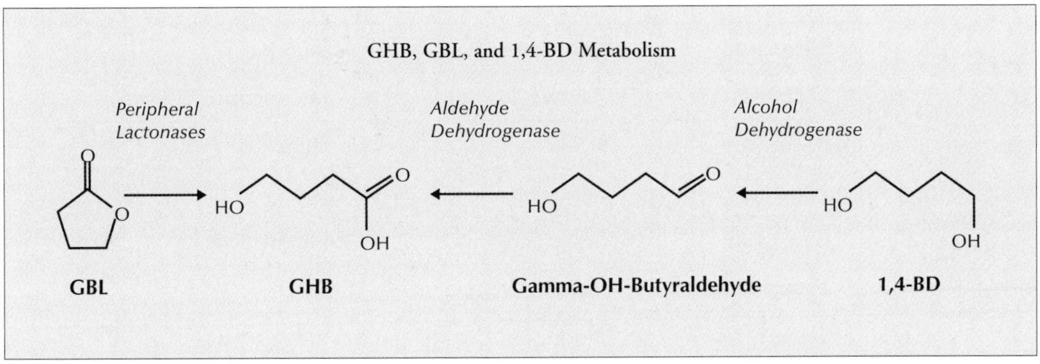

GHB, GBL, and 1,4-BD Metabolism

Benzodiazepines

The benzodiazepine drug class accounts for the most commonly used prescription medications in DFSA cases.[7,57] Benzodiazepines, one of the world's most widely prescribed drug classes, are primarily used as anxiolytics, anticonvulsants, anesthetic adjuncts, hypnotics, and muscle relaxants and to treat obsessive-compulsive disorders.

Prescription drug use in DFSA is important to consider, as the perpetrator of DFSAs may have personal experience with the drug's effects. It is quite common to see benzodiazepines abused in combination with illicit drugs (ie, opiates and cocaine), so the personal experiences may also be through recreational use. The most popular benzodiazepines used for DFSA are listed in **Table 15-3**.

In the 1990s, flunitrazepam (Rohypnol) was reported as a popular drug to use in DFSA. This potent drug is typically used as an adjunct to general anesthetics in surgical procedures because it can cause muscle relaxation and anterograde amnesia. While flunitrazepam has never been approved for use in the United States, it has been approved in many other countries and is smuggled into the United States for illicit use.

In 1997, the manufacturer of Rohypnol responded to concerns about its use in DFSA by changing the formulation to include a blue dye in its core. This dye releases if the tablet is dissolved into a light-colored liquid; however, the dye was not added to generic versions of the drug. Additionally, the maximum amount of flunitrazepam in a Rohypnol tablet was decreased from 2 to 1 mg to further minimize its potential use in DFSA cases.

Table 15-3. Benzodiazepines and Their Elimination Half-Lives

Benzodiazepine	Examples of Trade Name(s)	Half-Life*
Alprazolam	Xanax	Intermediate
Bromazepam	Lectopam, Lexotan	Intermediate
Chlordiazepoxide	Librium	Intermediate
Clonazepam	Clonopin, Klonopin	Long
Clorazepate	Tranxene	Short
Diazepam	Valium, Ducene	Long
Estazolam	ProSom, Eurodin	Intermediate
Flunitrazepam	Rohypnol, Hypnodorm	Long
Flurazepam	Dalmane	Long†
Halazepam	Paxipam	Long‡
Lorazepam	Ativan	Intermediate
Midazolam	Versed	Short
Nitrazepam	Mogadon	Long
Oxazepam	Serax, Serepax	Intermediate
Prazepam	Centrax, Vertran	Short
Temazepam	Normison, Restoril	Intermediate
Triazolam	Halcion	Short

* *Short: < 6 hours; Intermediate: 6-24 hours; Long: > 24 hours.*

† *Flurazepam has a very short elimination half-life, but its metabolite's half-life is long.*

‡ *Halazepam has an intermediate elimination half-life, but the half-life of its metabolite is long.*

Evidence now indicates there were relatively few proven cases of flunitrazepam's use in DFSA. Numerous studies and reports show other benzodiazepines used in DFSA at a greater frequency than Rohypnol, probably because of availability.

Clonazepam (Clonopin, Klonopin, Rivotril) is another highly potent benzodiazepine. Unlike flunitrazepam, clonazepam is available in the United States as a Schedule IV drug. Interestingly, the chemical structure of clonazepam is similar to flunitrazepam and its pharmacological effects are similar. Certain clonazepam tablets look similar to those of generic flunitrazepam, so it is common for clonazepam to be misrepresented as flunitrazepam when illegal purchases are made.[58]

Diazepam (Valium) was first approved for use in 1963 and was the top-selling pharmaceutical in the United States from 1969 to 1982. Newer benzodiazepines have become more popular than diazepam, but it is still considered an essential core drug by the World Health Organization and continues to be widely prescribed. Diazepam can cause deep sedation and amnesia.[59,60] Because diazepam has a lower potency than flunitrazepam, about 10 times more diazepam must be ingested to achieve the same effect.

Alprazolam (Xanax) is very popular both as a prescription medication and as a drug of abuse. It is primarily prescribed for anxiety disorders, but is also used as an adjunct to treat depression. It is considered a high-potency benzodiazepine, so only a small dose is required to achieve the desired pharmacological effect.[61]

Triazolam (Halcion) is generally prescribed for its sedative properties to treat acute insomnia or jet lag. It causes rapid sedation, but lacks the prolonged drowsiness that accompanies many other benzodiazepines.[62] As with the other benzodiazepines, triazolam also causes anterograde amnesia.

In DFSA cases, benzodiazepines are usually administered orally, but intravenous and intramuscular administration is also possible. With oral benzodiazepine ingestion, absorption into the bloodstream is nearly 100% because of the very high lipid solubility. However, the rate of absorption (and thus rate of activity) depends on the benzodiazepine itself. Generally speaking, most benzodiazepines reach peak blood concentrations within 30 minutes to 6 hours after ingestion. If the tablet formulation of a benzodiazepine is dissolved in an alcohol or aqueous solution, the absorption rates will likely be faster and peak effects should be felt significantly earlier than if exposure occurs via normal tablet administration.

Benzodiazepines are classified according to their elimination half-lives (**Table 15-3**). In pharmacology, the elimination half-life refers to the time that it takes 50% of the drug to be removed from the bloodstream. After 4 half-lives, only 6% of the original amount of ingested drug remains in the bloodstream. This means that the shorter the half-life, the faster the drug is eliminated from the body. Therefore, the short-acting benzodiazepines (eg, midazolam, triazolam) cannot be detected as long as the long-acting benzodiazepines (eg, diazepam, clonazepam). Additionally, the long-acting benzodiazepines tend to exhibit a more severe "hangover" side effect than do their short-acting counterparts.

Hepatic metabolism of benzodiazepines is extensive. The hydroxyl products are further metabolized by conjugation with glucuronic acid and are the major urinary products of benzodiazepines. The cytochrome P450 3A (CYP3A) enzyme family is involved in the metabolism of many benzodiazepines, so it is important to recognize the effects of coingestion of drugs that inhibit this enzyme system and their effects on benzodiazepine metabolism. For example, cimetidine, diltiazem, fluoxetine, verapamil, antifungals, antibiotics (eg, erythromycin and clarythromycin), and protease inhibitors are all known to inhibit the CYP3A enzymes.[63-65] Grapefruit juice also inhibits these enzymes.[66,67] If inhibition occurs, normal benzodiazepine metabolism will be altered and the resulting pharmacological effects enhanced.

Ketamine

Ketamine (Ketaset, Ketanest, Ketalar) is a dissociative anesthetic with analgesic properties and is structurally similar to the more recognized recreational drug, phencyclidine (PCP). Like GHB, ketamine has also become a popular drug of abuse and is considered a club drug.[68] Because of its popularity in veterinary medicine, ketamine is often stolen from veterinarian clinics.

Ketamine may be administered through intravenous, subcutaneous, intramuscular injections; nasal insufflation; smoking; or oral ingestion. Most users abuse ketamine for its hallucinogenic, dissociative properties, which they describe as being less connected to a sense of self and the reality around them. If large enough amounts are taken, the user may go into a "K-hole": a state of wildly dissociated experiences in which other worlds or dimensions are perceived while the user is unaware of what is actually going on. An individual's memories of events while under the influence of this drug can be altered or shaped by an outsider telling the person what is happening. While an individual is under the influence of this drug, they may appear to be awake, but in a trance-like state.

Some users may not remember the experience after regaining consciousness, much the way that a person may forget a dream. The process of emerging from under the influence of ketamine is slow, with the user gradually becoming aware of surroundings, initially being unable to remember his or her name. Movement may be extremely difficult.

Ketamine is quickly metabolized to norketamine and dehydronorketamine. Conjugates of hydroxylated derivatives of the parent drug, as well as its metabolites, may be excreted in the urine for at least 72 hours after ingestion.[69]

Cannabis

Cannabis (marijuana, hashish, kief, bhang, hash oil) continues to be the most widely abused illicit drug worldwide. It has been estimated that cannabis is used by 4% of the world's adult population each year, making it more popular than all other illicit drugs combined.

Cannabis is a product of the *Cannabis sativa* plant—particularly its flowers and buds. The primary psychoactive analyte is delta-tetrahydrocannabinol[9] (THC). Improvements in breeding and cultivation of the plant have produced much more potent strains of cannabis. The drug is typically smoked or ingested orally.

When smoked, the technique (ie, number, duration, and spacing of puffs; hold time; and inhalation volume) strongly influences the concentration of THC that reaches the user's brain. THC can be measured in plasma within seconds after inhaling the first puff of a marijuana cigarette, so the brain is rapidly exposed to THC following smoking.

While the behavioral effects of euphoria and relaxation are generally what is desired by cannabis users, an acute toxic effect of marijuana is CNS depression, including lethargy and reduction in short-term memory. The effect is enhanced when cannabis is coingested with alcohol.

The major metabolic route of THC is via hydroxylation by the hepatic cytochrome P450 enzyme system. This results in the production of the active metabolite, 11-OH-THC, which is oxidized to an inactive metabolite, THCCOOH. THCCOOH forms a conjugate with glucuronic acid, which enhances the compound's water solubility. THCCOOH, both free and conjugated, is the primary metabolite seen in urine samples.

Due to its high lipid solubility, THC accumulates in fat where it slowly releases back into the bloodstream. This allows for extended detection times for THC and metabolites when laboratories are using highly sensitive analytical methods. THCCOOH excretion into the urine can occur for days after ingestion. Its long elimination half-life, as well as its enterohepatic recirculation, makes it very difficult to estimate the time of drug exposure when analyzing a urine sample. It becomes even more challenging when the sample is from a chronic marijuana user. Generally, a urine sample from a naïve user of marijuana may have measurable amounts of THC metabolites for 1 to 5 days after smoking a single marijuana cigarette. As is true for all drugs, the window of detection depends in part on the sensitivity of the analytical methods used.

Opiates

Opiates represent another large drug class used to facilitate crimes (**Table 15-4**). These drugs are potent analgesics and exhibit strong CNS depression as a major side effect. Analgesia is particularly important in DFSA cases. Many victims of these crimes report briefly waking during the assault, looking up to see the perpetrator assaulting them, but falling back into an unconscious state before they can fight off their attacker. These awakenings are believed to occur, in part, because of a sudden infliction of pain. Such pain may result when penetration first occurs or if their head or arm is suddenly injured by banging against the floor, a headboard, or a nightstand. The analgesic effects of the opiates minimize the likelihood of this awakening occurring; however, the effectiveness of individual opiates varies.

Due to poor bioavailability, many opiates are best absorbed via parenteral administration. Absorption after oral administration can also be effective, but the extent of the pharmacological effects varies. Many opiates ultimately form glucuronide metabolites for elimination in the urine. Detection of opiates in the urine after a single administration is generally between 1 to 5 days, depending on the opiate consumed and the sensitivity of the testing method.

Table 15-4. Narcotic and Nonnarcotic Analgesics

Drug	Examples of Trade Name(s)	Half-Life*
Buprenorphine	Buprenex, Subutex	Short
Butorphanol	Stadol	Intermediate
Codeine	Codral forte	Short
Dextromethorphan	DM, DXM	Short
Dihydrocodeine	DHCplus, Synalgos-DC	Short
Fentanyl	Actiq, Duragesic, Sublimaze, Innovar	Short-Intermediate
Heroin		Short

(continued)

Table 15-4. Narcotic and Nonnarcotic Analgesics *(continued)*

Drug	Examples of Trade Name(s)	Half-Life*
Hydrocodone	Anexsia, Hycodan, Lorcet, Lortab, Norco, Pancet, Vicodin, Zydone	Short
Hydromorphone	Dilaudad, Palladone	Short
Levorphanol	Dromoran, Levo-Dromoran	Intermediate
Meperidine (Pethidine)	Demerol, Mepergan	Short
Methadone	Dolophine, Physeptone	Long
Morphine	Avinza, Astramorph, Duramorph, Kadian, MS Contin, Oramorph, Roxanol	Short
Nalbuphine	Nubain	Short-Intermediate
Oxycodone	Oxycontin, Oxyir, Roxicodone, Percodan, Percocet, Percolone, Roxicet, Tylox	Short
Oxymorphone	Numorphan	Short
Pentazocine	Talacen, Talwin	Short
Propoxyphene	Darvocet, Darvon, Wygesic	Intermediate

* *Short: <6 hours; Intermediate: 6-12 hours; Long: >12 hours.*

Antihistamines

In allergic reactions, mast cells in our bodies release histamine, causing itching, vasodilation, flushing, headaches, and other symptoms. Antihistamine drugs serve to reduce or eliminate the effects of histamine.

In recent years, the abuse of some antihistamine drugs—the first generation antihistamines—has increased. These drugs are the oldest members of the antihistamine class, are relatively inexpensive, and have widespread availability as over-the-counter medications. They are attractive because of their strong CNS depressant effects that lead to sedation, euphoria, dizziness, blurred vision, ringing in the ears, hallucinations, and psychosis. **Table 15-5** lists the first-generation antihistamines grouped by chemical structure. Antihistamines with similar chemical structures have equivalent effects.

Antihistamines are readily absorbed after oral administration with an onset of action generally within an hour after ingestion. The half-life of antihistamines varies considerably, so detection times after administration may range from hours to days, depending on the antihistamine consumed. Laboratories that primarily test for drugs of abuse may not screen for over-the-counter medications such as antihistamines.

Table 15-5. Antihistamines Grouped by Chemical Structure

CHEMICAL STRUCTURE: ANTIHISTAMINE
Ethylenediamines: First group of effective antihistamines.
— *Mepyramine*
— *Antazoline*
Ethanolamines: Cause significant sedation.
— *Diphenhydramine*
— *Carbinoxamine*
— *Doxylamine*
— *Clemastine*
— *Dimenhydrinate*
Alkylamines: More prone to paradoxical CNS stimulation than the others.
— *Pheniramine*
— *Chlorpheniramine*
— *Dexchlorpheniramine*
— *Brompheniramine*
— *Triprolidine*
Piperazines: Produce significant anticholinergic effects.
— *Cyclizine*
— *Chlorcyclizine*
— *Hydroxyzine*
— *Meclizine*
Tricyclics: Produce mild to moderate sedation.
— *Promethazine*
— *Trimeprazine*
— *Cyproheptadine*
— *Azatadine*
— *Ketotifen*

Tricyclic Antidepressants

Tricyclic antidepressants (TCAs) were first used in the 1950s. Their name is derived from their chemical structure, which contains 3 rings of atoms. Common TCAs include amitriptyline (Elavil), clomipramine (Anafranil), desipramine (Norpramin), doxepin (Adapin), imipramine (Tofranil), nortriptyline (Pamelor), protriptyline (Vivactil), and trimipramine (Surmontil).

In addition to treating depression, these drugs are used clinically to treat a number of other conditions, including pain, bedwetting, and attention-deficit hyperactivity disorder. TCAs enhance the effects of alcohol, barbiturates, and other CNS depressants.[70] As newer antidepressants have become available, the popularity of TCAs has declined.

The "Z" Drugs

The "Z" drugs–zolpidem, zolpiclone, and zaleplon–are sedative/hypnotics that have become popular prescription medications. While not of the benzodiazepine class, these drugs act on the same receptors as benzodiazepines and produce similar pharmacological effects.

Zolpidem (Ambien, Stilnox, Stilnoct, Hypnogen) is typically prescribed as a short-term treatment for insomnia.[71] At higher doses, it can also cause euphoria, muscle relaxation, hallucinations, and amnesia. This makes it popular as a recreational drug of abuse. As with other CNS depressants, zolpidem is also used to counter the unwanted effects experienced by abusers of stimulants such as cocaine or methamphetamine. The US Air Force uses zolpidem as "no-go" pills to help pilots fall asleep after a mission.

Like zolpidem, zopiclone (Imovane, Zimovane) is typically prescribed to treat insomnia. It is sold worldwide as a racemic mixture of 2 stereoisomers, with only one pharmacologically active. The active stereoisomer—eszopiclone—is marketed in the United States as Lunesta. Typical pharmacological effects include drowsiness, amnesia, dizziness, coordination difficulties, and hallucinations. Zopiclone has a bitter, metallic taste to it, increasing the challenge of surreptitious administration.

When ingested, zaleplon (Sonata, Starnoc) causes anterograde amnesia, hallucinations, severe confusion, unsteadiness, and strong sedation. It is extensively metabolized to 5-oxo-zaleplon and 5-oxo-desethylzaleplon so that less than 1% of the parent drug is excreted unchanged in urine.

Chloral Hydrate

Chloral hydrate (Aquachloral, Somnos, Noctec, Equithesin) was discovered in 1832 and was widely abused through the end of the 19th century. It is a strong sedative/hypnotic medication typically used to treat insomnia or as a sedative before minor surgeries. Since the development of the benzodiazepines, its use has largely declined. Higher doses can cause confusion, unconsciousness, and respiratory depression.

Chloral hydrate is rapidly metabolized in the liver into trichloroethanol. Neither the parent drug nor its metabolite is routinely tested for in most toxicology laboratories.

Chloral hydrate is historically important in the development of the slang phrase, "slipping a Mickey." Mickey Finn was the owner or a bartender of a Chicago establishment called the Lone Star Saloon and Palm Garden Restaurant in the late 19th century and early 20th century. Finn or one of his employees would slip chloral hydrate into the drink of unsuspecting patrons. Once the victim was incapacitated, he was escorted into a back room, robbed, and then dumped into a back alley. When he awoke, he had no recollection of the events that occurred. In December 1903, the bar was closed by Chicago authorities, yet the phrase "slipping a Mickey" lives on today.

Miscellaneous Drugs

Many other drugs are used to facilitate crimes. Included are muscle relaxants such as cyclobenzaprine (Flexaril), carisoprodol (Soma), and meprobamate (Equanil); barbiturates; and some antipsychotics (eg, clozapine [Clozaril], thioridazine, chlorpromazine [Thorazine]). Chemical solvents have been used to incapacitate a person to commit a crime against her. As new sedative medications (or prescription medications with sedative effects) continue to emerge, the list of drugs that have or can be used to facilitate sexual assaults will expand.

Conclusion

While DFSA cases have occurred for hundreds of years, recent times have seen a concerted effort by law enforcement, medical professionals, the media, and toxicologists to raise the public's awareness of these crimes. While the true prevalence of DFSAs will never be fully recognized, acknowledgement of the many challenges that come with these cases provides insight as to how to improve the chances of successfully investigating allegations of a DFSA.

References

1. LeBeau M, Andollo W, Hearn WL, Baselt R, Cone E, Finkle B, Fraser D, Jenkins A, Mayer J, Negrusz A, Poklis A, Walls HC, Raymon L, Robertson M, Saady J. Recommendations for toxicological investigations of drug-facilitated sexual assaults. *J Forensic Sci.* 1999;44:227-230.

2. Schwartz RH, Milteer R, LeBeau MA. Drug-facilitated sexual assault ('date rape'). *South Med J.* 2000;93:558-561.

3. Juhascik MP, Negrusz A, Faugno D, Ledray L, Greene P, Lindner A, Haner B, Gaensslen RE. An estimate of the proportion of drug-facilitation of sexual assault in four U.S. localities. *J Forensic Sci.* 2007;52:1396-1400.

4. ElSohly MA, Salamone SJ. Prevalence of drugs used in cases of alleged sexual assault. *J Anal Toxicol.* 1999;23:141-146

5. Ferrara SD, Frison G, Tedeschi L, et al. Gamma-hydroxybutyrate (GHB) and related products. In: LeBeau MA, Mozayani A, eds. *Drug-Facilitated Sexual Assault: A Forensic Handbook.* San Diego, CA: Academic Press; 2001:107-126.

6. LeBeau MA, Christenson RH, Levine B, Darwin WD, Huestis MA. Intra- and interindividual variations in urinary concentrations of endogenous gamma-hydroxybutyrate. *J Anal Toxicol.* 2002;26:340-346

7. Scott-Ham M, Burton FC. Toxicological findings in cases of alleged drug-facilitated sexual assault in the United Kingdom over a 3-year period. *J Clin Forensic Med.* 2005;12:175-186

8. Gee D, Owen P, McLean I, Brentnall K, Thundercloud C. Operation Matisse: Investigating Drug Facilitated Sexual Assault. London: Association of Chief Police Officers; 2006.

9. Hurley M, Parker H, Wells DL. The epidemiology of drug facilitated sexual assault. *J Clin Forensic Med.* 2006;13:181-185.

10. McGregor MJ, Lipowska M, Shah S, Du MJ, De Siato C. An exploratory analysis of suspected drug-facilitated sexual assault seen in a hospital emergency department. *Women Health.* 2003;37:71-80.

11. Questel F, Sec I, Sicot R, Pourriat JL. Drug-facilitated crimes: prospective data collection in a forensic unit in Paris [in French]. *Presse Med.* 2009;38(7-8):1049-1055.

12. Adamowicz P, Kala M. Date-rape drugs scene in Poland. *Przegl Lek.* 2005;62:572-575.

13. Society of Forensic Toxicologists. Recommended Maximum Detection Limits for Common DFSA Drugs and Metabolites in Urine Samples. http://www.soft-tox.org/docs/SOFT%20DFSA%20List.pdf. Updated October 2005. Accessed December 8, 2009.

14. Smith KM. Drugs used in acquaintance rape. *J Am Pharm Assoc (Wash).* 1999;39:519-525.

15. Haller C, Thai D, Jacob P, III, Dyer JE. GHB urine concentrations after single-dose administration in humans. *J Anal Toxicol.* 2006;30:360-364.

16. Negrusz A, Moore CM, Stockham TL, Poiser KR, Kern JL, Palaparthy R, Le NL, Janicak PG, Levy NA. Elimination of 7-aminoflunitrazepam and flunitrazepam in urine after a single dose of Rohypnol. *J Forensic Sci.* 2000;45:1031-1040.

17. Abarbanel G. The victim. In: LeBeau MA, Mozayani A, eds. *Drug-Facilitated Sexual Assault: A Forensic Handbook.* San Diego, CA: Academic Press; 2001:1-37.

18. LeBeau M, Mozayani A. Collection of evidence from DFSA. In: LeBeau MA, Mozayani A, eds. *Drug-Facilitated Sexual Assault: A Forensic Handbook.* San Diego, CA: Academic Press; 2001:197-209.

19. Society of Forensic Toxicologists. Fact Sheet: Drug-Facilitated Sexual Assault. http://www.soft-tox.org/docs/DFSA%20Fact%20Sheet.pdf. Published 2009. Accessed December 8, 2009.

20. Negrusz A, Moore CM, Hinkel KB, Stockham TL, Verma M, Strong MJ, Janicak PG. Deposition of 7-aminoflunitrazepam and flunitrazepam in hair after a single dose of Rohypnol. *J Forensic Sci.* 2001;46:1143-1151.

21. Negrusz A, Moore CM, Kern JL, Janicak PG, Strong MJ, Levy NA. Quantitation of clonazepam and its major metabolite 7-aminoclonazepam in hair, *J Anal Toxicol.* 2000;24:614-620.

22. Villain M, Cheze M, Dumestre V, Ludes B, Kintz P. Hair to document drug-facilitated crimes: four cases involving bromazepam. *J Anal Toxicol.* 2004;28:516-519.

23. Villain M, Cheze M, Tracqui A, Ludes B, Kintz P. Windows of detection of zolpidem in urine and hair: application to two drug facilitated sexual assaults. *Forensic Sci Int.* 2004;143:157-161.

24. Chaikomin R, Russo A, Rayner CK, Feinle-Bisset C, O'Donovan DG, Horowitz M, Jones KL. Effects of lipase inhibition on gastric emptying and alcohol absorption in healthy subjects. *Br J Nutr.* 2006;96:883-887.

25. Wu KL, Chaikomin R, Doran S, Jones KL, Horowitz M, Rayner CK. Artificially sweetened versus regular mixers increase gastric emptying and alcohol absorption. *Am J Med.* 2006;119:802-804.

26. Hahn RG, Norberg A, Jones AW. 'Overshoot' of ethanol in the blood after drinking on an empty stomach. *Alcohol Alcohol.* 1997;32:501-505.

27. Jones AW. Interindividual variations in the disposition and metabolism of ethanol in healthy men. *Alcohol.* 1984;1:385-391.

28. Jones AW, Jonsson KA, Kechagias S. Effect of high-fat, high-protein, and high-carbohydrate meals on the pharmacokinetics of a small dose of ethanol. *Br J Clin Pharmacol.* 1997;44:521-526.

29. Norberg A, Jones AW, Hahn RG, Gabrielsson JL. Role of variability in explaining ethanol pharmacokinetics: research and forensic applications. *Clin Pharmacokinet.* 2003;42:1-31.

30. Martin CS, Moss HB. Measurement of acute tolerance to alcohol in human subjects. *Alcohol Clin Exp Res.* 1993;17:211-216.

31. Kalant H. Current state of knowledge about the mechanisms of alcohol tolerance. *Addict Biol.* 1996;1:133-141.

32. Widmark EMP. *Principles and Applications of Medicolegal Alcohol Determination (Translation of Widmark's 1934 monograph).* Davis, CA: Biomedical Publications; 1981.

33. Snead OC, III, Liu CC, Bearden LJ. Studies on the relation of gamma-hydroxybutyric acid (GHB) to gamma-aminobutyric acid (GABA). Evidence that GABA is not the sole source for GHB in rat brain. *Biochem Pharmacol.* 1982;31: 3917-3923.

34. Couper FJ, Logan BK. Determination of gamma-hydroxybutyrate (GHB) in biological specimens by gas chromatography—mass spectrometry. *J Anal Toxicol.* 2000;24:1-7.

35. Laborit H, Jouany JM, Gerard J, Fabiani F. Generalities concerning the experimental study and clinical use of gamma hydroxybutyrate of Na [in French]. *Agressologie.* 1960;1:397-406.

36. Scharf MB, Fletcher KA, Jennings SW. Current pharmacologic management of narcolepsy. *Am Fam Physician.* 1988;38:143-148.

37. Scharf MB, Fletcher KA. GHB—new hope for narcoleptics? *Biol Psychiatry.* 1989;26:329-330.

38. Scharf MB, Lai AA, Branigan B, Stover R, Berkowitz DB. Pharmacokinetics of gammahydroxybutyrate (GHB) in narcoleptic patients. *Sleep.* 1998;21:507-514.

39. Scharf MB, Brown D, Woods M, Brown L, Hirschowitz J. The effects and effectiveness of gamma-hydroxybutyrate in patients with narcolepsy. *J Clin Psychiatry.* 1985;46:222-225.

40. US Xyrem Multicenter Study Group. Sodium oxybate demonstrates long-term efficacy for the treatment of cataplexy in patients with narcolepsy. *Sleep Med.* 2004;5:119-123.

41. Food and Drug Administration. Xyrem approved for muscle problems in narcolepsy. *FDA Consum.* 2002;36:7.

42. Abad VC, Guilleminault C. Emerging drugs for narcolepsy. *Expert Opin Emerg Drugs.* 2004;9:281-291.

43. Fuller DE, Hornfeldt CS. From club drug to orphan drug: sodium oxybate (Xyrem) for the treatment of cataplexy. *Pharmacotherapy.* 2003;23:1205-1209.

44. Kalra MA, Hart LL. Gammahydroxybutyrate in narcolepsy. *Ann Pharmacother.* 1992;26:647-648.

45. Price PA, Schachter M, Smith SJ, Baxter RC, Parkes JD. Gamma-hydroxybutyrate in narcolepsy. *Ann Neurol.* 1981;9:198.

46. Jazz Pharmaceuticals. Xyrem (sodium oxybate) [prescribing information]. Palo Alto, CA: Jazz Pharaceuticals; 2005.

47. Helrich M, Mcaslan TC, Skolnik S, Bessman SP. Correlation of blood levels of 4-hydroxybutyrate with state of consciousness. *Anesthesiology.* 1964;25:771-775.

48. Miotto K, Darakjian J, Basch J, Murray S, Zogg J, Rawson R. Gamma-hydroxybutyric acid: patterns of use, effects and withdrawal. *Am J Addict.* 2001;10: 232-241.

49. Palatini P, Tedeschi L, Frison G, Padrini R, Zordan R, Orlando R, Gallimberti L, Gessa GL, Ferrara SD. Dose-dependent absorption and elimination of gamma-hydroxybutyric acid in healthy volunteers. *Eur J Clin Pharmacol.* 1993;45:353-356.

50. Metcalf DR, Emde RN, Stripe JT. An EEG-behavioral study of sodium hydroxybutyrate in humans. *Electroencephalogr Clin Neurophysiol.* 1966;20:506-512.

51. Ferrara SD, Zotti S, Tedeschi L, Frison G, Castagna F, Gallimberti L, Gessa GL, Palatini P. Pharmacokinetics of gamma-hydroxybutyric acid in alcohol dependent patients after single and repeated oral doses. *Br J Clin Pharmacol.* 1992;34:231-235.

52. Arena C, Fung HL. Absorption of sodium gamma-hydroxybutyrate and its prodrug gamma-butyrolactone: relationship between in vitro transport and in vivo absorption. *J Pharm Sci.* 1980;69:356-358.

53. Lettieri J, Fung HL. Absorption and first-pass metabolism of 14C-gamma-hydroxybutyric acid. *Res Commun Chem Pathol Pharmacol.* 1976;13:425-437.

54. Jamieson MA, Weir E, Rickert VI, Coupey SM. Rave culture and drug rape. *J Pediatr Adolesc Gynecol.* 2002;15:251-257.

55. Galloway GP, Frederick-Osborne SL, Seymour R, Contini SE, Smith DE. Abuse and therapeutic potential of gamma-hydroxybutyric acid. *Alcohol.* 2000;20:263-269.

56. Galloway GP, Frederick SL, Staggers FE Jr, Gonzales M, Stalcup SA, Smith DE. Gamma-hydroxybutyrate: an emerging drug of abuse that causes physical dependence. *Addiction.* 1997;92:89-96.

57. Hindmarch I, Brinkmann R. Trends in the use of alcohol and other drugs in cases of sexual assault. *Hum Psychopharmacol Clin Exp.* 1999;14:225-231.

58. Calhoun SR, Wesson DR, Galloway GP, Smith DE. Abuse of flunitrazepam (Rohypnol) and other benzodiazepines in Austin and south Texas. *J Psychoactive Drugs.* 1996;28:183-189.

59. Lauven PM, Stoeckel H, Schwilden H, Schuttler J. Clinical pharmacokinetics of midazolam, flunitrazepam and diazepam [in German]. *Anasth Intensivther Notfallmed.* 1981;16:135-142.

60. Linnoila M, Stapleton JM, Lister R, Moss H, Lane E, Granger A, Eckardt MJ. Effects of single doses of alprazolam and diazepam, alone and in combination with ethanol, on psychomotor and cognitive performance and on autonomic nervous system reactivity in healthy volunteers. *Eur J Clin Pharmacol.* 1990;39:21-28.

61. Ciraulo DA, Barnhill JG, Boxenbaum HG, Greenblatt DJ, Smith RB. Pharmacokinetics and clinical effects of alprazolam following single and multiple oral doses in patients with panic disorder. *J Clin Pharmacol.* 1986;26:292-298.

62. Kroboth PD, Juhl RP. New drug evaluations. Triazolam. *Drug Intel Clin Pharm.* 1983;17:495-500.

63. Devane CL, Donovan JL, Liston HL, Markowitz JS, Cheng KT, Risch SC, Willard L. Comparative CYP3A4 inhibitory effects of venlafaxine, fluoxetine, sertraline, and nefazodone in healthy volunteers. *J Clin Psychopharmacol.* 2004;24:4-10.

64. Park JY, Kim KA, Park PW, Lee OJ, Kang DK, Shon JH, Liu KH, Shin JG. Effect of CYP3A5*3 genotype on the pharmacokinetics and pharmacodynamics of alprazolam in healthy subjects. *Clin Pharmacol Ther.* 2006;79:590-599.

65. von Moltke LL, Tran TH, Cotreau MM, Greenblatt DJ. Unusually low clearance of two CYP3A substrates, alprazolam and trazodone, in a volunteer subject with wild-type CYP3A4 promoter region. *J Clin Pharmacol.* 2000;40:200-204.

66. Bailey DG, Malcolm J, Arnold O, Spence JD. Grapefruit juice-drug interactions. *Br J Clin Pharmacol.* 1998;46:101-110.

67. Yasui N, Kondo T, Furukori H, Kaneko S, Ohkubo T, Uno T, Osanai T, Sugawara K, Otani K. Effects of repeated ingestion of grapefruit juice on the single and multiple oral-dose pharmacokinetics and pharmacodynamics of alprazolam. *Psychopharmacology (Berl).* 2000;150:185-190.

68. Smith KM, Larive LL, Romanelli F. Club drugs: methylenedioxy-methamphetamine, flunitrazepam, ketamine hydrochloride, and gamma-hydroxybutyrate. *Am J Health Syst Pharm.* 2002;59:1067-1076.

69. Adamowicz P, Kala M. Urinary excretion rates of ketamine and norketamine following therapeutic ketamine administration: method and detection window considerations. *J Anal Toxicol.* 2005;29:376-382.

70. Tanaka E, Misawa S. Pharmacokinetic interactions between acute alcohol ingestion and single doses of benzodiazepines, and tricyclic and tetracyclic antidepressants—an update. *J Clin Pharm Ther.* 1998;23:331-336.

71. Hoehns JD, Perry PJ. Zolpidem: a nonbenzodiazepine hypnotic for treatment of insomnia. *Clin Pharm.* 1993;12:814-828.

Chapter 16

Intimate Partner Violence: Assessment, Forensic Documentation, and Safety Planning

Daniel J. Sheridan, PhD, RN, FNE-A, SANE-A, FAAN
Katherine Nash Scafide, PhD(c), RN, FNE-A, FNE-P, SANE-A, SANE-P
Jill Kapur, MSN, RN
Angelo P. Giardino, MD, PhD, MPH, FAAP

Nearly 2 million injuries and 1300 deaths occur annually in the United States as a result of intimate partner violence (IPV).[1] A National Violence Against Women Survey indicated that 31% of women who sustained injuries from their most recent intimate partner rape and 28.1% with injuries from physical assault received some form of medical treatment.[2] Women affected by IPV are likelier to have unmet medical needs and overuse health care services because providers fail to properly assess the underlying cause.[3] Because IPV is a psychosocial health concern, it cannot easily be managed by a disease-based approach.[4] In this chapter, the authors will review issues related to the prevalence of intimate partner violence in health care settings and provide a practical review of assessment tools used surrounding IPV that may be of assistance to the health care provider. Useful tips on conducting accurate physical assessments are provided, and advice is given related to how to construct forensically sound written documentation of IPV evaluations. Among the issues to be addressed is the use of pictorial documentation of IPV injuries, the basic tenets of safety planning in health care settings, and community-wide IPV prevention strategies.

Background

Prevalence

Every year, an estimated 4.5 million women are physically abused by an intimate partner.[5] Approximately 1 in 4 women has experienced IPV in her lifetime.[6] Sheridan succinctly defines IPV as the physical, emotional, sexual, or financial abuse of a former or current intimate partner.[7,8] According to the Centers for Disease Control (CDC), IPV includes physical or sexual violence, threats of violence, psychological/emotional abuse, or coercive tactics between persons who are spouses or nonmarital partners or former spouses or nonmarital partners.[9]

Nearly 10% of women will experience IPV in the next 2 years.[10] These statistics are not just limited to the United States. Globally, the World Health Organization (WHO) found that in many countries, over half of the women experienced physical or sexual abuse by a current or former partner in their lifetime.[11] Women represent the majority of IPV victims.[12] Young adults, adolescents, and ethnic minorities, such as African Americans, Native Americans, and Hispanics, were found to be at greater risk of IPV victimization.[2]

Health Implications

When women attempt to leave abusive relationships, the level of violence and psychological abuse will often increase.[13,14] This risk also includes homicide. Nearly one-third of female homicide victims are killed by an intimate partner annually.[15,16] The risk of women being killed by an intimate partner is 9 times that of being killed by a stranger with the most common factor being prior IPV.[17]

In addition to acute physical injuries, IPV has been significantly linked to numerous physical, psychological, and obstetric health outcomes. Women who experience IPV report greater levels of gastrointestinal disorders, chronic pain, central nervous system symptoms, diabetes, hypertension, and immune system suppression.[18-21]

Psychological effects of exposure to IPV include posttraumatic stress disorder, anxiety, depression, suicide attempts, hostility, substance abuse, and sleep disturbance, and some have been linked through circulating proinflammatory cytokines to cardiovascular disease and metabolic syndrome.[19,20,22] Pregnancy health outcomes of IPV during the perinatal period include increased risk for neonatal demise, preterm labor, and low birth weight.[23] Poor sexual health indicators have been linked to IPV, such as sexual risk-taking behaviors, sexually transmitted infections including human immunodeficiency virus/acquired immunodeficiency syndrome (HIV/AIDS), unwanted pregnancy and elective abortion, and pain disorders associated with sexual dysfunction.[24]

Barriers to Care

Health care practitioners must recognize additional barriers that exist for IPV victims of different cultural, societal, and ethnic backgrounds. These include individual, institutional, and systemic barriers.[16] Such individual cultural barriers may include feelings of shame or secrecy and seeking help through local community members (eg, priests) instead of formal authorities. Women of different ethnic backgrounds may experience difficulties with stereotyping, language, and cultural competence on an institutional level that can prevent them from seeking help from health care providers. Finally, system-wide societal hurdles include poverty, illegal immigration status, and suspicion of the health care system.

Assessing for Intimate Partner Violence

In recent years, there has been controversy about using the term *screening* for IPV versus *assessing* for IPV. In 2004, the US Preventive Services Task Force (USPSTF) did not support universal screening for IPV since its review of the research did not uncover measurable health benefits at reasonable costs. Many have challenged the USPSTF findings.[25-29] Research on the cost-benefit analysis for elder abuse and child abuse screening has served as criticism of the USPSTF report.[26]

Traditional screening tools used to diagnose and treat medical diseases ideally minimize false-positive and false-negative results, and IPV does not fit nicely into a traditional medical disease model.[29] Chamberlain advocates that the USPSTF revisit its analysis and grade existing research on IPV within its guidelines for evaluating counseling services around lifestyle choices such as smoking.[26] She believes screening for IPV would then receive a score similar to the high marks tobacco screening receives from the USPSTF.[26]

Despite the controversy among medical researchers, IPV assessments continue to be made in everyday clinical settings. The Joint Commission (formerly the Joint Commission on Accreditation of Healthcare Organizations) has not changed its guidelines that all hospitals and regulated clinics have protocols and staff training to assist in the identification and documentation of IPV.[30]

There are at least 33 tools developed to assess for IPV.[31] There are at least 2 reliable and valid assessment tools that are clinically useful: (1) The Abuse Assessment Scale (AAS)[28,32-34] and (2)The Partner Violence Scale (PVS).[35]

There are at least 3 versions of the AAS in use: (a) 6-question version[36] (b) 3-question version[32] and (c) 2-question version[37] (see **Tables 16-1, 16-2,** and **16-3**). The 6-question AAS asks questions regarding fear, emotional abuse, control, physical abuse, and sexual abuse. The 3-question and 2-question AAS only ask about physical and sexual abuse. Women experiencing IPV state the pain from being emotionally abused hurts more and takes longer to heal than the physical abuse.[38] Therefore, whenever time permits, providers should use the 6-question AAS to gain a better understanding of emotional abuse and control.

Shorter assessment tools were developed because busy practitioners said they did not have time to ask a lot of questions.[37] Some standardized IPV assessments in health care settings include only one question, "Do you feel safe in your home?" This question has been shown to be ineffective in identifying IPV.[29] It can also lead to false IPV positives since someone living in a high-crime area may be in a healthy and loving relationship but is afraid of being victimized by street crime.

Table 16-1. Abuse Assessment Scale: 6-Question Version[36]

VIOLENCE AFFECTS MANY PEOPLE; THEREFORE PATIENTS SHOULD BE ROUTINELY ASKED THE FOLLOWING QUESTIONS ABOUT VIOLENCE IN THEIR LIVES.

— These questions should be introduced by saying something like, "All couples argue now and again, even the best of couples…"

1. When you and your partner argue, are you ever afraid of him or her?
2. When you and your partner verbally argue, do you think he or she tries to emotionally hurt/abuse you?
3. Does your partner try to control you? Where you go? Who you see? How much money you can have?
4. Has your partner (or anyone) ever hit, slapped, kicked, choked, pushed, shoved, or otherwise physically hurt you?
5. Since you have been pregnant (or when you were pregnant), has your partner ever hit, slapped, kicked, choked, pushed, shoved, or otherwise physically hurt you?
6. Has your partner ever forced you into sex when you did not want to participate?

— Whenever a patient answers yes, the doctor should thank him or her for sharing and ask, "Can you give me an example? Can you tell me about the last time it happened?"

Adapted from the Nursing Research Consortium on Violence and Abuse. *The* Nursing Research Consortium on Violence and Abuse *(1988) encourages the reproduction, modification, and/or use of the Abuse Assessment Screen in routine domestic violence assessments.*

Table 16-2. Abuse Assessment Scale: 3-Question Version[32]

Questions to Ask
1. Within the last year, have you been hit, slapped, kicked, choked, pushed, shoved, or otherwise physically hurt by someone? If yes, by whom? Total number of times?
2. Since you've been pregnant, have you been hit, slapped, kicked, choked, pushed, shoved, or otherwise physically hurt by someone? If yes, by whom? Total number of times?
3. Within the last year, has anyone forced you to have sexual activities? If yes, by whom? Total number of times?

Table 16-3. Abuse Assessment Scale: 2-Question Version[37]

Questions to Ask
1. Within the last year, have you been hit, slapped, kicked, choked, pushed, shoved, or otherwise physically hurt by someone?
2. Have you ever been forced to have sexual activities?

The PVS is a 3-question assessment tool that asks about physical abuse, if persons feel safe in their current relationship, and if someone from a previous relationship is making a person still feel unsafe (see **Table 16-4**). The last question is very important, especially for women who are being stalked, or are divorced, estranged, or separated but still have to interact with a former abusive partner because of their children.

Women in ongoing abusive relationships present to health providers for a plethora of reasons that are not directly related to injuries from physical abuse. A woman may not volunteer that she is in an abusive relationship unless directly asked by her provider.[3] Various studies have demonstrated women overwhelmingly (76% to 96%) support being asked about abuse in medical, obstetrics, and gynecologic settings.[39,40]

Table 16-4. Partner Violence Screen[35]

Questions to Ask
1. Have you been hit, kicked, punched, or otherwise hurt by someone within the past year? If so, by whom?
2. Do you feel safe in your current relationship?
3. Is there a partner from a previous relationship who is making you feel unsafe now?

When women present with physical injuries, especially injuries that do not match the given history, health providers should ask directly if the injuries were from being physically assaulted. It is critical that providers perform a complete physical exam, not only on the presenting injury, but to assess for other current injuries and injuries in various stages of healing. The following section reviews the physical assessment of IPV with a focus on the types and locations of most IPV injuries.

Physical Assessment

Mechanism of Injury

Mechanism of injury is defined as "the exchange of physical forces that result in injury, whether from the force of a fist, a bottle, or a bullet."[41] Knowing the mechanism of injury can help identify the type and location of injury that may be expected. Often, victims of IPV suffer multiple mechanisms of injury resulting in multiple locations and types of injury.[42,43] Among victims of IPV, the most common mechanism of injury is being struck by a hand; however, a punch with a fist can result in substantially different and more severe injuries than being slapped with an open hand.[41] Often a slap will leave little more than a patterned, painful contusion that will likely not result in medical treatment. A close-handed punch, on the other hand, is the most common cause of maxillofacial or ocular injuries.[44] Traumatic brain injury, no matter how mild, is frequently underdiagnosed among victims of IPV.[45]

Weapons (eg, gun, knife) are an infrequent mechanism of injury in nonfatal IPV, occurring between 0.5% and 2.5%.[46,47] More often than a weapon, a household object is used to inflict the injury, perhaps due to its accessibility.[41] Being hit with an object is found to result in 30% of IPV injuries.[48] Strangulation is frequently underrecognized due to lack of screening or presence of symptoms. Over half of IPV victims report suffering strangulation, and, overwhelmingly, hands are used to compress the neck versus a ligature.[49-51]

Reported sexual assault among IPV victims ranges from 40% to 50%.[52,53] Injuries are dependent on the object(s) used and orifice(s) penetrated. The posterior fourchette remains the most frequently injured site of the female genitalia resulting from sexual assault, but injuries to other areas of the body, especially the lower extremities, are common.[54,55] Depending on examination technique (eg, colposcopy, dye application), the frequency of genital injuries following sexual assault varies greatly from 33% to 90%.[54,56] Genital injuries may be associated with an increased homicide risk.[57] Injuries, in general, are less frequent when the assailant is known to the victim.[55]

Other, less frequent, mechanisms of injury include kicking, biting, burns, and hair pulling. Kicking can result in substantial injury to the victim, whereas biting can cause anything from transient, patterned bite impressions to a complete amputation or avulsion of a body part.[41] Among IPV survivors, burns are relatively rare.[6] Often the pattern of the heat implement (eg, cigarette, electric stove) can be observed on the skin. Hair pulling is frequently reported clinically and can result in traumatic alopecia and, in severe cases, cervical spine injury.[41]

Location of Injury

Areas of the head, neck, and face (HNF) are not only the most frequently reported sites of injury resulting from IPV, but have been found to be predictive of IPV (**Figures 16-1** and **16-2**).[41,58,59] Women with HNF injuries are 11.8 times likelier to have been injured as a result of IPV then other injuries to the body.[60] The importance of assessing for IPV is imperative with women seeking health care for HNF injuries. The next most common injury location is to the upper extremities, frequently associated with defensive wounds (**Figures 16-3** and **16-4**).[41] The least common location of injuries to IPV patients is to the stomach and back.[61]

However, during pregnancy, the location of injury may change based on the intent of the batterer. The most common location of injury continues to be the HNF during the prenatal and postnatal periods.[62] Because of frequent visits to the health care provider during pregnancy, it is not surprising that more hidden areas, such as extremities, are the second most common location. However, if the pregnancy is unexpected or the abuser holds rage against its existence, he may target the patient's abdomen. Nannini et al found that the number of IPV-related physical injuries to the torso dropped from 21.5% to 8.7% after the victim gave birth.[62]

The visibility of the injuries is often a motive for their location on the part of the assailants. To keep victims isolated, assailants may choose to injure a visible area, since victims will self-isolate until the injuries heal or victims develop fictitious explanations, but the reverse can also be true. Injuries to the chest, breast, abdomen, pelvic, buttocks, genitals, and thighs that are IPV-related can be the result of assailants attempting to hide the injuries from view.

Types of Injury and Injury Patterns

Patterned injuries have characteristics whereby providers have a reasonable idea a specific object was used to create the injury or the injury was caused by a particular mechanism of injury (**Figures 16-5** through **16-6**).[36,41]

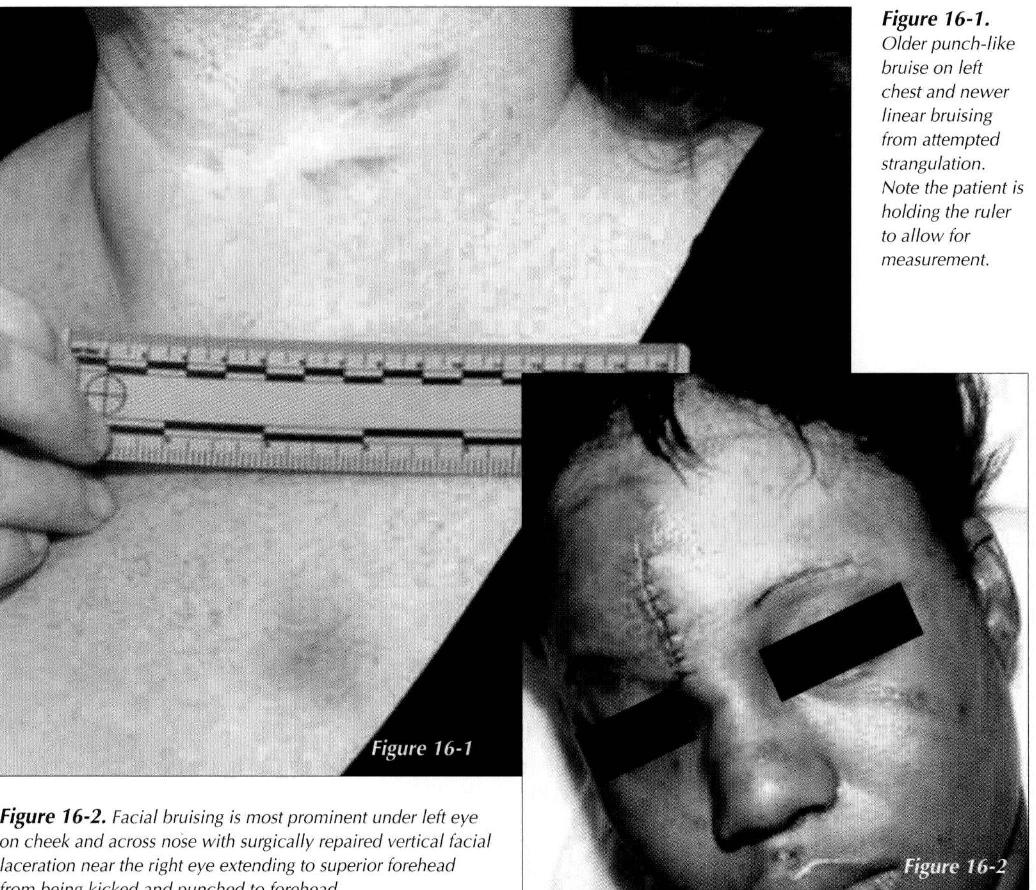

Figure 16-1. *Older punch-like bruise on left chest and newer linear bruising from attempted strangulation. Note the patient is holding the ruler to allow for measurement.*

Figure 16-2. *Facial bruising is most prominent under left eye on cheek and across nose with surgically repaired vertical facial laceration near the right eye extending to superior forehead from being kicked and punched to forehead.*

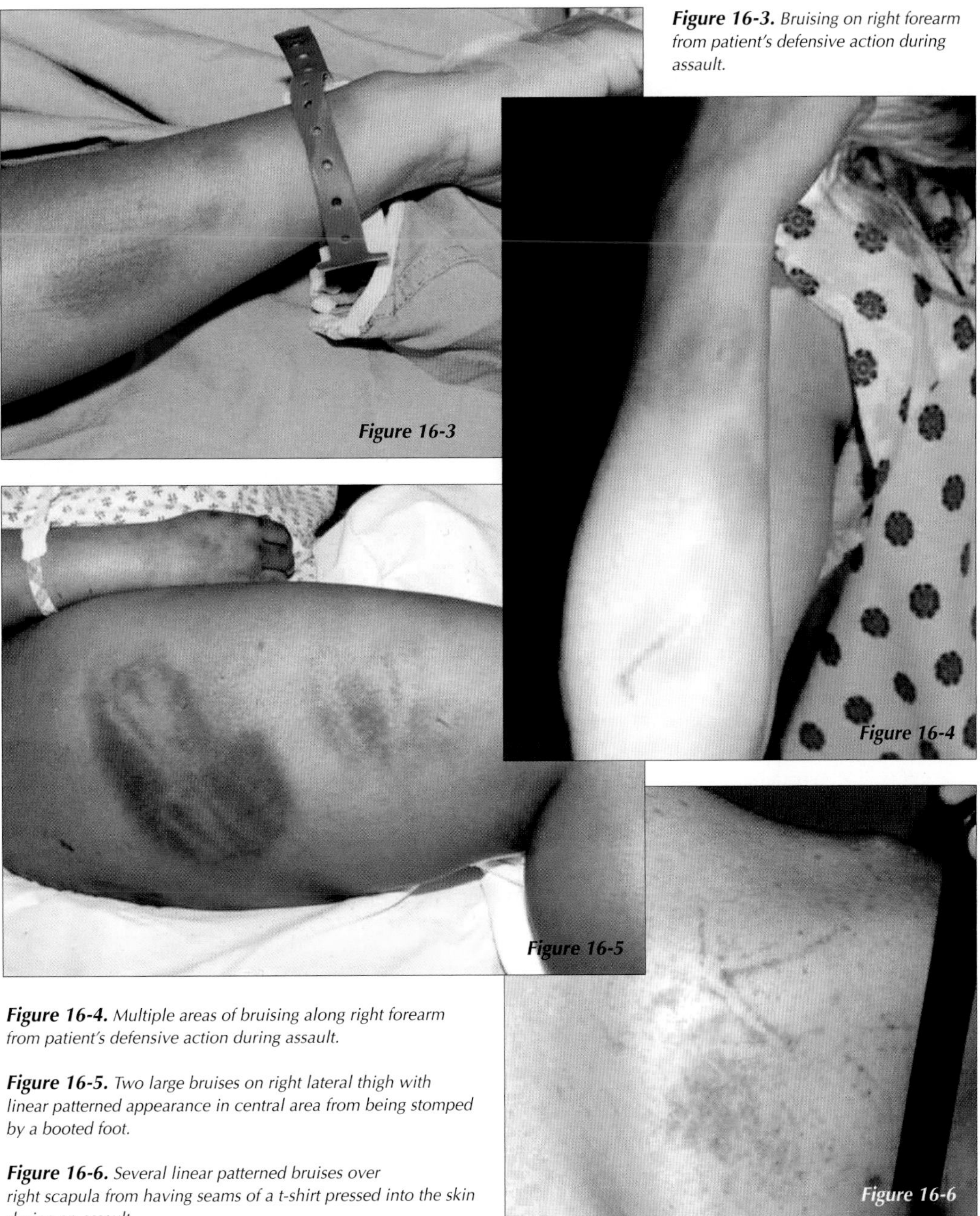

Figure 16-3. *Bruising on right forearm from patient's defensive action during assault.*

Figure 16-4. *Multiple areas of bruising along right forearm from patient's defensive action during assault.*

Figure 16-5. *Two large bruises on right lateral thigh with linear patterned appearance in central area from being stomped by a booted foot.*

Figure 16-6. *Several linear patterned bruises over right scapula from having seams of a t-shirt pressed into the skin during an assault.*

A pattern of injury is a collection of internal or external injuries in various stages of healing demonstrating injuries of a period of time (**Figures 16-7** and **16-8**).[7,63] The following injuries may be a sign of ongoing abuse.

Abrasions

Abrasions are caused by rubbing, grinding, wearing, and/or scraping.[64] In IPV, abrasions usually involve the skin from being dragged over a rough surface or the vaginal mucous membranes from forced sexual assault.[36,41] When one is dragged along a carpeted surface, providers may mistakenly document this as a "rug burn" when it would be more correct to call it an abrasion.

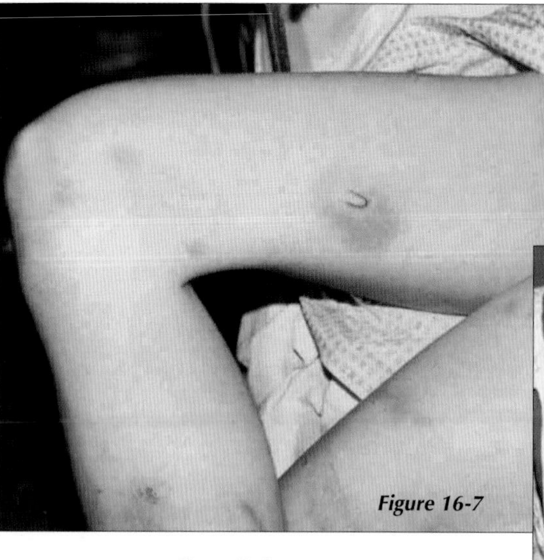

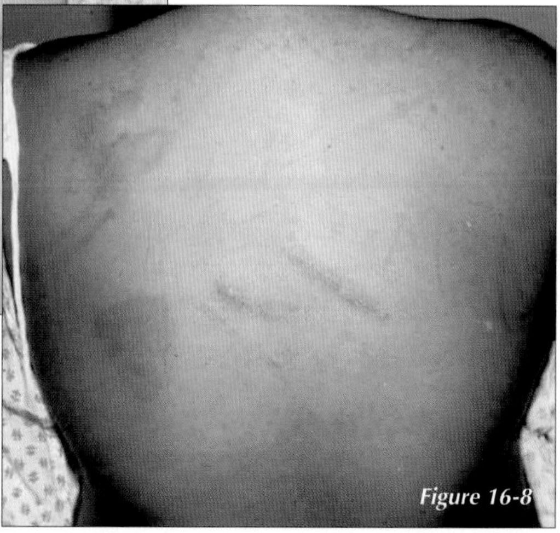

Figure 16-7. *Bruising at different stages of healing on thighs and right shin with ring-like abrasion to circular punch-related bruise to medial right thigh.*

Figure 16-8. *Several patterned bruises at different stages of healing, supporting a history of being kicked by a healed boot and whipped with a looped cord.*

Burn Injury

Though burns are relatively uncommon among IPV victims, the injuries can be painful and disfiguring.[6] Intentional burns often show a clear demarcation or pattern, such as an iron or cigarette/cigar burns. The terms *sock burn* or *glove burn* are used to describe patterned, forced, immersion burns more often seen in pediatric patients.[65] Glove burns can occur in the kitchen when a hand is forced into a pan of hot fluid on the stovetop. If the hand touches the bottom of the pan, there may be a more severe area of contact burn. Skin may adhere to the bottom of the pan leaving trace evidence. Sock (stocking) burns can occur in bathtubs when feet are forced into hot tap water. If the skin sloughs off, skin may remain in the tub or the drain and possibly be retrieved as evidence.

Splash burns can be accidental or intentional in nature. Splash burns do not have well-defined margins. Rather, the burn follows the flow of the hot fluid. When trying to determine if a splash-burn was caused accidentally or intentionally, a thorough history is essential, regardless if the injury is consistent or not.

Bite Injury

Being bitten by a human being can result in a distinct patterned injury.[36,41] In sexual assault and IPV, the location of the bite wound is often to the breasts; however, Le et al found only 3 of 236 domestic violence patients presenting to a Level I trauma center had bite injuries.[44] Bite injuries can result in punctuate wounds, skin abrasions, and patterned bruises in the shape of the assailant's teeth. While not among the more common IPV injuries, when present, bite injuries should be swabbed with sterile cotton-tipped applicators moistened with sterile water. Once dried, the swabs should be placed in either a paper envelope or cardboard tube, sealed, labeled with patient identifiers, and preserved as evidence for DNA sampling.[7,36] Bite wounds should be photographed with a right-angle ruler, which may aid forensic odentologists to identify the assailant.

Bruise/Contusion

A bruise is synonymous with a contusion. When a person is bruised, she has experienced blunt or squeezed force trauma that has injured tissues under the skin resulting in bleeding.[7,36,41,64] Being punched (**Figure 16-9**), kicked, forcefully grabbed, and struck with an object are among the most commonly reported mechanisms of injury to IPV patients (**Figures 16-10, 16-11,** and **16-12**).[44,66] These mechanisms often result in bruising to the skin and, if enough force is used, lacerations to the skin and fractures of the underlying bones (**Figure 16-13**). Fresh bruises are painful and indurated (ie, slightly firm) to touch and have fairly distinct outer margins.

If one is struck with a solid object, especially a solid cylindrical object, the bruise may have evidence of central clearing, whereby the extravasated blood is forced to the outer edges of the impact area, leaving the center of the bruise less discolored than the edges. Examples of objects that can leave centrally cleared bruises include canes, broom and mop handles, rods, baseball bats, and pipes. If one is slapped forcefully with a hand, the initial injury will appear as reddened raised welts. As the welts resolve, there may be a series of patterned parallel bruises with central clearing distinguishing the fingers.

While it is tempting for trained health professionals to evaluate a bruise's age based on its discoloration, the existing research on the subject is inconsistent and limited.[67-70] The accuracy of determining the age of a bruise within 24 hours in vivo is only 40%, which is no better than chance.[68] Recent research has shown that describing the subtle color changes of bruises via the naked eye is a subjective and unreliable practice.[71,72] This practice has also led to disparity in the recognition of the seriousness of injuries in dark-skinned individuals.[54]

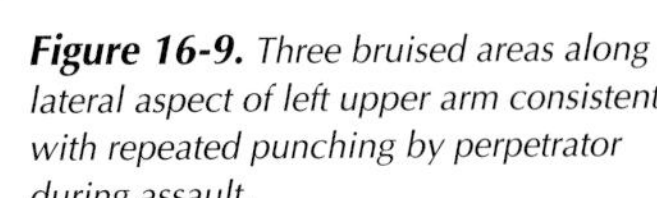

Figure 16-9. *Three bruised areas along lateral aspect of left upper arm consistent with repeated punching by perpetrator during assault.*

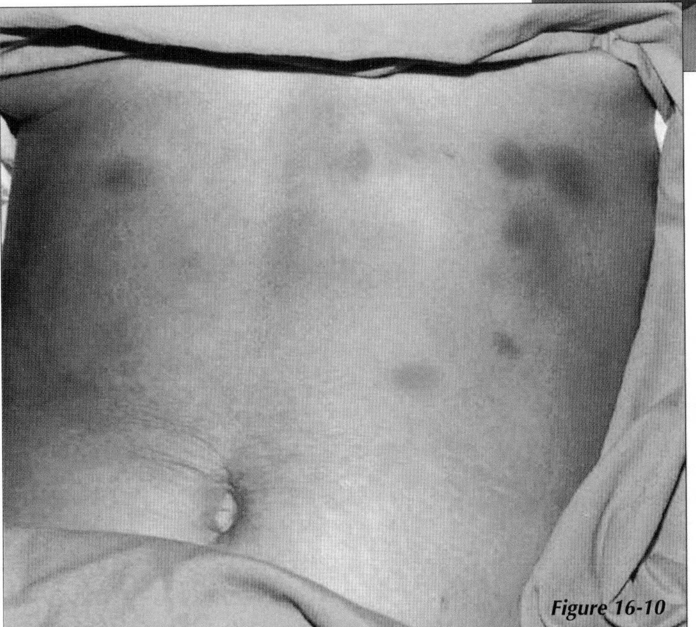

Figure 16-10. *Multiple rounded bruises on chest and abdomen consistent with history of perpetrator inflicting injuries via jab-like punches during attack in area of the victim's body that would be covered by clothing.*

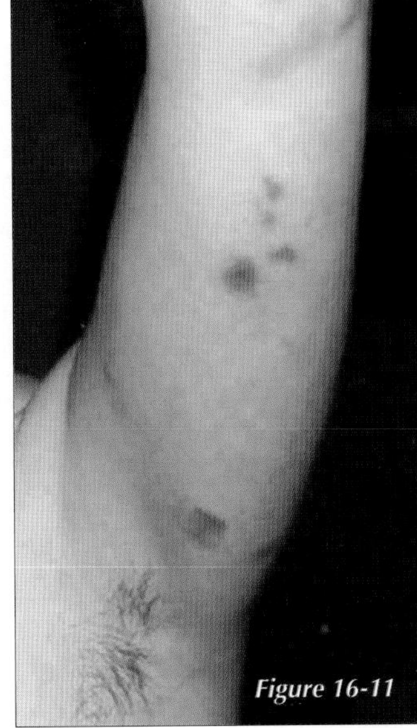

Figure 16-11. *Multiple rounded fingertip-like bruises on relatively protected area of left arm consistent with history of victim being grabbed by perpetrator during assault.*

Figure 16-12. *Linear array of finger-tip bruises on underside of right arm consistent with victim being forcefully grabbed by perpetrator.*

Figure 16-13. *Left temple bruise with overlapping abrasion with spread of blood under the skin resulting in bilateral periorbital ecchymoses secondary to an accidental fall from a bed onto a carpeted floor in a nursing home.*

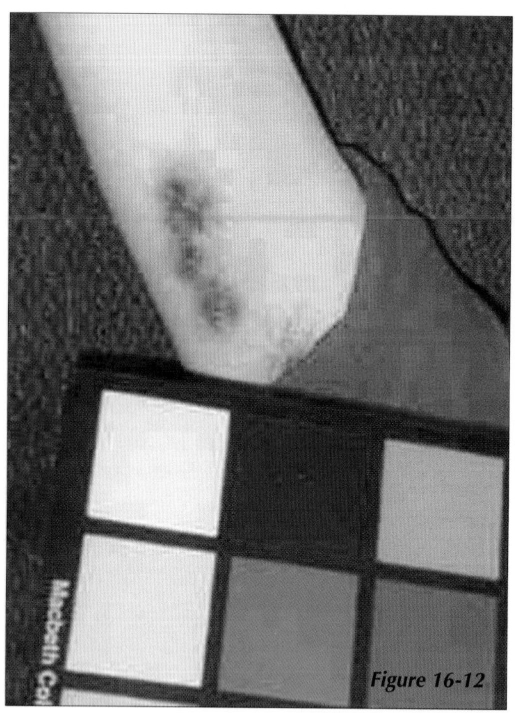

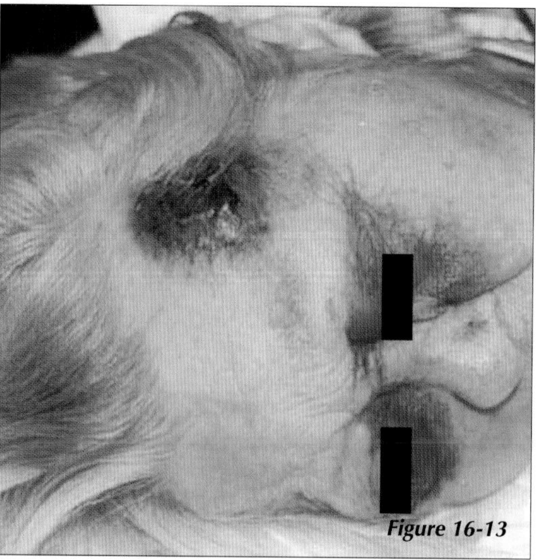

Ecchymosis

Ecchymotic lesions are not synonymous with bruising. Ecchymosis is the escape of blood, usually very slowly, under the skin into subcutaneous tissues.[36,64] Ecchymotic lesions are generally not painful to touch, are just as soft on palpation as the adjacent nondiscolored skin, and do not have well-defined margins. The elderly are prone to developing ecchymotic lesions to arms and hands. Blood under the skin from a bruise will often spread downward (gravity-dependent) producing an ecchymotic lesion. For example, being punched to the mid-face will result in bilateral periorbital ecchymoses (**Figure 16-14**). Being punched to one eye will result in a bruise at the point of impact; however, blood from that bruise may leak down the side of the face into the neck. The discoloration down the side of the face and neck is best described as ecchymotic spread (**Figures 16-15** and **16-16**).[36]

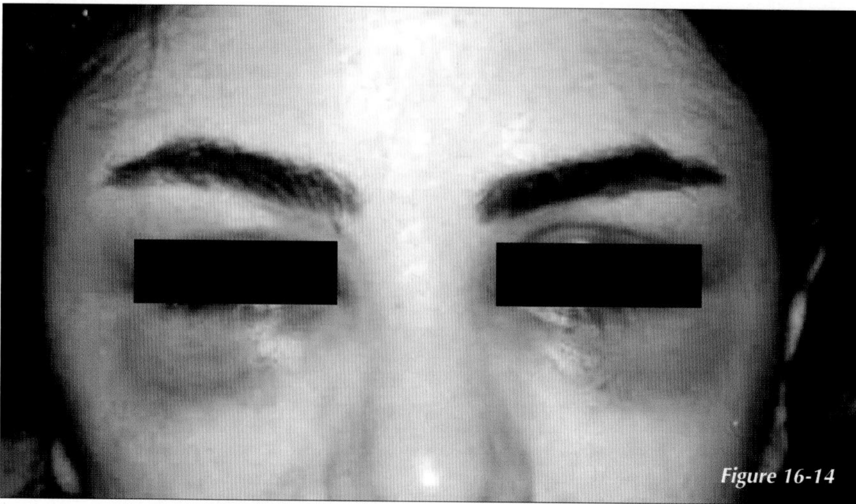

Figure 16-14. *Bilateral periorbital ecchymoses from direct blow to the mid-forehead.*

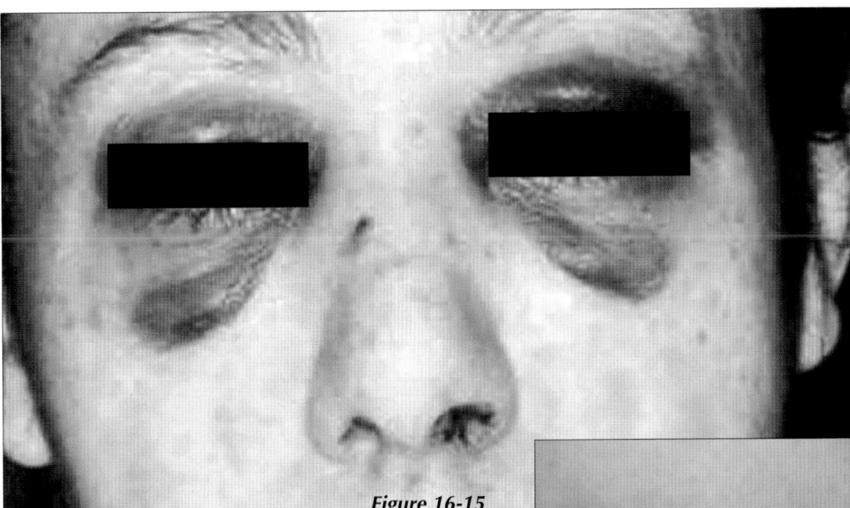

Figure 16-15

Figure 16-15. *Bilateral periorbital ecchymoses from a direct blow to the mid-forehead. Please note the small bruise to the right nose suggesting the patient was wearing glasses when struck. Also note the dried blood in the nares suggesting recent facial trauma.*

Figure 16-16-a

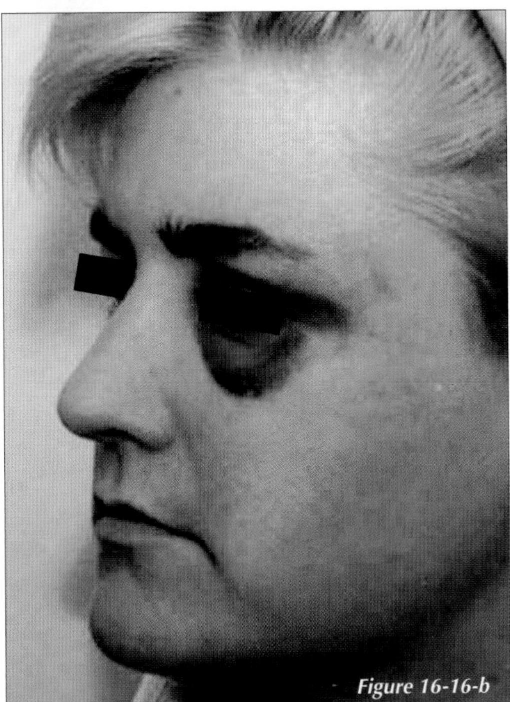

Figure 16-16-b

Figure 16-16-a. *Direct blow to left eye causing bruise and collection of draining blood to dependent area below eye above cheek.*

Figure 16-16-b. *A different view of the injuries in the same patient.*

Figure 16-16-c. *In the same patient, a ruler is held to allow for measurement.*

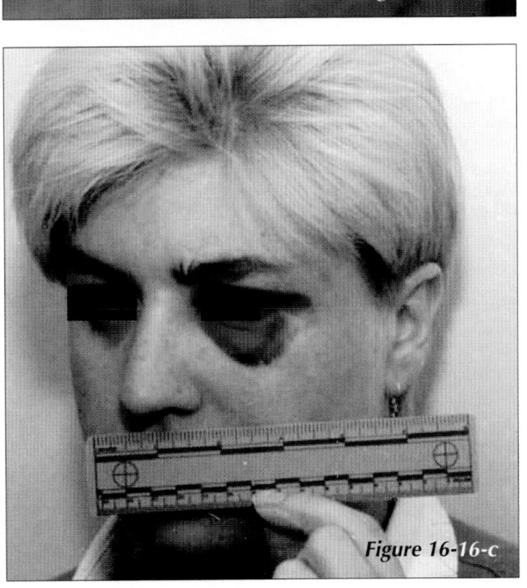

Figure 16-16-c

Incision/Cut

An incision is synonymous with a cut. Both mean an opening made by a sharp instrument.[64,73,74] When an incision is examined, the internal edges are generally very smooth and equidistant in depth. Incisions are often described as being clean since there is seldom any gross foreign matter in the wound. A cut that is deeper than it is wide is called a stab wound. See **Figures 16-17** through **16-19** for examples of incisions and cuts.

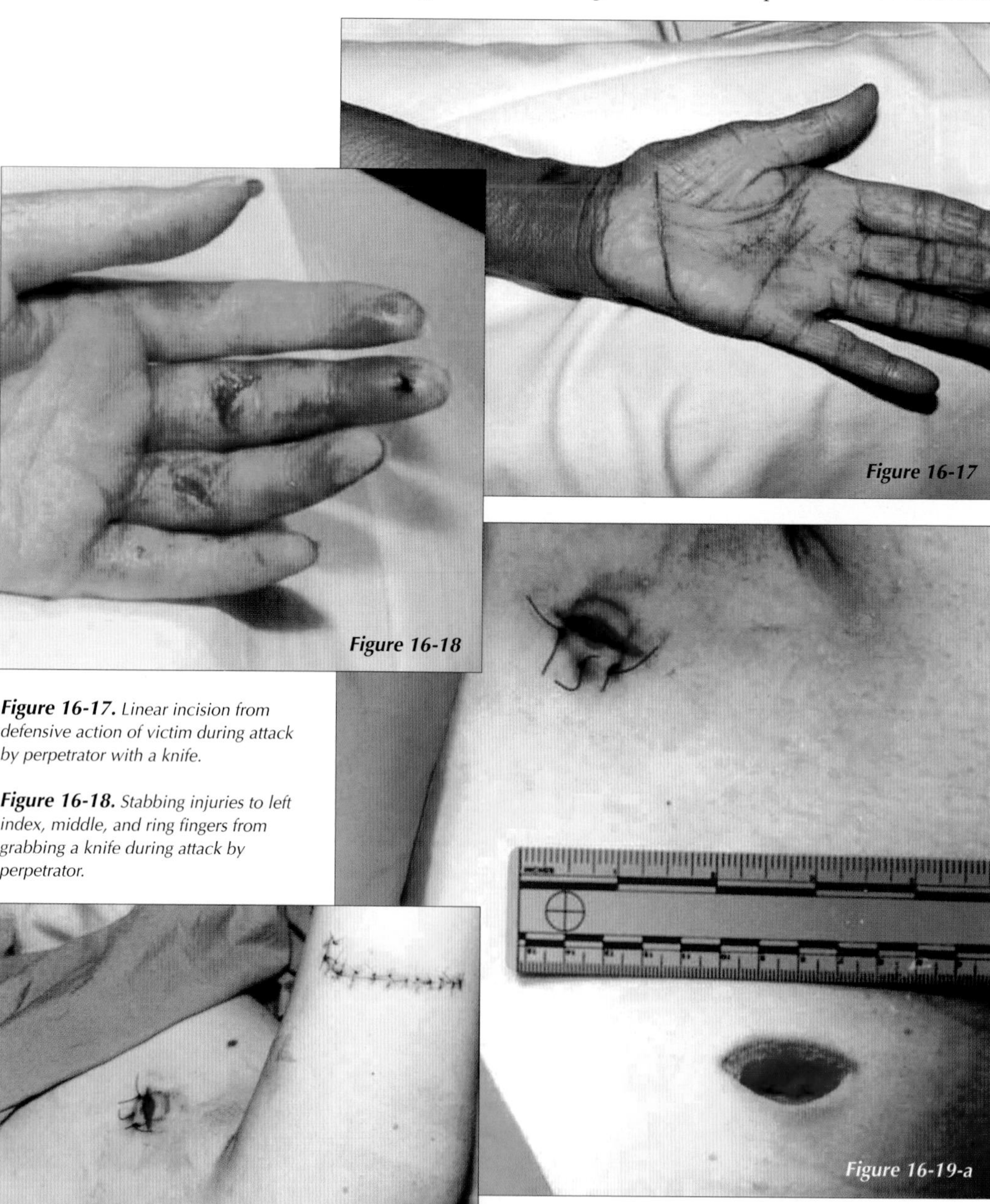

Figure 16-17. *Linear incision from defensive action of victim during attack by perpetrator with a knife.*

Figure 16-18. *Stabbing injuries to left index, middle, and ring fingers from grabbing a knife during attack by perpetrator.*

Figure 16-19-a. *Chest and axilla stab wounds, one has been surgically repaired, the other healing by primary intention secondary to being contaminated when knife entered lung.*

Figure 16-19-b. *In the same patient, there is a linear incision from being assaulted with a knife to left upper arm that is sutured.*

Laceration

Many health providers have developed a bad habit of calling all wounds that are open and bleeding a laceration, including wounds made by sharp, cutting implements.[7,36,75] To lacerate means to tear jaggedly.[64] Blunt or shearing forces applied to the skin, especially over boney surfaces will result in jagged tearing of the skin (**Figure 16-2**).[7,36,41,75] When a laceration is examined, the skin is opened in a jagged fashion and inside edges are not smooth. The wound has multiple depths, can show tissue bridging, and can tunnel under the skin from stretching the skin from the mechanism of blunt impact. Lacerations can often contain trace evidence from the scene of the trauma. While the medical treatment of lacerations and cuts is very similar, lacerations from blunt trauma may traumatize underlying structures and organs as compared to cuts, which usually only involve the area contacted by the sharp object.[63]

Petechiae

Petechiae are small, usually circular, reddish or purplish discolorations under the skin caused by ruptured capillaries. Strangulation can cause petechiae formation in and around the eyes and face. Other causes of facial petechiae include severe vomiting and severe coughing. Severe sneezing and childbirth have also been reported to cause facial petechiae.[36]

Traumatic Alopecia

Traumatic alopecia is hair loss from a traumatic event. During assaults, IPV patients may have been pulled or dragged by their hair. Unless a section of the scalp is completely pulled away from the head, visualizing and documenting traumatic alopecia can be clinically challenging. On exam, patients who experienced hair pulling will have pain on palpation to areas of the scalp corresponding to the areas of hair that were pulled. These areas can be documented on an injury map. If reported hair-pulling events were very recent, examiners can run combs through patients' hair.[36] The comb may contain a large number of hairs that can be photographed and sent to a crime lab to support a history of traumatic hair-pulling since most of the hairs will contain roots.

Firearm Injury

One of the most common causes of IPV homicide is being shot, usually with a handgun.[16] Patients with fatal gunshot injuries are often rushed to the emergency/trauma department by emergency medical personnel only to be pronounced dead on arrival. Sometimes the IPV patient with a gunshot injury presents with vital signs but dies within a few minutes. Other IPV patients are shot but recover. Besant-Matthews cautions providers to avoid efforts to determine entrance and exit wounds solely based on the size of the wounds.[63]

The presence of powder and soot in and around the wound and clothing may suggest an entrance wound as well as stippling or tattooing of the skin from gunpowder residue imbedded in the skin.[63]

Fractures

Being struck by a fist, kicked with a foot, struck with an object, or thrown to the ground can result in fractures and joint dislocations, especially to the face.[43,44,59,65,76,77] Rib fractures and fractures to arms and hands to IPV patients are relatively common.[44] Two studies found 11% of female IPV victims had fractures.[6,49]

Strangulation

There are 3 types of strangulation: (a) manual, (b) ligature, and (c) mechanical.[36] Manual strangulation is the most common and includes using any part of a person's body to compress the neck of another person. When persons place their hands around the neck (especially if there is shaking) it is commonly called throttling. Headlocks are also very common as well as using a person's legs to place another person's neck in a scissor hold. Stepping on the neck or leaning a person's arm into a neck are also forms of manual strangulation. Compressing the neck, especially the sides of the neck can compress the venous and arterial flow of blood out of and into the brain. When venous return from the head (and brain) is impeded or stopped by constricting the neck and its vessels, blood will back up and increase pressure in the capillary beds above the constriction, which may lead these small fragile vessels to rupture and create petechial bleeding that may be seen on visual examination. Continued pressure with prolonged compression of the major veins and arteries in the neck can result in rapid death.

Manual strangulation can be potentially deadly but leave little to no external evidence.[50,51] When there are physical findings, they include patterned fingertip-like contusions, minor bruising, and scratch abrasions from fingernails, clothing, or jewelry (**Figure 16-1**).

Thumb imprint bruises from being grasped and squeezed tend to be square-like in appearance, while the imprints from the index, middle, and ring fingers tend to be more circular in shape.[7] When a hand is used to grasp a neck or other body part, the little finger does not generate much force and seldom leaves a compression bruise. Care should be taken in determining the handedness of an assailant solely by looking at the location of the circular fingertip bruises and the opposing thumb bruises.

Ligature strangulation occurs when any object is wrapped around the neck and compressed. This could include everyday household items such as electrical and telephone cords, ropes, and clothing.[78] Ligature strangulation will often leave ligature marks to the neck.

Mechanical strangulation occurs when the neck is compressed between objects or machinery. It is generally more accidental or neglect-related in nature and involves getting the neck caught in equipment or a device not designed for necks such as hospital bedrails, machinery, step rails, and everyday furniture. In addition to compressing the structures of the neck, mechanical strangulation can result in neck fractures.

All forms of strangulation can result in symptoms not usually identified as injuries such as headaches, shortness of breath, sore throats, difficulty swallowing, headaches, loss of consciousness, memory loss, voice changes, loss of consciousness, and the involuntary loss of control of bladder and bowels.[41]

Accidental versus Intentional Injuries

In general, accidental injuries are more likely to occur to distal parts of the body (fingers/toes and hands/feet) and to boney prominences such as knees, hips, chins, and elbows.[36,74] Abuse-related injuries tend to be more proximal than distal in location as well as on more central areas of the body (trunk, abdomen, back, chest, breasts, and genitalia).[41] Injuries in various stages of healing, especially in the absence of a credible history, should always be suspicious of intentional injury.[36,74]

Documentation

Thorough documentation of histories of intimate partner abuse in the medical record is a critical part of holistic care. Documentation needs to be in written and photographic formats.

Written Documentation

Abused patients' history should be documented as verbatim as possible using quotation marks, or the history of abuse should be thoroughly paraphrased in the medical record.[41] The written note needs to include specific actions that resulted in physical and/or emotional injury. It is best to start with a basic description of the events of the reported assault.[74] Patients need to be asked specific questions about the assault, which will then guide the physical exam. Answers to these questions need to be documented. For example, it is crucial to know the following:

— Time of the assault

— Place of the assault

— Names, if known, of those involved in the assault

— Witnesses of the assault

— Manner in which the patient was assaulted

— If punched, whether it was open-handed or close-fisted

— If kicked, whether it was barefoot, with gym shoes, or with work boots

— If bitten, where, number of times, whether the area has been washed (swab for DNA)

— If spat upon, where (swab for DNA)

— If strangled, whether it was manual, ligature, or both

  — If there was loss of consciousness

  — If there were voice changes

  — If there was difficulty swallowing

  — If there was loss of bowel/bladder control

  — If there was difficulty breathing

  — If there was presence or absence of petechial hemorrhages to eyes/face

— If they were struck with an object, where were they struck

— If they were struck with an object, how many times were they struck

— With which specific weapon were they injured

  — For example, knife, firearm, taser

— Where on the body the injuries were inflicted

— If there were verbal threats of harm

— If there were verbal threats of death

Written documentation needs to be accurate, objective, and free of bias. For example, when battered persons seek medical care, the charting needs to describe them as "patients" rather than "victims." It is preferable to document "patient states" or "patient reports" versus charting "patient claims" or "patient alleges." The latter is biased and suggests the health provider did not believe the patient was providing a truthful history. The health provider needs to avoid charting-biased and potentially patient-blaming statements such as "patient refuses" or "patient noncompliant" or "patient uncooperative."

Documentation of the patient's statements related to the assault should not be "sanitized" even if the reported assault occurred days or weeks prior to seeking health care.[41] It is forensically useless to document, "Patient hit, kicked, and threatened by known assailant five hours PTA [prior to admission]." It would be more accurate to write:

> Patient states she was punched five times to the face and head with a closed fist and kicked twice to the mid back by her husband, George Miller, who was wearing steel-toed shoes. Patient states her husband also said he would "blow her fucking head off if she fought him for custody of the kids." Patient was tearful throughout history. Negative loss of consciousness...

Every injury needs to be measured and described accurately in the medical record. In the United States, the measurements should be in inches and ounces versus millimeters and milliliters to facilitate easier understanding by the police, prosecutors, and juries. Every injury needs to be measured, not just approximated. Documentation of an injury needs to include a description of its color and if it is painful. As previously discussed, providers need to be careful to not date bruises purely by their color. There is no science to guide providers to accurately date bruises.[79] On the contrary, several studies demonstrate efforts to date bruises by their color are no more accurate than chance throughout the life-cycle.[67,68,70]

Photographic Documentation

In addition to detailed written notes, the health provider needs to document injuries from intimate partner violence pictorially using body maps and photographs.[36,41,74] Body maps need full anterior, posterior, and lateral views. If patients have facial injuries and/or report strangulation, full-size head and neck body maps are helpful when drawing the location of the injuries.

Critical to medical documentation of injuries from IPV are photographs.[36] Until recently, easy to use, "instant" (Polaroid) cameras were readily available and used in many health care settings.[41,36] However, these cameras are no longer being sold nor can one buy film for Polaroid cameras. Other camera options include 35 mm film cameras and digital cameras. Because of difficulties sending 35 mm film out to be developed, digital cameras are the most practical for documentation of abuse-related injuries.

Facilities should have current policies guiding forensic photographic documentation and include items such as the following:

- — Obtaining signed informed consent to photograph
- — Using a scale in every image
  - — For example, ruler, coin
- — Taking 3 views of each injury:
  - — Far view (6 feet away)
  - — Mid-range view (4 feet away)
  - — Close-range view (2 feet away)
- — Transferring, printing, labeling, and storing the digital images in a confidential manner
- — Releasing the images to law enforcement agencies via:
  - — Release of information forms signed by the patient
  - — Court order

Evidence Collection

Whenever assault patients present to health care settings, the crime scenes arrive with them. Health care providers can provide quality emergent care and preserve valuable evidence. Suspected or reported perpetrators also present to health care settings for either injuries received during the assault or for DNA testing. They, too, are a source of valuable forensic evidence. Every health care facility needs to have a clearly written policy and protocol for evidence collection that has been reviewed by the facilities legal counsel as well as local police and prosecutors.

Dr. Edmund Locard, a French pathologist, founded the first police laboratory in 1910.[80] Locard postulated at the turn of the century, long before the concept of DNA existed, when 2 objects touch there is an exchange of matter and materials providing potential evidence.[81] His theories earned him the reputation as the "father of trace evidence" and have given rise to the oft-stated term–*Locard's Principle*.[80]

Most health care settings have very specific protocols concerning evidence collection when patients report sexual assault. In most communities, there are specialized forensic evidence collection kits specifically designed in collaboration with input from the police, the prosecutor's office, the area crime laboratory, and the medical/nursing specialists who conduct the exams. These kits are very useful when a patient is reporting sexual assault and intimate partner abuse.

However, few hospitals have available ready-made kits when a patient is only reporting intimate partner abuse. In collaboration with local police, health care settings can still collect valuable trace evidence from patients using common, readily available medical supplies as follows:

- Gloves need to be worn at all times when handling potential evidence to avoid mixing the examiner's DNA with the evidence. Changing gloves frequently is recommended.
- New paper bags (large, medium, and small) need to be available to individually package clothing collected as evidence.
- Sterile cotton tip applicators and sterile water need to be available to swab for possible DNA from the reported assailant (saliva, blood). The first swab should be moistened with sterile water (not sterile saline) and rolled over the site. The second swab should be rolled over the same site dry. The swabs need to be air-dried then packaged in either cardboard tubes or new envelopes. Each packaged swab needs to be labeled with the patient's name, date, and time of collection and sealed.
- Miscellaneous debris can be collected in clean envelopes or a sterile cup, labeled, and sealed.
- When official evidence tape is not available, envelopes and paper bags can be sealed with medical tape. Paper bags should not be closed with staples since staples present finger-stick risks.

Each facility needs an evidence storage locker and a "sign-in/sign-out" evidence sheet. The evidence locker could be a locked closet with shelves and dividers or a basic locking file cabinet with holes drilled into the sides and back to improve ventilation and enhance drying. Each drawer of the file cabinet can be used for an individual case. Small hospitals may only need a 2-drawer file cabinet, while busier facilities may need a 4-drawer or large lateral file cabinet to store evidence until retrieved by the police.

In general, evidence collected from patients victimized by intimate partner abuse should be transferred to the police as soon as possible. Historically, the health care setting was not designed as a long-term evidence storage facility. This is being challenged by the emergence of anonymous reporting (ie, Jane Doe cases) for sexual assault cases. Changes in federal law now allow patients reporting sexual assault to receive, at no cost to them, a medical forensic evidentiary exam without involving the police.

Hospitals in some communities, in collaboration with local police and crime labs, have agreed to store the anonymous kits for an agreed upon length of time. For example, various hospitals in Maryland have agreed to store evidence from 30 days to 1 year. At the end of that time, the evidence is destroyed if the patient still does not want the police involved. Evidence should never be given to the police without either a signed consent form from the patient giving permission to release the evidence to law enforcement or a valid court order from the police.

Safety Planning

Health care providers must be able to develop and provide patients affected by IPV with a safety plan prior to hospital discharge. A safety plan may either assist the patient in preparing protective strategies for subsequent incidents of violence or may provide useful information to aid in escaping from an abusive partner.[82] According to Goodkind, Sullivan, and Bybee, women who experience severe abuse are likelier to obtain assistance from formal sources and participate in the development of emergency escape–planning strategies.[83] Providers should convey to patients their ability to provide assistance, regardless of whether they decide to stay with or leave their abuser.[4] "Women's choices are never solely autonomous decisions; they are made within relationships, norms, and circumstances that sustain and constrain what is acceptable and feasible."[84] Effective providers must express concerns to patients in a supportive, sincere manner.[85] Collaboration between patients and providers in combination with appropriate resources may increase patient certainty of their own competency.[86]

Four-Step Safety Plan

Safety planning provides patients with the necessary information required to protect themselves in a variety of situations. The risks and benefits of all possible options must be weighed when developing intervention strategies.[85] Providers who care for patients affected by IPV must be knowledgeable in available resources and state laws of interest to this population. The 4-step safety plan developed by the Family Violence Prevention Fund (FVPF) is designed to assist providers in formulating strategies with their patients. These steps include (a) safety during a violent incident, (b) safety when preparing to leave, (c) safety within the residence, and (d) safety with a protection order.[4] A similar personalized safety plan created by the National Center on Domestic and Sexual Violence expands on those same 4 strategies to also include (a) safety on the job and in public, (b) safety and drug or alcohol use, (c) safety and emotional health, and (d) items to take when leaving.[86]

Patients planning to maintain relationships with their abusers should collaboratively work with their health care providers to develop safety measures in case of future violent incidents. Providers must educate patients that with time, abuse tends to increase in frequency and severity.[85] In health care settings staffed with family violence counselors or advocates, providers should immediately activate these services if patients are agreeable.[85]

National Domestic Violence Hotline

If these services are not available on-site, providers should contact local advocacy groups by telephone and provide patients with their number for use at a later time. Patients should also be provided with the telephone number for the National Domestic Violence Hotline (1-800-799-7233), which they can access for 24-hour advocacy assistance. The establishment of a code word or signal with family, friends, and/or neighbors can be used to indicate the need to call for help in a violent situation. They can also alert their neighbors to call law enforcement upon hearing any suspicious noises coming from the home. Patients have the option to teach their children how to dial 911 in case they are unable. Providers confronted with situations that put children at risk for abuse and neglect have an ethical and legal obligation to file reports with appropriate child protection agencies.[87]

Providers should advise patients to avoid rooms lacking outside exits or that contain possible weapons during arguments, such as kitchens and garages. Providers should also assist patients in identifying all methods of safely exiting the home, such as through windows, doors, and fire escapes. Patients also should devise methods to placate abusers in a serious situation to protect themselves until they are safe. Providers should advise patients to determine a location where they may readily access their keys or purse to quickly exit the home and establish a safe location where they can stay. Providers should also discuss what time of day may be safest to leave the home. For example, if abusers work evening shifts, it may be best to leave shortly after they go to work. Patients and providers must discuss methods by which to keep all written resource material concealed from the abuser.[4]

Providers should offer to call law enforcement if patients are agreeable. It is also important for patients to determine a safe location where they may stay if they choose to leave the abusive relationship. For individuals with limited social resources, providers may assist in arranging temporary housing for these patients and their children at a battered women's shelter. Shelters provide their residents with a variety of services that address their complex needs. Shelter services include lodging, food, clothing, counseling, and health care access and provide residents with legal, financial, employment, and housing resources.[85] Providers must be aware that shelter space is limited, which may contribute to overcrowding and waiting lists.[85]

Safety Tips When Leaving

Providers can prepare patients for leaving an abusive relationship by exploring methods that will increase independence, such as opening a savings account solely in their name.[4] Patients also have the ability to withdraw funds from and close all joint bank accounts.[86] Patients should gather copies of important documents, phone numbers, keys, clothes, and money, and store these items in a secret location within the home or with a trusted individual. Patients should review their safety plan as needed to maintain familiarity with their strategies. Upon leaving, patients must avoid using any cellular phones or telephone cards that would produce billing statements sent to the abuser. To maintain confidentiality, patients should be instructed to use coins or borrow a phone to place calls.[4] Encourage patients to avoid all contact with abusers after leaving the abusive environment.

In cases where abusers have been removed from the home, patients and providers can develop strategies to increase safety within the residence. Patients should be encouraged to change all door locks and add additional locks if necessary. Patients should consider changing their phone number or screening their phone calls. If possible, patients may also consider electronic security systems, metal doors, window bars, and motion lights. Providers can suggest the use of rope ladders for second floor escapes and reinforce the importance of functional smoke detectors and fire extinguishers. Patients may want to inform neighbors that their partner is no longer welcome in the home and to alert law enforcement if they are observed at the residence. Child care providers and schools must be notified that partners do not have permission to access the children. Patients should teach their children how to make collect phone calls or dial 911 in the event that this happens.[4]

Providing Legal Advocacy

Health care providers can supply patients with legal service contacts to facilitate obtaining an order of protection. It will be important for patients to disclose abusers' possession of firearms so that all weapons are confiscated. Providers should also instruct patients to carry a certified copy of the order with them at all times and to provide the police department in areas of residence and employment with a copy to keep on file. Providers must confirm that patients have referrals for advocates and/or legal services to follow-up with any protection order concerns prior to discharge.[4]

Providers should discuss important items that patients should collect and bring with them when leaving an abusive relationship. Important documents that patients will need include identification, birth certificates, vaccination records, welfare records, work permits, green cards, social security cards, protection orders, divorce papers, passports, medical records, bank books, insurance papers, house deed/rental agreements, and driver licenses and registrations. Patients should also take money, credit cards, medications, extra pairs of eyeglasses, sentimental items, and children's items. Telephone numbers of importance include the local police department, prosecutor's office, battered women's program, advocacy group, protection order registry, and numbers associated with patients' place of employment.[86]

Prevention

Health care providers play an important role in primary prevention because of their responsibility to promote the health of their patients. Providers routinely talk to and educate their patients about topics such as healthy relationships and parenting skills.[88] Elliott, Haller, and Peterson found that providers who participate in educational opportunities pertaining to IPV significantly improve their screening and intervention behaviors.[89] It is essential that all providers identify characteristics that may increase patients' risk for IPV. Patients who have been exposed to violence in childhood, abuse alcohol, are in highly stressful situations, are unemployed, or have partners who display macho characteristics are at risk.[90] Although assertiveness and leadership training are interventions that better suit middle-class patients at risk, instructors may creatively adapt these concepts to fit the needs of all women.[90]

Violence prevention education must be developed and implemented within the community setting. Providers may become invaluable educational resources to the public, as well as activists, in the movement to change societal norms and structure that promotes violence.[88] By doing this, public awareness of IPV will also be heightened. For example, the Hands & Words Are Not For Hurting organization developed their HANDS Pledge (Pledge) to educate adults and children about violence and what can be done on an individual basis to end the cycle of abuse. The Pledge is performed in a variety of settings such as schools, businesses, shelters, and government agencies. Educating children early mitigates the perpetuation of violent behavior in intimate relationships.[91]

Involved partnering is a vital element of primary prevention by acting to change male roles that promote aggression, as well as supporting characteristics associated with caring.[88] By challenging dominant standards of masculinity, men with the ability to mentor young boys facilitate the development of gender equality and healthy relationships.[92] Crooks et al suggest implementing interventions that identify clear goals regarding gender equality, oppose bystander apathy, and develop self-efficacy as an involved bystander to prevent acts of violence.[92] Effective IPV interventions should include public education emphasizing a zero-tolerance policy. Mass media may also be used to raise public awareness and reinforce the message that behaviors associated with IPV are unacceptable.[88]

Secondary prevention involves skillful screening by health care providers to detect and intervene with patients in the early stages of IPV.[90] Universal violence screening provides patients with an opportunity to disclose abuse and develop strategies intended to improve both health and safety.[93] Health care providers have a professional responsibility to screen for and identify violence within their patient population, as well as provide appropriate service referrals. Providers should ask patients simple, direct questions in an empathetic manner, ensuring that the interview is conducted in a safe and confidential area.[86] However, research may indicate that women prefer self-report questionnaires compared to direct clinician questioning.[39,94] A study by McFarlane, Groff, O'Brien, and Watson found little difference in the effectiveness of referral card distribution versus 20-minute nurse case management sessions.[28] Both groups adopted more safety behaviors and reported fewer threats, assaults, danger risk for homicide, and work harassment.[28] Unfortunately, while universal screening is supported, very few women are actually screened, indicating the need for further improvement by health care providers.[95]

Helping severely abused patients achieve safety and begin the recovery process are included in tertiary prevention.[90] Once patients have disclosed the abuse, providers should assess the individual's degree of danger. Patients should be encouraged to complete the Danger Assessment (DA) and the Harassment in Abusive Relationships: A Self-Report Scale (HARASS) tool. Providers and patients may use this information to develop appropriate safety planning strategies and resource referrals.[36]

Conclusion

IPV is clearly a complex problem, with both social and public health dimensions, involving large portions of our population. The material in this chapter shows why a traditional disease-based approach is inadequate. Because of the myriad social dimensions, there are health care aspects that require the informed attention of health care providers in order to assure the appropriate identification and management of potential IPV victims. Staying informed, following the best practices, and meticulously documenting one's evaluations are essential responsibilities for health care providers in today's health care environment, and the staggering numbers of potential victims who are likely to be seen by a health care provider during even a typical practice day certainly speak to the importance of developing competence in this area. In addition to accurate identification and management for existing victims, a shared goal among health care providers is to engage in community efforts that build the type of society where IPV is prevented long before it has the opportunity to wreak the havoc it is known to cause among its many victims.

References

1. Centers for Disease Control and Prevention. Costs of intimate partner violence against women in the United States. http://www.cdc.gov/ncipc/pub-res/ipv_cost/IPVBook-Final-Feb18.pdf. Published March 2003. Accessed April 20, 2008.

2. Tjaden PJ, Thoennes N. *Extent, Nature, and Consequences of Intimate Partner Violence: Findings from the National Violence Against Women Survey.* Washington, DC: US Dept of Justice; 2000A. NCJ 181867.

3. Plichta SB. Interactions between victims of intimate partner violence against women and the health care system: policy and practice implications. *Trauma Violence Abuse.* 2007;8(2):226-239.

4. Family Violence Prevention Fund. *National Consensus Guidelines on Identifying and Responding to Domestic Violence Victimization in Health Care Settings.* San Francisco, CA: Family Violence Prevention Fund; 2004.

5. National Center for Injury Prevention and Control (NCIPC). *Costs of Intimate Partner Violence Against Women in the United States.* Atlanta, GA: Centers for Disease Control and Prevention; 2003.

6. Tjaden PJ, Thoennes N. *Full Report of the Prevalence, Incidence, and Consequences of Violence Against Women: Findings from the National Violence Against Women Survey.* Washington, DC: National Institute of Justice; 2000B. NCJ 183781.

7. Sheridan DJ. Treating survivors of intimate partner abuse: forensic identification and documentation. In: Olshaker JS, Jackson MC, Smock MS, eds. *Forensic Emergency Medicine.* Philadelphia, PA: Lippincott, Williams, and Wilkins; 2001:203-228.

8. Sheridan DJ. Legal and forensic responses to family violence. In: Humphreys J, Campbell JC, eds. *Family Violence and Nursing Practice.* Philadelphia, PA: Williams and Wilkins; 2004:385-406.

9. Saltzman LE, Fanslow JL, McMahnon PM, Shelley GA. *Intimate Partner Violence Surveillance: Uniform Definitions and Recommended Data Elements, version 1.0.* Atlanta, GA: National Center for Injury Prevention and Control, Centers for Disease Prevention; 1999.

10. Walton-Moss BJ, Manganello J, Frye V, Campbell JC. Risk factors for intimate partner violence and associated injury among urban women. *J Community Health.* 2005;30(5):377-389.

11. World Health Organization (WHO). *WHO Multicountry Study on Women's Health and Domestic Violence Against Women: Initial Results on Prevalence, Health Consequences, and Women's Responses.* Geneva, Switzerland: Author; 2005.

12. United States Department of Justice. Criminal Victimization, 2005. In: *Bureau of Justice Statistics Bulletin.* Washington, DC: Author; 2006. NCJ 214644.

13. Campbell JC, Sharps PW, Sachs C, Yam ML. Medical lethality assessment and safety planning in domestic violence cases. *Clin Fam Pract.* 2003;5(1):101-112.

14. Campbell JC, Soeken KL, McFarlane J, Parker B. Risk factors for femicide among pregnant and nonpregnant battered women. In: JC Campbell, ed. *Empowering Survivors of Abuse: Health Care for Battered Women and Their Children.* Thousand Oaks, CA: Sage; 1998:90-97.

15. Rennison CM. Intimate partner violence, 1993-2001. Bureau of Justice Statistics Crime Data Brief. http://www.ojp.usdoj.gov/bjs/pub/pdf/ipv01.pdf. Published February 2003. Accessed April 20, 2008. NCJ 197838.

16. Bent-Goodley TB. Health disparities and violence against women: why and how cultural and societal influences matter. *Trauma Violence Abuse.* 2007;8(2):90-104.

17. Campbell JC, Glass N, Sharps PW, Laughon K, Bloom T. Intimate partner homicide: Review and implications of research and policy. *Trauma Violence Abuse.* 2007;8(3):246-269.

18. Campbell JC. Health consequences of intimate partner violence. *Lancet.* 2002; 359:1331-1336.

19. Coker AL, Davis KE, Arias Il, Desai S, Sanderson M, Brandt HM, Smith PH. Physical and mental health effects of intimate partner violence for men and women. *Am J Prev Med.* 2002;23(4):260-268.

20. Fisher JW, Shelton AJ. Survivors of domestic violence demographics and disparities in visitors to an interdisciplinary specialty clinic. *Fam Community Health.* 2006; 29(2):118-130.

21. Leserman J, Drossman DA. Relationship of abuse history to functional gastrointestinal disorders and symptoms. *Trauma Violence Abuse.* 2007;8:331-343.

22. Kendall-Tackett KA. Inflammation, cardiovascular disease and metabolic syndrome as sequelae of violence against women: the role of depression, hostility, and sleep disturbance. *Trauma Violence Abuse.* 2007;8(2):117-126.

23. Sharps PW, Laughon K, Giangrande SK. Intimate partner violence and the childbearing year: maternal and infant health consequences. *Trauma Violence Abuse.* 2007;8(2):105-116.

24. Coker AL. Does physical intimate partner violence affect sexual health? A systematic review. *Trauma Violence Abuse.* 2007;8(2):149-177.

25. Burnett LB, Adler J, Conrad S, Talavera F, Harwood RC, Halamka J. Domestic Violence. http://www.emedicine.com. Updated 2008. Accessed November 10, 2009.

26. Chamberlain L. The USPTSTF recommendation on intimate violence: what we can learn from it, and what we can do about it. *Fam Violence Health Pract.* 2005;1(1):1-24. http://www.endabuse.org/health/ejournal/archive/1-1/. Accessed November 10, 2009.

27. McFarlane JM, Groff JY, O'Brien JA, Watson K. Behaviors of children following a randomized controlled treatment program for their abused mothers. *Issues Compr Pediatr Nurs.* 2005;28(4):195-211.

28. McFarlane JM, Groff JY, O'Brien JA, Watson K. Secondary prevention of intimate partner violence. *Nurs Res.* 2006;55(1):52-61.

29. Phelan MB. Screening for intimate partner violence in medical settings. *Trauma Violence Abuse.* 2007;8:199-213.

30. Joint Commission on Accreditation of Healthcare Organizations (JCAHO). Hospital accreditation program, provision of care, treatment, and services: Standard PC.01.02.09. The Joint Commission. http://www.jointcommission.org/NR/rdonlyres/73E965C5-6718-4CD7-AEBD-4A79F9D5F058/0/HAP_PC.pdf. Accessed May 30, 2008.

31. Waltermaurer E. Measuring intimate partner violence (IPV): you may only get what you ask for. *J Interpersonal Violence.* 2005;2(4):501-506.

32. McFarlane J, Parker B, Soeken K, Bullock L. Assessing for abuse during pregnancy. *J Am Med Assoc.* 1992;267(3):3176-3178.

33. McFarlane JM, Parker B, Scoken K, Silva C, Reel S. Safety behaviors of abused women after an intervention during pregnancy. *J Obstet Gynecol Neonatal Nurs.* 1998;27(1):64-69.

34. McFarlane JM, Soeken K, Wiist W. An evaluation of interventions to decrease intimate violence to pregnant women. *Public Health Nursing.* 2000;17(6):443-451.

35. Feldhaus KM, Koziol-McLain J, Amsbury HL, Norton IM, Lowenstein SR, Abbott JT. Accuracy of 3 brief screening questions for detecting partner violence in the emergency department. *J Am Med Assoc.* 1997;277(17):1357-1361.

36. Sheridan DJ, Nash KR, Hawkins SL, Makely JL, Campbell JC. Forensic implications of intimate partner violence. In: Hammer RM, Moynihan B, Pagliaro EM, eds. *Forensic Nursing: A Handbook for Practice.* Sudbury, MA: Jones and Bartlett; 2006:255-278.

37. McFarlane J, Greenberg L, Weltge A, Watson M. Identification of abuse in emergency departments: effectiveness of a two-question screening tool. *J Emerg Nurs.* 1995;21(5):391-394.

38. Sheridan DJ. *Measuring Harassment of Abused Women: A Nursing Concern* [unpublished dissertation]. Portland, OR: Oregon Health Sciences University; 1998.

39. Glass N, Dearwater S, Campbell J. Intimate partner violence screening and intervention: data from eleven Pennsylvania and California community hospital emergency departments. *J Emerg Nurs.* 2001;27:141-149.

40. Renkin RP, Tonkin P. Women's views of prenatal violence screening acceptability and confidentiality issues. *Obstet Gynecol.* 2006;107(2):348-354.

41. Sheridan DJ, Nash KR. Acute injury patterns of intimate partner violence victims. *Trauma Violence Abuse.* 2007;8(3):281-289.

42. Reijnder UJ, Van der Leden ME, De Bruin KH. Injuries due to domestic violence against women: sites on the body, types of injury and the methods of infliction [in Dutch]. *Nederlands Tijdschrift Voor Geneeskunde.* 2006;150(8):429-435.

43. Amar AF, Gennaro S. Dating violence in college women: associated physical injury, healthcare usage, and mental health symptoms. *Nurs Res.* 2005;54:235-242.

44. Le BT, Dierks EJ, Ueeck-Homer LD, Potter BF. Maxillofacial injuries associated with domestic violence. *J Oral Maxillofac Surg.* 2001;59:1277-1283.

45. Banks ME. Overlooked but critical: traumatic brain injury as a consequence of interpersonal violence. *Trauma Violence Abuse.* 2007;8(3):290-298.

46. Greenfeld LA, Rand MR, Craven D, Klaus PA, Perkins CA, Ringel C, et al. *Violence by Intimates: Analysis of Data on Crimes by Current or Former Spouses, Boyfriends, and Girlfriends.* Washington, DC: Bureau of Justice Statistics; 1998. NCJ 167237.

47. Celbis O, Gokdogan MR, Kaya M, Gunes G. Review of forensic assessments of female referrals to the branch of legal medicine, Malatya region, Turkey—1996-2000. *J Clin Forensic Med.* 2006;13:21-25.

48. Muelleman RL, Lenaghan PA, Pakieser RA. Battered women: injury locations and types. *Ann Emerg Med.* 1996;28(5):486-492.

49. Sutherland CA, Bybee DI, Sullivan CM. Beyond bruises and broken bones: the joint effects of stress and injuries on battered women's health. *Am J Community Psychol.* 2002;30(5):609-636.

50. Wilbur L, Higley M, Hatfield J, Surprenant Z, Taliaferro E, Smith DJ, et al. Survey results of women who have been strangled while in an abusive relationship. *J Emerg Med.* 2001;21(3):297-302.

51. Strack GB, McClane GE, Hawley D. A review of 300 attempted strangulation cases part I: criminal legal issues. *J Emerg Med.* 2001;21:303-309.

52. Bergen RK. *Wife Rape: Understanding the Responses of Survivors and Service Providers.* Thousand Oaks, CA: Sage; 1996.

53. Campbell JC, Soeken K. Forced sex and intimate partner violence: effects on women's risk and women's health. *Violence Against Women.* 1999;51:1017-1035.

54. Sommers MS. Defining patterns of genital injury from sexual assault: a review. *Trauma Violence Abuse.* 2007;8(3):270-280.

55. Jones JS, Wynn BN, Kroeze B, Dunnuck C, Rossman L. Comparison of sexual assaults by strangers versus known assailants in a community-based population. *Am J Emerg Med.* 2004;22(6):454-459.

56. Anderson S, McClain N, Riviello R. Genital findings of women after consensual and nonconsensual intercourse. *J Forensic Nurs.* 2006;2(2):59-65.

57. Wadman MC, Muelleman RL. Domestic violence homicides: ED use before victimization. *Am J Emerg Med.* 1999;17(7):689-691.

58. Carey JW, Perciaccante VJ, Dodson TB. Predicting domestic violence based on injury location and screening questions. *J Oral Maxillofac Surg.* 1999;57(suppl 1):42-43.

59. Centers for Disease Control and Prevention. Intimate partner violence injuries—Oklahoma, 2002. *MMWR.* 2005;54(41):1041-1045.

60. Ochs HA, Neuenschwander MC, Dodson TB. Are head, neck and facial injuries markers for domestic violence? *J Am Dent Assoc.* 1995;127:757-761.

61. Brismar B, Bergman B, Larsson G, Strandberg A. Battered women: a diagnostic and therapeutical dilemma. *Acta Chirurgica Scandinavica.* 1987;153:1-5.

62. Nannini A, Lazar J, Berg C, Barger M, Tomashek K, Cabral H, et al. Physical injuries reported on hospital visits for assault during the pregnancy-associated period. *Nurs Res.* 2008;57(3):144-149.

63. Besant-Matthews PE. Blunt and sharp injuries. In: Lynch VA, Duval JB, eds. *Forensic Nurs.* St. Louis, MO: Elsevier Mosby; 2006:189-200.

64. *Merriam-Webster's Medical Desk Dictionary.* Springfield, MA: Merriam-Webster Inc; 1996.

65. LaSala KB, Lynch VA. Child abuse and neglect. In: Lynch VA, Duval JB, eds. *Forensic Nurs.* St. Louis, MO: Elsevier Mosby; 2006:249-259.

66. Beck SR, Freitag SK, Singer N. Ocular injuries in battered women. *Ophthalmol.* 1996;103:148-151.

67. Mosqueda L, Burnight K, Liao S. The life cycle of bruises in older adults. *J Am Geriatr Soc.* 2005;53(8):1339-1343.

68. Bariciak ED, Plint AC, Gaboury I, Bennett S. Dating of bruises in children: an assessment of physician accuracy. *Pediatrics.* 2003;112(4):804-807.

69. Stephenson T, Bialas Y. Estimation of the age of bruising. *Arch Dis Child.* 1996;74:53-55.

70. Langlois NEI, Gresham GA. The ageing of bruises: a review and study of the colour changes with time. *Forensic Sci Int.* 1991;50:227-238.

71. Hughes VK, Ellis PS, Langlois NEI. The perception of yellow in bruises. *J Clin Forensic Med.* 2004;11:257-259.

72. Munang LA, Leonard PA, Mok JYQ. Lack of agreement on colour description between clinicians examining childhood bruising. *J Clin Forensic Med.* 2002;9:171-174.

73. Rooms RR, Shapiro PD. Approach for emergency medical personnel. In: Lynch VA, Duval JB, eds. *Forensic Nursing.* St. Louis, MO: Elsevier Mosby; 2006:341-350.

74. Brockmeyer DM, Sheridan DJ. Domestic violence: a practical guide to the use of forensic evaluation in clinical examination and documentation of injuries. In: Campbell JC, ed. *Empowering Survivors of Abuse: Health Care for Battered Women and Their Children.* Thousand Oaks, CA: Sage; 1998:23-31.

75. Sheridan DJ. Forensic identification and documentation of patients experiencing intimate partner violence. *Clin Family Pract.* 2003;5(1):113-143.

76. Biroscak BJ, Smith PK, Roznowski H, Tucker J, Carlson G. Intimate partner violence against women: finds from one state's ED surveillance system. *J Emerg Nurs.* 2006;32:12-16.

77. Balci YG, Ayranci U. Physical violence against women: evaluation of women assaulted by spouses. *J Clin Forensic Med.* 2005;12(5):258-263.

78. Maryland Network Against Domestic Violence. Investigation of strangulation cases: a model protocol for Maryland law enforcement officers. http://marcpi.jhu.edu/marcpi/DVProtocols/InvestigationandProsecutionofStrangulationCasesforMDProsecutors.pdf. Accessed October 15, 2008.

79. Nash K, Sheridan DJ. Can one accurately date a bruise? State of the science. *J Forensic Nurs*. 2009;5(1):31-37.

80. Cabelus NB, Spangler K. Evidence collection and documentation. In: Hammer RM, Moynihan B, PagliaroEM, eds. *Forensic Nursing: A Handbook for Practice*. Sudbury, MA: Jones and Bartlett; 2006:489-518.

81. Inman K, Rodin N. *Principles and Practice of Criminalistics: The Profession of Forensic Science*. Boca Ratan, FL: CRC Press; 2001.

82. Schornstein SL. *Domestic Violence and Health Care: What Every Professional Needs to Know*. Thousand Oaks, CA: Sage; 1997.

83. Goodkind JR, Sullivan CM, Bybee DI. A contextual analysis of battered women's safety planning. *Violence Against Women*. 2004;10(5):514-533.

84. Pennell J, Francis S. Safety conferencing. *Violence Against Women*. 2005;11(5):666-692.

85. Parker B, Bullock L, Bohn D, Curry M. Abuse during pregnancy. In: J Humphreys, JC Campbell, eds. *Family Violence and Nursing Practice*. Philadelphia, PA: Lippincott Williams & Wilkins; 2004:307-360.

86. National Center on Domestic and Sexual Violence. *Domestic Violence Personalized Safety Plan*. http://www.ncdsv.org/publications_safetyplans.html. Accessed April 20, 2008.

87. Moynihan BA. Domestic violence. In: Lynch VA, Duval JB eds. Forensic Nurs. St. Louis, MO: Elsevier Mosby; 2006:260-270.

88. Coker AL. Opportunities for prevention: addressing IPV in the health care setting. *Fam Violence Prev Health Pract*. 2005;1(1). http://www.endabuse.org/health/ejournal/archive/1-1/Coker.pdf. Accessed April 20, 2008.

89. Elliott BA, Haller IV, Peterson JM. Targeted IPV education: sustained change in rural and mid-sized medical settings. *Fam Violence Prev Health Pract*. 2005;1(2). http://www.endabuse.org/health/ejournal/archive/1-2/Elliott.pdf. Accessed April 20, 2008.

90. Campbell JC, Torres S, McKenna LS, Sheridan DJ, Landenburger K. Nursing care of survivors of intimate partner violence. In: Humphreys, Campbell JC, eds. *Family Violence Nursing Practice*. Philadelphia, PA: Lippincott Williams & Wilkins; 2004:77-96.

91. Gundersen L. Intimate partner violence: the need for primary prevention in the community. *Ann Intern Med*. 2002;136(8):637-640.

92. Crooks CV, Goodall GR, Hughes R, Jaffe PG, Baker LL. Engaging men and boys in preventing violence against women. *Violence Against Women*. 2007;13(3):217-239.

93. Family Violence Prevention Fund. *Preventing Domestic Violence: Clinical Guidelines on Routine Screening*. San Francisco, CA: Family Violence Prevention Fund; 1999.

94. MacMillan HL, Wathen CN, Jamieson E, Boyle M, McNutt L, Worster A, et al. Approaches to screening for intimate partner violence in health care settings. *J Am Med Assoc*. 2006;296(5):530-536.

95. Walton-Moss BJ, Campbell JC. Intimate partner violence: implications for nursing. *Online J Issues Nurs.* 2002;7(1). http://www.nursingworld.org/MainMenuCategories/ANAMarketplace/ANAPeriodicals/OJIN/TableofContents/Volume72002/No1Jan2002/IntimatePartnerViolence.aspx?css=print. Accessed April 20, 2008.

Chapter 17

HUMAN TRAFFICKING

Imelda Buncab, BA
Annie Heirendt, LCSW

No one shall be held in slavery or servitude; slavery and the slave trade shall be prohibited in all their forms.[1]

Human trafficking is a significant human rights issue on both the global and national stages. Trafficked persons are subjected to physical, sexual, and psychological abuse through forced labor, commercial sex, and slavery-like practices. Traffickers are opportunistic exploiters, essentially abusers who lure potential victims with false pretenses or use coercion to take advantage of individuals' vulnerabilities. To understand human trafficking is to understand the various structural and proximate factors that increase vulnerability to human trafficking; these factors have social, cultural, and political dimensions.[2] Trafficked persons include forced or voluntary foreign migrants motivated by a desire to escape poverty, improve their economic situation, leave behind abusive relationships, flee war torn countries, escape gender discrimination, evade religious persecution, or simply seek opportunities for a better life. Trafficked persons can also be born into exploitation through a practice known as inherited-debt bonded labor, which is perpetuated through widely tolerated societal and cultural beliefs. In the United States, trafficked persons can be documented or undocumented foreign migrants, legal permanent residents, or US citizens. Trafficking takes place within a given nation-state (also known as internal or domestic trafficking) and across international borders. Because of these dynamics, human trafficking is a complex and multifaceted crime—as a field, the response to trafficking is still in its infancy and poses unique challenges to practitioners.

First, existing statistics do not necessarily provide a comprehensive picture of the problem. The numbers available to us today may be incomplete, demographically insufficient (ie, exclusive to only women and children), or based on varying definitions of trafficking in persons, resulting in inconsistent methodologies of data gathering.[3] The prevailing research focuses primarily on sex trafficking of women and children. A study on forced labor in the United States documented that nearly half of human trafficking cases did not involve sexual exploitation but were rather crimes such as forced domestic service, agricultural work, sweatshop or factory labor, restaurant service, or hotel work and victimized men as well as women and children.[4] Globally, the International Labor Organization (ILO) found that the vast majority of forced labor cases (64% of 12.3 million cases) were economic exploitation, including bonded labor, forced domestic work, or forced agricultural labor and other work in remote rural areas.[5] When cases not involving commercial sexual exploitation are not included, opportunities to identify victims of trafficking are missed; equal attention to all forms and contexts of trafficking is needed.

Second, human trafficking as a public health issue is not yet widely recognized. Many trafficked persons are sexually assaulted and abused during the course of their exploitation and oftentimes labor in dangerous and unregulated work environments.[4]

They are vulnerable to contracting human immunodeficiency virus (HIV) and other sexually transmitted infections (STIs), undergoing forced abortions, experiencing chronic health problems (eg, back pain, hearing, cardiovascular, or respiratory problems), contracting infectious diseases, developing alcohol or substance addictions, and developing other health-related problems in addition to mental health issues. Trafficked persons may endure existing health impairments and may not have access to services while in captivity. If they do receive services, the standard of care most often lacks the quality necessary to address the myriad presenting health issues of victims. Within the trafficking situation, victims often develop new health problems without routine medical care and other clinical interventions. Posttrafficking prevention and intervention opportunities are also often missed, particularly when victims decide to repatriate. Recent research highlights victim repatriation as a conduit for the spread of HIV and other STIs. For example, a study of 257 girls and women trafficked for sexual exploitation found that 38% were infected with HIV.[6] Repatriated victims faced ostracism within their communities, barriers to treatment access, and a lack of knowledge regarding HIV. This leads to a higher risk for partner transmission and mother-child transmission in rural, less developed regions. Experts have indicated that there is a strong association between migration and the spread of disease; thus, trafficking victims' health is an increasingly important public health matter for countries of origin, transit, and destination.[7]

Human trafficking is distinctive in the level of exploitation endured by victims and the length of enslavement.[8] The exploitation endured by victims of trafficking encompasses multiple types of victimization and meeting the unique needs of trafficking victims requires a comprehensive and collaborative response from medical providers, social service providers, law enforcement officers and agents, and community resource managers. The initial trafficking cases in the United States engendered reactive responses that provided valuable practical experience to address this crime and created baseline data from which to work. Additionally, it has helped to further shape national and state policy for victim protection, criminal prosecution, and prevention efforts. The field has borrowed heavily from research on sexual assault and domestic violence victimology to better understand and therapeutically engage with trafficking victims, as clinical research within the antitrafficking field is insubstantial as of 2009.[9]

The antitrafficking field—at least in the United States—requires more empirical data and continued development of promising practices for effective policies, victim response, and service model approaches. A contextualized empowerment approach to survivor services is fundamental. For example, debate over the terminology of *survivor* and *victim* ascribed to trafficked persons is of current discourse within the antitrafficking field. Some contend that to label a trafficked person a victim is a disservice, because it ignores the structural aspects (push-pull factors) that encourage trafficking and deprives the trafficked individual of their own agency[10]; however, the term *victim* is used by law enforcement to ensure that the individual is treated as a victim of a crime. Advocates within the antitrafficking field have followed the trend of sexual assault and domestic violence advocates and have chosen to utilize the term *survivor* to acknowledge trafficked individuals' resiliency. To respect both the trafficked individual's resiliency and victimization, this narrative will ascribe the general term *trafficked person* to account for the trafficked individual's experiences as well as *victim* and *survivor* when appropriate.

This narrative will draw from the writers' experiences in working in the antitrafficking field both domestically and internationally, through a culturally competent empowerment model and a victim-rights perspective. This chapter will provide an introductory overview of human trafficking, present the possible impacts and clinical implications of human trafficking on both female and male adults, and provide guidance in working with trafficked persons, in addition to recommended resources for practitioners.

Overview of Human Trafficking

Fundamentally, human trafficking is a violation of a person's human rights in which a person's individual freedoms are denied. Human trafficking is an inherently violent form of modern-day slavery; a crime in which women, men, and children are treated as expendable commodities. Traffickers sell, trade, and exploit victims, using violence as a means of control.[11] The clandestine black market of human trafficking nets tens of billions of dollars annually and is one of the top 3 illegal activities of organized criminal syndicates, following drugs and weapons trafficking.[12] Unlike drugs and weapons—commodities that can only be sold once—trafficked persons become a constant source of revenue through continuous exploitation. Sex trafficking alone pockets $7 to $19 billion annually.[13] The business of human trafficking is lucrative for the exploiters, providing wealth at the expense of trafficked persons' physical and mental health and leading to the disruption of sustainable living practices within communities of origin, transit, and destination; public health concerns through widening disease prevalence; increased criminal activities; and the disruption of the rule of law within societies.

Worldwide, 27 million people are enslaved.[8] Forced to make rugs in India, pick coffee beans in Africa, work coal mines in Brazil, and subjected to domestic work in Saudi Arabia, "entertaining" in Japan, and forced prostitution and labor in the United States, these are the world's current slaves. There are an estimated 12.3 million people subjected to forced labor globally.[5] While at any one time there are 2.5 million victims of human trafficking.[12] The US Department of State's annual Trafficking in Persons (TIP) report estimates as many as 600 000 to 800 000 people are trafficked around the globe; of this number, 80% are women and girls.[13] The United States ranks as a top destination country, receiving 14 500 to 17 500 trafficked persons annually.[13] These statistics provide a glimpse of the prevalence and magnitude of human trafficking.

Human Trafficking as Contemporary Slavery

Human trafficking is contemporary slavery with defining attributes. What makes this modern-day slavery different from historical institutionalized slavery is that slaves are cheaper and more affordable to "maintain" due to the localization of the trafficking phenomenon. Currently, the length of enslavement is generally shorter and the global trend of slavery demonstrates similar patterns of enslavement that incorporate shared structural and proximate factors.

Furthermore, human trafficking is a nondiscriminatory crime. The tendency of enslaving a person is not based heavily on ethnic or racial discrimination.[8] Rather, trafficking follows the trend of intraethnic exploitation, where the trafficker is often of the same ethnicity as his or her victims. They speak the same languages, come from the same communities, and may know one another through friends or relatives. Traffickers can also be from a privileged group (eg, religious leaders, business owners, community leaders, diplomats) within the community; this power inequity creates an environment conducive to exploitation. Through power and control, the trafficker lures victims into a web of false promises, compounded debts, and egregious violence. As Bales points out, human trafficking is a dynamic relationship between the trafficker or slaveholder and the trafficked person, a relationship of power, resources, and economic differentials perpetuated through violence.[11] Traffickers can be individual males or females, small operations of friends, family members or acquaintances, owners of small to medium-sized businesses, or brokers.

The criminal act of human trafficking relies on vulnerabilities of potential trafficking victims. Any person can be a trafficking victim; victims can be adults, young females, or males. The likelihood of becoming trafficked is increased by certain vulnerabilities that include poverty, civil strife, natural disaster, political instability, religious persecution, family violence, and marginalization resulting from ethnic minority status, sexual orientation, gender, or the presence of physical or mental health disabilities.

Individuals with disabilities are at an increased risk of exploitation. One study demonstrated that 64% of individuals with disabilities experienced multiple perpetrators of sexual assault; 76% experienced multiple assault incidences; and 28% experienced both sexual assault and domestic violence, including abuse from care providers. Another study found that 52% of abusers were acquaintances, family members, and peers with disabilities.[14] For example, one trafficking case involved multiple disabled trafficked persons who were recruited by a family acquaintance from a rural village in Mexico. Trafficked persons were forced to peddle trinkets and beg along subway lines and at bus stations and were regularly subjected to physical violence.[15]

Unlike other types of crimes, human trafficking involves multiple victims at one time. According to statistical findings from the Human Trafficking Reporting System (HTRS), an average of 3 victims per incident of confirmed human trafficking were reported by federally funded task forces addressing the crime.[16] As the field continues to evolve, multiple victims' cases are investigated and prosecuted and social service agencies are building the capacity and resources to respond to their needs. A single human trafficking case that is discovered, confirmed, and prosecuted could involve as many as 6 or more trafficking victim-survivors.

When a multiple-victim trafficking case occurs, it poses many challenges for law enforcement and social service providers in meeting the various needs of victims. These challenges can involve lack of experience responding to human trafficking incidents, lack of shelter for discovered victims, lack of antitrafficking service providers, and generally, lack of protocols within a state or local level for when a human trafficking incident is reported. For example, between 2007 and 2008, 71% of human trafficking incidents were reported by a state or local law enforcement entity. Furthermore, nearly one-third of these cases involved multiagency collaboration.[16] Collaboration is key to creating an effective human trafficking response system. For example, one federally funded task force in Los Angeles has developed an emergency response protocol for when a trafficking incident is reported from various outlets, such as a local human trafficking hotline, a national hotline, from community organizations, or from task force members.[17] The task force rotates on-call responsibility for investigating reported incidents between local and federal law enforcement agencies. A local antitrafficking organization specializing in serving trafficked persons is then contacted for victims' crisis care needs. Crisis care is necessary to establish trust between the service provider and the trafficking victim. When victims' basic needs for shelter, food, and safety are met expeditiously, they become empowered. Information and education detailing options available to victims enable individuals to make an informed choice when requesting social and legal services.

Legal Framework

US Law

Countries of origin, transit, and destination have made efforts to combat this transnational crime. The Protocol to Prevent, Suppress, and Punish Trafficking in Persons, especially Women and Children (the Protocol), supplements the UN Convention Against Transnational Organized Crime, which was adopted in November 2000 by the UN General Assembly.[18] The Protocol makes the following definitions:

(a) "Trafficking in persons" shall mean the recruitment, transportation, transfer, harboring or receipt of persons, by means of the threat or use of force or other forms of coercion, of abduction, of fraud, of deception, of the abuse of power or of a position of vulnerability or of the giving or receiving of payments or benefits to achieve the consent of a person having control over another person, for the purpose of exploitation. Exploitation shall include, at a minimum, the exploitation of the prostitution of others or other forms of sexual exploitation, forced labor or services, slavery or practices similar to slavery, servitude or the removal of organs;

(b) The consent of a victim of trafficking in persons to the intended exploitation set forth in subparagraph (a) of this article shall be irrelevant where any of the means set forth in subparagraph (a) have been used;

(c) The recruitment, transportation, transfer, harboring or receipt of a child for the purpose of exploitation shall be considered "trafficking in persons" even if this does not involve any of the means set forth in subparagraph (a) of this article;

(d) "Child" shall mean any person under eighteen years of age

This international framework helped inform the US antitrafficking policy model. In 2000, the US Congress enacted the Trafficking Victim Protection Act (TVPA) through bipartisan efforts. The law federally criminalized human trafficking through increased penalties, created new statutes to address the crime, provided for victim services (including legal status to foreign nationals), and engaged in prevention work with countries of origin. The TVPA can be summarized as a 3-pronged approach of prosecution, protection, and prevention. The 2000 TVPA defines "severe forms of trafficking in persons" as[19]:

(a) Sex trafficking in which a commercial sex act is induced by force, fraud, or coercion, or in which the person induced to perform such act has not attained 18 years of age; or

(b) The recruitment, harboring, transportation, provision, or obtaining of a person for labor or services, through the use of force, fraud, or coercion for the purpose of subjection to involuntary servitude, peonage, debt bondage or slavery.

Coercion is defined as "threats of serious harm to or physical restraint against any person; any scheme, plan, or pattern intended to cause a person to believe that failure to perform an act would result in serious harm to or physical restraint against any person; or the abuse or threats of the legal process." Additionally, the movement of a person from one place to another is not necessary to meet the violation of human trafficking.[20] This is important to note, as the term *trafficking* implies required movement of a person, which often creates confusion in assessing human trafficking cases.

The law differentiates between human trafficking and smuggling of persons. Human trafficking is considered a crime against a person, and involves exploitation through compelled services or labor. Trafficked persons are considered victims of a crime under the US TVPA. Smuggling is considered a crime against the country entered, and usually involves illegal crossing of international borders. Smuggling can be viewed as a business transaction; the smugglers provide a service and are paid for their service once the border is crossed. The relationship between the smuggler and smuggled ends at the border, and the smuggled person is free to leave. Smuggling situations can become trafficking situations, should the smuggler maintain control or sell or transfer the individual to other exploiters for compelled services or labor after the border is crossed. Last, a smuggled person is considered a criminal under US immigration laws. See **Table 17-1** for an explanation of human trafficking versus smuggling distinctions within the United States.

Table 17-1. Human Trafficking versus Smuggling within the United States

Trafficking	Smuggling
Violates a person's civil/human rights	Violates country/international immigration laws
Involves force, fraud, coercion	Involves self-initiation
Relationship with trafficker of exploitation and violence for compelled services	Relationship facilitated with smuggler as business transaction for a service
Trafficked person is considered a victim of a crime	Smuggled person is considered a criminal

The TVPA is also a victim-centered law. Trafficking victims are entitled to the right to safety, privacy, access to information, legal representation, court hearings, and compensation for damages, and to seek protection through US residency. Victims of trafficking are offered various protections that aim to assist in their rehabilitation and reintegration into the community or repatriation to their country of origin. Access to these protections is by way of victim certification from the US Department of Health and Human Services. Trafficking victims are certified for eligibility to receive government refugee benefits for up to 8 months, including refugee cash and medical assistance, food stamps, and employment assistance.[21] Additionally, survivors and their immediate family members are eligible for various nonimmigrant legal visas, which will be further discussed later in this chapter.

State Law

Because the TVPA is a federal antitrafficking law, law enforcement jurisdiction fell on federal agencies. However, local law enforcement officials have indicated that they have also encountered human trafficking. Examples of local law enforcement calls that uncovered human trafficking included instances of sexual assault, domestic violence, burglary, illegal immigration, wage disputes, attempted suicide, prostitution, kidnapping, information from antitrafficking advocacy organizations, and informants on criminal cases. The creation of state antitrafficking legislation is therefore imperative to aid in investigation and prosecution of trafficking offenders by local and state law enforcement agencies. States have begun enacting criminal statutes addressing human trafficking, thereby localizing law enforcement responses. Some states have legislatively implemented statewide task forces that provide recommendations for antitrafficking policy. **Tables 17-2** and **17-3** detail US states with antitrafficking laws and legislated statewide interagency task forces on human trafficking, respectively.

Federally funded law enforcement antitrafficking task forces complement statewide task forces. These federally funded task forces are required to establish at least one memorandum of understanding (MOU) indicating partnership with a nongovernmental organization (NGO), and are generally comprised of local and federal law enforcement agencies in addition to non–law enforcement local and federal agencies like the Department of Labor, the Internal Revenue Service, and the Departments of Adult and Child Protective Services. Forty-two of these collaborative task forces are operating throughout the United States and take on activities such as creating public awareness campaigns, improving efforts in proactive law enforcement investigations of human trafficking, implementing trafficking in persons emergency response teams, and conducting law enforcement training events. Ultimately, the overall goals of the task force are to: (1) continue to enhance law enforcement's ability to identify and rescue victims of human trafficking, (2) provide law enforcement with the resources and training to identify and rescue victims of trafficking, and (3) ensure that comprehensive services are available wherever trafficking victims are found.[22]

Community-based organizations, such as rape crisis centers, are valuable members of these task forces in both the sharing of expertise and developing insights. One task force in Southern California was referred a trafficking case from their local rape crisis center that involved a significant number of possible victims. With the collaborative response of task force members, the identified trafficked persons received social services support, legal support, and law enforcement investigation that were comprehensively victim sensitive. This collaborative approach is essential in helping to ease the many coercive fears that trafficked persons experience—especially distrust of law enforcement and the outside community—and that are often used as tools of control by traffickers.

Table 17-2. US States with Antitrafficking Laws

State	Criminalization Statute	Effective Date
Alaska	SB 12	July 1, 2006
Arizona	SB 1372	August 12, 2005
Arkansas	HB 2979	August 11, 2005
California	AB 22	September 21, 2005
Colorado	SB 207	July 1, 2006
Connecticut	SB153	July 1, 2006
Florida	SB 1962, SB 250	October 1, 2006
Georgia	SB 529	July 1, 2007
Idaho	HB 536	July 1, 2006
Illinois	HB 1469	January 1, 2006
Indiana	HB 1155	July 1, 2006
Iowa	SF 2219	July 1, 2006
Kansas	SB 72	July 1, 2005
Kentucky	SB 43	July 26, 2007
Louisiana	HB 56	August 15, 2005
Maryland	SB 606	October 1, 2007
Michigan	HB 5747	August 24, 2006
Minnesota	HB 1	August 1, 2005
Mississippi	HB 381	July 1, 2006
Missouri	HB 1487	August 28, 2004

(continued)

Table 17-2. US States with Antitrafficking Laws *(continued)*

State	Criminalization Statute	Effective Date
Montana	SB 385	April 2007
Nebraska	LB 1086	July 14, 2006
Nevada	AB 383	October 1, 2007
New Jersey	AB 2730	April 26, 2005
New York	SB 5902	November 1, 2007
North Carolina	HB 1896	December 1, 2006
Oregon	SB 578	June 26, 2007
Pennsylvania	HB 1112	January 9, 2007
Rhode Island	SB 692	June 27, 2007
South Carolina	HB 3060	May 2, 2006
Texas	HB 2096	September 1, 2003
Washington	HB 1175	July 27, 2003

Adapted from Center for Women Policy Studies. Fact Sheet on State Anti-Trafficking Laws from US Policy Advocacy to Combat Trafficking. Available at: http://www.centerwomenpolicy.org/documents/FactSheeton StateAntiTraffickingLawsJanuary2010.pdf. Published in January 2010. Accessed February 16, 2011.

Table 17-3. States with Legislated Statewide Interagency Task Forces on Human Trafficking

State	Statute	Effective Date
California	SB 180	September 21, 2005
Colorado	HB 1143	April 5, 2005
Connecticut	HB 5358	October 1, 2004
Hawaii	HB 2051	July 1, 2006
Idaho	HCR 8	April 1, 2005
Iowa	SF 2219	July 1, 2006
Maine	HP 893	April 28, 2006
Minnesota	HB 1	July 1, 2005
Washington	HB 2381	May 14, 2003

Adapted from Center for Women Policy Studies. Fact Sheet on State Anti-Trafficking Laws from US Policy Advocacy to Combat Trafficking. Available at: http://www.centerwomenpolicy.org/documents/FactSheeton StateAntiTraffickingLawsJanuary2010.pdf. Published in January 2010. Accessed February 16, 2011.

Immigration Relief and Psychosocial Implications

Under the TVPA, protections are provided for trafficked persons who are potential witnesses in the investigation or prosecution of human trafficking crimes. An immediate form of victim protection is Continued Presence (CP). Trafficked persons are able to obtain temporary status to stay in the United States and to legally work with a government-issued work authorization card. Also, immediate family members are able to obtain CP. Continued Presence is granted shortly after the trafficking incident and renewed annually by a federal law enforcement agency (eg, the Federal Bureau of Investigations, Immigration and Customs Enforcement), but it can be revoked at any time at the discretion of the issuing investigating federal agency. In state or local human trafficking cases, local and state law enforcement agencies cannot request CP without federal law enforcement endorsement.[44]

Nonimmigrant T-visas allow survivors to remain in the United States for a longer period of time and provide a path to permanent legal residency through a green card. The T-visa is valid for 4 years; on the third year, the survivor can apply for a green card. Under the T-visa, survivors can bring their immediate family members (also called **derivatives**) to the United States and are also eligible for green card status. Applying for the T-visa requires that adult trafficking survivors cooperate in the investigation or prosecution of their traffickers and that the survivors establish that extreme hardship will be met upon removal from the United States. T-visa provision has also been expanded to include those in the United States to assist in the investigation or prosecution of a crime, and is no longer limited to human trafficking.[45] Additionally, victims of qualifying crimes, including trafficking, are eligible for a U-visa. The qualifying crimes include "rape; torture; trafficking; incest; domestic violence; sexual assault; abusive sexual contact; prostitution; sexual exploitation; female genital mutilation; being held hostage; peonage; involuntary servitude; slave trade; kidnapping; abduction; unlawful criminal restraint; false imprisonment; blackmail; extortion; manslaughter; murder; felonious assault; witness tampering; obstruction of justice; perjury; or attempt, conspiracy, or solicitation to commit any of the above mentioned crimes."[46] U-visa holders are also eligible for employment authorization and can adjust their status after 3 years to become legal permanent residents. Legal advocates and private immigration attorneys assist victim-survivors in the T- and U-visa application processes.

Obtaining long-term immigration relief is often a lengthy process and can affect the ability of the trafficked person to participate in criminal or civil legal proceedings and to reintegrate into posttrafficking life. Oftentimes, trafficked persons' T-visa applications are delayed at the request of the investigating law enforcement agency until full adjudication of the criminal case. Requests for delay, coupled with delay in family reunification, can have an adverse psychological impact on survivors. Immigration assistance and family reunification give survivors hope. However, survivors may distrust the legal system based upon socialization within their countries of origin, where biased systems uphold the rich (and therefore powerful) and often make finding adequate representation difficult for the poor.[47] Trafficked persons who choose to pursue criminal charges or civil suits against their former traffickers can experience additional emotional trauma. The process of cooperating with law enforcement investigation and prosecution of traffickers forces victims to recount their trafficking experiences. Additionally, victims must often face their trafficker in either criminal or civil court. Due to high levels of trauma, victims may not perceive the courtroom as a safe space and may experience distrust and extreme anxiety while undergoing multiple cross-examinations.[4] These processes increase the trafficked person's risk of retraumatization.

In addition, the effects of trauma impact trafficked persons' ability to accurately recall the trafficking experience, which may be exacerbated when victims are required to testify before their recovery process is complete. Due to the extreme difficulty victims face in accepting the reality of the abuses perpetrated against them, they may unconsciously reconstruct their stories, experience amnesia, or experience alterations in memory recall as they adjust to their posttrafficking life.[42] Over time, and with supportive assistance, victims may have the ability to recall an accurate representation of historical facts; however, for some victims, this process may take a significant amount of time—a luxury not currently afforded to victims. Supportive assistance is therefore important to help trafficked persons navigate through complex and often lengthy legal proceedings.

Safety issues arise when trafficked persons choose to repatriate to their country of origin. Trafficked persons must make weighted decisions when considering their ability to return due to potential safety risks. These risks often include traffickers' knowledge of the victims' addresses in their locations of origin, threats against family members, relatives that are associated with the traffickers, or ostracization within the community due to incurred abuses, thus risking further victimization—including becoming retrafficked.

Public health issues associated with repatriation should not be overlooked. Trafficked persons who have contracted STIs (particularly HIV) may risk lack of access to medical treatment and protective barriers upon return to their communities of origin. Due to social stigma, victims may find accessibility to resources and disclosure difficult and, in some cases, dangerous. Within structured patriarchal communities, female victims may face a power imbalance making it difficult for them to negotiate safer sex practices and therefore risk future partner transmission and mother-to-child transmission.

Those who choose voluntary repatriation often return to their communities with unmet expectations of the life they dreamed they would live in the United States. The United Nations reports, "Reunification is never a return to the situation that preexisted before the trafficking incident."[48] Returning trafficked persons face adjustments related to family, psychological, safety, financial, legal, and health domains.[48] The International Organization for Migration (IOM), an intergovernmental agency, helps facilitate voluntary repatriation for trafficked persons and reintegration in their communities of origin.

Community-based organizations that provide services to trafficked persons can be referred repatriating individuals and can assist with these individuals' reintegration and access to care. One nonprofit organization in Thailand's northernmost province utilizes stabilized repatriated trafficked persons to increase education about the dangers associated with trafficking. Repatriated individuals in surrounding source countries such as China, Laos, and Cambodia were welcomed back by the nonprofit and provided education and leadership training to become antitrafficking advocates in their home communities. Creative interventions such as this counter victimization by creating constructs of meaning for victims to engage in advocacy and deter trafficking in source countries, in addition to increasing service provision for trafficked persons in hard-to-reach rural areas. While some repatriated individuals are empowered to become advocates in their home communities, many trafficked persons return with a "new normal," utilizing resiliency to engage in daily living. The adjustment of life skills is expressed among trafficked persons in a variety of contexts.

Mental Health Impacts of Trafficking

Trafficked persons have experienced high levels of trauma and may present with depression, anxiety, PTSD, and co-occurring disorders.[49] A study assessing the health needs of trafficked persons entering rehabilitation services in Europe found that over half the sample scored within the range of severe distress, indicating a possible PTSD diagnosis, while 39% of participants acknowledged suicidal thoughts within the past 7 days.[23] This finding is similar to other international studies that demonstrate increased levels of anxiety and depression, indicating that trafficked persons have profound mental health needs that necessitate immediate intervention.[50]

Research in the field of trauma supports the theory that one specific event does not cause trauma; rather, the traumatic reaction is a culmination of personal and environmental factors that either contribute to or defuse an individual's trauma reaction.[51] On one end of the spectrum would be a single traumatic incident, such as a car accident, in which the individual's experience involved "actual or threatened death or serious injury, or a threat to the physical integrity of self or others."[52] Normal childhood development and no preexisting mental health impairments would defuse the effects of the traumatic event. On the other end of the spectrum are individuals who experience pervasive (multiple and extended or chronic), invasive trauma with environmental and personal stressors. A typical trafficked person rests at this end of the spectrum, at risk for suffering severe trauma reactions due to personal, interpersonal, and environmental contributors inherent to human trafficking (see **Figure 17-2**).

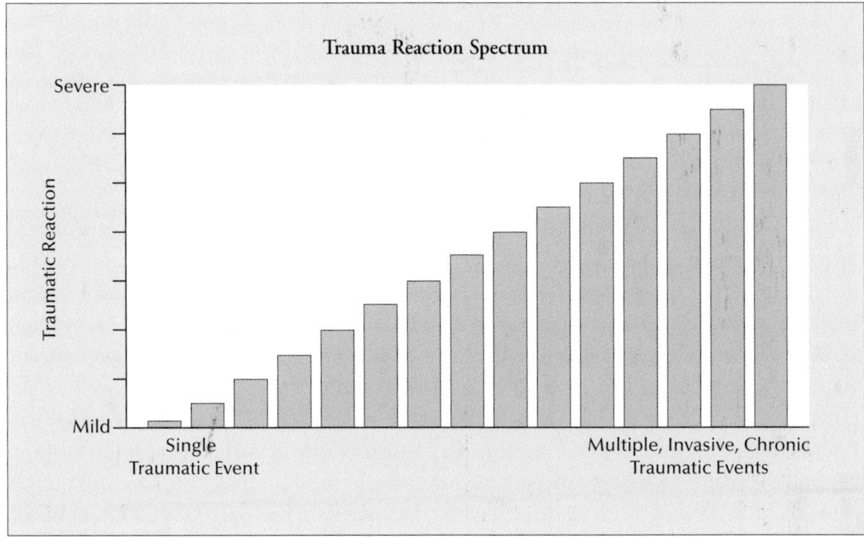

Figure 17-2. *A typical trafficked person rests at the end of the spectrum and is at risk for suffering severe trauma reactions due to personal, interpersonal, and environmental contributors inherent to human trafficking.*

Trafficking survivors may have experienced a variety of factors that increase their trauma reaction and few buffers to minimize traumatic reactions (see **Table 17-7**). Both personal and environmental factors may increase trafficked persons' traumatic reactions.

The trafficking experience, in addition to the individual's experiences prior to trafficking, have important implications for practitioners working with trafficked persons. Resiliency, or the ability to "spring back" after trauma, is impaired by a history of previous victimization, the chronic nature of a trafficking experience, the repetition of traumatic incidents, and the resulting moral dilemmas (eg, "If I escape, will my family be harmed?"), which leads to important treatment implications.[53]

Anxiety among the trafficked population is common. Panic attacks are frequent and may culminate in agoraphobia. Trafficked persons may limit their activities in public or restrict their movement to specific safe locations. This behavior helps victims to feel safe in a world perceived to be unsafe or even hostile. Over time, victims may expand their safe zone until few psychological restrictions inhibit their movement.

Trafficked persons may present with symptoms congruent with PTSD. Posttraumatic stress disorder is marked by symptoms of increased arousal, avoidance of stimuli related to the traumatic event, and reexperiencing the traumatic event. While PTSD is considered a natural response to an abnormal situation,[54] trafficked persons often wonder if they are going insane and fear they are losing control.

Table 17-7. Factors That Increase Traumatic Reaction

Personal	Environmental
— Childhood trauma	— Inadequate legal support and complicity
— Mental health disorder	— Marginalization
— Genetic predisposition	— Environmental deprivation
— Low education level	— Low socioeconomic status
— Personality	— Community violence
— Drug/alcohol use	— National disaster
— Gender status	— Inadequate social support
— Cognitive deficits	— Family violence
	— Stigma within culture regarding traumatic incident

While no empirical data exploring the relationship between chronic trauma experienced in the trafficking situation and victims' mental health are available in early 2009, a diagnosis of PTSD or acute stress disorder may not be the most appropriate diagnosis for trafficked persons who experience severe distress. Literature shows that PTSD symptomatology is not pervasive enough in its scope to account for the experiences of chronic trauma victims, whom experience trust, safety, and self-esteem issues as well as the possibility of revictimization. Posttraumatic stress disorder is classified as an anxiety disorder and, therefore, does not account for regulatory disturbances that often result from chronic trauma.[55,56] Victims experiencing interpersonal and prolonged trauma at younger ages present with symptoms associated with affect deregulation, aggression, disassociation, and somatization.[55] In relation, trafficked persons may experience chronic PTSD or disorders of extreme stress not otherwise specified (DESNOS), which is characterized by interpersonal trauma, multiple traumatic events, or prolonged trauma.[57] Disorders of extreme stress not otherwise specified have been associated with individuals with severe interpersonal trauma in a dose response.[56] Literature is unclear on whether DESNOS is a form of extreme PTSD or if it is co-morbid with PTSD.[56] DESNOS is not listed in the DSM-IV-TR as its own classification; rather, DESNOS symptoms are classified as associated features of PTSD.[57] DESNOS includes alterations in self-regulation and interpersonal functioning in 7 key areas as detailed in **Table 17-8**. Treatment for DESNOS progresses slower, has a longer duration, and calls for a more structured treatment environment than does conventional PTSD.[30]

Table 17-8. Disorders of Extreme Stress Not Otherwise Specified Characteristics

Self-Perception
— Trafficked person may view self as damaged, ie "damaged goods"
— Trafficked person may feel sense of guilt or responsibility, eg "I must have done something to deserve this" or "I trusted that person, so I am to blame."
— Trafficked person may feel a profound sense of shame

(continued)

Table 17-8. *(continued)*

DISSOCIATION
— Trafficked person may experience derealization, which is experienced as the unreality of surroundings.
— Trafficked person may experience depersonalization, which is experienced as the unreality of self, eg "I feel like I am in a dream."
EMOTIONAL SELF-REGULATION
— Trafficked person may experience reduction in the ability to control impulses, ie anger management, eating disorders
— Trafficked person may report feelings of persistent distress
— Trafficked person may engage in self-harm behaviors, eg cutting
— Trafficked person may engage in risky behaviors, eg drug use
— Trafficked person may experience strong suicidal and/or homicidal urges
SOMATIZATION
— Trafficked person may experience chronic pain in addition to symptoms that may affect or be observed to affect sexual, digestive, and cardiopulmonary domains
UNSTABLE RELATIONSHIP PATTERNS
— Trafficked person may experience distrust of others
— Trafficked person may re-create trauma by victimizing others
— Trafficked person may make self vulnerable to revictimization, such as accepting jobs with unsafe work conditions, engaging in high-risk sexual behaviors, and placing self in environments that have high risk for abuse
PERCEPTION OF PERPETRATOR(S)
— Trafficked person may adopt distorted beliefs towards the perpetrator(s)
— Trafficked person may idealize the perpetrator(s)
— Trafficked person may have revenge fantasy and sense of wanting to get even with perpetrator(s)
SHIFT IN SYSTEMS OF MEANING
— Trafficked person may experience loss of faith in previous belief, eg "How can I believe that God is good if this happened to me?" or "What did I do in a past life to deserve this?"
— Trafficked person may experience sense of hopelessness and despair for the future resulting from traumatization

Adapted from Van der Kolk B, et al.[55]

Research supports the idea that trauma experienced during childhood increases traumatic reactions later in life.[58] Furthermore, there is an association between childhood abuse and borderline personality disorder (BPD).[59] One study assessing trafficked persons reported that over half the sample experienced physical or sexual assault prior to the trafficking occurrence.[23] Due to the high levels of trauma experienced by trafficked persons, they may present with a higher incidence of borderline personality traits than the general population. Borderline personality disorder criteria overlaps with DESNOS symptomatology, making differential diagnosis a challenge—especially as these diagnoses can co-occur. Whereas DESNOS is viewed as a self-regulation disorder, BPD is viewed as a disorder resulting primarily from attachment.[57]

Interpersonal relationships can be difficult for trafficked persons to negotiate. The trafficked individual may experience difficulty trusting others due to the victimization. Trafficked persons are at risk for revictimization through engagement in unhealthy and abusive relationships that mirror exploitation inflicted by the trafficker. Sex trafficking victims may engage in independent sexual solicitation or avoid sexual expression altogether. For trafficked persons who were sexually exploited, achieving sexual health may be a challenge both psychologically and physically. Sexual health is a target for practitioners' interventions with the trafficked population, as individuals may negatively associate sexual encounters from their trafficking experience and lack pleasure in sexual activity or experience hypersexuality as a result of the abuse.

Trafficked persons are challenged by diverse stressors in the form of intrapersonal conflict, interpersonal issues, and environmental stressors. When individuals' coping ability becomes overwhelmed by emotional distress, individuals may resort to impulsive self-injurious behaviors. Acts like cutting, repetitious pinching, burning, scraping, or hair pulling may be utilized so that the trafficked person can experience painful stimuli. Tension-reduction behaviors can be understood as trauma victims' attempts to externalize their internal trauma reaction to avoid their emotional distress.[51] These acts are means by which the survivor can cope with the numbness associated with dissociation or the painful feelings that overwhelm the victim's coping capacity. Trafficked persons may also engage in coping through substance abuse. Substances overcome the numbing effects associated with traumatic responses, allowing the individual physical and emotional feeling (**Figure 17-3**).[51] Additionally, self-harm behaviors may be reenactments of the abuse experienced by trafficked persons.[42] While self-injury externalizes the victim's internal distress, this behavior is often accompanied by feelings of shame and guilt and often results in isolation.[60]

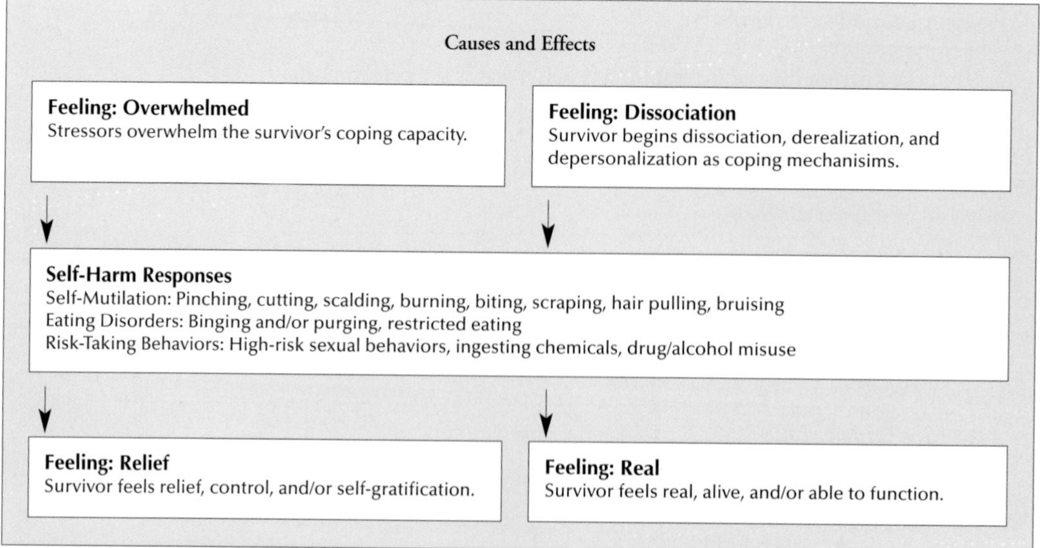

Figure 17-3. *This figure displays the different types of self-harm that a survivor may carry out and the emotions felt upon inflicting that self-harm. Adapted from: FirstSigns. What self injury is. http://www.firstsigns.org.uk/. Accessed February 16, 2011.*

Gender Differences and Trauma Reaction

While literature addressing the mental health outcomes of trafficked females is scarce, studies assessing the mental health of male victims of trafficking are virtually nonexistent. If women constitute 80% of all those trafficked, the remaining 20% are male victims. If the US Department of State statistics are correct, there should be roughly 2900 to 3500 male trafficking victims entering the United States annually.[13] Research specific to male victims of trafficking needs to be conducted to better guide practitioners, advocates, and policymakers to ensure that the identification, needs, and service delivery to male victims of trafficking are acknowledged. Currently, service provision for trafficked persons is tailored for women.

Culturally bound ideas of gender roles such as male dominance may deter trafficked males from disclosing the mental heath consequences of their trafficking experiences to others. Preconceptions of masculinity based on cultural ideas of "maleness" may also deter reporting of sexual assault within the trafficking situation. Research among the general population purports that women are twice as likely to develop PTSD sequelae from trauma than are men.[30] However, little is known about male traumatic reaction specific to trafficking. One study assessing male victims of trafficking from Eastern Europe reported that, while some men experienced depression and traumatic reactions, men showed a tendency to resist mental health treatment due to concern over confidentiality and stigma.[40]

Male victims may experience self-esteem issues related to culturally condoned ideals of being a "provider," which is grossly undermined in the trafficking situation. Male victims may feel they need to compensate for their experience by undoing what was done to them in the trafficking situation. For example, male victims may rush to join the workforce and begin sending money home so that they feel a renewed sense of productivity. Men who cannot locate work may suffer from feelings of failure and believe that they are not doing their part to help their families, which can compound the inner turmoil experienced while they were being exploited and lead to deflated self-esteem and poor self-image.

In general, males tend to utilize avoidance as a coping mechanism and develop lower levels of PTSD than women. Male trafficking victims may also rely on alcohol or illicit substances as a coping method, as substance abuse is more culturally accepted among men than sharing painful feelings.[40] Manifestation of mental health issues as physical symptoms may also occur. Additionally, male victims of sexual assault have higher levels of self-harming behaviors.[61] While self-harm has not yet been conclusively studied among male victims of trafficking, practitioners may see these behaviors.

While female victims of trafficking are often pitted against one another while being victimized,[33] male victims of trafficking may be treated differently, thereby increasing the solidarity and camaraderie among a group of trafficked men. In the writers' experience, male victims of trafficking utilize alternative coping techniques centered on ideals of community and interdependence between the victims that assist them in their recovery processes. In general, men may be more hesitant to accept services due to shame. The IOM suggests male victims may be more likely to accept assistance if it is offered by another man.[40]

Existential Task of Trafficking Survivors

Trauma has physiological, spiritual, emotional, cognitive, social, and interpersonal effects.[62] While culture impacts the way an individual will process grief and loss, the existential task that trafficked persons generally face is to assign meaning to their trafficking experience and to normalize their lives. The task of the trafficked person is to incorporate 2 polarized worldviews—that the world is a safe place and that the world is an unsafe place—into a new, healthy worldview that incorporates truths from both aspects of the individual's being.

In general, trauma victims maneuver through 3 phases in the course of their recovery. The first phase entails establishing both physical and environmental safety. In the second phase, victims focus on grieving, while the third phase marks reestablishing a normal daily life.[42] Victims who have endured chronic and extended trauma may devote a prolonged period of time to establishing safety. Repeated acts of self-harm such as suicide attempts or ideation, self-injury, substance use, eating disorders, and exploitative relationships prolong the first phase of recovery.[42]

Victims tend to either be brought closer to or driven further from their religious ties in the course of recovery as they construct meaning around their mistreatment and the resulting questions of morality (ie, "Why do bad things happen to good people?", "How can I live in a world with such hatred?", "Why did God let this happen to me?"). Spirituality can be utilized as a source of strength that may help trafficked persons to connect and integrate with their communities and ultimately aid the recovery process. For those who were manipulated using religious discourse or who were trafficked by a religious figure, spirituality may become a source of confusion. During the course of recovery, trafficked persons may come to believe that the trafficking incident was a form of punishment from their respective religious tradition. This signifies that the individual is processing the traumatic incident and incorporating it into a new worldview without denying or dissociating from the event, and this is part of the second stage of the recovery process.

All trauma involves loss, which may be primary or secondary. Secondary losses result from the primary loss in a ripple effect.[63] Trafficked persons who choose to remain in the United States may experience secondary losses related to their home communities, family members, cultures, and traditions. Trafficked persons may feel they have been uprooted and may struggle with the reality that returning to their home communities may not be safe. They may struggle with cultural stigmas associated with being a trafficking "victim" and fear or avoid disclosure, often at the cost of community engagement.

Some trafficked persons may experience cultural bereavement.[64] Originally coined for refugees forced to suddenly flee their homeland, trafficked persons may also undergo this phenomenon in which an individual experiences traumatic losses related to their culture and location of origin.[65] Alternatively, persons trafficked from marginalized groups within their communities of origin may perceive the United States as a fresh start, and feel a renewed sense of hope.

Trafficked individuals' perceptions of the trafficking event emanates from their experiences in their countries of origin. An individual's culture (race, class, ethnicity, and nationality),[66] family ties, religion, and political climate lay the foundation for the way in which the trafficked person will interpret and ultimately process the trafficking experience. Trafficked persons' cultures, when viewed as a source of strength, can be utilized to buffer stress resulting from trafficking. Trafficked persons may be able to provide examples of rituals from their cultural traditions that can be solicited, incorporated, and engaged in therapeutically by practitioners to help facilitate the healing processes.[67] Utilizing ethnographic interviewing to better understand the world from the trafficked person's points of reference is especially therapeutic, as it allows the practitioner to understand the individual's description and perception of his presenting problem. For example, one indigenous trafficked survivor from Mexico selected the word *asusto* to explain her feelings. This word, translated to English, means "scared" or, more precisely, "soul loss." When asked what this word meant to the survivor, she explained that after waking from nightmares and when thinking of her trafficking experience she would feel as if her soul was leaving her body. She would then experience great fear and at these times believed that she was going to die. Understanding the cultural beliefs that shape each individual's experience is essential to the healing process and the incorporation of culturally appropriate interventions.

Trafficked persons may choose not to engage in therapy due to associated social stigma. In general, they often feel therapy is for "crazy" people, feel uncomfortable with traditional Western talk therapy, or avoid mental health treatment due to unfamiliarity with such assistance or negative mental associations between mental health care and ideas of mental dysfunction. Education on the benefits of therapy for trauma victims is ethically optimal, but their right to self-determination must ultimately be respected. Trafficked persons may choose to seek out shaman or other natural healers for holistic healing or seek religious figures within their respective faith traditions for support. Alternative interventions, such as body movement therapy, can help trafficked persons reconnect with their bodies and reduce shame and are therapeutically and physically beneficial. Creative writing, performance, or other artistic expressions are healthy coping techniques that can be encouraged.[47] Survivor-led support groups and mentoring are especially beneficial to trafficked persons because such interventions help strengthen self-efficacy, which is often diminished within the trafficking situation. Interacting with other trafficked persons can reduce feelings of isolation and shame. Additionally, the opportunity to mentor affords stabilized trafficked persons the chance to give back based on their own lessons of loss, which is a positive, altruistic coping strategy trauma victims can employ.[64]

For trafficked persons who choose to engage in therapy, language barriers sometimes necessitate a need for interpretation services. Special care should be taken to ensure that interpreters do not impinge on clients' confidentiality and safety, especially if they are from the same ethnic community as the victim or the victim's trafficker. Interpreters create a triangulating effect within the therapeutic relationship, and should therefore be trained regarding affect regulation, direct interpreting, confidentiality, and the effects of vicarious trauma. Also, the presence of the interpreter can deter trafficked persons from engaging in trauma work, as they must recount their experience to 2 individuals instead of only to one. Use of interpretation services, while sometimes necessary, can reduce the effectiveness of the helping environment due to the nature of trafficking victims' trauma.

The final stage of recovery entails the victim's ability to "establish a new normal." In this phase, trafficked persons have processed their grief reactions and mourned the myriad primary and secondary losses resulting from their maltreatment. As a result, the trafficked person has undergone significant personal change. The individual is now ready to ascribe meaning to the trafficking experience. The individual may reinvest in self-care and begin hoping and planning for the future at this time.[42] In this stage, trafficked persons have regained the ability to trust others; interpersonal relationships have a quality of depth and intimacy that was unattainable before. In this stage, trafficked persons come to understand that trauma is irreversible.[42] Trafficked persons may become motivated to engage in advocacy or may hold their trafficker accountable through civil recourse.

Physical Health Impacts of Trafficking

Physical health concerns trafficked persons present with are similar to those experienced by domestic violence victims, sweatshop workers, seasonal workers, internally displaced persons (IDPs), and torture victims.[26] Trafficked persons may present to the medical practitioner with infectious diseases such as hepatitis or tuberculosis or with STIs, including HIV, and may also present with external injuries caused by physical assault or neglect.

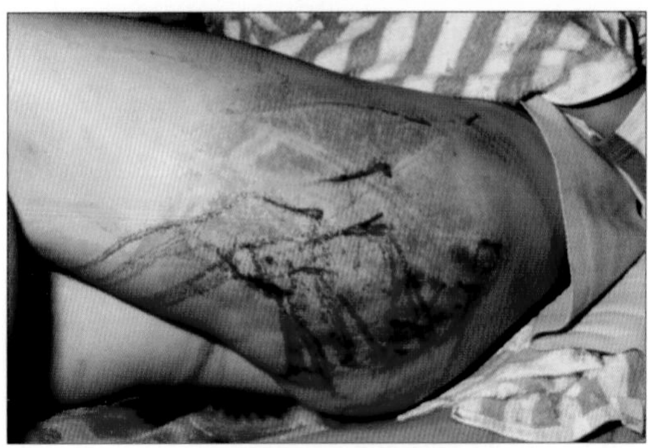

Figure 17-4. *This woman has lacerations on her left upper thigh after being severely beaten with a wire coat hanger as punishment for her disobedience to the trafficker. Provided with permission by Detective Rick Castro.*

Physical Injuries

Traffickers frequently use violence as a means to control trafficked persons, causing them to present with signs of physical abuse. Sex trafficking victims may show signs of physical assault in areas of their body that do not alter their physical appearance, such as the lower back.[38] **Figure 17-4** depicts a woman who was severely beaten with a wire coat hanger as punishment for her disobedience to the trafficker. This beating was carried out in front of other female trafficking victims, reinforcing the dominance of the perpetrator to the witnesses as well as to the victim suffering the abuse. Her injuries included lacerations on her left upper thigh, an area easily concealed by clothing.

The experience of this victim is not an isolated incident; rather, trafficker-perpetrated violence, as a means to instill fear and maintain control, is a global trend that victims of human trafficking encounter. For example, a trafficking survivor in Thailand gave the following report:

> We talked about running away. But, we couldn't see any possibility because we didn't know where we could run to, how far from our home we were. We also worried that if they knew that we were planning to run away they would kill us, because they always said that they would kill us if we did not obey them. One girl they burnt her face with a hot iron.[26]

Other signs of physical abuse include cigarette burns[32] and chemical or heated liquid burns (eg, boiling water). Studies suggest trafficked persons often present with trauma to the head[33] resulting from head bashing, falls from being shoved, and beatings with household appliances. Therefore, diagnosing possible untreated internal injuries is an important intervention for health care practitioners.

Labor trafficking victims are forced to work in high-risk environments. Due to these sub-standard conditions, individuals may present with muscle and joint pain in addition to severe injuries.[4,68] Unregulated work environments, such as trafficking for sweatshops and construction work, expose individuals to unsafe chemicals, broken bones, heat stroke, skin damage, stab wounds, oral injuries, skin infections, and respiratory disease.[4] Within the agricultural sector, trafficked persons are exposed to high levels of pesticides and chemicals that have been linked to depression, headaches, and neurological disorders.[40]

Victims may have been subjected to inadequate living conditions for prolonged periods and, therefore, may present with a variety of physical symptoms of neglect. In general, trafficking victims' environment is controlled, meaning that their access to basic needs is limited by the volition of the trafficker. Victims may have food withheld, may be subjected to inadequate diets, and may experience sleep deprivation. Additionally, they may experience overcrowding and improper sanitation.[4] These abuses, over a prolonged period, may have a significant physical impact, increasing trafficked persons' vulnerability to illness.[4]

Trafficking pulls from vulnerable populations within societies. Due to a lack of access to medical care and treatment in countries of origin and within the trafficking situation, trafficked persons may present with a variety of chronic care needs. Trafficked persons may not have had access to immunizations in their countries of origin, increasing disease prevalence.[4] Human trafficking often circumvents formal migration channels; therefore, trafficked persons may have a higher prevalence of tuberculosis, malaria, hepatitis, and other infectious diseases.

Sexual Health

While being victimized, individuals often lack the ability to negotiate for safer sex practices. Therefore, STIs among the trafficking population are overwhelmingly common.[69] Even when condoms are available for use, trafficked persons may not utilize them for all high-risk behaviors due to a lack of education. Additionally, customers may pay higher prices for not wearing a condom, thus reducing the trafficked persons' ability to negotiate for safer sex.[26] One study found the majority of female trafficking victims reported experiencing pelvic pain, vaginal discharge, and gynecological infections, with pain ranging in intensity from little to extreme discomfort.[23]

The United Nations and World Health Organization have identified trafficking victims as a population at increased risk for HIV infection.[70] Internationally based human trafficking studies cite high levels of HIV prevalence in developing countries including India, Nepal,[7,71] and within Southeast Asia.[72] No statistics are available that quantify HIV transmission and human trafficking within the United States; however, trafficked persons are at an increased risk for HIV seroconversion due to the inherent nature of trafficking. CDC data suggests HIV seroconversion for persons who experience sexual assault alone is low[73]; however, trauma resulting from violent intercourse and repeat exposure through multiple partners increases HIV prevalence.[73] Additionally, the presence of other STIs increases victims' susceptibility to seroconversion.[70] In one health study, HIV-positive trafficked persons in Southeast Asia were shown to have higher co-morbidities with hepatitis B and syphilis than trafficked persons not infected with HIV.[23]

Trafficked persons may be at increased risk for HIV and other STIs not only because of sexual abuse, but also because of psychological conditions resulting from that abuse. Individuals with a history of trauma are at an increased risk for HIV transmission due to their likely engagement in higher-risk behavior. In general, trafficked persons have little to no education in regards to safer sex practices. In one study, half of the individuals self-reported having little to no knowledge about STIs before they were trafficked.[26] Therefore, trafficked persons benefit from continued education regarding STIs, safer sex practices, and reproductive health. For example, a group of trafficked persons attending a reproductive health workshop expressed that seeing a model of their reproductive organs was their first exposure to those elements of their anatomy.

Trafficked persons who are HIV-positive may struggle with the stigma of that diagnosis, which may be exacerbated by socialization within communities of origin. For example, a study in Mexico reported that 57% of respondents divulged that they would not live in the same house with someone who had HIV/AIDS.[74] Additionally, trafficked persons may feel that they have been given a death sentence due to observations of those with HIV in their home communities and lack of access to treatment. Trafficked persons may have a variety of misconceptions regarding HIV and may benefit from bolstered support, education, and assistance in accessing resources, including treatment options.

After trafficking, individuals may resist STI testing due to potential marginalization within their respective communities. Additionally, trafficked persons may fear testing due to retraumatization. They may negatively associate gynecological care with abuses incurred within the trafficking situation, as trafficked persons sometimes undergo painful gynecological procedures and are subsequently forced to return to work without adequate recovery time. Furthermore, trafficked persons may have been subject to forced and unsanitary procedures. A study of 55 sex workers in Israel, half of whom were trafficked, found that more than half of the sample underwent at least one abortion.[50] For trafficked persons who experienced invasive traumas that may include unwanted pregnancies, forced abortion, repeated sexual assault, and inadequate or unsanitary health care, accepting health care postemancipation may pose challenges.

Patience in educating the individual and following the trafficked person's lead to minimize risk to self or others until the individual chooses testing ultimately benefits trafficked persons most. When an individual accepts medical testing, returning as much control as possible to the trafficked persons is paramount, as the individual is ultimately surrendering bodily control into the hands of another they may distrust. Negotiating a way for the trafficked person to stop the procedure if she becomes distressed and talking the individual through the procedure supports the individual both physically and emotionally. Utilizing this collaborative approach to care empowers the trafficked person by returning control and enables the individual to regain body autonomy.

Sexual Assault Forensic Exam

In the writers' experience, most trafficked persons do not undergo forensic sexual assault examinations, and other reports also indicate that sexual assault forensic exams related to human trafficking cases are infrequent (C. Nelli, personal communication, May 2009). When exams are conducted, they often involve only single victims and a known perpetrator, such as in a domestic servitude case where the victim is sexually assaulted by the trafficker or by a member of the trafficker's family. Lack of documentation on trafficked persons who may have undergone forensic exams is one barrier to identifying possible benefits of this exam for trafficked persons.

The greatest benefit of a forensic exam is to establish a criminal case against the trafficker or other abuser. Exams forensically confirm and document that a sexual encounter has occurred and examine physical abuse such as cigarette burns, current or past bruising, and branding (eg, tattoos, other types of marks of ownership). However, trafficked persons who experience multiple sexual encounters over a prolonged period do not typically benefit from such an exam, as their abuse is not due to one particular incident of sexual assault or rape. Rather, trafficked persons have experienced prolonged periods of sustained abuse by their trafficker and those procured by the trafficker. As exams are intrusive and can be an overwhelming experience, trafficked persons should be told that having one is optional.

Language, culture, and disabilities can hinder the ability of trafficked persons to fully participate in the sexual assault exam process. Some may feel embarrassed, scared, or overwhelmed by the exam's tools and procedures for evidence collection. Inclusion of properly vetted translators before, during, and after the exam should be considered for trafficked persons whose English is limited or nonexistent.

Health Consequences of Trafficking

Injuries suffered by trafficking victims and the resulting physical and mental health consequences are pervasive. They range in severity from chronic symptomatologies to death. Trafficked persons must negotiate the compounded health consequences from their exploitation into their posttrafficking lives (**Table 17-9**).

Table 17-9. Trafficking in Women: Health Consequences and Forms of Risk and Abuse

Forms of Risk and Abuse	Potential Health Consequences
Physical Abuse	**Physical Health**
— Murder — Physical attacks (beating with or without an object, kicking, knifing, whipping, and gunshots)	— Death — Acute and chronic physical injuries (contusions, lacerations, head trauma, concussion, scarring)

(continued)

Table 17-9. *(continued)*

Forms of Risk and Abuse	Potential Health Consequences
Physical Abuse *(continued)*	**Physical Health** *(continued)*
— Torture (ice-baths, cigarette burns, suspension, salt in wounds) — Physical deprivation (sleep, food, light, basic necessities) — Physical restraint (ropes, cuffs, chains) and confinement — Withholding medical or other essential care	— Acute and chronic physical disabilities, (nerve, muscle, or bone damage; sensory damage, dental problems) — Fatigue, exhaustion — Poor nutrition, malnutrition, starvation — Deterioration of preexisting conditions leading to disability or death
Sexual Abuse	**Sexual and Reproductive Health**
— Forced vaginal, oral, or anal sex; gang rape; degrading sexual acts — Forced prostitution, inability to control number or acceptance of clients — Forced unprotected sex and sex without lubricants — Unwanted pregnancy, forced abortion, unsafe abortion — Sexual humiliation, forced nakedness — Coerced misuse of oral contraceptives or other contraceptive methods	— HIV/AIDS — Sexually transmitted infections (STIs) and related complications, including pelvic inflammatory disease (PID), urinary tract infections (UTIs), cystitis, cervical cancer, and infertility — Amenorrhea and dysmenorrhea — Acute or chronic pain during sex; tearing and other damage to vaginal tract — Negative outcomes of unsafe abortion, including cervical incontinence, septic shock; unwanted birth — Irritable bowel syndrome, stress-related syndromes — Inability to negotiate sexual encounters
Psychological Abuse	**Mental Health**
— Intimidation of and threats to women and their loved ones — Lies, deception, and blackmail to coerce women, to discourage women from seeking help from authorities or others; lies about authorities, local situation, legal status, family members — Emotional manipulation by boyfriend-perpetrator — Unpredictable and uncontrollable events and environment — Isolation and forced dependency (see "social restrictions and manipulation")	— Suicidal thoughts, self-harm, suicide — Chronic anxiety, sleep disturbances, frequent nightmares, chronic fatigue, diminished coping capacity — Memory loss, memory defects, dissociation — Somatic complaints (eg chronic headache, stomach pain, trembling), immune suppression — Depression, frequent crying, withdrawal, difficulty concentrating — Aggressiveness, violent outbursts, violence against others — Substance misuse, addiction — Loss of trust in others or self, problems with or changes in identity and self-esteem, guilt, shame, difficulty developing and maintaining intimate relationships

(continued)

Table 17-9. Trafficking in Women: Health Consequences and Forms of Risk and Abuse *(continued)*

Forms of Risk and Abuse	Potential Health Consequences
Forced and Coerced Use of Drugs and Alcohol	**Substance Abuse and Misuse**
— Nonconsensual administration and coercive use of alcohol or drugs in order to: — Abduct, rape, prostitute women — Control activities, coerce compliance, impose long work hours, coerce women to engage in degrading or dangerous acts — Decrease self-protective defenses, increase compliance — Prevent women from leaving or escaping	— Overdose, self-harm, death, suicide — Participation in unwanted sexual acts, unprotected and high-risk sexual acts, high-risk activities, violence, crime — Addiction — Brain or liver damage, including precancerous conditions — Needle-introduced infection, including HIV and hepatitis C — Dependence on drugs, alcohol, or cigarettes to cope with abuse, stress, anxiety, and fear, work, long hours, pain, and personal disgust; cold and physical deprivation, insomnia, fatigue
Social Restrictions and Manipulation	**Social Well-Being**
— Restrictions on movement, time, and activities; confinement; surveillance; manipulative scheduling in order to restrict contact with others and formation of helping relationships — Frequent relocation — Absence of social support, denial or loss of contact with family, friends, ethnic and local community — Emotional manipulation by boyfriends-perpetrators — Favoritism or perquisites with the goal of causing divisiveness between coworkers and discouraging formation of friendships — Denial of or control over access to health and other services — Denial of privacy or control over privacy	— Feelings of isolation, loneliness, exclusion — Inability to establish and maintain helping or supportive relationships, mistrust of others, social withdrawal, personal insecurity — Poor overall health from lack of exercise, healthy socializing, health-promoting activities — Vulnerability to infection from lack of information, deteriorating conditions from restricted health screening, lack of treatment — Vulnerability to infection and abuse due to restricted access to work advice from peers — Difficulty with (re)integration, difficulty developing healthy relationships, feelings of loneliness, alienation, helplessness, aggressiveness — Shunned, rejected by family, community, society, boyfriends — Retrafficked, reentry into high-risk labor and relationships

(continued)

Table 17-9. *(continued)*

Forms of Risk and Abuse	Potential Health Consequences
Economic Exploitation and Debt Bondage	**Economic Related Well-Being**
— Indentured servitude resulting from inflated debt — Usurious charges for travel documents, housing, food, clothing, condoms, health care, other basic necessities — Usurious and deceptive accounting practices, control over and confiscation of earnings — Resale of women and renewal of debts — Turning women over to immigration or police to prevent them from collecting wages — Forced or coerced acceptance of long hours, large numbers of clients, and sexual risks in order to meet financial demands	— Inability to afford: — Basic hygiene, nutrition, safe housing — Condoms, contraception, lubricants — Gloves, protective gear for factory work or domestic service — Pharmaceuticals (over-the-counter or prescription) — General health care, reproductive health care, prenatal care, safe termination of pregnancy (TOP) — Heightened vulnerability to STIs, infections, work-related injuries from high-risk work practices — Potentially dangerous self-medication or foregoing of medication — Punishment (eg physical abuse, financial penalties) for not earning enough or for withholding tips or earnings — Physical or economic retribution for trying to escape (eg, abduction of other female family members to pay off debts) — Rejection by family for not sending money or returning home without money
Legal Insecurity	**Legal Security**
— Restrictive laws limiting routes of legal migration and independent employment — Confiscation by traffickers or employers of travel documents, passports, tickets, other vital documents — Threats by traffickers or employers to expose women to authorities in order to coerce women to perform dangerous or high-risk activities — Concealment of women's legal status from the women themselves — Health providers requiring identity documents	— Acceptance of dangerous travel conditions, dependency on traffickers and employers during travel and work relationships — Arrest, detention, long periods in immigration detention centers or prisons; unhygienic, unsafe detention conditions — Inability or difficulty obtaining treatment from public clinics and other medical services — Anxiety or trauma as a result of interrogation, cross-examination, or participation in a criminal investigation or trial — Deportation to unsafe, insecure locations; risk of retrafficking and retribution — Ill health or deterioration of health problems as a result of reluctance to use health and other support services

(continued)

Table 17-9. Trafficking in Women: Health Consequences and Forms of Risk and Abuse *(continued)*

Forms of Risk and Abuse	Potential Health Consequences
High-risk, Abusive Working and Living Conditions	**Occupational and Enviromental Health**
— Abusive work hours, practices — Dangerous work and living conditions (including unsafe, unhygienic, overcrowded, or poorly ventilated spaces) — Work-related penalties and punishment — Abusive work employer-employee relationships, lack of personal safety — Abusive interpersonal social and coworker relationships — Nonconsensual marketing, sale, and exploitation of women	— Vulnerability to infection, parasites (lice, scabies), communicable diseases — Exhaustion and poor nutrition — Injuries and anxiety as a result of exploitation by employers, risky and dangerous work conditions — Injuries and anxiety as a result of domestic or boyfriend-pimp abuse

Reprinted with permission by Cathy Zimmerman, PhD, MSc, MA from Zimmerman C, Yun K, Watts C, et al. The Health Risks and Consequences of Trafficking in Women and Adolescents; Findings from a European Study. *London, England: London School of Hygiene and Tropical Medicine (LSHTM); 2003.*

Trauma-Informed Practice

Some trafficked persons experience violence within their families, communities, or violence motivated by political issues after their trafficking episodes. Gushulak and MacPherson note that, "Individuals who have been subjected to violence may have consequential health or medical problems, both organic and psychological, that may be exacerbated by trafficking."[75] Operating from a trauma-informed model of care is imperative,[49] as survivors often experience multiple forms of abuse that have physiological ramifications. For example, arthritis and diabetes are associated with trauma in men.[76] Among women, both cancer and digestive diseases are linked to trauma.[76] Posttraumatic stress disorder is associated with an increased health risk for cardiac, respiratory, nervous, and digestive diseases, as well as arthritis.[76] Additionally, PTSD has a high rate of comorbidity with somatization and substance abuse.[77] Substance abuse before, during the trafficking situation, and after exiting the trafficking environment should be assessed. Trafficked persons may present with health concerns related to smoking and alcohol consumption, which have been utilized as coping methods.[40] In extreme cases, drug or alcohol detoxification may be necessary.[69]

Cultural Competency

Cultural competency is an important consideration in providing medical treatment.[23] A study found that trafficked persons utilizing medical clinics in the United Kingdom felt discriminated against and blamed by practitioners.[26] Providers may become frustrated when trafficked persons tell practitioners what the trafficked person thinks the clinician wants to hear rather than providing actual symptoms. Trafficked persons need to feel secure in the helping environment[4]; therefore, ethnic identity factors that incorporate cultural value should be included in health care practice.[64] Trafficked persons may not perceive Western health practice as what they need for their ailment. Additionally, trafficked persons may take longer to trust health services due to unfamiliarity with service provision.[4] Trafficked persons may feel more comfortable engaging in non-

Western techniques such as acupuncture, acupressure, cupping, Reiki, herbal teas, natural vitamin supplements, and reflexology. Awareness of how such techniques can complement mainstream medical care can help the provider in facilitating the trafficked persons access to holistic health, thus helping to establish trust with trafficked persons by creating a supportive professional relationship.

Self-Care

Practitioners engaging with the human trafficking population should be aware of the pervasive effects of vicarious trauma, which those assisting traumatized populations are prone. As a helper empathically engages with a traumatized individual, the fear, horror, and intense helplessness the traumatized individual experienced can transfer over, thereby vicariously traumatizing the helper. Symptoms characteristic of a traumatized individual include difficulty trusting, a shift in worldview, fear, hyperarousal, numbing, avoidance of stimuli related to traumatic events, and reoccurring thoughts and imagery are typical to both the traumatized and the vicariously traumatized. Vicarious trauma affects a practitioner's personal life by altering an individual's perception of the world. Alterations may include "the ability to manage strong feelings, maintain a positive sense of self and connect to others; and in spirituality or sense of meaning, expectation, awareness, and connection; as well as in basic needs and schemata about safety, esteem, trust and dependency, control and intimacy."[78]

Untreated vicarious trauma has professional ramifications. Within the workplace, vicarious trauma can include a loss of objectivity, attempts to rescue the client, difficulty problem solving, and blurring of professional boundaries.[42] In addition, vicarious trauma can be an ethical dilemma, as unresolved vicarious trauma can negatively impact the helping relationship by undermining a helper's ability to be present with the client in their trauma.[78] It can also lead to the helper literally abandoning the client.[42] Over time, symptoms may escalate to burnout, premature resignation, or feelings of professional failure.[79]

Coping techniques to minimize vicarious traumatic reactions include humor, exercise, recreational activity, spirituality, a supportive work environment, supportive friends, therapy, and support groups. Within the workplace, the use of supervision, self-care, social support, and training counteracts vicarious trauma symptomatology.[80] The most important coping technique practitioners can utilize is balance within the workplace as time spent in direct contact with trafficked persons is significantly correlated with symptoms of vicarious trauma.[81]

Trafficked persons bear witness to the art of human resiliency. Many navigate through trauma and loss to live lives different than ever imagined. Many are reunited with their family members, are able to obtain and hold formal jobs, and experience psychological healing. Trafficked persons' strength should ultimately be a beacon for practitioners in our own struggles to minimize the effects of vicarious trauma within our respective practices (see **Table 17-10**).

Conclusion

Human trafficking is a dynamic crime that calls for dynamic solutions. The anti-trafficking field—at least in the United States—needs more empirical data to better inform practitioners. The trafficking field is in continuous development of promising practices for victim response and service model approaches to comprehensive care that encompass the unique legal, safety, medical, educational, and mental health needs of trafficked persons. Data from a 2008 national survey of reported incidents from January 1, 2007 to September 30, 2008 on law enforcement responses to human trafficking support the importance of multiagency task forces for identifying and investigating human trafficking incidents. Multiagency task forces tended to have response protocols and procedures in place, more investigations (36 on average by task forces compared to 15 on average by non–task force agencies), more arrests (12 by task forces compared to 8 by non–task force agencies), and more cases resulting in formal charges that were identified by local law enforcement (75% of task force agency cases compared to 45% non–task force agency cases) and were twice as likely to result in federal charges (55% versus 25% for non–task force agencies).[82]

Collaboration is essential in addressing the crime of human trafficking. Sexual assault victim advocates, domestic violence victim advocates, sexual assault forensic nurse examiners, various health care professionals, law enforcement officers, and other community social services providers are important agents in identifying and assisting trafficked persons. Promising practices include establishing a proactive multiagency task force that provides training to its members and outreach to the target population through each participating agency's existing service protocols and procedures. The development of model task force response protocols and procedures and an increased understanding and continuous dialogue of human trafficking legal and definition issues are additional promising practices.[82]

Table 17-10. Additional Resources

ORGANIZATIONS

Department of Justice Worker Exploitation and Trafficking
Complaint Line: 1-888-428-7581. The department can assist practitioners if a potential victim of trafficking is identified.

Department of Human Services (DHHS) Rescue & Restore Campaign
DHHS has toolkits available at http://www.acf.hhs.gov/trafficking/. They also manage a 24-hour National Human Trafficking Resource Center: 1-888-373-7888.

World Health Organization (WHO)
WHO has published guidelines for interviewing trafficking survivors, entitled "WHO Ethical and Safety Recommendations for Interviewing Trafficked Women" available at http://www.who.int/gender/documents/en/final%20recommendations%2023%20oct.pdf.

Family Violence Prevention Fund
This organization has a report on human trafficking geared for health care practitioners entitled "Turning Pain into Power: Trafficking Survivors Perspectives on Early Intervention Strategies" available at http://www.endabuse.org/programs/immigrant/files/PaintoPower.pdf.

Free the Slaves and the Human Rights Center
Downloadable report on Human Trafficking, entitled "Hidden Slaves: Forced Labor in the United States;" available at: http://www.hrcberkeley.org/download/hiddenslaves_report.pdf.

BOOKS

Rothshild B, Rand M. *Help for the Helper: The Psychology of Compassion Fatigue and Vicarious Trauma.* New York, NY: W.W. Norton & Company, Inc; 2006.

Bryant-Davis T. *Thriving in the Wake of Trauma: A Multicultural Guide.* Westport, CT: Praeger Publishers; 2005.

Members of a multiagency task force embody their discipline's respective philosophies of criminal and victim directed interventions. For example, law enforcement agencies may find the presence of a legal advocate unnecessary during a trafficked person's interview, though a legal advocate's presence may be necessary to ensure that the rights of the trafficked person are respected, especially if the trafficked person is foreign-born or a legal permanent resident. At times, differing philosophies present barriers to collaboration and can hinder formation of positive working relationships.

Building relationships of trust, respecting one another's varied roles and responsibilities, and maintaining systems accountability are important steps in creating an effective response to the crime of human trafficking and ensuring the well being of trafficked persons.[83] We know from practical experience that human trafficking often leaves its victims physically, psychologically, and spiritually broken. Therefore, an empowerment approach that is culturally sensitive and centered on the needs of trafficked persons is critical to overcoming the diverse challenges inherent in the crime of human trafficking.

REFERENCES

1. United Nations. The Universal Declaration of Human Rights. http://www.un.org/en/documents/udhr. Accessed May 27, 2009.
2. Cameron S, Newman E. Introduction: Understanding human trafficking. In: Cameron S, Newman E, eds. *Trafficking in Human$: Social Cultural and Political Dimensions*. Tokyo, Japan: United Nations University Press; 2008.
3. Gozdziak E, Collett E. Research on human trafficking in North America: a review of literature. *Int Migration*. 2005;43:99-128.
4. Bales K, Fletcher L, Stover E. *Hidden Slaves: Forced Labor in the United States*. Washington DC: University of California, Berkeley; 2004.
5. International Labor Organization. *A Global Alliance Against Forced Labor*. Geneva, Switzerland: International Labor Office; 2005:12.
6. Silverman J, Decker M, Gupta J, Maheshwari A, Patel V, Raj A. HIV prevalence and predictors among rescued sex-trafficked women and girls in Mumbai, India. Epidemiology and social science. *J Acquired Immune Defic Syndrome*. 2006;43:588-593.
7. World Health Organization. Health of migrants. *Secretariat Report*. EB122/11; 2007.
8. Bales K. *Disposable People*. Berkeley, CA: University of California Press; 2004.
9. Shigekane R. Rehabilitation and community integration of trafficking survivors in the United States. *Human Rights Q*. 2007;29:112-136.
10. Buckland B. More than just victims: the truth about human trafficking. *Public Policy Res*. 2008;15:42-47.
11. Bales K. *Understanding Global Slavery: A Reader*. Berkeley, CA: University of California Press: 2005.
12. United Nations Office on Drugs and Crime. http://www.unodc.org/undoc/en/human-trafficking/faqs.html. Accessed May 31, 2009.
13. US Department of State Trafficking in Persons (TIP) Report. Washington, DC: US Dept of State; 2006-2008.

14. Rape Abuse Incest National Network. STOP the Violence, Break the Silence: Sexual Assault Against Individuals with Disabilities [Webinar]. http:// www.rainn train.org/course/view.php?id=35. Accessed May 21, 2009.

15. King G. *Woman, Child for Sale: The New Slave Trade in the 21st Century*. New York, NY: Chamberlain Press; 2004.

16. US Department of Justice. Characteristics of Suspected Incidents, 2007-2008. Washington, DC: US Dept of Justice; 2009.

17. Los Angeles Metro Task Force on Human Trafficking (LAMTF-HT). Los Angeles Police Department Robbery Homicide Division.

18. The Protocol to Prevent, Suppress, and Punish Trafficking in Persons, Especially Women and Children. www2.ohchr.org/english/law/protocoltraffic.htm. Accessed May 30, 2009.

19. Trafficking Victims Protection Act (2000) Pub. L. No. 106-386, 114 Stat. 1473.

20. Trafficking Victims Protection Act, Pub. L. 106-386, Section 103.

21. US Department of Health and Human Services. The Campaign to Rescue & Restore Victims of Human Trafficking. Washington, DC: US Dept of Health and Human Services. http://www.acf.hhs.gov/trafficking/about/index.html. Accessed October 14, 2009.

22. US Department of Justice. Bureau of Justice Assistance. BJA Program Initiatives Information Sheet. Washington, DC: US Dept of Justice; 2008.

23. Zimmerman C, Hossain M, Yun K, et al. The health of trafficked women: a survey of women entering posttrafficking services in Europe. *Am J Public Health*. 2008;98(1):55-59.

24. Su J. El Monte Thai Garment Workers: Slave Sweatshops. Sweatshop Watch. http://www.sweatshopwatch.org/index.php?s=68. Accessed June 6, 2008.

25. US Department of Justice. Labor Contractor Admits He Enslaved African-American Worker in Florida, Pleads Guilty to Federal Charges [Press Release]. http://www.usdoj.gov/opa/pr/2001/February/069crt.htm. Published February 15, 2001. Accessed June 15, 2008.

26. Zimmerman C, Yun K, Watts C, et al. The Health Risks and Consequences of Trafficking in Women and Adolescents: Findings from a European Study. London, England: London School of Hygiene and Tropical Medicine (LSHTM); 2003.

27. Tudorache D. General considerations on the psychological aspects of the trafficking phenomenon. In: Schinina G, Guthmiller A, Nikolovska M, O'Flaherty L, Janskijevic I, eds. *Psychosocial Support to Groups of Victims of Human Trafficking in Transit Situations*. Geneva, Switzerland: International Organization for Migration (IOM); 2004.

28. Herman J. *Trauma and Recovery: The Aftermath of Violence—From Domestic Abuse to Political Terror*. New York, NY: BasicBooks; 1997.

29. Biderman's Chart of Coercion. http://www.nwrain.net/~refocus/coerchrt.html. Accessed February 1, 2009.

30. Haley J, Stein W, Kittleson M, ed. *The Truth About Abuse*. New York, NY: Book Builders LLC; 2005.

31. Bales K. The social psychology of modern slavery. *Sci Am.* 2002;286:80-88.

32. Aghatise E. Trafficking for prostitution in Italy: possible effects of government proposals for legalization of brothels. *Violence Against Women.* 2004;10:1124-1155.

33. Turning Pain into Power: Trafficking Survivors Perspectives on Early Intervention Strategies. San Francisco, CA: Family Violence Prevention Fund; 2005.

34. *Dreams Die Hard: Survivors of Slavery in America Tell Their Stories* [DVD]. Free the Slaves and Crisis House; 2005.

35. US Attorneys Office. Five Defendants Convicted of International Sex Trafficking for Forcing Guatemalan Girls and Women into Prostitution [Press Release]. http://www.justice.gov/usao/cac/pressroom/pr2009/011.html. Accessed January 25, 2010.

36. US Department of Justice Part V. Halting Human Trafficking with a Record Number of Successful Investigations and Prosecutions FY 2001-2005. US Department of Justice. http://www.ojp.usdoj.gov/bjs/abstract/fpht05.htm. Accessed May 10, 2008.

37. Gajic-Veljanoski O, Stewart D. Women trafficked into prostitution: determinants, human rights and health needs. *Transcultural Psychiatry.* 2007;44:338-359.

38. US Department of Health and Human Services. Look Beneath the Surface: Role of Healthcare Providers in Identifying and Helping Victims of Human Trafficking [Rescue & Restore Campaign Tool Kits PowerPoint Presentation for Health Care Providers]. http://www.acf.hhs.gov/trafficking/campaign_kits/index.html. Accessed January 25, 2010.

39. Hughes D. *Hiding in Plain Sight: A Practical Guide to Identifying Victims of Trafficking in the U.S.* http://www.uri.edu/artsci/wms/hughes/hiding_in_plain_sight.pdf. Published October 2003. Accessed January 25, 2010.

40. Surtees R. *Trafficking of Men—A Trend Less Considered: The Case of Belarus and Ukraine.* Geneva, Switzerland: International Organization for Migration (IOM); 2008.

41. US Department of State. US Agents Crack West Coast Human Smuggling, Trafficking Ring [Press Release]. http://www.america.gov/st/washfile-english/2005/July/20050701182254cmretrop0.2110865.html. Published July 2005. Accessed January 25, 2010.

42. Herman J. Recovery from psychological trauma. *Psychiatry Clin Neurosci.* 1998;52:145-150.

43. Green L, Burke G. Beyond self-actualization. *J Health Human Serv Administration.* 2007;30(2):116-128.

44. 22 USC §§ 7102, 7105.

45. 22 USC §§ 7105 (c) (3), 1595.

46. National Network to End Violence Against Women. U Visa Interim Regulations Fact Sheet and Guidance. http://www.povertylawsection.com/uploads/U_Visa_Bulleted_Summary.pdf. Accessed January 25, 2010.

47. Bryant-Davis T. *Thriving in the Wake of Trauma: A Multicultural Guide.* Westport, CT: Praeger Publishers; 2005.

48. United Nations Office on Drugs and Crime. Toolkit to Combat Trafficking in Persons. Vienna, Austria: Vienna International Center; 2006.

49. Clawson H, Salomon A, Goldblatt G. Treating the Hidden Wounds: Trauma Treatment and Mental Health Recovery for Victims of Human Trafficking. US Department of Health and Human Services. http://aspe.hhs.gov/hsp/07/Human Trafficking/Treating/ib.htm. Accessed May 11, 2008.

50. Chudakov B, Ilan K, Belmaker R, Cwikel J. The motivation and mental health of sex workers. *J Sex Marital Ther*. 2002;28:305-315.

51. Briere J, Spinazzola J. Phenomenology and psychological assessment of complex posttraumatic states. *J Trauma Stress*. 2005;18:401-412.

52. American Psychiatric Association. *Diagnostic and Statistical Manual of Mental Disorders-DSM-IV-TR*. Arlington, VA: American Psychiatric Association; 2000.

53. Danis F. Introductory Workshop on Crime Victims' Rights and Service Trainer's Manual. US Department of Justice, Office of Victims of Crime. Texas: NASW;2006. http://www.ojp.usdoj.gov/ovc/assist/NASW_Kit/pdf/01_trainer_manual.pdf. Accessed October 12, 2008.

54. Parkinson F. *Post-trauma Stress: A Personal Guide to Reduce the Long-term Effects and Hidden Emotional Damage Caused by Violence and Disaster*. 2nd ed. Cambridge, MA: DeCapo Press; 2000.

55. Van der Kolk B, Roth S, Pelcovitz D, Sunday S, Spinazzola J. Disorders of extreme stress: the empirical foundation of a complex adaptation to trauma. *J Trauma Stress*. 2005;18:389-399.

56. Ford J, Stockton P, Kaltman S, Green B. Disorders of extreme stress (DESNOS) symptoms are associated with type and severity of interpersonal trauma exposure in a sample of healthy young women. *J Interpersonal Violence*. 2006;21:1399-1416.

57. Luxenburg T, Spinazzola J, Hidalgo J, Hunt C, VanderKolk B. Complex trauma and disorders of extreme stress (DESNOS) diagnosis, Part one: assessment. *Dir Psychiatry*. 2001;21:373-393. http://www.traumacenter.org/products/pdf_files/DESNOS.pdf. Accessed June 6, 2008.

58. Ford K, Kidd P. Early childhood trauma and disorders of extreme stress as predictors of treatment outcome with chronic posttraumatic stress disorder. *J Trauma Stress*. 1998;11-2:743-761.

59. Modestin J, Furrer R, Malti T. Different traumatic experiences are associated with different pathologies. *Psychiatr Q*. 2005;76:19-32.

60. Hicks MK, Hinck SM. Concept analysis of self-mutilation. *J Adv Nurs*. 2008; 64(4):408-413.

61. Mezey G, King M. *Male Victims of Sexual Assault*. Oxford, England: Oxford University Press; 2000.

62. Wheeler K. Psychotherapeutic strategies for healing trauma. *Perspect Psychiatr Care*. 2007;43:132-141.

63. Harvey J. *Perspectives on Loss and Trauma: Assaults on the Self.* Thousand Oaks, CA: Sage Publications, Inc; 2002.

64. Davis R, Kennedy M, Austin W. Refugee experiences and southeast Asian women's mental health. *West J Nurs Res.* 2000;22:144-168.

65. Pathak N. Ethnic and cultural components responses to cultural bereavement of immigrant Tibetans in India. *Tibet J.* 2002; 28(3):53-60.

66. McKinney K. Culture, power, and practice in a psychosocial program for survivors of torture and refugee trauma. *Transcultural Psychiatry.* 2007;44:482-504.

67. Dyregrov A, Gupta L, Gjestad R, Raundalen M. Is the culture always right? *Traumatology.* 2002;8:135-145.

68. Skolnik L, Boontinand J. Traffic in women in Asia. *Pacific Forum Appl Res Public Policy.* 1999;14:76-81.

69. Ugarte M, Zarate L, Farley M. Prostitution and trafficking of women and children from Mexico to the United States. In: Farley M, ed. *Prostitution, Trafficking and Traumatic Stress.* Binghamton, NY: The Hawthorne Maltreatment & Trauma Press; 2003.

70. World Health Organization. *Guidelines for Surveillance of Sexually Transmitted Diseases.* New Delhi, India: Regional Office for Southeast Asia; 2000.

71. Silverman J, Decker M, Gupta J, Maheshwari A, Willis B, Raj A. HIV prevalence and predictors of infection in sex-trafficked Nepalese girls and women. *J Am Med.* 2007;298:536-542.

72. Huda S. Sex trafficking in south Asia. *Int J Gynecol Obstet.* 2006;94:374-381.

73. Centers for Disease Control and Prevention. Sexually transmitted diseases treatment guidelines, 2006. Atlanta, GA: Centers for Disease Control and Prevention, US Dept of Health and Human Services. *MMWR.* 2006;55(RR-12).

74. Encuesta Nacional de Cultura Política y Prácticas Ciudadanas 2001. Revista Cambio, 17 de Agosto del 2002. http://www.inegi.gob.mx/est/contenidos/espanol/proyectos/metadatos/encuestas/encppc_239.asp?c=4887#Antecedentes. Accessed May 23, 2008.

75. Gushulak B, MacPherson D. Health issues associated with the smuggling and trafficking of migrants. *J Immigrant Health.* 2000;2:67-78.

76. Norman S, Means-Christensen A, Craske M, Sherbourne C, Roy-Byrne P, Stein B. Associations between psychological trauma and physical illness in primary care. *J Trauma Stress.* 2006;19:461-470.

77. Sbordone R. Post-traumatic stress disorder: an overview and its relationship to closed head injuries. *Neuro Rehabil.* 1999;13:69-78.

78. Pearlman L, Saakvitne, K. Treating therapists with vicarious traumatization and secondary traumatic stress disorders. In: Figley C, ed. *Compassion Fatigue: Coping with Secondary Traumatic Stress in Those Who Treat the Traumatized.* New York, NY: Brunner/Mazel; 1995:150-175.

79. Sexton L. Vicarious traumatization of counselors and effects on their workplaces. *Br J Guidance Counseling.* 1999;27:393-403.

80. Way I, Van Deusen K, Marin G, Apllegate B, et al. Vicarious trauma: a comparison of clinicians who treat survivors of sexual abuse and sexual offenders. *J Interpers Violence.* 2004;19:49-71.

81. Heirendt A. *The Presence of Vicarious Trauma, the Impact of Empathy and the Intervening Effect of Coping Among Anti-Trafficking Service Providers* [master's thesis]. Los Angeles, CA: California State University Los Angeles; 2006.

82. Farrell A. McDevitt J, Fahy S. Understanding and Improving Law Enforcement Responses to Human Trafficking. US Department of Justice. Washington, DC: The Institute on Race and Justice at Northeast University; 2008.

83. Family Violence Prevention Fund. *Collaborating to Help Trafficking Survivors: Emerging Issues and Practice Pointers.* San Francisco, CA: Family Violence Prevention Fund; 2007.

Chapter 18

ELDER SEXUAL ABUSE

Ann Wolbert Burgess, DNSc, APRN, BC, FAAN
Kathleen M. Brown, RN, MSN, CRNP, PhD, FAAN*

Although sexual abuse is well established as a major social and health problem with significant physical and psychological consequences for its victims under age 60, the literature has neglected addressing the reporting, assessment, treatment, and impact of sexual abuse on adults over age 60. While prevention programs are making a difference in child sexual abuse, there is no prototype in elders' (ie, adults over age 60) sexual abuse arena for several reasons: (1) anecdotal and research data are scarce as to the efficacy of assessment and treatment programs in the area of elder sexual abuse; (2) there is a history of discrimination against elders as well as misperceptions and stereotypes against older adults that has put elders at an increased risk for sexual assault; (3) barriers to effective health care interventions include delayed reporting of the sexual abuse that results in failure to obtain a timely forensic evidentiary examination and treatment for injuries and infection; (4) there are few resources available for educating seniors and others about the prevention of sexual abuse; and (5) there is little information on the motivation of offenders who sexually assault elders to provide direction for early detection to reduce offending behavior.

This chapter is for sexual assault forensic examiners, mental health clinicians, and sexual violence advocates with the goal to provide them with ideas, practices, and solutions to the issues presented when helping older victims. The issues with seniors are quite varied and include helping persons with cognitive and physical disabilities and elders who have specific belief systems about sex and sexual violence in general. This chapter presents actual cases of elder sexual victimization and offers advocates suggestions to treating this group throughout the process of moving client from victim to survivor. It discusses early detection and reporting of elder sexual abuse, treatment services for elders who are living independently, in assisted living facilities, or in nursing homes and educational prevention programs for seniors.

EARLY DETECTION AND REPORTING

Early recognition and detection of abuse and reporting of cases means knowing the physical and behavioral indicators of sexual abuse in elders, being able to ask the right questions of elders, and to report all suspected cases to the proper agency (eg, law enforcement, protective services, hospital for forensic services). Two major barriers that reduce reporting elder sexual abuse include the victims' reluctance to report incidents and the disbelief of others that elder sexual abuse occurs. In the case of victim reluctance, the senior may be frightened or embarrassed to report or the offender may be a domestic partner—a situation often noted in domestic violence cases. In such situations, elders may fear being sent to nursing homes and losing their independence and/or financial base from the partner. In such a case, advocates need to work with

* *Acknowledgement is made for support and cases obtained through NIJ Grant #2003-WG-BX-1007.*

elders on plans that will not jeopardize their home security by identifying the resources and social support available to help elders remain in the home. This may require talking with law enforcement and/or the prosecutor regarding charges that can be brought on offending partners.

The second barrier in reporting elder sexual abuse is that of the disbelief of others. Caregivers, staff, and family may believe the elder is fantasizing, in a cognitively disorganized state, or inventing a story. As with all ages of victims, staff members need to take seriously all reports of sexual abuse. It will be up to the person's expert in the area of elder sexual abuse to determine the credibility of the allegation and up to the prosecutor as to the viability of the case in the criminal justice system. Even if the prosecutor does find adequate evidence to "make the case," the elder should be respected and receive advocate services.

Literature on Elder Sexual Abuse

There is a paucity of research on elder sexual abuse due, in part, to the definition of elderly. There is no generally accepted age that defines it; therefore, studies that look at the elderly may be hard to find or tease out. There are no reliable estimates of the incidence or prevalence of elder sexual abuse in the community or in facilities; however, for over 30 years, statistics have been reported on sexual abuse of older individuals.[1] Statistics from early studies on sexual assault victims seen in hospital emergency rooms (ER) and rape crisis centers were noted. MacDonald reported that 7% of 200 sexual assault victims in Denver were aged 50 and older.[2] Amir reported that 3.6% of rape victims in Philadelphia were over age 50.[3] Fletcher found that 5.2% of victims referred to a Syracuse rape crisis center were over 55 years of age.[4] Victims over 61 years comprised 2.1% of the 1162 cases seen during the first 19 months of operation of the Miami rape crisis center, and 5.8% were ages 41 to 60.[5] Cartwright and Moore found that 2.7% of sexual assault victims treated at an inner city hospital were 60 years and older and a Texas study found that 2.2% of the reported sexual assault victims were women over age 50.[6,7]

Data from cases reported to adult protective services (APS) were another source of information about elder abuse. In 1991, Ramsey-Klawsnik surveyed APS case workers in Massachusetts and identified 28 cases of women believed to have been sexually assaulted in the home primarily by family members including adult sons and husbands.[8] In a similar study drawing on Ramsey-Klawsnik's work, Holt reported 90 suspected elder sexual assault victims in England, 86% of whom were female.[9] The majority were over the age of 85, had dementia, and were frail. Most abuse occurred in the elder's domicile, and 90% of the offenders were males upon whom the victim was dependent.

Nursing homes are not immune from elder sexual abuse, as both staff and other residents have been identified as perpetrators. Teaster and colleagues reported 42 Virginia APS cases of sexual abuse in both domestic and institutional settings.[10] They found that 75% of the identified offenders were residents in the same nursing home as their victims. Facility staff members were also identified as offenders. In a study of 20 cases of 18 women and 2 men referred for civil litigation, Burgess, Dowdell, and Prentky identified 3 methods of reporting an assault: informing a family member, sexual abuse that was witnessed, and clues detected by staff or family.[11] In 10 cases, sexual assault examinations were not conducted due to delayed reporting, elder resistance, difficulty communicating with the elder, and difficulty obtaining accurate information. Of the 10 cases that had an examination, 6 revealed positive evidence. Elder response was identified in terms of expressions of fear and/or avoidance of male staff, change in behavior to withdrawal or lying in fetal position, and development of new behaviors. All but 3 perpetrators were identified. Nursing home victims generally had documented symptoms of compounded and silent rape trauma.[12] Compounded conditions include preexisting factors such as a physical disorder or dementia. Silent rape trauma is where the individual has not told anyone of the sexual abuse.

In continuing her study of APS data, Ramsey-Klawsnik identified 5 types of elder sexual abuse: stranger or acquaintance assault, abuse by unrelated care providers, incestuous abuse, marital or partner abuse, and resident-to-resident assault in elder care settings.[13] She further delineated subtypes of marital and incestuous abuse.[14] Three patterns of marital abuse seen in clinical samples are (1) long-term domestic violence, (2) recent onset of sexual abuse within a long-term marriage, and (3) sexual victimization within a new marriage. Incestuous elder abuse involves cases perpetrated by adult children, other relatives, and quasi-relatives. Resident-to-resident sexual abuse has been substantiated in nursing homes, assisted living facilities, board and care homes, and other settings, which care for elder persons.[15]

In a study of forensic markers in 125 elder female sexual abuse cases, Burgess, Hanrahan, and Baker reported that the offender's hand was the primary mechanism of physical injury to the nongenital area of the elder's body and the offender's hands, fingers, mouth, penis, or foreign object caused injury to the genital area.[16] Over half of the elder victims had at least one part of their body injured and nearly half had signs of vaginal injury. Of the 46 cases with forensic results from a rape examination, 35% had positive evidence for the presence of sperm in the vagina, anus, or mouth.

Reporting and Investigating Alleged Elder Sexual Abuse

The clandestine nature of elder sexual abuse has been a major barrier in case detection and in developing interventions for victims and perpetrators. Two key agencies have responsibilities for investigating alleged cases: the criminal justice system (CJS) and APS.

Criminal Justice System

Local law enforcement is the agency of first report in the CJS for sexual behaviors considered criminal by state or federal law for all aged victims. Criminal sexual behavior such as rape usually requires that the act was nonconsensual, with penetration and under force or threat of force. State or federal laws define additional criminal sexual acts and special circumstances when the victim is unable to consent.

Elder sexual abuse cases can be reported to the criminal justice system through a local law enforcement agency in much the same route as a younger victim report. Elders can self-report to police, a rape crisis center, or a hospital. In cases reported to rape crisis centers or hospitals, elders are offered the choice to report the crime to the police, thus entering the CJS, but third parties may also observe or suspect sexual abuse and report to law enforcement.

Adult Protective Service

APS is typically the agency of first report for the mistreatment of vulnerable adults and elders.[17,18] Across the country, laws exist requiring mandated professionals (such as those in medicine, nursing, social services, law enforcement, and aging services) to report suspected abuse of vulnerable adults, including elders, to APS. Reports can also be made by non-mandated individuals such as family members and friends, as well as by victims themselves. Reports of abuse, neglect (including self-neglect), and financial exploitation of adults who are unable to protect themselves due to a physical or mental limitation, are investigated by APS, as they operate under a mandate to protect safety, health, and civil liberties.[19] They also assess the need for protective services and provide services to reduce risk to identified victims. When APS receives a report of abuse, workers investigate and address substantiated cases with referrals for medical, psychological, legal, and social services.[20] Although all state APS programs have the authority to investigate in domestic settings, only 68.5% investigate in institutional settings.[18] During 2003, 192 243 cases of alleged elder abuse were investigated by APS in 29 states.[17] Nearly half were substantiated, one percent of which were confirmed for sexual abuse.

Nursing Home Victimization

The sexual victimization of older adults in nursing homes is underrecognized and underreported. Even when an incident is identified, reporting is delayed and treatment and postrape services are often inadequate.[21] Furthermore, prosecution of these crimes is fraught with problems related to poor quality evidence because of delays in reporting.[22] Older adults residing in nursing homes often require assistance with basic activities of daily living such as bathing, dressing, and feeding because of physical and cognitive impairments. These disabilities make an individual dependent upon others and an easy target for a sexual predator.[11] The cases presented in this paper were selected to draw attention to factors that hinder the detection and substantiation of elder sexual abuse.

There are approximately 17 000 nursing homes in the nation with 1.5 million older adult residents.[21] In a study of 5297 nursing homes in Pennsylvania, New Jersey, and New York, a quarter of these nursing homes had serious complaints alleging situations that harmed residents or placed them at risk of death or serious injury.[21] Concerns about the quality of care have mostly been focused on malnutrition, dehydration, and other forms of neglect. However, there is mounting concern about physical violence by those whom have been entrusted with their care, particularly sexual abuse.[11]

While experts acknowledge that elder sexual abuse exists, the lack of attention to these victims is long standing. In October 1976, the National Center for the Prevention and Control of Rape of the National Institute of Mental Health awarded a 1-year grant to the Philadelphia Geriatric Center to prepare a report on the sexual assault of elder women. In the report issuing from that grant, Davis and Brody observed that, "There was virtually no information about rape and older women, nor had programs been developed."[23] It is more remarkable that after over 20 years of progress in identifying precursors, course, and treatment of sexually aggressive and coercive behavior, little more is currently known about the sexual abuse of elders, especially in nursing homes, than in the 1970s.[24]

In a pilot study of 20 elder women, the most profound result of sexual assaults against these victims was that 11 of the 20 victims died within 12 months of the assault.[11] Because more than half of these victims were ages 80 to 96 at the time of the assault, it obviously cannot be asserted that death was a distal effect of the assault. Although it is not possible to determine in each case whether the assault accelerated death, the fact that more than half of the victims died, not from the assault itself but within months of the assault, is clearly noteworthy, if not alarming.

Little empirical evidence exists about the physical and psychological correlates of older adult sexual victims. Furthermore, the prosecution and conviction of a perpetrator of sexual abuse is confounded by cognitive and physical impairments common to the resident of a nursing home. The issues and case studies in this chapter will show the difficulties in differentiating intentional injuries from unintentional injuries.

Intentional versus Unintentional Injury

Assessing injury in the older adult as intentional or unintentional is the first step in the critical assessment of allegations. Often the events are not witnessed and accidental explanations are offered. The scenario is further complicated when there is more than one caregiver spanning over the period that injuries might have occurred. Additionally, there can be conflicting opinions between various health care specialties regarding the nature of the injury. All of these factors combined make the detection and substantiation of elder sexual abuse extremely difficult.

Nursing homes do not promptly report allegations of sexual or physical abuse, which results in delays in the investigation.[11] Often, evidence has been compromised and investigations delayed, which results in a reduced likelihood of a successful prosecution.[21] Reasons for untimely reporting of allegations include (a) residents may fear retribution if they report the abuse, (b) family members are troubled with having to find a new place because the nursing home may ask the resident to leave, (c) staff do not report abuse promptly for fear of losing their jobs, and recrimination from coworkers and management, (d) nursing homes want to avoid negative publicity and sanctions from the state. The following cases show the difficulty in sorting out intentional versus unintentional injury.

Before it can be concluded that an elder's condition is the result of an intentional sexual injury, the possibility that bruising or injury is unintentional needs to be considered. There are several significant conditions, some of which are confined to the period of aging that can mimic bruising and genital bleeding. The propensity to hemorrhage may result from specific clotting factor deficiencies, platelet defects, or capillary fragility. Collagen defects and bone dystrophies such as osteoporosis need to be considered as well as blood conditions of anemia and medications such as Coumadin or Heparin.

There are unique physiologic factors associated with aging (such as multiple medical problems, increased prevalence of depression, and cognitive and sensory impairment) that can confound the assessment, investigation, and prosecution of elder sexual abuse crimes. Also, methods for data collection and measuring the consequences of elder sexual abuse are complicated by these unique physiologic factors associated with aging.

Case Study 18-1 Trauma Masquerading as Accidental Bruising

Ms. D began showing signs of progressive dementia at age 77. She had minimal affect, wandering behavior, less interaction with people, was less meticulous of her hygiene, and was agitated around her grandchildren. She was admitted to a nursing home with the complaint of diarrhea, weakness, and fainting. She had a history of hypertension for 15 to 20 years and progressive dementia, Alzheimer's type for the past 1 to 2 years. She had thyroid surgery in 1976 and right eye cataract surgery in 1990. She was described as unable to communicate well, forgetful, and sometimes very hard to manage. On admission, she was noted to be cooperative, ambulatory, eating independently, incontinent of bowel and bladder, and needing total care for all activities of living. Her daughter and other family members visited frequently and were primary supports to Ms. D.

The daughter began to notice bruising and brought it to the attention of staff. A record review over a 5-month period noted multiple recording of bruising to her temple, hand, lip, thigh; excoriated skin to her genital area; bright blood to her mouth; discomfort to raising left arm; chest wall tender when hugged; purple lump to back of head; and greenish-yellow bruise to left upper hip.

The staff suggested 2 explanations: first, Ms. D had a history of falling or missing a chair in attempting to sit, and second, she was combative to staff intervention. The daughter reminded staff that the facility advertised itself as able to handle Alzheimer's patients. The daughter next noted her mother's mouth was cut; then she noticed a serious pelvic rash and her mother moaning and holding her knees together. This inattention to her mother prompted the daughter to begin to do personal care for her mother. Her suspicions were founded. She marked the diaper in the morning and when she checked in the evening, it had not been changed all day.

An aide reported seeing another aide hit her mother on the thigh and volunteered that she had reported this to the administrator. The aide also said other patients were being abused in the nursing home, and she suspected someone was abusing her mother's roommate.

The daughter continued to believe someone was handling her mother inappropriately, especially after a black eye appeared. She appealed to the new director of nursing but was dismayed when the solution was to place "bumper guards" on her mother's bed. The director also told the daughter that no resident was getting enough care because staffing was inadequate. When the daughter continued to notice bruises on her mother's thighs and legs, she was told "to remember that her mother was in a nursing home." The daughter felt intimidated, worried that she was being paranoid, as well as placated.

The daughter began providing all the care to her mother except for the night shift. She had narrowed the time period that the bruises seemed to originate. She decided to set up a video camera. She locked a camera in a cabinet she bought (because things were also disappearing at the nursing home), put a 10-hour tape in the camera, turned the tape on with a remote control, which she then put into her pocket, and left.

When she viewed the tape, 6 hours elapsed with no care being given despite the fact orders were for her mother to be turned every 2 hours. Then the tape later revealed a nursing aide entered the room, flung the mother's diaper to the floor, and began to physically provoke her mother with her hand. The aide then went to a closet, returned with a coat hanger, and repeatedly hit and poked the mother. The videotape captured 13 minutes of abuse. Of surprise to the daughter was the identity of the aide. She was the aide who had previously reported other aides abusing patients hitting her mother with her hands, a hanger, and a teddy bear. The videotape, however, showed the aide spitting on her mother, slapping her feet with a hanger, poking at her vaginal area, and other acts of abuse.

After the aide was arrested, state investigators determined that a criminal history check was not done on this aide when she was hired. A criminal history noted she had been fired 6 months earlier from another nursing home for abusive behavior to residents.

In addition to the physical signs of abuse to Ms. D, there were symptoms or changes in her behavior. She complained of lower back and leg pain, and her agitation increased. She was withdrawn and fearful; she had completely changed from the person she was before entering the nursing home. The daughter reported that for several weeks after taking her mother home, when she would go in at night, her mother would startle, look like a scared animal, and put her hands up to protect herself. She refused to walk in narrow corridors, and had lost her independence, and her spirit appeared to have been broken.

There are situations in which sexual injury is suspected, but there is no outcry, witness, or forensic evidence to make a legal determination. However, measures should be taken to provide safety for the elder as in the following case.

Case Study 18-2 Incommunicable Elder Victims

An 89-year-old widow with Alzheimer's disease would open her eyes but not speak. She had been in a nursing home for 3 years. She was sent to a hospital ER because of a hematoma in her inguinal area. The nursing home staff stated the hematoma was from her straining because of constipation and that developed into an inguinal hematoma. Her prior history included a left hip fracture, dementia, and cerebral atrophy.

She was taken by ambulance to the ER after her son noticed bruising to her lower abdomen. Staff was not aware of any fall or injury. The report from the ER stated, "ecchymosis is a few days old; abdomen soft and nontender. Legs drawn up and resists any movement of legs. Bruising was noted to the labia majora and the groin was also bruised with purulent vaginal discharge." A rape kit was negative for the presence of sperm; however, a test for chlamydia was suspicious and ordered to be repeated. X-rays in the ER revealed separation of the pubic symphysis. She was treated for a urinary tract infection and released back to the nursing home.

An X-ray taken 10 months previously was compared to the ER X-ray and revealed a 4.4 cm diastasis of the symphysis pubis. Examination of the inguinal area showed a triangular-shaped subcutaneous hematoma approximately 20 cm x 10 x 10, with the base towards the umbilicus of the triangular area. There was no definite area of pain.

The nursing home administration suggested that the injury was caused either by restraints used to hold her in a chair or from pushing her legs open to do perineal care (peri-care). However, there was no evidence that the woman's pelvic and labial bruising could occur from the use of a seatbelt restraint. Such a restraint fastens around a waist and not the hips. Similarly, a Posey Hugger (Posey Company) is to secure the patient within the wheelchair and could not cause bruising to the lower pelvic area. Also, the resident wore soft diapers that acted, in part, as padding to her pelvic region.

This elder had severe contractures of her legs, whereby she held her legs together and her knees pulled up toward her body. That no one knew if she could straighten her legs suggests no range of motion was ever done with her. Perineal/pelvic injuries were caused by force to the area not through changing a diaper or bathing her. She would have pain as noted in the ER exam when her stomach was palpated.

Leg muscles do shorten when unused; however, stretching of muscles would not cause bruising. It would cause a tonic reflex of shaking. Bruising is caused by the breaking of blood vessels and capillaries, not by stretching.

This case had signs (bruising, separation of symphysis pubis) and symptoms (vaginal discharge, urinary tract infection, protest behavior when touched) of sexual injury. The separation of the symphysis pubis is considered normal only during childbirth. Such a condition in an elder would be a red flag for extreme pressure being placed on the abdomen as in someone lying on top of her. There was a pattern of bruising that could be from migrating blood into tissue indicating extent of injury.

The logical question was who had sexual access to this woman. It was learned that an employee—a maintenance supervisor—had keys to the facility. The staff rumor was that this man would make sexual advances to residents. There were 2 reports that said he had made advances, and one resident, whom he offered to drive somewhere, had to flee from the car. He was hired after being fired from another facility for sex with a mentally ill resident. His son was seen on the floor the day before the bruising was noted, looking for his father. The son had been fired for sex with residents at another nursing facility.

Police were unable to make an arrest in this case despite the suspicion that a sexual assault had occurred. The son, however, did remove his mother from that nursing home to one he believed provided safety and protection. The outcome was that the woman died within 6 months of the discovery of the injury.

Case Study 18-3 Unwitnessed Events

Most sexual assaults are not witnessed. However, when the victim is infirm as through cognitive deficits, the lack of an eyewitness is a complicating issue in the assessment and investigation of these cases. The skill and challenge is to reconstruct the events surrounding the possible sexual injury. A forensic examiner can conclude whether a particular account is possible, or likely, or which of two accounts is more likely to be true. Without such an account, without some starting point, the reconstruction of the circumstances is likely to be characterized by generalities.

A 91-year-old nursing home resident had a 3-week history of increasing falls, refusal to be bathed, ordering staff out of her room, refusing medications, and telling her daughter she wanted a gun "to shoot someone." Her health deteriorated with the major concern focusing on her distended abdomen. She was taken to the ER where a colonoscopy was ordered. In a routine urine analysis, 5 non-motile sperm were observed. The patient died 2 days later, and no autopsy was performed.

The conclusion that, more likely than not, this woman suffered a sexual injury is based on several theories. First, the urine was obtained from catheterization, suggesting that poor catheter technique introduced the sperm from the perineal area into the catheter. Blood cells were also noted in the urine suggesting trauma or infection. Second, the acute abdomen could be associated with vaginal trauma. Unestrogenized vaginas tend to bruise in the fornix area when penetrated. Vaginal/bowel trauma can produce adhesions and with poor catheter technique, pooled seminal products in the vulva area can be picked up in the supposedly clean catheter. Trauma to the vaginal/bowel wall can bruise the intestine, producing an erythema and ulcerative process as described in the surgeon's report. Third, the elder had symptoms of emotional trauma with evidence of protest behavior, a history of falls, and trying to control who entered her room. She advised caregivers she did not want to be "messed with," and her requesting a gun suggests the perpetrator was known and had access to her.

Compounding the issue of a criminogenic environment is the tendency of an elder to either deny sexual assault or recant an allegation. Sexual assault victims with cognitive impairments are unable to consent to sex, unable to defend themselves, and often delay in reporting a rape. The neurobiology of trauma suggests that traumatic memories with the attendant emotion cannot be totally extinguished, and sleep disturbance and mood instability of angry outbursts, withdrawal, and depression often follow.

Case Study 18-4 Elder Victim Recantation

A 71-year-old woman was admitted to a nursing home with a diagnosis of paranoid disorder and depressive disorder with psychotic features, oriented only to name. Psychiatric consultation documented her to be demented, disoriented, and forgetful. She had a history of depressed mood and recent history of agitated confusion.

A psychiatrist noted her to have become more emotionally labile, quarrelsome, disagreeable, uncooperative, and agitated 6 months after admission. Her nurse's notes documented her being found lying on the floor or under her bed in fetal position numerous times. Her daughter questioned why her mother was falling so much. The resident began refusing medications, meals, having vital signs taken, and allowing the nurses to treat her decubitus ulcer. She would cry, moan, ask to sit by the nursing station, insist on staying in her wheelchair, or ask to go home. She was given a psychiatric diagnosis of major depressive disorder, recurrent with a recommendation of psychotherapy; however, this was not instituted due to memory deficits. No other treatment, such as supportive counseling or reminiscent therapy, was ordered.

The resident then reported to a charge nurse that she was raped. She was subsequently referred to her physician, who transferred her to a hospital for a rape examination where she then denied that a rape had occurred.

Several points are important in this case. First, with an elder oriented only to name, it cannot be assumed that the resident has the ability to accurately relate to time. She was correct in answering the examiner's question that a rape had not just occurred. She had made a delayed report that was not understood until she was more carefully interviewed.

Second, this particular nursing home ignored red flags of predatory employees. The nursing home had demonstrated a general acceptance of the risks associated with the hiring of staff with criminal records and inattention to the state requirement that criminal histories be checked. A review of employee records revealed 46% of the male employees had histories of being convicted of a crime. Some employees had no personnel file. No drug testing was performed on new applicants, thereby increasing the risk of active employee involvement in the drug culture. No reference checks to confirm the quality of applicants were performed on the majority of the personnel files.

Another red flag involved 2 male employees with prior histories of sexual abuse. One was arrested and convicted when caught at another nursing home with his pants down and penis exposed to the buttocks of a 96-year-old female resident. A second male employee was also arrested for the assault of a 72-year-old woman who was mentally retarded at another nursing home. This employee had a criminal history that included an indictment 8 years prior for aggravated sexual assault of a child. Additionally, he pled guilty 2 years prior to his working at this nursing home to another charge of assault for which he received one-year probation. This employee subsequently confessed to sexually assaulting this resident.

As previously noted, elders may bruise easily and physical signs are misinterpreted as the consequence of aging. Similarly, emotional symptoms of anxiety and depression with accompanying feelings of fear and confusion are not uncommon complaints of elders. The cause of the distress may not be known and the elder is treated for the symptom. A sexual assault, either acute or chronic, may be missed. The defining criteria, as in child sexual abuse cases, are the presence of genitourinary symptoms or bruising and/or sexually related commentary. Consider the following case.

Case Study 18-5 Evidentiary Signs and Symptoms

Ms. B, age 94, a never-married Caucasian woman worked as a bank teller prior to retirement. She lived independently until she required surgery at age 91 and was subsequently placed at a nursing home. Her medical diagnoses included atrial fibrillation, diabetes, osteoporosis, cataracts, hypothyroidism, and senile dementia.

Her great-nieces, visiting one day, observed bruises on Ms. B's thighs and pubic region. They notified the nursing staff, who said the bruises came from a recent catheterization. The niece, not satisfied with the explanation, had her aunt transferred to an ER where an examination revealed ecchymosis and bruising on her pubic mons, a linear region of ecchymosis on her left inner thigh, and some ecchymosis and bruising on her buttocks. While Ms. B was hospitalized she was noted to be crying out "help me" at intervals, yelling, "Somebody help me. I'm scared to be alone. Please stay with me," and holding on to staff when they came close.

Before discovery of the sexual abuse, nursing notes documented withdrawn behavior through decreased mobility, increased sleeping, depression, lack of appetite, weight loss, and genitourinary tract infections. Ms. B was reported not to be her usual self; she was confused, disoriented to place and time, and would hide under her bed. She complained of rectal pain and refused examination. She continued to have increased agitation, was looking for the exit door, asked for her dead sister and parents, and asked, "What's done with a girl who gets pregnant?" She would yell for a nurse, grab on to staff, and remove her clothing in the lobby. She became tearful and frightened and said some boy was going to hurt her. She did not eat well and lost 17 pounds.

Ms. B had 3 geropsychiatric consultations prior to the confirmation of the sexual assault. She was seen for increased anxiety over a 6-week period, diagnosed with an underlying dementia, and started on an antidepressant for mood elevation. A psychiatrist described her increased anxiety, decreased functional level, verbally abusive language, thought disorganization, paranoid ideation, agitation, pacing, and self-admitted depression.

She was again seen for "anxiety and attention-seeking behavior; a recent fall and resultant hip pain; a recently completed antibiotic treatment for a urinary tract infection; her constant calling for staff and helpless behavior; her stated depression and boredom; and preoccupation with finances." She was diagnosed with dementia with delusions, and her medications were changed again. A consulting psychiatrist next diagnosed Ms. B with organic anxiety disorder secondary to dementia and recommended another medication change to control her repeated "yelling out 'worthy matron.'" After the sexual assault was confirmed, a review of records noted repeated references to "sex, pregnancy, a young man, and fear."

Elder victims of sexual assault are less likely to have a complete sexual assault examination including the collection of an evidence kit, an internal exam, and tests for sexually transmitted infections (STIs). Part of the difficulty may be in the examination of the elder as in the following case.

Case Study 18-6 Inadequate Evidentiary Examination

Ms. G, age 85, had lived in a nursing home for 2 years. Although diagnosed with dementia, she was able to walk, feed, and bathe herself. Medical records indicated that she was not able to communicate intelligently with others, which was the main reason she was in the nursing home.

Court testimony revealed that on a Thursday, around 4:15 PM, a medical aide went to Ms. G's room to give her medication. The door was closed, which was contrary to the norm. The aide knocked lightly on the door 2 times and received no answer. She entered the room and noticed the privacy curtain pulled around the farthest bed in the room, a bed designated with the letter "C" and that didn't belong to Ms. G. The medication aide pulled back the curtain on bed C and observed Ms. G lying totally nude, with her legs up in the air near her shoulders. A male aide was bending over Ms. G with his penis out of unzipped pants. The male aide attempted to cover himself. The medication aide reported that on prior occasions when she gave Ms. G her medication, she would grab her vaginal area and spoke one word to her, "hurts." The medication aide reported the incident to the charge nurse saying that she could not believe what she had seen.

Ms. G was transported to a hospital for a sexual assault examination; however, the nurse was unable to complete the exam or collect specimens due to Ms. G's agitation and discomfort. The case was plea-bargained due, in part, to the inability of the victim to testify, the lack of forensics, and the lack of evidence that there had been sexual contact.

The difficulties in the forensic examination include the resistance of the elder to the pelvic position, difficulty in visualizing the pelvic area due to leg contractures, difficulty in communicating and explaining the procedure to a cognitively impaired elder, and difficulty obtaining a reliable and accurate victim report of the assault, injuries sustained, and regions of pain and discomfort.

The presence of an STI is usually a hallmark of sexual abuse in a child. However, when it is an elder, the argument can be made that it was the result of a preexisting condition or, as in the next case, it was transmitted by health care staff.

Case Study 18-7 Sexually Transmitted Infection

A twice-widowed 80-year-old black woman, who was living in a nursing home, had been living with one of her children prior to being hospitalized with urinary tract infection and increased blood sugar. She was diagnosed with progressive dementia upon admission to the nursing home and also had a history of congestive heart failure, diabetes, and hypertension.

A review of the nursing notes indicated unexplained bruises on her inner right lower arm (2.5 cm) and right upper outer arm (3 cm) and being found on the floor with swelling to the right side of the head. Six days later her right hand and arm were noted to be swollen. Three weeks later, blisters were noted on her right inner knee, and right upper arm and abrasions on both knees. Her daughter was concerned about her loss of weight, and nursing plan notes confirmed poor to no intake of foods/fluids. Because of the edema to her right hand and wrist, X-rays were ordered. Two weeks later, a large amount of white odorous vaginal discharge was noted and treated for 7 days, but no cultures were ordered.

The next month, 4+ edema was noted. The resident was complaining and moaning in pain; blisters noted to inner aspect of right arm, hand edema. She was described as being very lethargic with drooping right side of mouth and unopened right eye; a bruise to fifth finger found to be a fracture. Blood clots were noted in her catheter, guaiac noted in stool, she had diarrhea, and weight loss, and bright red blood noted from anal area. A urinary tract infection was discovered with blood-tinged urine 3 months later, followed by a report of vaginal warts. She was moved for contact isolation and staff in-serviced on venereal warts. She was diagnosed with condylomata acuminata in the perianal and right labia majora sites.

Her daughter transferred her to another nursing home. A neuropsychological evaluation report 6 months after transfer indicated she had marked improvement in her cognitive functioning.

Condylomata acuminata is transmitted through sexual contact, and it is a recurring condition. There is no evidence that the elder resident ever had any prior history of venereal warts. However, on the same floor, a 15-year-old comatose accident victim also was diagnosed with condylomata acuminata. The nursing home administrator implied that poor hand-washing technique was the cause of the sexually transmitted disease.

To counter the nursing home theory for trial, symptoms of emotional trauma were argued. The daughter testified at deposition that her mother was coherent off and on, slept a great deal, was worse at night, and was treated with medication for depression. She was able to communicate only by withdrawn behavior, depressed affect, sleep disturbance, crying spells, and depression. She was fearful at night of the "boy in her closet." No suspect was identified for a criminal trial, but both civil suits were settled in favor of the plaintiffs.

Case Study 18-8 Resident-on-Resident Sexual Abuse

The issue of elder sexual activity is sometimes addressed in policy manuals of nursing homes with a section on the sexual rights of elders. There is an attitude that sexual activity should even be encouraged among elder residents. However, the part about consent between the 2 elders is less clear. In fact, sexual harassment, fondling, and even intercourse is often viewed as "no big deal" and certainly not harmful to the elder. In some nursing homes, nursing home staff is said to ignore the pleas for help by resident females. The cases in this category all involved elder women who tried to reject the sexual advances of elder males who, in most cases, preyed on many elder victims. There was no history of a developing relationship but rather a predatory style to the act.

A 91-year-old widow was admitted to the nursing home after having been treated for chest pain of several weeks duration. Her admission diagnoses included left chest pain, etiology undetermined but pleuritic in nature, rheumatoid arthritis, history of congestive heart failure treated with a pacemaker, history of diverticulitis, severe obesity, status post–total knee arthroplasty, status post-ovarian cancer, bilateral lens implants, large hiatus hernia, and atrial fibrillation. She had not been declared incompetent by any court and had a living will and a do not resuscitate (DNR) order on file. She was alert and oriented to person, and partially to place, but not oriented to time. She could make decisions about her health care. The chart noted she "was able to communicate her needs and wants, understands what is said to her, and makes herself understood. She comes out and socializes with other residents but not to a great extent.

She remains uninvolved in activities. She appears to be sad and is being medicated for depression. She requires assistance with ADLs; side rails used for safety and requires assistance to toilet."

Her son received a call, on a Friday, that his mother was in great distress, had suffered a mental breakdown, that they had to medicate her heavily, and perhaps they should order a psychological evaluation. He went to see her the next morning and found her depressed, regressed, in a weak state, and very drowsy. He next received a telephone call from the director of nursing on Monday to say that his mother had been sexually abused by a resident but that it probably (in her opinion) didn't amount to a whole lot. He went to the nursing home immediately and was told the police had been called.

On Tuesday, he went to visit his mother. While talking to the charge nurse in the hallway, she pointed out a man in a wheelchair as "the guy who assaulted your mother." She then walked over to the man and told him that messing around with old women would get him "five to ten."

The son was shocked to learn from the police report that a nurse saw the resident with his hand under his mother's gown fondling her breast. He learned that the doctor had not been notified of the assault and that nothing substantive had happened to the offender as he was still on the same floor as his mother.

The mother's health quickly deteriorated, and she died 7 months later. Her son reported she looked depressed, regressed like she was in a stupor, was not eating well, and began having gastroenteritis symptoms.

Staff did not take the sexual assault seriously. It took a significant amount of time for the nurse to separate the abuser from the woman, and he was not transferred off the floor until the son complained. A 2-year review of complaints regarding this nursing home revealed there were at least 17 complaints of rough handling/physical abuse, of which there were 3 citations issued on quality of care. His mother had at least 15 notations of skin tears in a 6-month period. She suffered a serious gash to her leg and her broken leg was not diagnosed in a timely fashion.

Detecting Injury in Elders

The cases described previously emphasize the importance of a careful assessment and examination of elders for signs of injury. As already noted, the detection of sexual injury in elders is underrecognized. **Table 18-1** illustrates the minimal data available on sexual injury to elder victims of rape and sexual assault.

Studies indicate that injured elders differ from the younger population in terms of (a) cause of injury, (b) response to injury, and (c) outcome.[25-27]

Cause

For elders, falls are the most common cause of injury followed by motor vehicle accidents, pedestrian accidents, and stab and gunshot wounds.[28] For the younger population, motor vehicle accidents are the number one cause of injury followed by stab and gunshot wounds, falls, and pedestrian accidents.

Elders can also be injured intentionally as victims of assault and sexual abuse. Although not as well published as child assault and abuse, elder abuse and assault does occur in alarming numbers. The Centers for Disease Control report that in 1999, 32 219 people over the age of 65 died of unintentional injury. An unknown percentage of these cases were believed to be related to abuse or assault.[29]

Response to Injury

Because age affects the body's ability to respond to injury and disruptions in physiologic balance, elders recover at a slower rate from minor injury than do their younger counterparts. Elders may have preexisting diseases, but several studies suggest that chronic disease does not influence survival from trauma. It is the trauma itself that creates morbidity and mortality.

Table 18-1. Comparison of Studies of Older Women Who Were Sexually Victimized

	Forensic Markers Study*	NCVS 1992-2002 Rape victims >60 years old†	The National Women's Study (15)‡	Elder Victim/ Offender Study (cases with data)§
	N=125	N=8642	N=549	N=284
Victims				
Mean age	78.4	72.2	67	78.2
% Female	100	74.6	100	93.2
% Caucasians	83.1	100.0	83	82.3
% Black	11.9	12.3	8.5	12.2
Setting				
% Domestic	42.5	40	ND	72.0
% Institutional	38	ND	ND	23.2
% Other	19.5	ND	ND	4.8
Perpetrators % male	92.4	100	ND	90.9
Forced vaginal rape	78	ND	5.3	59.0
Forced oral rape	13.4	ND	.5	15.7
Forced anal rape	23.9	ND	.2	18.0
Forced digital rape	11.6	ND	2.2	ND
Physical assault with weapon	15.7	0	3.5	10.0
Physical assault without weapon	84.3	100	2.6	90.0
Perpetrator known to the victim	58.3	52.3	9.1	70.8
Rape reported to authorities	96.7	44	9.1	100
Charges or referred to district attorney	55.2	50	ND	45.8

* *Forensic Marker Study based on contributed cases by experts.*
† *National Crime Victimization Study (NCVS) is a weighted sample from 1992-2002 of women 60 years and older who were sexually abused or assaulted.*
‡ *The National Women's Study (NSW) is a subgroup of 549 women 55 years and older from the larger sample of 4009.*
§ *Elder Victim/Offender Study based on contributed cases by experts; % by cases with data.*

Outcome

Elder victims demonstrate decreased survival rates when compared to younger counterparts with the same or similar injuries.[26] A disparity is also noted for minor injury. Elders are twice as likely to suffer serious injury in the commission of a crime as their younger counterparts, and they require more hospitalization after a crime than any other age group.[30]

The practitioner who conducts a forensic examination of an elder victim must obtain consent from the victim and/or caregiver, provide emotional support to the victim during the exam, and follow the protocol for an evidentiary exam (photograph injuries and collect evidence). This section focuses on the detection of injury component of the evidentiary exam and describes sexual abuse as the type of injury analyzed in the study, the effects of aging on injury, and the physical assessment of geriatric victims of sexual assault.

Forensic Detection of Injury

The reporting of a suspected case of recent elder sexual abuse requires that forensic evidence be collected. The goal of the forensic examination is the systematic and comprehensive collection of evidence from the victim that has been transferred from the perpetrator. It is conducted in a psychologically supportive manner by explaining and requesting consent for each step in the process. Often a family member will be with the elder to help in this process, especially if it is a nursing home case. Photographs will need to be taken, clothing worn during the assault collected, and slow, careful examination of the victim's body for any transfer of evidence. Saliva and semen will be of prime importance. Hairs and fabrics must be collected and placed on paper for folding. Fingernail scrapings and hairs may be collected. Evidence will be collected from body orifices. The use of a high-intensity light (eg, colposcope) will be used and photographs taken. A standard rape kit will be used, and all evidence will be air-dried and submitted to a police crime laboratory for analysis.

Evidence collection may be different in elders than in adult victims. Assistance may be required for supporting elders' legs during inspections. Legs that are contracted from muscle atrophy require gentle pressure for abduction from assistants. Severe contractures may require the legs being held upwards toward the ceiling in order to accomplish external visualization. The fragility of skin and the lack of estrogenized vaginal tissues require very careful handling of elders' bodies. Also, a small pediatric speculum is recommended for the internal examination.

Assessment

The following therapeutic tasks are important to develop trust with elders in order to do accurate assessments of the sexual abuse:

— Tell elders what to expect. Talk slowly and clearly. Advise victims they will be going to a hospital for an examination and for the collection of evidence.

— Assess victims' sensory systems. Can they hear and see people? A quiet and well-lit area should be used and the staff persons' faces should be well in line of vision of elders. If there are sensory problems, learn how the elder adjusts to the deficit by asking him or her or their family or caregivers.

— Observe the victims' demeanors. Are they quiet, crying, angry, or distressed? Ask how they are feeling and if they have any questions about what shall happen. Allow adequate time for elders to express their emotions.

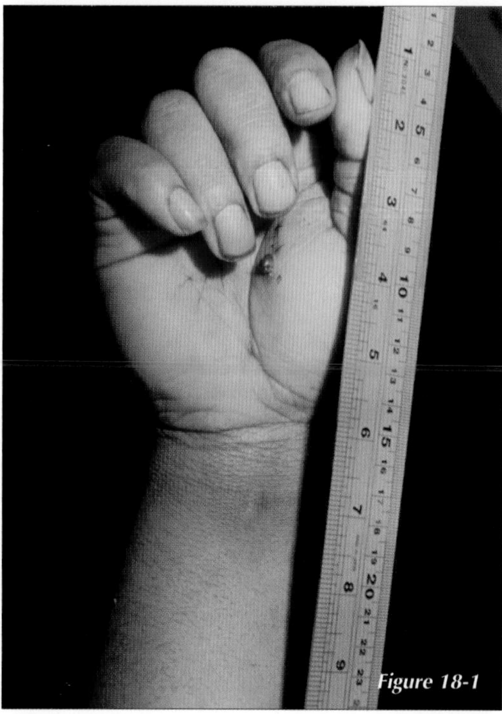

Figure 18-1. *Defensive injuries of the hand and bruising of the wrist are visible on this elder victim.*

Skin and Mucous Membrane

Skin, as people age, becomes thin, loose, transparent, and its vascularity decreases. The skin of elders is atrophic, making it more fragile. The lighter the skin of the elder, the more it tends to look pale and opaque with age. The elder victim has more skin and mucous membrane injury than the younger victims of assault due to the fragility of the skin and mucous membranes (**Figure 18-1**).

Fragility of the vessels in and under the skin creates bruising in elders. Elders bruise under force or pressure that would not create bruising in younger adults. As with younger adults, the color of a bruise changes with time. A purplish-red discoloration is seen first, often accompanied by swelling. A change to darkish-purple occurs within days followed by a greenish-yellow color as the bruise heals.

Assessment for Bruises

The entire body of elders who are the victims of assault must be examined for signs of bruising (**Figure 18-2**). Fingertip bruising from restraint is frequently noted on the neck, the arms, and/or the legs. Bruising from punching can be seen on the face, the breasts, the chest, the abdomen, and the extremities. Bruising from punches resembles an area the shape of a fist with a somewhat clear area in the center of the bruise. This clear area is called the area of central clearing and is created by the blow forcing the blood from the capillaries out and away from the targeted area.

Assessment for Abrasions

Elders' bodies must be examined for abrasions and skin transferred from one area to another (**Figure 18-3**). If elder victims are pulled or dragged across a surface, the skin will abrade (ie, be rubbed off). This can be seen when elder victims are dragged across

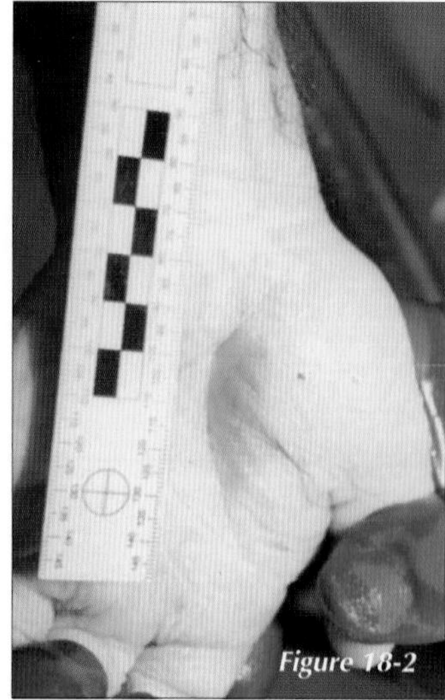

Figure 18-2. *This victim displays bruising of the hand.*

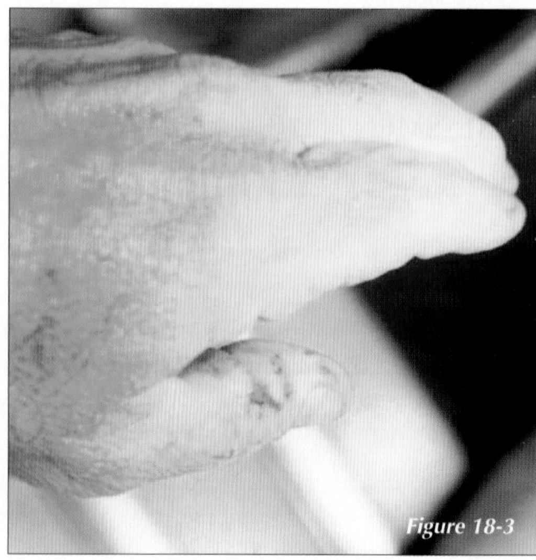

Figure 18-3. *Abrasions on the victim's hand that are the result of defensive actions are visible.*

pavement or grass, but it can also be seen, because of the fragility of the skin on elder victims, on those who have been dragged across a sheet or a carpet. If pillows or similar objects are held over elder victims' faces, injury to the skin on the face is likely to occur.

Assessment for Lacerations

Cutting can occur if a knife or similar weapon is utilized in the commission of the crime. Lacerations from blunt force trauma are much more common in sexual assault and may occur from splitting of the skin due to force applied. If elder victims are punched, pulled, or restrained, the fragile skin will often tear creating a laceration (**Figure 18-4**).

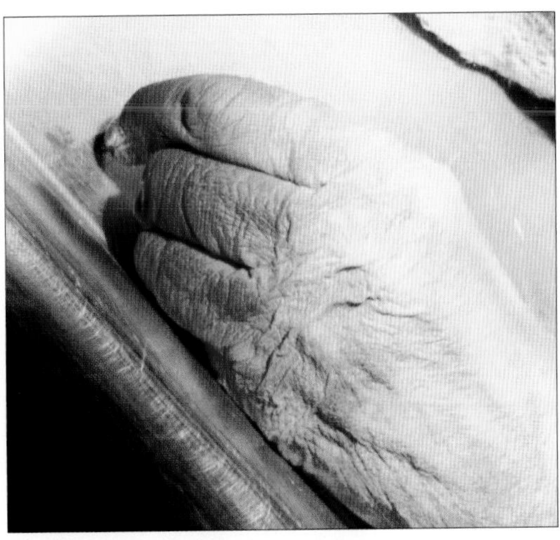

Figure 18-4. *This victim has a laceration on the hand that is the result of defensive actions.*

Methodical and meticulous examination of the skin and genitalia of elder sexual assault victims is necessary. An excellent light source is a requirement. All injury must be noted whether or not it requires medical intervention. Each injury must be described in writing and drawn on a body map. Photographs of each injury must be obtained to ensure documentation of each injury.

Response to Trauma

The skin of elders has a slower healing rate due to aging that causes changes in circulation. The slower healing wounds of elders cause an increased risk of infection. Instructions should be given to victims and/or victims' caregivers on how to keep injuries clean and infection-free.

All injuries should be photographed. Early bruising is difficult to detect in any victim. A follow-up visit 24 hours after the assault may be necessary for continued forensic documentation.

Head Injury

Traumatic brain injury extracts a high morbidity and mortality in any age group. In elders, mortality following severe brain trauma is 90%.[31,32] In this study, over one-third (38%) of the elder victims had injury to their head.

If elder victims experience trauma to the head during the assault, they are likelier to experience subdural hematomas than younger victims are. Elders have increased fragility of the veins in the head, increased cerebral atrophy, and increased stretching of the bridging veins, making them more susceptible to this injury.

In studies focusing on geriatric trauma, an absence of a history of head trauma in elders with confirmed subdural hematoma was 35% to 50%.[33] Because even minor head trauma can lead to mortality in elders, all elder victims of assault should be evaluated for head injury whether they have symptomatology or not.

It is clear that any elder victim of sexual assault who complains of headache has a change in mental status or a disturbance in gait should be evaluated for head injury. If victims do not display any of these symptoms, history of the attack must be carefully solicited and decisions made as to the possibility of head trauma. Elder victims often have hearing deficit, sight deficit, and altered equilibrium and reaction time, making assessment for central nervous system (CNS) injury difficult.

If assaults involved force that may have included the head and/or neck, a computed tomography (CT) scan should be obtained. Lower thresholds are needed for elders

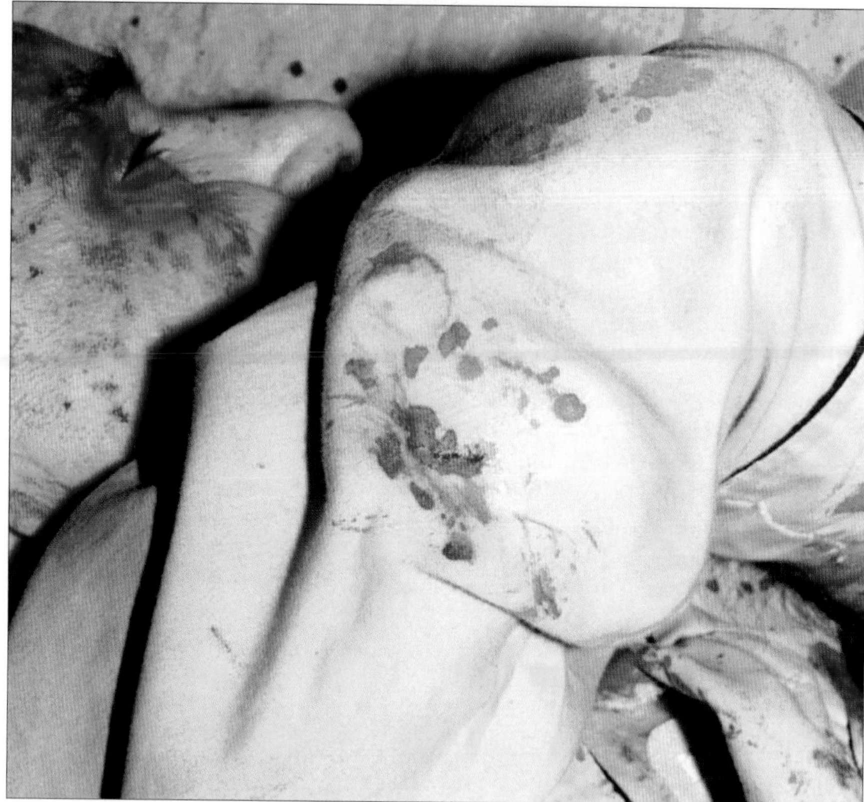

Figure 18-5. *Bruising of the face and blood spatter on the victim's face and clothing are shown in this image.*

given their fragility. Subdural hematomas shown in CT scans may be hyperdense for the first 5 to 10 days, followed by isodense days 7 to 20, and finally hypodense. Sexual assault usually occurs in reclining or "down" positions as on a bed. If victims are forced down and into a reclining position, head injury can occur. If the assault occurred in the victims' homes or on the street and victims were forced onto the ground or floor by offenders, head injury must be considered. Victims can be forced from a standing or sitting position onto the ground or floor as part of a blitzing attack. Head injury can also occur via blows to the head from offenders. The heads of victims can be violently shaken by offenders creating injury, or the heads of the victims can be slammed into beds or floors or the ground by offenders, creating injury (**Figure 18-5**).

Neck Injury

Neck injury can occur when the neck is compressed as in strangulation. Assailants may try to silence the screams of victims. Inquiry needs to be made as to how the assailant controlled the victim and whether or not the neck was held. Positioning of the victim during the assault and amount of force used may cause injury especially in victims with underlying medical conditions such as rheumatoid arthritis. Markings on the neck need to be photographed. In this sample, strangulation occurred in the majority of sexual homicides. Careful and complete physical assessment coupled with knowledge of the crime is necessary for decision on neck injury evaluation.

Chest Wall Injury

Elder victims are more susceptible to fractures. The thoracic cage can be brittle and susceptible to fracture during an assault. Rib fractures, pulmonary contusions, and cardiac contusions can be detected via radiographs. If the facts of the case indicate the possibility of such injuries, a radiograph should be obtained. Fractured ribs can create hemothorax or pneumothorax, both of which may be detected by chest X-ray or CT scan. Chest trauma creates more morbidity and mortality in elders than it does in younger populations; therefore, elder victims with rib fractures should be considered for hospital admission.

Fracture of the ribs occurs when force is applied to the chest. Force can be applied when offenders overcome victims in order to gain control of them. If victims are forced to the floor or ground and fall onto their chest area, fracture can occur. Force can be applied to the chest and ribs fractured, especially if perpetrators are lying on top of their victims during the assault. Blows from hands and arms or legs can fracture ribs as can assailants holding victims in the chest area as a means of restraint.

Abdominal Injury

Of all elder patients who are multiple trauma victims, an estimated 35% have abdominal injury.[26] If abdominal injury is suspected, a CT scan should be obtained. Bedside ultrasonography, focused abdominal sonography in trauma (FAST), may reveal hemoperitoneum suggesting solid organ injury and hemorrhage. Abdominal injury in elders creates mortality 5 times more often than it does in the younger population.[26]

Abdominal injury occurs most commonly from blows to the abdomen by offenders. Abdominal injury can occur from being on top of victims, grabbing, restraining, or moving them with force during the assault.

Extremities

The arms and legs of elders are most vulnerable to bruising. In this study, 31.6% had injuries to their arms and 23.4% had at least one bruise noted to their legs (**Figure 18-6**).

Injury on the inner thighs, especially fingerprint bruising from forcing the legs open or scratches on the inner thighs, is a common finding in sexual assault victims. Bruising on the outside of the thigh can be seen if the legs were forced open and pushed against something firm such as a bedrail or a wall. If the elder victims' extremities are restrained, bruising of the extremities and tearing of the skin is likely to occur (**Figure 18-7**).

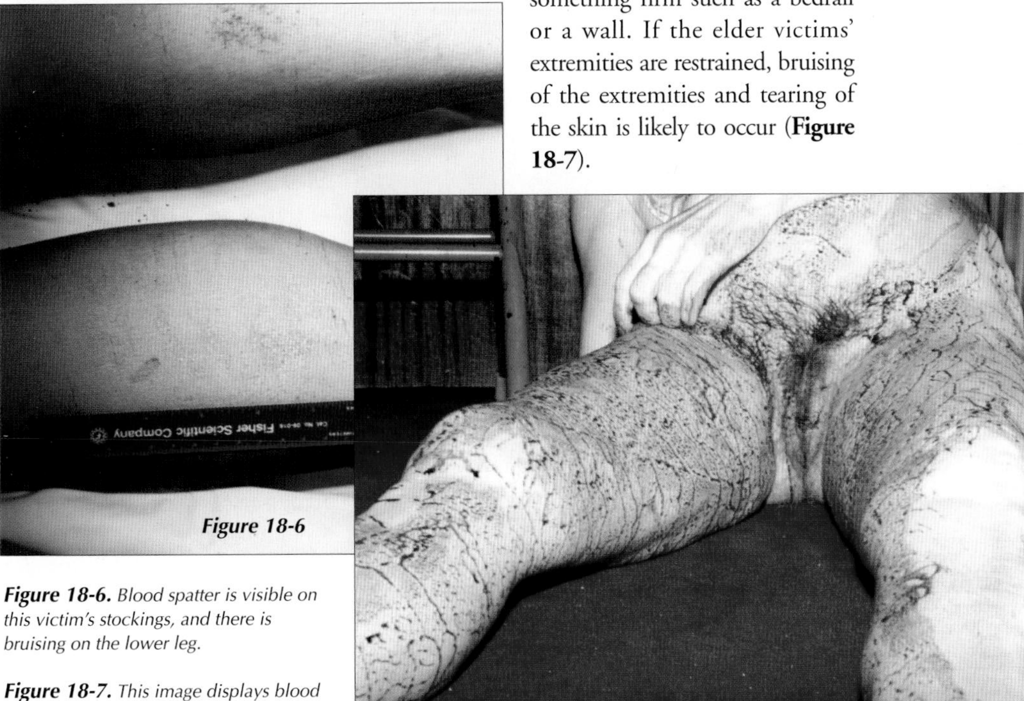

Figure 18-6. *Blood spatter is visible on this victim's stockings, and there is bruising on the lower leg.*

Figure 18-7. *This image displays blood spatter on the victim's thighs, abdomen, and genitals.*

Genital Injuries

Penetration of the vulva, mouth, and anus are the primary sites of genital injury. Bruises, abrasions, and lacerations need to be assessed. The few studies on elder rape victims are equivocal regarding injury. Genital trauma, evident even without colposcopy, is more evident in the postmenopausal sexually assaulted woman than it is in their younger counterparts.[34] However, as with those 65 and younger, rape may occur without obvious injury.[6,35] Medical and forensic records were reviewed between 1986-1991 from 129 women older than 50 years and 129 women from a comparison group ages 14 to 49. Trauma, in general, occurred in 67% of the older group and 71% in the younger group. Genital trauma was more common in older than younger victims (66% versus 49%). Forensic findings were similar in both groups; however, in the older group motile spermatozoa were seen only in those examined within 6 hours of the assault.[7]

In the Burgess, Hanrahan, and Baker study, almost half (45%) of the elder victims who were examined within 72 hours had vaginal trauma (20%), anal trauma (17%), or oral penetration (13%).[16] It is to be noted, however, that elder residents in nursing homes did not necessarily have timely examinations due to delayed reporting.

The high rate of genital injury in this study is related to decreased estrogen and, therefore, less lubrication of the genital mucous membrane, and thinning of the tissue. Female genital mucous membrane in elders is susceptible to trauma because it is atrophic and fragile. The genital mucosa of elderly females is pale, thin, and dry. With the decline of estrogenic stimulus, the labia and clitoris become smaller. The vagina also narrows and becomes shorter adding to the increased probability of vaginal injury.

Inspection of the genitalia of an elder female is a clinical challenge. Many elder women cannot be placed into the traditional position utilized for pelvic examination. Contractures, arthritis, and many other medical conditions common to elders prohibit the use of this position. External genitalia can be examined in a supine position with legs supported by assistants. External genitalia must be carefully inspected utilizing a colposcope or high-intensity light source. Injury may occur at any genital location, but careful attention should be given to inspection of the posterior aspect of the entrance to the vagina and the perineum. Inspection of the vagina and cervix requires speculum inspection. A small narrow speculum (not a pediatric speculum because length is required to reach the cervix) should be utilized. Lubrication with sterile water is not desired but may be necessary with elder patients. Common genital injuries in elder victims of sexual assault are lacerations, abrasions, and bruises.

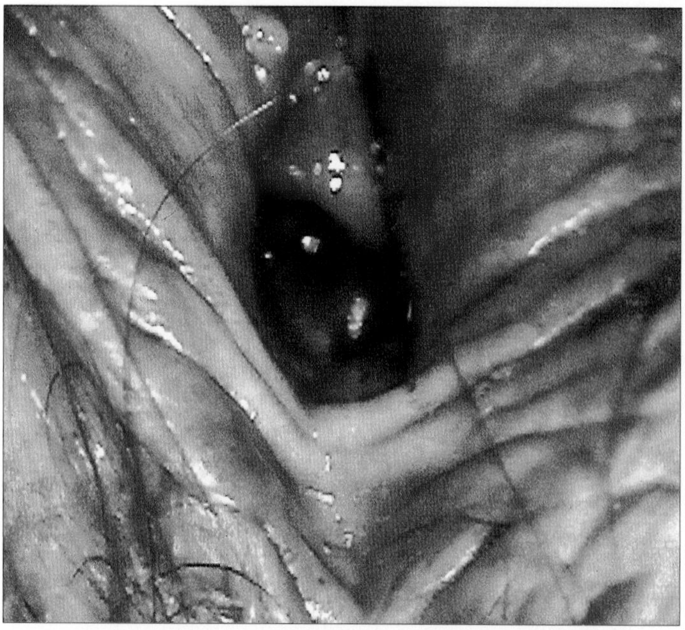

Figure 18-8. *80-year-old postmenopausal woman 5 hours after assault. Image contributed by Linda E. Ledray, SANE-A, PhD, FAAN.*

The time lapse between injury and examination is important to document (**Figures 18-8** through **18-11**).

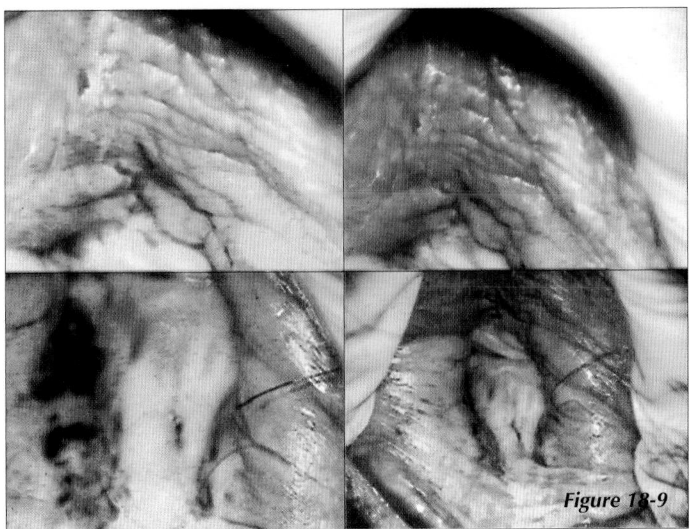

Figure 18-9. *60-year-old woman 5 hours after assault. Image contributed by Linda E. Ledray, SANE-A, PhD, FAAN.*

Figure 18-10. *80-year-old woman 10 hours after assault. Image contributed by Linda E. Ledray, SANE-A, PhD, FAAN.*

Figure 18-11. *57-year-old woman 5 hours after assault. Image contributed by Linda E. Ledray, SANE-A, PhD, FAAN.*

Orthopedic Injuries

Elder victims are more prone to orthopedic injuries from minor trauma than the rest of the population due to osteoporosis and decreased muscle mass. Fractures of the arms can occur while breaking a fall with arms or by raising the arms to ward off blows from the attacker. Fractured lower extremities may occur during an assault. Blows to the extremities, restraining extremities, as well as falls and pushes to the ground can create fractures. Diagnosis of a fracture requires radiographs. Cervical spine injuries in elders are commonly seen. The possibility of cervical spine injuries postassault should be considered during evaluation.

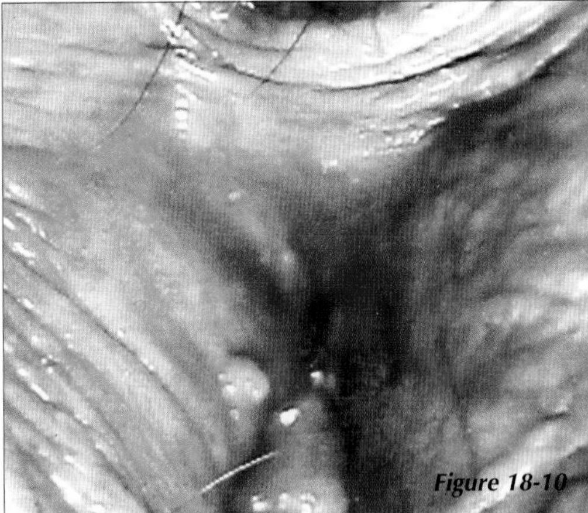

Following relatively minor trauma in elders, degenerative and arthritic changes make diagnosis difficult but necessary for appropriate treatment. Radiographs as well as CT, MRI, and/or bone scans may be required. Pelvic fractures in elders create morbidity and mortality. Closed pelvic fracture must be considered in elder victims of assault.

Pain Perception

Decreased pain perception is an issue in dealing with elder victims of sexual assault. Elder victims of trauma often have more injury than they report. Assessment cannot be confined to what the victim reports to be uncomfortable or painful. The entire body must be evaluated for injury.

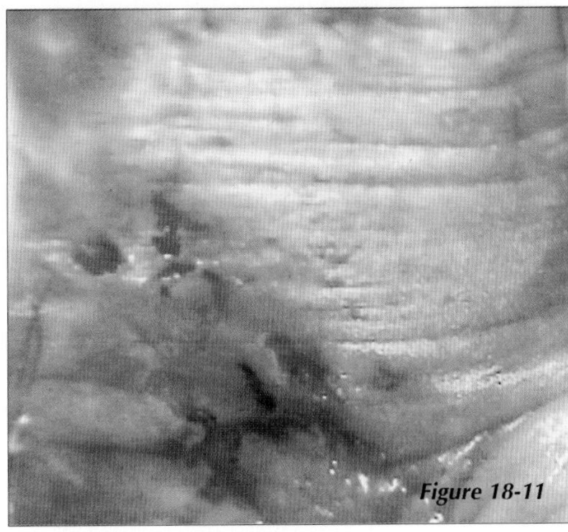

Memory Loss

Loss of short-term memory makes giving an accurate account of the events during the assault difficult for some elder victims. Victims may simply be unable to remember all the details. This possibility requires meticulous examination of the entire body for indications of injury and interview of the person accompanying the elder to the examination.

HOSPITAL ADMISSION

Sexual assault victims are typically evaluated and released provided that evaluation rules out medical necessity for admission. Considering the fragility of elder victims of assault, this routine practice should be revised for elder victims. Perhaps elder victims of assault should be admitted to a hospital facility to increase the possibility of more thorough medical evaluation of injury. The probability of detecting injury would be increased by increasing observation time and likewise allowing for additional testing. Admission would also allow for interviews in stages without pressure for total recall during one encounter.

It has been noted in studies of elder trauma, that elder trauma victims have better outcomes if admitted to trauma centers than if they are not.[26] Criteria for admission to trauma centers should be lowered for elder victims. If elder victims of assault have injuries requiring medical intervention, requirements for admission to trauma centers should be carefully considered to ensure a comprehensive evaluation and early initiation of treatment.

Mortality rates in the injured elder population are significantly higher than for younger adults. Even with correction for severity of injury, elders are still 5 to 6 times likelier to die of similar injuries than younger adults. Careful evaluation by skilled staff over time is required to ensure the health and safety of elder victims of sexual assault.

DOCUMENTATION

Sexual assault cases are forensic cases; that is, documentation may be used in criminal and/or civil litigation proceedings. It is recommended that forensic examinations be performed by those specially trained as sexual assault nurse examiners (SANE). Such training generally suggests documentation of physical injuries and signs using the acronym TEARS.[36] This acronym provides a consistent structure:

— Tears or lacerations and/or tenderness

— Ecchymosis

— Abrasions

— Redness

— Swelling

Signs of physical trauma include observable, objective evidence of injury such as bruises, abrasions, lacerations, and/or bleeding. The elder and accompanying family members need to be told that a comprehensive physical assessment will be conducted by the forensic examiner observing injury to the elder's general body condition and a separate genital examination will be conducted. Evidence of intentional injury is sought by asking the question as to how the injury occurred. Accidental injury needs to be ruled out. For example, nursing home staff has described genital bleeding as the result of "rough peri-care." This may or may not be accidental and needs further investigation. Symptoms of physical trauma include indications of trauma provided by elders. For example, elders may say they were slapped or held by their throat but no observable injury can be noted. The symptom would be noted as part of the forensic record.

Signs of emotional trauma include observable signs such as crying, rocking, hands shaking, flushed appearance, signs of perspiration. Elders may try to hide their feelings by being very quiet, guarded, or controlled in their demeanor. Symptoms of emotional trauma include reports by elders of what was done to them. The record might state that the assailant covered their eyes or held a knife to their throat or pinned them to the floor. One victim said she feared the assailant would try to smother her with pillows that were on her bed.

Documenting Contusions by Computer

A contusion (ie, a bruise) is an area of hemorrhage located under unbroken skin usually resulting from some form of blunt-force trauma. A great deal can be learned about the events surrounding violence by thorough visual examination of existing bruises and bruising patterns. The most common method of assessing a bruise is by (1) visually examining the contusion, (2) describing the area through a subjective observation and use of color words such as red, blue, yellow, green, etc, and (3) comparing the sequence of color changes by time to suggest the age of the contusion.

A key question regarding patterns of injury is whether or not bruises in elders follow the same color patterns as those that occur on younger victims. There is no consensus on color of bruises in any age group.

The dating of contusions has long plagued forensic examiners, especially in light of studies by Mosqueda and colleagues challenging the traditional color trajectory of aging bruises.[37]

Promising tools include the use of computer programs that detect subtle shading and color changes and thus are more discerning than the human eye. In computer analyses, color is described scientifically in terms of wavelength of light. For example, when the term *red* is utilized, it is specified as red-617.2, meaning a red color with a specific wavelength of 617.2 μm. With this approach, those who deal with colors have a common understanding and reference scale. An individual point of color in the computer is called a pixel. A picture is made up of a number of pixels. The computer software program calculates the average value of the primary colors of red, blue, and green in the total photo and then identifies each unique color and determines the number of pixels of that color in the photo and calculates the percentage of that color in the picture.

The ratio of number of colors to the total number of pixels provides some insight into how diverse the color of the bruising is relative to the human eye (**Figures 18-12** through **18-18**). **Figure 18-13** has the greatest number of different colors according to the computer but viewed by the human eye appears to be similar to the other 4 photos. **Figure 18-14** has the color bar and ruler and has a ratio of .412 colors to total pixels. **Figures 18-15** through **18-17** have a ratio of .243 to .245 unique colors to total pixels. The sensitivity of the computer to colors is quite large, ranging from 11 383 different colors in **Figure 18-13** (ratio of .706 to total pixels) to .243 in **Figure 18-16** (41 060 different colors).

Table 18-2. Ratio of the Number of Colors to the Total Number of Pixels

Figure 18-12

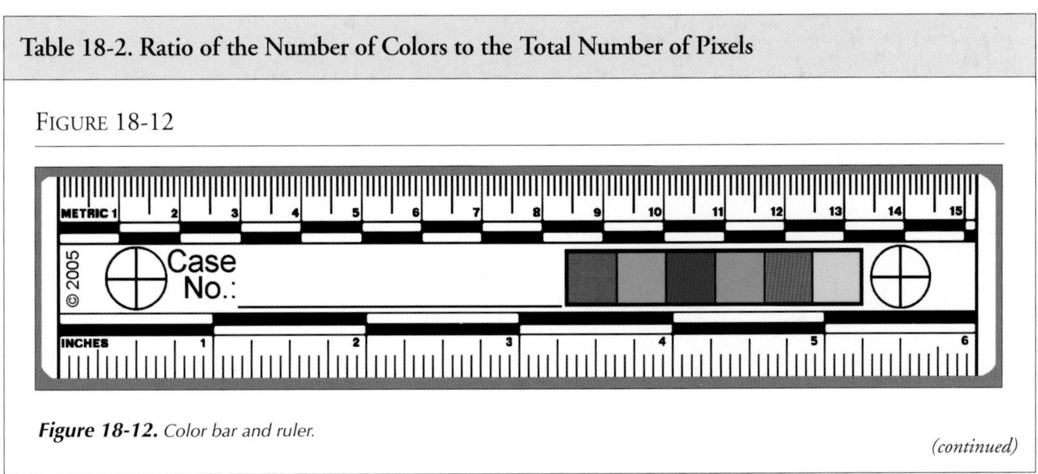

Figure 18-12. *Color bar and ruler.*

(continued)

Table 18-2. Ratio of the Number of Colors to the Total Number of Pixels *(continued)*

FIGURE 18-13

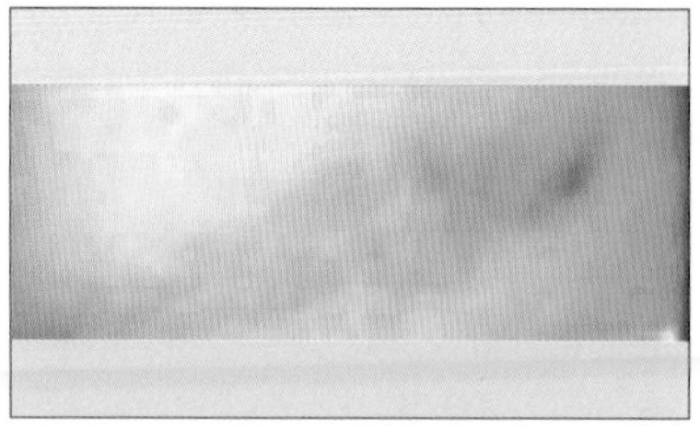

Figure 18-13. This is the bruise of a 50-year-old bumped on leg by snow blower.

Averages:
Red = 187
Green = 195
Blue = 177
Total pixels = 16112
Number of different colors = 11383
Ratio of number of colors to total number of pixels = 0.706

FIGURE 18-14

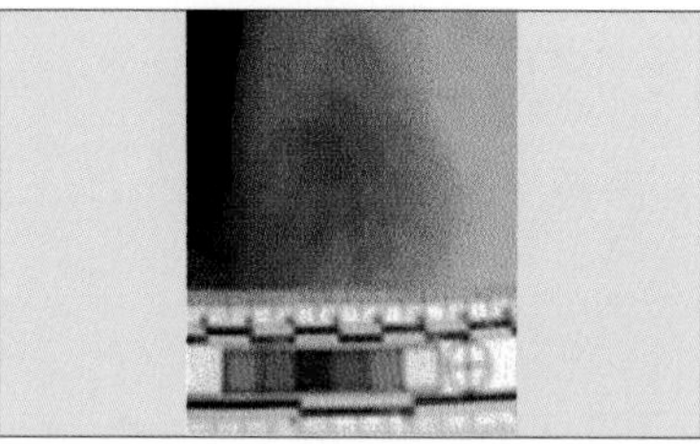

Figure 18-14. This is a bruise shown with a color bar and ruler.

Averages:
Red = 152
Green = 136
Blue = 139
Total pixels = 11770
Number of different colors = 4847
Ratio of number of colors to total number of pixels = 0.412

FIGURE 18-15

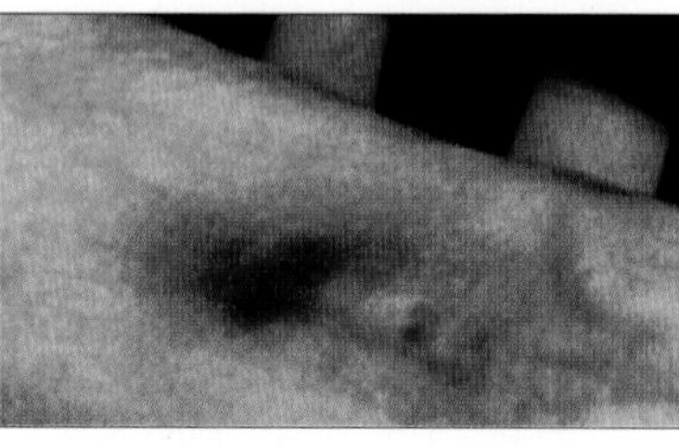

Figure 18-15. This is the bruise of a 50-year-old that is a result of drug use.

Averages:
Red = 148
Green = 110
Blue = 78
Total pixels = 76125
Number of different colors = 18669
Ratio of number of colors to total number of pixels = 0.245

FIGURE 18-16

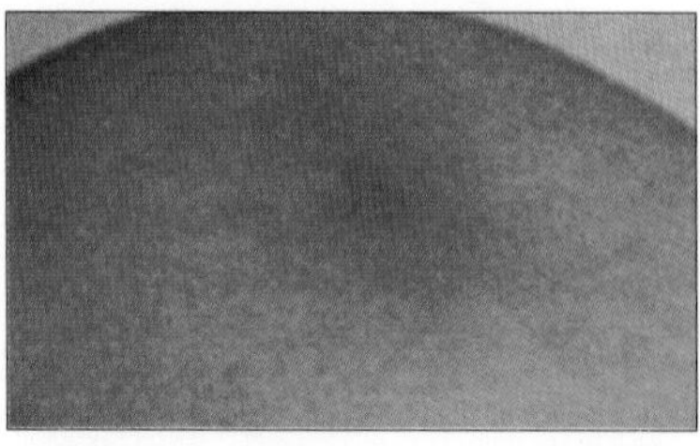

Figure 18-16. Bruise.

Averages:
Red = 188
Green = 139
Blue = 73
Total pixels = 168744
Number of different colors = 41060
Ratio of number of colors to total number of pixels = 0.243

(continued)

Table 18-2. *(continued)*

FIGURE 18-17

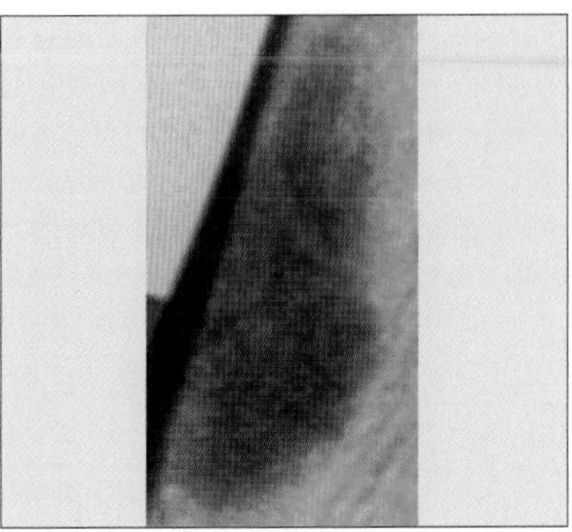

Averages:
Red = 188
Green = 139
Blue = 73
Total pixels = 168744
Number of different colors = 41060
Ratio of number of colors to total number of pixels = 0.243

Figure 18-17. *86-year-old female nursing home resident with bruising to leg.*

FIGURE 18-18

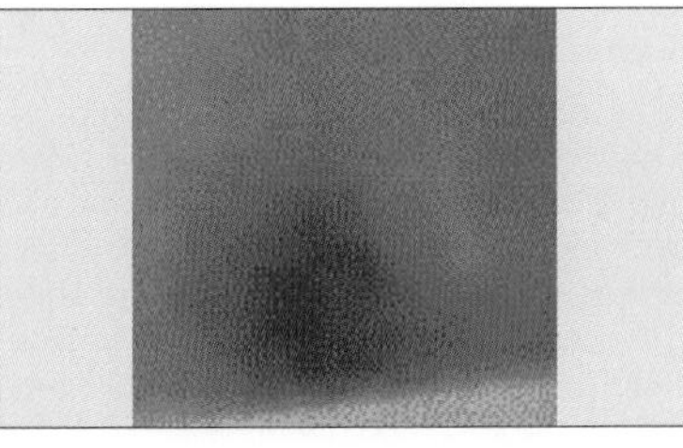

Averages:
Red = 141
Green = 120
Blue = 110
Total pixels = 5850
Number of different colors = 3366
Ratio of number of colors to total number of pixels = 0.575

Figure 18-18. *Bruise.*

Figures 18-12 through 18-18 are provided courtesy of Kohler S, Petrozzi D, and Data Integrity, Inc.

Intervention Services for Elders

Transitioning Elders from Victims to Survivors

Interventions aim to provide services to those already harmed and move them from a victim status to a survivor status and to an optimal level of health. All victims need follow-up for medical and psychological services.

Individual Counseling

There needs to be a list of counselors who have experience with elder victims for purposes of referral. The impact of sexual assaults on elders needs to consider the advanced age, general health status, and diminished cognitive processing. The latter explains why behavioral symptoms may be delayed and prolonged in elders. The following behavioral signs and symptoms have been documented in elders in terms of rape trauma syndrome and posttrauma symptoms. Advocates need to remember that some of the symptoms are muted in elders due to their declining ability to report problems.

Rape Trauma Symptoms

Elders who have been victimized have been noted to exhibit rape-related trauma symptoms, such as becoming fearful of the location of the rape (eg, bathrooms, showers); becoming fearful of males and male caregivers (if assaulted in nursing homes); experiencing flashbacks (eg, believing there is a boy in the closet); and being easily startled (ie, hyperarousal symptoms). They will also exhibit general symptoms of traumatic stress (eg, fear, confusion, hypersomnia, lack of appetite, withdrawal) and symptoms related to existing physical and prior mental conditions will be exacerbated. Elders with the presence of a preexisting cognitive deficit, such as a dementia, may have delay in information processing and impaired communication that potentially compounds the trauma of the sexual assault. The vulnerability of an elder due to physical and emotional fragility places victims at unusually high risk for severe traumatic reactions to assault. Elder victims simply are not equipped physically, constitutionally, or psychologically to defend against and cope with the proximal effects of sexual assault. One 87-year-old nursing home resident with severe dementia who was raped by an attendant, would cry constantly for weeks following the assault. Only her daughter's presence helped to relieve the sobbing.

Rape trauma syndrome, which includes both acute and long-term symptom responses to traumatic sexual assault, has 2 distinct variations: compounded rape trauma and silent rape trauma. In compounded rape trauma, victims have a past and/or current history of psychiatric, psychosocial problems that compound the effects of the sexual assault. In silent rape trauma, expression of assault-related symptomatology is muted, undetected, or absent. Elder sexual abuse victims are subject to both compounded and silent rape trauma.

Case Study 18-9

A 77-year-old victim of the Belmont Shore, California rapist was a cancer survivor with a colostomy bag. She testified that she was sleeping in her easy chair when she awoke suddenly to someone grabbing the crown of her head. She thought it might be an animal and tried to squirm around only to note the hand got tighter. He led her into the bedroom and raped her and told her to relax and enjoy it. The victim testified that the rapist spoke kindly, asked her about her life, offered her a glass of water at one point, and tucked her in before he left. The rapist returned and raped her in her bed 2 weeks later. He had disconnected her motion-detecting lights as well as her phone lines. The victim did not report the first rape due to fear and shame, but did report the second rape. The jury acquitted the defendant for the first assault claiming no DNA, but convicted for the second rape where there was DNA to match to the rapist. This serial offender was charged and convicted of the rape of 14 women, ages 39 to 77, over a 5-year period.

Group Counseling

As with younger victims of sexual assault, advocates should have a list of counselors skilled in conducting group work with victims. Elder victims living in the community often join groups with younger victims. The deciding factor is the choice of elders and whether or not they wish to join.

Music Therapy

Advocates visiting elder victims in an institution can use the technique of music therapy. It requires having tape recorders and tapes of music selected by elders. The goal of the therapy is to help victims learn to reduce the anxiety experienced during the assault and in the activation of rape trauma aftermath symptoms.

Living Situations of Elder Victims and the Process of Recovery

Independent Living

Seniors living independently include those living with their family and/or partners as well as those living alone. If the senior who is raped is alert, verbal, and with minimal memory deficits, the sexual violence advocates generally follow usual protocol for support services as they do for adult victims in general. That is, meet with the senior, assess social network support, provide crisis counseling, and work with the prosecutor's office if the case is scheduled for trial. The following case is an example.

Case Study 18-10

A 68-year-old woman was raped and robbed of $80 by an intruder who kicked down her door. The offender managed to get into the apartment building lobby and past a locked front door. The woman had just returned home and left the apartment door ajar. The man walked up to the woman's apartment and asked if he could use her phone. The woman answered that he could not and shut the door but he kicked open the door, pulled out a knife, and ordered her not to scream. An hour later the woman's husband returned home, found his wife in shock, and called 911. The husband's support and the encouragement provided by the sexual violence advocate and prosecutor enabled the victim to testify in court and help to win a conviction.

Assisted Living

An elder living in assisted living generally implies there is a protected environment that has safety features in place. That is, staff checks on them over 24-hour shifts, and meals and cleaning services are often provided.

When an elder is sexually assaulted in a perceived safe environment, such as assisted living and/or institution, it causes additional trauma because staff has been trusted and there is a breach in safety and security. Very often, the family feels guilty for not keeping the elder at home. Elder intervention needs to focus on verbal and nonverbal signs of stress, behavioral disorganization, aggression, functional ability, and health status. The traumatized elder needs careful observation and a good description of pre-assault behavior from family and staff members for a baseline to assess changes. The following case illustrates the permanent damage of a rape.

Case Study 18-11

A 41-year-old man entered the unsecured door of an assisted living facility and raped an 83-year-old woman in her room. The woman reported she was awakened to the man being in her room and that he stated, "Don't scream or I am going to kill you." She further stated that he held her down and assaulted her, taunting her, and ordering her to use profanity. She refused. After the assault, the man ran into a facility employee and asked her to help him find a friend who he said worked at the facility. He then put his hand over her mouth and wrestled her to the ground, grabbing her checkbook. He escaped and the employee called 911. The police arrived at 2:45 AM and found the perpetrator a few blocks away. When shown videos of himself at the facility, he admitted he entered the premises to sexually assault someone. The son reported that his mother's personality changed after the attack. She moved closer to him but remained withdrawn and reclusive, the opposite of her pre-assault lifestyle.

Nursing Home

Three common nursing home sexual abuse victim profiles include (1) physically disabled older resident, (2) cognitively impaired nursing home resident, and (3) physically impaired younger resident. The physically disabled older resident has no cognitive or mental impairment but requires assistance with mobility. The assistance may be short-term such as needing rehabilitation following surgery or long-term as in residents with complications from a stroke. The cognitively impaired resident has a primary diagnosis of Alzheimer's disease or other dementia, and the physically impaired younger resident may have a physical impairment due to a chronic neuromuscular disorder such as multiple sclerosis or amyotrophic lateral sclerosis (ie, ALS or Lou Gehrig's disease) or an impairment as a result of trauma from a motor vehicle accident or gunshot wound.

Nursing homes are, for the residents, precisely that—a home—and the staff function as the resident's caregivers (in both a literal and figurative sense). The nursing home and its staff are perceived as "safe" and violations represent a more profound betrayal of trust than violations committed outside the sanctity of the home.

Intervention for Family Members of Sexually Abused Elders

Family members need help when an elder is sexually abused whether it happens when the elder is living alone, living in assisted living, or living in a nursing home.

Case Study 18-12

A Queens, New York woman read about a man assaulting 2 elder patients in their hospital beds. She reported it was like reliving her own nightmare. She told a friend she thought it was the same man who assaulted her mother, then 79, in her bed at a New York Medical Center. The man had been taken into the hospital as a patient and admitted to the narcotics unit. Somehow he escaped from his bed and was lost for nearly an hour before hospital officials found him, dressed in scrubs in her mother's room. When her mother attempted to resist his attempts to abuse her, he slapped her face. The woman was quoted in the newspaper as saying, "Maybe when you are younger, you are more resilient, but my mother was never the same after that. She had nightmares three times a week until she died." The woman said her mother was subjected to over a dozen interviews with police, district attorneys, and hospital staff after the assault. The daughter wondered if it hastened her developing senility. She added, "I live with the guilt because I put her in the hospital originally." She also bemoaned the lack of support groups and organizations to address the problem.

It is common for family members to feel guilty when elders are sexually abused. They often feel responsible for decisions made for elders, especially if they are in a nursing home. Advocates can explore with family members decisions for living situations of elders, whether it is independent, assisted, or dependent living. Sometimes family members feel doubly guilty that elders are in nursing homes and then are raped. The exploration of this guilt in terms of realistic parameters is best accomplished in support group settings and is an important part of counseling. There are care provider support groups for persons who have to make decisions to put family members into nursing homes.

Case Study 18-13

A husband made the difficult decision to place his 64-year-old wife in a nursing home, as he was unable to care for her due to a developing dementia and her increasing agitation. Three months after her admission, the husband received a telephone call from a discharged employee stating her conscience was bothering her knowing that information was being withheld from him. The employee went on to relate that the wife had been sexually assaulted by another nursing home resident. When the husband inquired about the incident, the executive director told him that patients are allowed to hug, kiss, and fondle each other, even to the point of sex. When the husband talked directly to the care manager, he learned that his wife and the male resident were both found nude in bed and the male penetrating his wife. The husband argued it was rape (not consensual sex) given the fact that his wife could not dress or undress herself and could not get into bed by herself. The husband immediately removed his wife from the nursing home and contacted the state Ombudsman office and police to report the rape. Unfortunately, the case lacked forensic evidence and witnesses for a criminal case, but a civil suit was pursued and a settlement reached against the nursing home.

Outreach by sexual violence advocates would be critical for intervention both for the wife in the new nursing home and the husband for a family member support group. There was no service available in his state and arrangements were made for him to talk by telephone to another family member of a resident-on-resident nursing home sexual abuse case.

Prevention of Elder Sexual Abuse

Prevention programs of elder sexual abuse are aimed at public education to help people understand what elder sexual abuse is and how it can be prevented. The programs focus on educating seniors, front line workers, and the public about situations and behaviors indicative of abuse. Case examples from news media provide talking points for discussion. The following case illustrates police working with rape crisis staff to educate seniors.

Case Study 18-14

In a Georgia case, a man cut the back porch screen of a home and attacked an 80-year-old woman. The woman told police a man with a cloth over his head ripped off her pajamas and raped her. He then took her nightclothes and bed sheets with him. The victim took a shower after the man left. The police had little to work with on this case and thus the news media account published the following:

If you are raped, rape crisis organizations urge you not to take a shower or bathe before you are examined. You may have valuable evidence on you. Don't touch the crime scene if possible.

The rapist may have touched a surface and police could get a fingerprint. Save all your clothing from the crime and give them to police. Document any injury you have either by photograph or by showing them to investigators. All of these things will help investigators trying to solve the crime.

Prevention programs for elders living independently in the community, in assisted living facilities, or in nursing homes need to be part of all sexual violence community education programs. The program would include the traditional public education to teach elder safety as well as media ads to raise awareness and to increase reporting.

The senior safety education component requires an understanding of the level of the elder's independent functioning and the social network support. In addition, there should be emphasis on a safety checklist specifically designed for seniors. It is stressed that prevention is by safety awareness and not by unreasonable fear of attack.

For seniors living alone in a neighborhood, the safety questions are as follows: Does the senior have some connection with neighbors or family; is there an alert button; does someone check on her each day; does she have good safety locks; are the outside areas well lit so an attacker cannot hide in the yard or bushes; are ground windows secure and routinely examined; are workmen or handymen known to family and or neighbors? For suspected domestic violence cases, elders should be asked if they have been slapped, hit, or beaten in the last 6 months.

The following case examples illustrate elders living independently who were raped and the relationship of the offender.

Case Study 18-15 Victims of Strangers

In Texas, a 95-year-old great grandmother was trimming grass near some railroad tracks outside her home when she was pushed down by a stranger and raped. Her grandson discovered her after the security company telephoned him that his grandmother's alert button had discharged and she was not responding to her telephone. In this case, the elder's alert button saved her life even though it took many hours for her to be found.

Case Study 18-16 Domestic Violence Victims

Sometimes the offender is a family member in a domestic rape as in this case. In Florida, a 94-year-old widow called police to report that her 42-year-old grandson (who lived with his wife in his grandmother's home) had raped her. Police found the elder bleeding and badly bruised. The grandson was found asleep and drunk in the grandmother's bed. Forensic evidence linked him to the crime. Subsequently, the victim's health deteriorated. She became wheelchair bound, required oxygen, and was admitted to a nursing home 3 months after the attack.

Suggested Approaches to Elder Victims in Nursing Homes

Sexual Violence Advocates

Intervention services are much more difficult to provide for the physically handicapped and/or cognitively compromised patient. The critical first step to a traumatized elder in a nursing home is to try to establish contact and trust using a soothing approach and voice.

Sexual violence advocates need training to work with elder sexual assault victims. Talk therapy is usually not the treatment of choice. Expressive therapies, including music therapy and drawing, may be more useful to calm a frightened and anxious elder resident. The elder's favorite music tapes played on a cassette can be soothing and calming during a 30-minute session with an elder victim. Just sitting quietly with elders shows safety, compassion, and concern.

Advocates should not avoid expressing knowing that something happened to them. Even if victims have serious cognitive deficits as through a stroke, advocates should not assume that the victims do not understand. Staff sometimes fail at trying to understand the avenues of communication in persons with cognitive problems because they assume elders do not understand.

Advocates should develop a system of communication whereby elders can tell them "yes" or "no." Once established, a person can try to work with victims. It is important to use comforting measures, such as positioning pillows and adjusting covers, and to talk in a soft, soothing voice (but be sure elders can hear). Avoidance of what happened is not a comfort. It is not necessary to dwell on it but it should be addressed. Suggestions include saying, "I know something happened to you; that you were hurt on your body. Can you show me or tell me about it?" It is critical to emphasize persons who hurt them have been taken away; that they are now safe. The sensory link is important to establish. The advocate should say, "I want to try to understand and talk with you the best way you can. Squeeze my hand if you understand. Nod or blink your eyes to let me know you understand."

Consistency of visits is important. Try to schedule the visit to the nursing home at a consistent time each visit. Short frequent visits are most therapeutic. Try to visit when elders are not receiving nursing or other services. Avoid nap times. Many people are not trained to deal with elders. Centers and agencies need to have staff who have experience with elders. However, most people have elder relatives or have visited nursing homes. Have them draw on those experiences. Elder victims may have preexisting areas of weakness or vulnerability, primarily physical and cognitive, which serve to complicate or mute the assault symptom presentation. Observe behavior carefully for symptoms of trauma. If no one is available on staff to visit a victim in a nursing home, refer to a visiting nurse association that can provide a geropsychiatric nurse specialist for consultation and guidance. Sometimes staff are uncomfortable with elders and their physical and cognitive limitations. Schools are bringing children into nursing homes to help them feel more comfortable around elders. Rape crisis centers could do prevention programs in nursing homes to help their staff feel more comfortable dealing with an elder.

Nursing Home Staff

A thorough physical, cognitive, and psychosocial assessment should be completed by professional staff at the time of admission to the nursing home. These assessments provide nursing staff and other caregivers with a baseline from which to judge behavioral changes. They need training to detect noteworthy changes in baseline behavior in victims who are likely to exhibit symptoms in a muted or "silent" fashion.

All nursing home personnel should be trained rigorously to identify signs and symptoms of assault-related trauma and to be vigilant to suspicious, pre-assault behaviors, including the same grooming and manipulation observed with most sex offenders. Nursing home staff need to be sensitized to the gravity of the assaults on the residents. Stereotypes exist, including the cynical disbelief that anyone would sexually assault an elder to what can be described as a perverse sense of amusement. In conclusion, elder victims of sexual violence represent a vulnerable and poorly understood population of victims. Elders may be sexually assaulted in their homes or the community, in an assisted living facility, or in a nursing home environment. Offenders can be strangers, domestic partners, family members, another nursing home resident, or caregiver. As with all victims, the primary goal of prevention and intervention is safety for elders. Special adjustments need to be made for the interview and forensic examination process due to elders' physical and emotional health status. Trauma symptoms will be filtered through any cognitive deficits that are present and adjustments need to be made for any short-term memory issues.

The prosecution of offenders of elder victims is critical to decrease additional victims. Sexual violence advocates need to continue working as a team member with law enforcement, SANEs, medical and mental health staff, social service providers, and prosecutors. Most importantly, sexual violence advocates need to add elder sexual abuse to their community education programs, train their staff in detecting and reporting elder sexual abuse, and recruit staff who will provide crisis intervention services to traumatized elder victims.

Discussion

Advanced age is no defense against sexual assault. Elders victimized in the Burgess et al study spanned 4 decades from 60 to 100 years of age.[38] Offenders ranged in age from 13 to 90 years. Neither ages of victims nor offenders was a barrier to sexual abuse.

Study findings reveal the extreme vulnerability of elders to sexual assault. Elder women are likelier to be perceived by motivated offenders as suitable targets.[39] Those who do not require care often live alone due to their longer life expectancy over males and higher risk for widowhood. Vulnerability is related to physical size and strength and elder women are perceived as less capable than younger women to flee or resist attack. Age-related skeletal, neuromuscular, and other physical changes restrict mobility and reduce ability to self-defend. Significant physical and cognitive disabilities existed in the studied victims. Almost half were controlled by the mere presence of the offender, and a weapon was used in less than 4% of the cases. Based upon study findings, it appears that sexual offenders deem it unnecessary to restrain people with dementia during sexual assaults. This finding alone is powerful evidence of the high vulnerability of elders with cognitive loss to assault.

Fairly equal numbers of cases were reported to APS and CJS.[40] However, cases in which relationships existed between alleged victims and offenders tended not to be initially referred to CJS. These cases were less frequently investigated as potential crimes and less often referred for prosecution. In addition, the involved elders were less likely to receive physical examinations. All of these factors can jeopardize the particular elder as well as other potential victims. Of special concern are residents and staff members who offend in elder care facilities. Failure to notify law enforcement, collect forensic evidence, and prosecute when indicated puts other residents at risk due to the repetitive nature of sexual offending and the vulnerability of facility residents.

Typically, suspected sexual abuse victims coming to official attention are referred for a physical and rape examination and forensic evidence is collected. However, less than half of the studied suspected victims received forensic medical examinations. Several APS records indicated instances of caseworkers requesting sexual assault examinations for elders and medical personnel refusing to "put the elder through the trauma" or resisting the idea that an elder would require this type of exam. While this study found more visible physical injuries and genital trauma in the CJS elders, the fact that only 18% of APS elders were examined raises the possibility that undetected injuries existed.[40]

Elders who may have been sexually assaulted should routinely be offered the opportunity to undergo a forensic examination to assess injuries, arrange necessary treatment, and collect evidence. In cases in which elders are unable to grant informed consent, permission should be sought from substitute decision makers authorized by a court having jurisdiction. Impaired elders' assent should be elicited for all medical and forensic procedures. Examinations must be conducted by properly trained and compassionate forensic personnel who do not have a stake in the case; preferably SANEs experienced in working with elders. Clinical records reveal that some alleged victims are examined by staff employed in the facility in which alleged abuse occurred. They are not only forensically untrained but also have a potential vested interest in case outcome. Advanced age should not be a barrier to receiving competent and unbiased medical/nursing assessment and treatment following sexual assault.

Prosecutors were more successful in the cases initially reported to CJS than APS. One barrier to prosecution can be the familial relationship between victim and offender. In these cases, civil court orders of protection and other APS interventions help to protect victims. However, societal attention to promote increased prosecution of domestic violence elder offenders is recommended.

A second barrier in investigation and prosecution results because of the limited memory and lack of capacity for communication amongst elders. People with dementia frequently experience aphasia and other language difficulties.[41-43] Specialized training is critical to equip investigators to effectively interview elders with barriers to communication.[44] Behavior displayed by victims following abuse demonstrated psychosocial trauma regardless of whether or not they could verbally discuss the event(s). In fact, there was no significant difference between elders with and without dementia in terms of post-abuse behavioral symptoms of distress. Prosecutors might consider using as fact testimony the presence of behavioral indicators of distress in victims following assault.[38]

Presently, elder sexual abuse statistics are not included in criminal justice reporting. Expanding the national database to include details regarding forced intentional sexual injury of elders would address the under reporting issue and help encourage professional awareness of and education regarding elder sexual abuse.

Conclusion

In summary, when elders are victimized, they may suffer greater physical injuries than other age groups. Furthermore, the aging process brings with it a decreased ability to heal after injury. Elder victims may never fully recover from the trauma of victimization. Additionally, there may be disbelief that an elder has been sexually victimized. To counter this attitude, nurse practitioners are advised to examine and record all information as a forensic case. The only persons who are designated to determine sexual assault are the judge and jury.

Advanced age and disability are not protections from sexual abuse. In fact, these conditions increase vulnerability and reduce chances that a victim will be examined, will be able to disclose abuse experiences, and that her case will be successfully prosecuted.

All practitioners, family, and other caregivers need to be informed about sexual assault and other forms of interpersonal violence perpetrated against elders. They need to be able to implement prevention strategies, recognize forensic abuse markers, support victims, and provide opportunities for comprehensive assessment and medicolegal and psychosocial intervention. Information should emphasize that an elder's inability to demonstrate recall of sexual victimization via verbal disclosure does not necessarily indicate that an elder victim has not been psychosocially or physically traumatized by abuse.

References

1. Lachs M, Williams CS, O'Brien S, Pillemer KA, Charlson ME. The mortality of elder mistreatment. *J Am Med Assoc.* 1998;280:428-432.

2. MacDonald J. *Rape: Offenders and Their Victims.* Springfield, IL: CC Thomas Co; 1971.

3. Amir M. *Patterns in Forcible Rape.* Chicago, Il: University of Chicago Press; 1971.

4. Fletcher A. *Annual report of the Syracuse Rape Crisis Center.* Syracuse, NY: Syracuse Rape Crisis Center; 1978.

5. Hicks D. Medical treatment for the victim: the development of a rape treatment center. In: Walker M, Brodsky S, eds. *Sexual Assault.* Lexington, MA: Lexington Books; 1976:53-59.

6. Cartwright PS, Moore RA. The elderly victim of rape. *South Med J.* 1989;82:988-989.

7. Ramin SM, Satin AJ, Stone IC, Wendel GD. Sexual assault in postmenopausal women. *Obstet Gynecol.* 1992;80:860-864.

8. Ramsey-Klawsnik H. Elder sexual abuse: preliminary findings. *J Elder Abuse Negl.* 1991;3(3):73-90.

9. Holt MG. Elder sexual abuse in Britain: preliminary findings. *J Elder Abuse Negl.* 1993;5(2):63-71.

10. Teaster PB, Roberto KA, Duke JO, Kim M. Sexual abuse of older adults: preliminary findings of cases in Virginia. *J Elder Abuse Negl.* 2000;12(3/4):1-17.

11. Burgess AW, Dowdell EB, Prentky RA. Sexual abuse of nursing home residents. *J Psychosoc Nurs.* 2000;38(6):10-18.

12. Burgess AW, Holmstrom LL. Rape trauma syndrome. *Am J Psychiatry.* 1974;131:981-986.

13. Ramsey-Klawsnik H. Dynamics of sexual assault/abuse against people with disabilities and the elderly. In: Wisconsin Coalition Against Sexual Assault. *Widening the Circle: Sexual Assault/Abuse and People with Disabilities and the Elderly.* Madison, WI: Author; 1998:131, 981-986.

14. Ramsey-Klawsnik H. Elder sexual abuse within the family. *J Elder Abuse Negl.* 2003;15(1):43-58.

15. Ramsey-Klawsnik H. Elder sexual abuse perpetrated by residents in care settings. *Victimization Elderly Disabled.* 2004;6(6):81, 93–95.

16. Burgess AW, Hanrahan NP, Baker T. Forensic markers in female sexual abuse cases. *Clin Geriatr Med.* 2005;21(2):399-412.

17. National Center on Elder Abuse. Attitudes toward elder mistreatment and reporting: A multicultural study. Washington, DC: National Center on Elder Abuse; 1998.

18. Teaster PB. A response to the abuse of vulnerable adults: the 2000 survey of state adult protective services. Washington, DC: National Center on Elder Abuse; 2003.

19. US Department of Justice. Statistics on Adult Protective Services, Office of Justice Programs. Washington, DC: US Printing Office; 2000.

20. Roberto KA Teaster PB. Sexual abuse of vulnerable young and old women. *Violence Against Women.* 2005;2(4):473-504.

21. Bureau of Justice Statistics. Crimes against persons age 65 or older 1992-1997. Washington, DC: US Dept of Justice; 2002.

22. Resnick H, Acierno R, Holmes M, Kilpatrick DG, Jager N. Prevention of post-rape psychopathology: preliminary findings of a controlled acute rape treatment study. *J Anxiety Disord.* 1999;13:359-370.

23. Davis, L. & Brody, E. Rape and older women: a guide to prevention and protection (DHEW Publication No. 78-734). Bethesday, MD: National Institute of Mental Health; 1979.

24. Crowell N, Burgess AW. *Understanding Violence Against Women.* Washington, DC: National Academy Press; 1996.

25. Bobb J. Trauma in the elderly. *J Gerontologic Nurs.* 1995;13:8-15.

26. Levy D, Hanlon D, Townsend R. Geriatric trauma. *Geriatr Emerg Care*. 1993;9(3): 601-620.

27. Finelli F, et al. A case controlled study of major trauma in geriatric patients. *J Trauma*. 1989;29:541-548.

28. Champion E, et al. Medical intensive care for the elderly. *JAMA*. 1991;246:2052-2056.

29. Centers for Disease Control. Older population age 65 years and older: deaths and life expectancy. Washington, DC: National Center for Health Statistics; 2008.

30. Office of Victims of Crime. First response to victims of crime: a handbook for law enforcement officers on how to approach and help. Washington DC: US Dept of Justice; 2001.

31. Hogue C. Injury in later life: Part 1, Epidemiology. *J Am Geriatric Soc*. 1982;30: 183-190.

32. Pentland B, et al. Head injury in the elderly. *Aging*. 1996;15:193-201.

33. Fogelholm R, Heiskanen O, Waltimo. Chronic subdurals in adults: influence of patient age. *J Neurosurg*. 1995;42:43-46.

34. Cartwright PS. Factors that correlate with injury sustained by survivors of sexual assault. *Obstet Gynecol*. 1987;70:44-46.

35. Tyra P. Older women: victims of rape. *J Gerontol Nurs*. 1993;19(5):7-12.

36. Slaughter L, et al. Patterns of genital injury in female sexual assault victims. *Am J Obstet Gynecol*. 1997;176(3):609-616.

37. Mosqueda L, Mosqueda L, Burnight K, Liao S. The life cycle of bruises in older adults. *J Am Geriatr Soc*. 2005;53(8):1339-1343.

38. Burgess AW, Phillips SL. Sexual abuse, trauma and dementia in the elderly: a retrospective study of 284 cases. *Victims Offenders*. 2006;1:193-204.

39. Safarik ME. Elder female sexual homicide. In: Douglas JE, Burgess AW, Burgess AG, Ressler RK, eds. *Crime Classification Manual*. 2nd ed. San Francisco, CA: Jossey-Bass; 2006: 235.

40. Burgess AW, Ramsey-Klawsnik H, Gregorian SB. Comparing elder sexual abuse victims reporting patterns. *J Elder Abuse Negl*. 2008;20(4):336-352.

41. Gambassi G, Landi F, Peng L, Brostrup-Jensen C, Calore K, Hiris J, Lipsitz L, Mor V, Bernabei R. Comorbidity and drug use in cognitively impaired elderly living in long-term care. *J Am Geriatr Soc*. 1998;46:250-252.

42. Hawes C, Morris JN, Phillips CD, Mor V, Fries BE, Nonemaker S. Facility characteristics associated with hospitalization of nursing home residents: results of a national study. *Med Care*. 1999;37(3):228-237.

43. Phillips CD, Chu CW, Morris JN, Hawes C. Effects of cognitive impairment on the reliability of geriatric assessments in nursing homes. *J Am Geriatr Soc*. 1993;41(2):136-142.

44. Ramsey-Klawsnik H, Klawsnik L. Interviewing victims with barriers to communication. *Victimization Elderly Disabled*. 2004;2(4):49-50, 63-64.

Chapter 19

Sexual Homicide

Ann Wolbert Burgess, DNSc, APRN, BC, FAAN
Mark E. Safarik, MS, VSM (FBI Ret.)

The act of homicide draws public interest through the media as well as professional concern through scholarly publications. The homicide literature has specialized research areas by age of victim (eg, infanticide, elder murder), number of victims (eg, double, triple, mass, serial), type of victim(s) (family annihilators and co-dependent crimes [eg, felony, sexual]). Since the late 1960s, the reemergence of the women's movement has helped to focus attention on violence against women, primarily on the crimes of rape and domestic violence.

Sexual homicide results from one person killing another in the context of power, control, aggression, and sexuality. It has been difficult to gather dependable statistics on sexual homicide victims for several reasons. First, the victim is officially reported as a homicide statistic and not as a rape assault, and thus the sexual component is subsumed into the homicide. Second, there is often a failure by law enforcement investigators to recognize any of the underlying sexual dynamics in a murder without clear visual evidence of a sexual assault. The sexual dynamic is usually identified by injury to or activity that focuses on the sexual areas of the body (eg, breasts, buttocks, and genital areas), and the adjustment or removal of the victim's clothing in order to gain access to the sexual areas of the body. Third, often those agencies that investigate, apprehend, and assess the murderer fail to share their findings, curtailing the collective pool of knowledge on the subject. Fourth, there may be a failure to collect forensic evidence associated with the crime's sexual nature either because it is absent or not recognized as potential evidence. In a sexual assault homicide where the offender has pushed up the bra of the victim in order to gain access to her breasts, although investigators recognize the rape component, they may not swab her breasts for saliva, thereby eliminating the potential to collect crucial physical evidence.

The assessment of a sexual homicide utilizes a multidisciplinary approach. Depending on the specific attributes associated with the crime, information critical to assessing the offender can be obtained from various factions of the investigation. This chapter highlights a scale measure used to assess injury severity; the assessment process involved in a forensic autopsy, and the contribution of the forensic examiner to understanding the crime scene dynamics—specifically the interaction of the offender, the victim, and the scene. The findings from a large sample of sexual homicides of adults over the age of 60 are also discussed with case examples.

Measuring Injury Severity in Homicide

In homicide, death is the outcome in all cases and few additional measures of violence are studied. Safarik and Jarvis first noted this methodological gap in their search of literature and suggested researchers assumed the measurement of injury severity was of little value because the victim suffered a lethal injury.[1] Taking into account that measurement is a key component in any scientific pursuit, the literature on homicide in general was searched for instruments specific to assessing violent injury in homicides. Safarik and Jarvis argued that injury measurement could be used to further study the nature of violent crime in terms of the dynamics of homicidal behavior.[1] The measurement and coding of victim injuries can assist in assessing victim injury, and studying crime scene dynamics and offender behavior.

Cause of death may be useful because most homicide studies attribute weapon use in cause of death as characteristic of homicidal injury. Weapon use is commonly addressed in most national studies including the US Federal Bureau of Investigation's (FBI) Uniform Crime Reporting (UCR) data,[2] Supplemental Homicide Reports (SHR), and the National Incident-Based Reporting System (NIBRS). For all homicides and the majority of other autopsies performed each day throughout the United States, medical examiners identify and describe both qualitatively and quantitatively, the minutiae of each injury, its severity, and its relationship to the cause of death. Therefore, cause of death is the "...disease, injury, or abnormality that alone or in combination is responsible for initiating the sequence of functional disturbances, whether brief or prolonged, that eventually ends in death."[3] This is somewhat different than the mechanism of death, which is the process that causes one or more vital organs or organ systems to fail when a fatal disease, injury, abnormality, or chemical insult occurs. It is the functional or structural changes that make independent life no longer possible after a lethal event has occurred.[3] Due to the complexity and lack of specificity associated with the mechanism of death, medical examiners usually focus on identifying the primary cause of death. Analyzing the details of the medical examiners report generally provides the information necessary to differentiate between postmortem and antemortem injuries, assess the severity of an injury along a continuum from superficial to fatal, and determine the presence or absence of a nexus between a particular injury and a cause of death. These details range from an anatomical examination of the body and organ systems at the macro level to a histological review of tissue samples.

Table 19-1. Abbreviated Injury Scale

AIS Score	Injury
1	Minor
2	Moderate
3	Serious
4	Severe
5	Critical
6	Fatal

A number of methods for determining the injury severity of trauma patients have been developed over the years. These methods, based on both the type and anatomical distribution of injuries, have been generally classified in two ways. Some evaluations use anatomical scores such as the Abbreviated Injury Scale (AIS)* (**Table 19-1**) and the Injury Severity Score (ISS), while others use physiological scores, which measure the physiological responses to injury, such as the Glasgow Coma Scale (GCS). What is clear from these measurement instruments is that in the field of medical trauma, many injury metrics are used and constant revisions are underway to provide for more situationally specific schemes. As a consequence, the medical community has a long history of using injury metrics to improve both our ability to evaluate and to respond to trauma and injury.

* *The first useful anatomical scoring system was created under sponsorship of the American Medical Association.[4] This resulted in the development of an Abbreviated Injury Scale (AIS). The AIS and the scales derived from it are anatomical scales that score the injuries themselves and not the consequences of the injuries. The AIS is a consensus-derived anatomically based system that classifies individual injury severity on a 6-point ordinal scale ranging from 1 (minor injury) to 6 (lethal injury) using 9 body regions at more than 1300 individual anatomical sites. More details on coding anatomical injury using the AIS are discussed elsewhere.[5]*

The Homicide Injury Scale (HIS), developed by Safarik and Jarvis, can compare injuries across a large sample of cases for multiple causes of death and attendant levels of injury.[1] According to Safarik and Jarvis, the HIS attempts to capture the qualitative element of a victim's fatal injuries (within the context of homicide) in a quantitative manner.[1] This is done by quantifying the severity of only those injuries that are directly related to the cause of death through a detailed review of the medical examiner's autopsy report and related protocols.[1]

The HIS is designed to capture the number of causes of death and related injury severities as identified by the medical examiner. The proposed values and attendant interpretations for the HIS are shown in **Table 19-2**.

Most homicide studies examine weapon use or, more broadly, cause of death, as attributes of homicidal injury. These attributes are commonly addressed in most national studies including the UCR data 2, SHR, and NIBRS.[6] Other large studies, such as the Chicago Homicide Data Set, capture similar basic injury data. Despite these extensive data collections, little if any homicide research has examined the severity of injury as an independent variable to predict offender attributes. Most studies consider only the cause of death, which assumes no variation in injury since every victim suffered a lethal injury.

Characterization of injury severity has been shown to be critical to the scientific study of trauma. Extensive research has been conducted to assess trauma and injury severity in patients for various reasons.[7,8] One of the most important reasons concerns trauma care research and assisting in the scientific study of the epidemiology of trauma.[9] The work presented here applies similar methodologies to the study of injury severity in homicide cases. Since outcome (ie, death) is a constant value in all cases, it clearly carries no value in this assessment. Instead, injury severity is used to predict different dependent variables, which are offender attributes in this case. However, this approach was challenged because there are no established or empirically valid scales for quantifying

Table 19-2. The Homicide Injury Scale

Value	Attendant Interpretations
1	Single cause of death only: Internal injuries only with no visible related external injuries
2	Single cause of death only: Internal injuries have only minor or minimal associated external injuries (eg, smothered with related abrasions and/or contusions of mouth and face; strangled with related abrasions or ligature marks)
3	Single cause of death only: External injuries are described as moderate, serious, or severe but are not considered excessive
4	Two or more causes of death: External injuries for each respective cause of death are described as moderate, serious, or severe but are not considered excessive
5	Single cause of death only: The related external injuries are identified as excessive
6	Two or more causes of death: Related internal and external injuries in at least one of the causes of death are identified as excessive

injury severity in homicide victims. Therefore, proposed methodologies for constructing such scales are inspired by existing trauma scoring systems and were tested using data selected from sexual homicides of women who were 60 years of age or older. The victims of this demographic seemed particularly appropriate since their advanced age and related inability to effectively defend themselves generally ensured that the severity of their injuries was not likely to be related to the offenders' inability to gain or maintain control of them. As a result, it was likely that any severe injury would be related to the offender's intent to inflict such injuries. The level of injury exhibited in a number of the cases in this study was found to be excessive and is an attribute believed to be distinct from other violent crimes. Interestingly, in studies by both Groth and Pollock, similar results were found in earlier studies of older adult sexual assault and homicide.[10,11] Qualitative analysis of these cases further suggested that variation in the degree of injury suffered may be a useful measure to analyze offender behavior. Therefore, 2 scales previously noted, the HIS and the ISS, were created to quantify the severity of those injuries to identify a way these cases could be compared using the severity of the victim's injuries.

The HIS draws on available medical examiner data and ranks injury severity from 1 to 6. Not relying solely on this convention, the ISS is currently used by the US Centers for Disease Control (CDC) and is utilized by adapting an injury scale developed by Baker et al.[12] The ISS is an anatomical scoring system that provides an overall score for patients with multiple injuries (**Table 19-3**). Each injury is assigned an AIS score and is assigned to one of 6 body regions (head, face, chest, abdomen, external, and extremities, which includes pelvis). Only the highest AIS score in each body region is used. The 3 most severely injured body regions have their score squared and added together to produce the ISS score. The ISS score takes values from 0 to 75. If an injury is assigned an AIS of 6 (ie, fatal injury), the ISS score is automatically assigned to 75. The ISS score is virtually the only anatomical scoring system in use and correlates linearly with mortality, morbidity, hospital stay, and other measures of severity, including the New Injury Severity Score (NISS).

Both the HIS and ISS have proven easy and uncomplicated to use and appropriate for quantifying the qualitative components of homicide injury severity. While the HIS and

Table 19-3. Injury Severity Score: Example Calculation

Region	Injury Description	Abbreviated Injury Scale	Square Top Three
Head and Neck	Cerebral contusion	3	9
Face	No injury	0	0
Chest	Flail chest	4	16
Abdomen	Minor contusion of liver complex rupture spleen	5	25
Extremity	Fractured femur	3	0
External	No injury	0	0
Injury Severity Score:			**50**

ISS metrics both capture fatal injuries, they are slightly different. Both these measures provide quantitative evidence supporting the differentiation of levels of homicidal injury as an attribute of these cases.

These scales also revealed that many victims suffered multiple, severe, and excessive injuries. The mean for both injury metrics approximated the range of the scale synonymous with excessive injury. Finally, the HIS and ISS were then used in subsequent analyses in an effort to further the examination of offender characteristics. They were shown to be useful in providing statistically significant offender variable information within a limited data set reflecting homicides of older women. As such, an accurate method for quantitatively measuring injury severity has many potential applications. Consider the following case example drawn from the research that is illustrative of the homicidal injury–scoring scheme of the HIS.

Case Study 19-1

A 67-year-old female was found dead in the bathroom of her apartment. The apartment was located in an apartment complex that catered to the senior community. She was found lying on her bathroom floor. She was completely nude and had suffered numerous cutting and stabbing injuries to the sexual areas of her body as well as her abdomen and lower back. The medical examiner described at least 87 stabbing injuries to her chest and abdomen. Many of these injuries had been inflicted antemortem. The offender had partially disemboweled her, removing a portion of her colon and other internal organs. The incised injuries resulted in near complete destruction of the vagina and rectum. This made any attempt to secure vaginal or anal swabs as part of the sexual assault examination nearly impossible due to the significant bleeding that resulted from those injuries. Due to the lack evidence from swab collection, the attention by both investigators and medical personnel to the complete documentation of all injuries became paramount. The significant documented injuries included the bruising of the breasts and buttocks, resulting from being viciously grabbed by the offender. Those documented injuries became important in supporting the sexual assault component to the homicide charges. Scoring of the injury severity would adhere to the HIS scheme. The medical examiner identified the cause of death as exsanguination due to sharp force injuries (ie, cutting and stabbing). Because a single cause of death was identified and the injuries related to that cause of death were clearly excessive, the assigned scoring value would be identified as a 5.

See **Figures 19-1** and **19-2**, which illustrate Case Study 19-1.

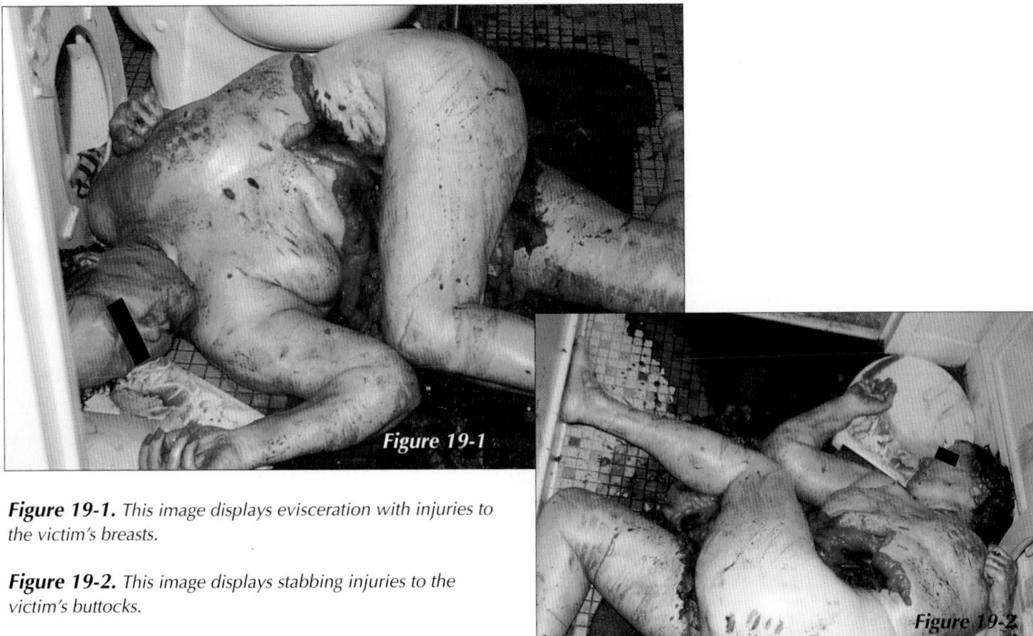

Figure 19-1. *This image displays evisceration with injuries to the victim's breasts.*

Figure 19-2. *This image displays stabbing injuries to the victim's buttocks.*

Other aspects not addressed by this work could also be considered (eg, the level of familiarity, the degree of psychosis).

To this end, the injury scales proposed and utilized were found to be useful; however, it should be cautioned that these measures represent a beginning, rather than an end, to metrics for analyzing injury severity in criminal behavior. Nonetheless, the findings discovered in the cases examined suggest that excessive homicidal injuries were indicative of an offender who was both younger and local to the crime scene. Extension of the methods and procedures to other types of homicide may find different results. In the meantime, this analysis clearly suggests that quantifying injury severity in homicides produces statistically viable metrics that may provide investigative direction as well as assist the police in identifying potential homicide suspects. This approach also suggests directions for future homicide research. Consider, for example, forensic or police field studies applying injury-scoring schemes along the lines suggested here to examine a wider variety of homicides. Still other areas that might be explored include examining the utility of injury scoring schemes in both lethal and nonlethal (typically aggravated assault) cases, and examination of injury scales as a solvability factor for law enforcement to utilize in efforts to increase clearance rates. In any event, the procedures suggested here for quantifying qualitative values of injury severity in homicide cases show promise for exciting avenues of future research.

Forensic Autopsy

The forensic pathologist first examines the outside of the body. A great deal can be learned in this way. Many pathologists use scalpels with rulers marked on their blades.

The body is opened using a Y-shaped incision from shoulders to mid-chest and down to the pubic region. If the skull is to be opened, the pathologist makes a second incision across the head, joining the bony prominences just below and behind the ears. When this is sewed back, the pillow on which the cadaver's head rests will conceal it.

The pathologist uses a scalpel for these incisions. There is almost no bleeding, since a cadaver has no blood pressure except that produced by gravity.

The incisions are carried down to the skull, thoracic wall, sternum, and abdominal cavity. The scalp and soft tissues of the anterior thoracic wall are then reflected. The pathologist observes for any abnormalities. The first dissection in the abdomen usually frees the large intestine. Some pathologists do this with a scalpel, while others use scissors. The skull vault is opened using 2 saw-cuts—one in front and one in back. These will not show through the scalp when it is sewed back together.

When the sternum and attached costal cartilages are removed, they are examined. Often, they are fractured during cardiopulmonary resuscitation. The top of the skull is removed, and the brain is very carefully cut free of its attachments from inside the skull. The chest organs, including the heart and lungs, are inspected. Sometimes pathologists take blood from the heart to check for bacteria in the blood and to run toxicological analyses for drugs and poisons. For this, they use very large hypodermic needles and syringes. They may also find something else that will need to be sent to the microbiology lab to search for infection. Blood, urine, bile, or even eye fluid will be sent to the lab for chemical study and to look for medicine, illicit drugs, alcohol, and poisons.

The pathologist weighs the major solid organs (eg, heart, lung, brain, kidney, liver, spleen) on a scale. The smaller organs (eg, thyroid, adrenals) get weighed on a chemist's triple-beam balance. Tissues are submitted to the histology lab to be made into microscopic slides. A sexual assault forensic exam is conducted to collect samples to test for the presence of semen as well as to document injuries to the vagina, anus, and internal organs. The procedure to follow is described in the chapter on collection of evidence in sexual assault cases.

Forensic Evidence

The sex crime investigator at the crime or death scene will need special equipment and special expertise. Recognizing the sexual nature of a homicide can be difficult. Unless the sexual component to the crime is obvious it can be subsumed within the homicide itself and investigators can overlook subtle indicators that reveal the true sexual nature of the crime. Offenders can engage in nonsexual behavior that in reality is servicing their sexual needs but often is not recognized as such by the investigators. Sexual sadism serves as an example of such behavior. Sexual sadists are sexually aroused by the suffering of their victims. The suffering results from the infliction of physical and/or psychological injury. Externally, though, what is observed by investigators in such cases are the physical injuries suffered by the victims. The investigator has no way to link the injuries to the sexual arousal of the offender. In these instances, the physical acts by the offender that inflict physical or emotional suffering, which in and of themselves cannot be construed as sexual behavior, service the sexual needs of the offender by intensifying his sexual or psychological arousal.[13] Conversely, offenders may engage in sexual behavior in the service of nonsexual needs. Because investigators must deal with the dynamics presented at the crime scene, the motive is less important than the offender's actions. The recognition of the sexual nature of the crime takes priority, and the type of evidence considered for collection must take into account the sexual aspect of the crime, regardless of the underlying motives. Forensic evidence often sought in sexual homicides can be difficult to identify and collect. Biological specimens, including semen, blood, saliva, urine, and sweat, as well as fingerprints, hairs, and fibers can all contain DNA or other nuclear material. The process of extracting fingerprints, debris, or DNA from duct tape or other binding material like rope knots is extraordinarily difficult. Locating and subsequently obtaining semen evidence, for instance, requires the use of forensic light sources. Semen has a faint fluorescence under a long-wave ultraviolet light (Wood's lamp), and many fibers have a strong fluorescence under this kind of light. Both the victim's body and her clothing should be subjected to forensic light analysis. The victim's clothing can reveal a great deal about the assault. Determining who removed the clothing based on its location at the scene, the victim, or offender; the physical condition of the clothes (eg, garment tearing or missing buttons); and if the clothes were removed fully or partially not only tell if a struggle ensued, but whether clothing worn after the assault may contain evidence (ie, from anal or vaginal discharge) (**Figures 19-3** and **19-4**).

Consideration should be given to examining deceased victims in much the same manner as for those who are survivors of sexual assault. The optimal procedure is to have a sexual assault examiner from a sexual assault nurse examiner (SANE) team or sexual assault response team (SART) conduct their examination in conjunction with any criminal investigation or autopsy. Law enforcement investigators should be cognizant of collecting forensic evidence that is most useful in a sexual assault case. Other evidence may be useful, such as footwear impressions or fingernail scrapings, but these are the standard trace items that are focused on in every "rape kit." The logical solution to a rape case among other investigative avenues should focus on matching trace evidence obtained from 3 distinct locations: crime scene, victim, and perpetrator.

Figure 19-3. *This victim died from blunt force trauma. The offender transported the body to this remote location; the sexual assault occurred elsewhere.*

Figure 19-4. *This is a different view of the same victim.*

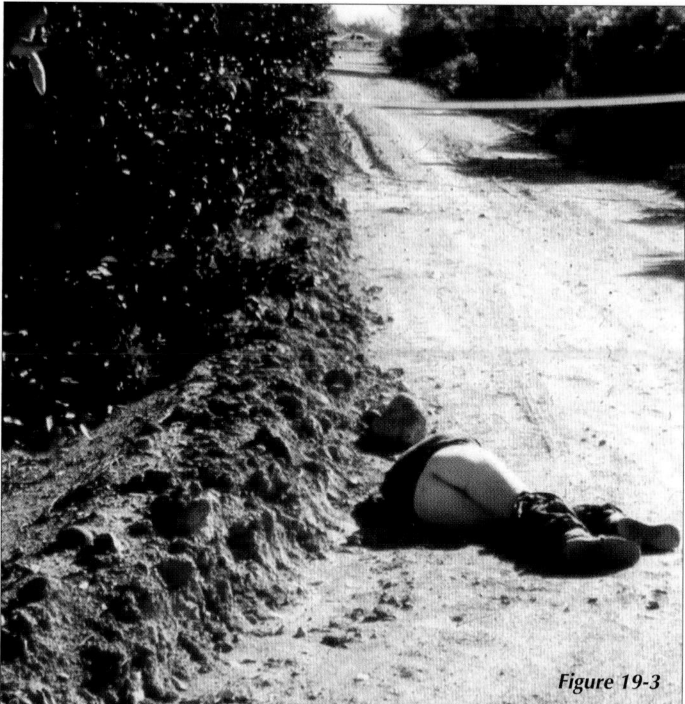

Figure 19-3

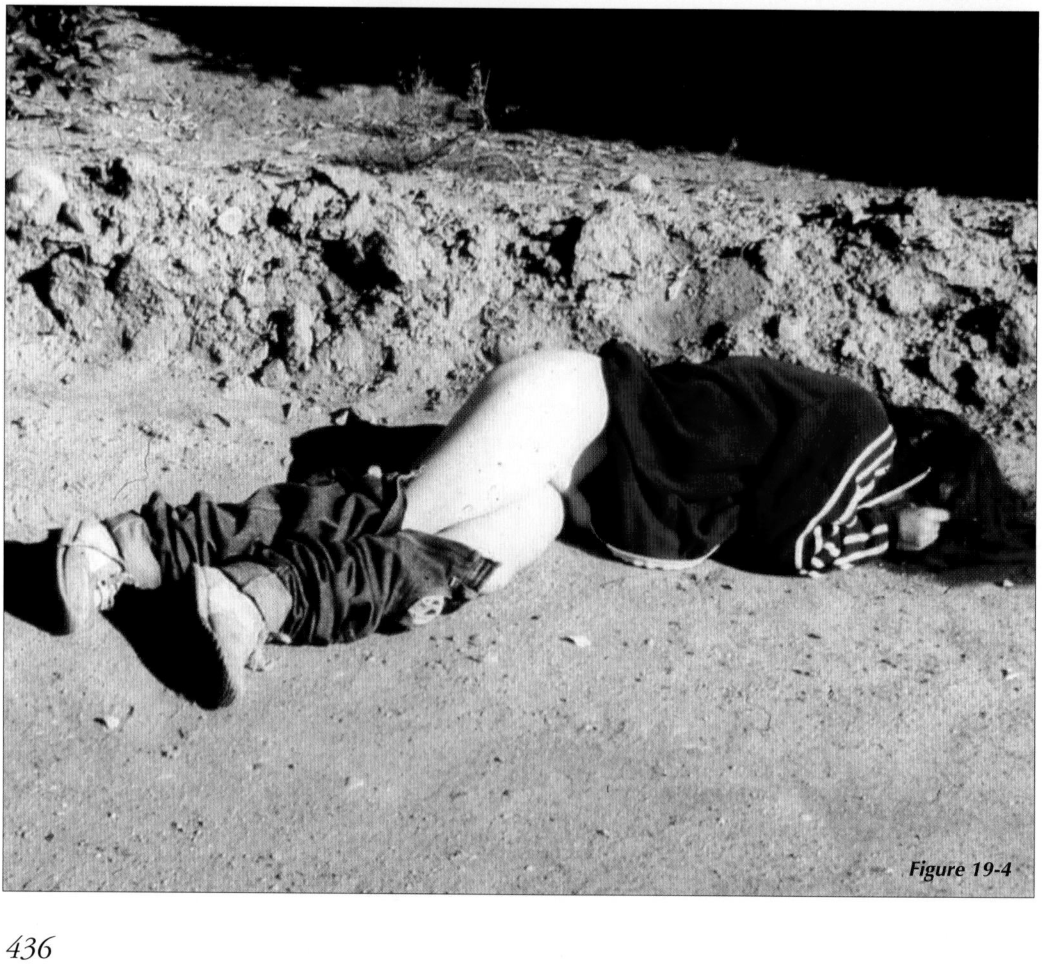

Figure 19-4

Crime Classification

An important measure in sexual homicide cases is the motive for murder. Forensic examiners can contribute important data to investigators searching for a suspect. Some of the crucial data points include the following:

— Time of death

— Postmortem interval

— Range of gunfire

— Type of blunt or sharp force weapon

— Identification of a pattern of injury that may reflect a particular weapon or instrument

— Findings indicating sexual assault

— Extent of force delivered

— Whether injuries were inflicted ante- or postmortem

— Defensive injuries

— Toxicological findings

Questions that forensic nurses might consider include the following: How much would it be expected for the victim to bleed with a wound of this type and in this location? Does the amount of blood on the victim's clothing or in the vicinity of the body provide information that may indicate whether the victim was killed at the location where she was found, or was she killed elsewhere and the body transported to this location? Another question from a case: Was the incised neck wound a postmortem injury, given the findings of petechiae as evidence of asphyxia and the belt mark on the neck, which might denote use of a ligature as a controlling device?

There have been a number of classification systems developed over the years for homicide. This chapter uses a crime classification typology developed by working groups at the Behavioral Science Unit of the FBI Academy.[14] Each of the homicides is classified according to one of the following homicide classifications: criminal enterprise (eg, contract killing, gang-motivated, criminal competition, kidnap murder, product tampering, drug murder, felony murder); personal cause (ie, erotomania-motivated) (eg, domestic, argument/conflict, authority killing, revenge killing, nonspecific killing, extremist homicide, mercy/hero homicide, hostage murder); sexual homicide (eg, organized, disorganized, mixed, sadistic); and group cause (eg, cult, extremist, group excitement). Sexual homicide involves a sexual element (activity) as the basis in the sequence of acts leading to death. Performance and meaning of this sexual element vary with offenders. The act may range from actual rape involving penetration (either pre- or postmortem) to a symbolic sexual assault such as insertion of foreign objects into a victim's body orifices.

Organized Offender

The term *organized*, when used to describe a sexual homicide offender, is based on assessment of the criminal act itself, comprehensive analysis of the victim, crime scene (including any staging present), and evaluation of forensic reports. These components combine to form traits common to organized offenders: those who appear to plan their murders, target their victims, and display control at the crime scene. A methodical and ordered approach is reflected through all phases of the crime.

Defining Characteristics

Victimology

The victim of a sexual homicide perpetrated by an organized offender is often an intraracial female. A single, employed person who is living alone is common to this victimology. Adolescent males are also targeted, as demonstrated by the case of John Wayne Gacy, who targeted young males for sexual assault and murder in Chicago, burying 33 of the bodies in the crawl space under his house.

The concept of victim risk is an important factor in assessing the victimology. Risk is a twofold factor. First, victim risk is determined by age, lifestyle, occupation, associates, and physical stature. Low-risk types include those whose daily lifestyle and occupation do not enhance their chances of being targeted as a victim. High-risk victims are ones who are targeted by a killer who knows where to find them and where engaging with these victims provides a relatively low risk for the offender of being identified or apprehended, for example, prostitutes or hitchhikers. Low-resistance capabilities as found in the elderly and young elevate the level of victim risk. Risk can also be elevated by locations where the victim becomes more vulnerable, such as isolated areas. A victim's attitude toward safety is also a factor that can raise or lower his or her risk factor. A naive, overly trusting, or careless stance concerning personal safety can increase one's chance of being victimized.

The second factor of victim risk is in the level of risk the offender takes to commit the crime. Generally, victims are at a lower risk level if the crime scene is indoors and at a higher risk level if it is outdoors. The time of day that the crime occurs also contributes to the amount of risk offenders take: Abduction at noon would pose more hazards to the offender than at midnight.

Victims are typically not known to offenders but are often chosen because they meet certain criteria important to the offender. These criteria will especially be seen if multiple victims are involved: They often will share common characteristics such as age, appearance, occupation, hairstyle, or lifestyle. Victims are targeted within a geographical region that is comfortable for the offender. They become victims because they enter his targeted area and possess the characteristics that he his looking for. The victims are targeted not for who they are personally but rather because they have entered the area within which the offender is looking for a victim and become a victim of opportunity. Consequently, investigators may not observe similarities in the victim characteristics.

Commonly Noted Crime Scene Indicators

There are often multiple crime scenes involved with organized killing: the locale of initial contact or assault, the scene of death, the method by which the offender transports the victim, and the body disposal site. If the victim is confronted indoors, the first crime scene where the contact occurs (confrontation) is commonly the first or second floor of a building or a single-family dwelling. The offender may then transport the victim or body from the site of confrontation, necessitating the use of the offender's or victim's vehicle.

Weapon use by the offender is an important investigative consideration. The offender generally brings a weapon with him. If the weapon has value or meaning to the offender, he will usually take it with him when he leaves. When weapons are obtained opportunistically from the scene, it usually signals a lack of planning on the part of the offender. It is always important to evaluate why an offender leaves the weapon at the scene or takes it with him. Another consideration is if the offender has utilized more than one weapon. Use of restraints is often noted by the presence of tape, blindfolds,

kits collected by physicians to include the proper sealing and labeling of specimen envelopes, the correct number of swabs and other evidence (pubic hairs and head hairs), the correct kind of blood tubes, a vaginal motility slide, and a completed crime lab form. The Sievers et al study provides the strongest evidence to date that SANEs collect forensic evidence correctly and, in fact, do so better than physicians. However, it is important to note that training and experience, not job title or professional degree, are the likely reasons behind these findings. Further underscoring the link between experience and evidence quality, DiNitto et al reported that prosecutors in Florida were "satisfied with evidence collected by nurse examiners, crediting the training of the nurse examiners.[8] Prosecutors tended to be more pleased with the quality of a physician's evidence "when the examiner had conducted many exams and thus had perfected the techniques."[8] Because SANEs have made it a professional priority to obtain extensive forensic training and practice, it is not surprising that both case study and empirical data suggest they are better forensic examiners than physicians and nurses who have not completed such training.

Legal Effectiveness

Law enforcement personnel and prosecutors are provided with detailed forensic evidence from SANEs documenting crimes of sexual assault. Police officers, detectives, prosecutors, nurses/SANEs, and victim advocates are brought together by SARTs to coordinate the community response to rape, which raises the question: Do SANE-SART programs have an impact on prosecution rates in their communities? As with the literature on the quality of forensic exams, case studies suggest that SANE programs increase prosecution.[4,5,9,12,13] For example, there are reports that SANE programs specifically increase the rate of plea bargains because when confronted with the detailed forensic evidence collected by the SANEs, assailants will decide to plead guilty (often to a lesser charge) rather than face trial.[5,12-14] Other reports indicate that when cases do go to trial, the expert witness testimony provided by SANEs is instrumental in obtaining convictions.[2,15] Canaff notes that the "value of SANE expert witness testimony often lies in its ability to explain the absence of injury rather than its presence" because sexual assault often does not cause bodily injury.[16]

Yet, there have been few studies that have rigorously tested the hypothesis that SANE, SART, and SANE-SART programs increase prosecution, and so far findings across studies have been mixed. With respect to research on SANE programs specifically, Crandall and Helitzer compared prosecution rates in a New Mexico jurisdiction before and after the implementation of a SANE program.[17] Their results indicated that significantly more victims treated in the SANE program reported to the police than before the SANE program was launched in this community (72% versus 50%) and significantly more survivors had evidence collection kits taken (88% versus 30%). Police filed more charges of sexual assault post-SANE as compared to pre-SANE (7.0 charges per perpetrator versus 5.4). The conviction rate for charged SANE cases was also significantly higher (69% versus 57%), resulting in longer average sentences (5.1 versus 1.2 years). However, this New Mexico community may be somewhat atypical in its pre-SANE responses to sexual assault survivors. The pre-SANE conviction rates were substantially higher than published reports, and post-SANE numbers were higher still, which raises the question whether such effects are possible in communities with lower starting conviction rates.

Studies of SART-only approaches have yielded mixed findings. In a study of a Rhode Island SART, Wilson and Klein found that SART cases were no more likely to be prosecuted than non-SART cases.[18] By contrast, in Campbell and Ahrens' national-scale study, victims in communities with SARTs were more likely to have their cases prosecuted than victims in communities without coordinated response teams.[19] However, the Campbell and Ahrens study did not specifically assess the involvement of SANEs in the different community SART models, and, therefore, these data may reflect SANE-SART interventions in many instances. Nugent-Borakove et al directly compared prosecution rates across 3 jurisdictions—one with only a SANE, one with a SANE-SART, and one having no SANE or SART.[20] The SANE-SART cases were more likely to have forensic evidence and were most likely to result in arrest and charges being filed.

Psychological Effectiveness

Although the forensic and legal aspects of SANEs have been a primary research focus in literature to date, a fundamental role of forensic nurses includes providing patients with physical and emotional care.[21-23] As Lynch noted, "As a professional nurse, the SANE's role encompasses all aspects of the bio-psycho-social needs of all patients, including the survivor of sexual assault."[24] Providing comprehensive medical care and responding to patients' psychological distress is essential for their long-term emotional well-being. Early intervention is particularly important with sexual assault survivors because most do not seek follow-up care.[25,26] As a result, if sexual assault survivors' medical and psychological needs are not addressed immediately postassault, they are at risk for longer-term health problems.

Although emotional care is a primary goal of SANE-SART programs, there have been few studies that have systematically evaluated the psychological impact of SANE programs. In a study of the Memphis SANE program, Solola et al found that 50% of victims in their study were able to return to their usual vocation within one month, and, in 3 to 6 months, 85% felt secure alone in public areas.[27] After 12 months, more than 90% of the survivors were entirely free of their initial assault-related anxieties and emotional discomposure.[27] Unfortunately, this publication did not provide sufficient details regarding the methodology of this study to assess whether the recovery gains were attributable to the SANE program or to "normal" recovery processes. Other research suggests that, at the very least, rape survivors perceive SANEs as helpful and supportive. In an evaluation of the Minneapolis SANE program, Malloy surveyed 70 patients in crisis, and found that 85% of the survivors identified the nurses' listening to them as one thing that helped them the most during their crisis period.[28] Similarly, Campbell et al's evaluation with 52 sexual assault patients in a Midwestern SANE program found that survivors felt very supported, respected, believed, and well-cared for by their SANE nurses.[29] In a qualitative study with 8 survivors treated in a Canadian "specialized sexual assault service," Ericksen et al also substantiated that specialized care helps patients feel respected, safe, reassured, in control, informed, and well cared for in their postassault crisis period.[30]

Medical/Health Care Effectiveness

Many rape survivors treated in hospital EDs do not receive needed medical services, which was another problem that SANE programs sought to address. As with the literature on psychological outcomes, there are few published reports documenting rates of medical service delivery in SANE programs, but available data suggest victims treated in SANE programs receive consistent and broad-based medical care. In a national survey of SANE program staff, Ciancone et al found that 97% of programs reported that they offer pregnancy testing, 97% provide emergency contraception, and 90% give sexually transmitted disease (STD) prophylaxis.[31] The SANE program staff indicated that services such as conducting STD cultures, human immunodeficiency virus (HIV) testing, toxicology, and ethanol screening are not routinely performed, but are selectively offered to survivors. A larger-scale study by Campbell et al substantiated rates similar to those of Ciancone et al, but also found that SANE programs affiliated with Catholic hospitals were significantly less likely to conduct pregnancy testing or offer emergency contraception.[32] In addition, Patterson, Campbell, and Townsend examined the interrelationships between patient care practices and organizational goals and mission.[33] Also, SANE programs that were highly focused on improving legal prosecution outcomes were less likely to provide patient education medical services such as information on sexually transmitted infection (STI) risk, safe sex practices with consensual partners, pregnancy risk, emergency contraception, and postexam assistance. However, in spite of these gaps in service delivery, medical provision is still far more comprehensive than what has been found in studies of traditional ED care.[25,34,35]

In the most comprehensive and methodologically rigorous study to date on medical service delivery in SANE programs, Crandall and Helitzer compared the services received for sexual assault cases seen at the University of New Mexico's Health Sciences Center for the 2 years prior to the inception of a SANE program (1994-1996) (N=242) and 4 years afterwards (1996-1999) (N=715).[17] Statistically significant changes in medical services delivery rates were found from pre-SANE to post-SANE. For example, the rate of pre-SANE pregnancy testing in this hospital was 79% and increased to 88% post-SANE. Providing emergency contraception was also more common after the SANE program was created (66% to 87%). Also more routinely provided in the SANE program was STD prophylaxis, as compared to the traditional hospital ED care (89% to 97%). Given the quasi-experimental design of this study, these increases are likely attributable to the implementation of the SANE program, but it is worth noting that the pre-SANE rates of service provision found at this hospital were already substantially higher than what has been found in prior studies of medical service delivery. For instance, service delivery rates for emergency contraception in hospital EDs are typically 20% to 38%, and at the University of New Mexico's Health Sciences Center they were 66% before the SANE program even started. Even though this hospital may have already been providing reasonably comprehensive care to rape survivors, their rates of service delivery still significantly increased post-SANE. However, it is not clear whether a SANE program could make such headway in hospitals with lower starting rates of service delivery.

Community Change Effectiveness

The effectiveness of SANE-SART programs in multiple domains—psychological, medical, forensic, and legal—suggest that something profoundly different happens when survivors are treated in these alternative programs. The successes of SANE-SART programs may be attributable not only to the work of the individual nurses, but also to the kind of community-level change that comes about in forming and sustaining a SANE-SART.[36] As discussed previously, rape survivors need help from multiple service providers and SANE-SART programs provide a structure for comprehensive, integrated care. Some programs may deliberately identify community change as a founding goal and purpose, but others may find that such change happens along the way as part of the process of implementing a SANE-SART. Indeed, case reports from local SANE programs suggest that these programs increase interagency collaboration and cooperation, which improves care for survivors.[37-39] For example, interagency collaboration may include developing policies and procedures or funding development to sustain the SANE program.[4]

In the only empirical study of the effectiveness of SANE programs in creating community change, Crandall and Helitzer interviewed 28 key informants from health care, victim services, law enforcement, and prosecution who had been involved in the care of sexual assault survivors both before and after a SANE program was implemented in their community.[17] The informants stated that before the SANE program, community services were disjointed and fractionalized, but, afterwards, care for survivors was centralized because there was a point of convergence where multiple service providers could come together to help victims. Informants also noted that the SANE program increased the efficiency of law enforcement officers by reducing the amount of time they spent waiting at the medical facility. As a result, officers could spend more time investigating the case. Moreover, the informants believed that police officers were better able to establish positive rapport with survivors, which increased the quality of victim witness statements.

In addition to improving the services provided to survivors, the informants indicated that since the SANE program was implemented, working relationships and communication between medical and legal professionals had improved substantially. For instance, prior to SANEs, law enforcement had difficulty communicating with health care providers because their working relationship lacked consistency. The SANE program created standardized response protocols and hosted regular interagency meetings to review cases and engage in ongoing quality improvement (see http://www.ncdsv.org/publications_sanesart.html for example community protocols). One important benefit of this direct communication was that officers were able to identify trends in similar assaults and perpetrator types more quickly and accurately, which was instrumental in discovering a pattern rapist in their community.

Evaluating the Effectiveness of Sexual Assault Nurse Examiners and Sexual Assault Response Teams

Evaluating the effectiveness of SANE-SARTs is challenging because, as already presented, there are many ways to define their effectiveness. In addition, the work of SANE-SARTs is complex and multidisciplinary, requiring that the evaluation team be knowledgeable in diverse substantive areas. As a result, we argue that a participatory evaluation model[40-42] may be a particularly useful approach for examining the effectiveness of SANE-SARTs. This approach stands in stark contrast to traditional program evaluation paradigms whereby evaluators function as independent "outsiders," planning and conducting projects on their own with minimal input and involvement from program staff.[43-45] Within the past 10 years, there has been growing use of more collaborative approaches in evaluation scholarship.[46] For example, in participatory evaluation methods, the evaluation is organized as a team project with researchers-evaluations and program stakeholders.[40-42] Program staff are directly involved in planning and conducting the evaluation.[47] Two key advantages of participatory evaluation make this an appropriate evaluation paradigm for working with SANE-SARTs. First, this approach values and capitalizes on the experience and expertise of program staff,[41] which is particularly important in SANE evaluations given the complexities of their work. Second, Patton noted that participatory evaluation tends to increase utilization.[48] The more stakeholders participate, the more likely they are to use the evaluation's findings to improve programs. Given the strengths of the participatory evaluation model, the latter half of the chapter outlines a 6-step participatory model for evaluating the work of SANE-SART programs (**Table 20-1**).

Table 20-1. Six-Step Process for Planning and Conducting Program Evaluations

Evaluation Step	Description of Step
Step 1: Define outcomes and narrow scope	— The scope of an evaluation must be narrowed because it is impossible to evaluate all program activities within a single project. In SANE programs, clarify whether evaluation will address forensic, legal, psychological, or medical/health outcomes. Whereas it is possible to evaluate multiple outcomes in one project, it is better to focus on only one outcome and then expand over time to include multiple outcomes.
Step 2: Define evaluation goals and objectives	— An evaluation **goal** states the desired effect program services will have on clients/patients. — An evaluation **objective** states in specific terms the intended effect on clients/patients. — Each **outcome** can have multiple goals, and each goal will have multiple objectives.
Step 3: Design program evaluation	— The design of an evaluation comes from the intersection of 4 main elements. These elements can be framed as 4 planning questions and the answers to these questions determine design: 1. Who to collect data from? Directly from patients? Records? 2. How many times to collect data? Once? More than once? 3. Data as numbers or words? Quantitative (rating scales)? Qualitative (in own words)? Both? 4. How to collect data? Survey? Interview? Observational record?
Step 4: Conduct evaluation and collect data	— The evaluation design (Step 3) provides a template for how and when to collect data. Evaluation data collection should not interfere with program services. Data can be collected by program staff, but preferably the person who provided service should not be the one to collect the evaluation data (possible response bias).
Step 5: Analyze data and present findings	— Quantitative data can be analyzed with SPSS or Excel. Data should be checked prior to analysis for data entry errors or coding mistakes. Qualitative data can be grouped into themes; software such as Ethnograph, NVivo, or AtlasTi can be used, or grouping can be done "by hand" with 2 coders working independently.
Step 6: Use findings for improvement	— Share findings with program stakeholders and develop action plan for using results to improve program functioning. Share findings with scientific and practice community.

Steps 1 and 2: Identification of Evaluation Outcomes, Goals, and Objectives

Consistent with the participatory evaluation framework, the first tasks are to jointly identify the primary *outcomes*, *goals*, and *objectives* for the evaluation (see **Table 20-1** for definitions). As discussed previously, there are 5 main ways to define the effectiveness of SANE-SARTs, and it would be very difficult to examine multiple outcomes within a single evaluation, so it may be necessary to focus on a single outcome type (eg, psychological effectiveness). However, it is important that the decision of which outcome will be evaluated be made jointly by all members of the evaluation team. Once the outcome has been identified, the overall goals and specific objectives of the program with respect to that outcome must be specified. It can be useful to codevelop a logic model to articulate the process by which the SANE-SART program works to achieve these goals and objectives for the focal outcome. Logic models can be constructed at multiple levels of analysis from entire programmatic functioning across multiple outcomes (eg, psychological, medical/health, forensic, legal, etc) to narrower foci on specific outcomes (eg, only psychological outcomes).[49-51]

Step 3: Development of Evaluation Design and Evaluation Questionnaire

The evaluation design should reflect the chosen outcome, goals, and objectives. One of the first decisions to make about the evaluation design is whether data need to be collected directly from sexual assault survivors/patients. The rest of this chapter focuses on evaluations that involve direct patient feedback (see Greeson, Campbell, and Patterson, in preparation for information on other evaluation design options). For some outcomes, it is not necessary to ask survivors directly about their experiences. For example, if the evaluation focus were legal outcomes, the evaluation design would center on collecting police and prosecution records, preferably before and after the implementation of the SANE-SART. Similarly, an evaluation focused on forensic outcomes would entail analysis of the collected kits after patient care had been completed.[10,11] However, for psychological and medical outcomes (and possibly community change outcomes, if survivors are defined as a key stakeholder group), it may be necessary to survey survivors directly. Return rates are often very low for mail surveys (often < 10%), so it may be necessary to explore whether evaluation data could be collected with patients at the time of their exam or very soon thereafter.[52,53] Campbell et al found that SANE-program advocates were an excellent partner in the evaluation process for collecting data directly from patients.[29] In addition, they found that response rates were highest when advocates completed the evaluation assessment on-site at the SANE program (compared to phone follow-up) after exam procedures were complete. Whatever approach used, it is critically important that the evaluation not interfere with patient care. If data are to be collected directly from patients, it is helpful if the evaluation questionnaire was codeveloped by the evaluators and SANE-SART program personnel so that it accurately reflects the goals and objectives of their program. There are 4 sections to develop when designing a questionnaire: (a) introduction, (b) instructions for those completing the questionnaire, (c) questions, and (d) conclusion. The introduction section provides patients with background information about the evaluation including the purpose of the survey (eg, "we would like your feedback on…"). In addition, the introduction section should include an explanation of patient rights as evaluation participants (eg, providing them with a choice to fill out the survey, explaining how their privacy will be maintained). The instructions section should provide clear direction on how to fill out the questionnaire (eg, please circle your response). Questions can be closed (ie, rating-type numerical scales), open (ie, patients write their answers in their own words), or a combination of both. In developing questions, keep the questions simple and unambiguous, avoiding jargon or words that have multiple meanings. Questions should reflect the literacy level of your patient population and be culturally sensitive. Questions should be arranged in a logical order, putting sensitive questions towards the end. This allows patients to become comfortable with the questionnaire prior to answering sensitive questions. Existing questionnaires may also be used and adapted to reflect your program and community. Finally, the questionnaire should be concluded with a show of gratitude to the patient for completing the questionnaire. Once a draft is completed, solicit feedback from SANE-SART program personnel and other colleagues to assess for any of the problems outlined in this paragraph. Once the draft is revised, the questionnaire should be piloted with a small group of patients to uncover any potential problems (eg, unclear questions).

Step 4: Collecting the Data

There are 2 primary decisions with collecting data: a) what level of privacy will be offered to patients, and who will collect the data from patients. There are 2 levels of privacy: anonymous and confidential. Collecting data anonymously means patients cannot be identified. Thus, dates of exams, patient medical records, and patient initials cannot be recorded on the questionnaire. Data collection is considered confidential when patients can be identified because the questionnaire is linked to a medical record or other type of identifier. However, these patients' identities are still protected by not divulging names in evaluation reports (eg, data is synthesized) and limiting staff access to evaluation data (eg, locking completed forms in a filing cabinet).

The second issue of data collection is who should collect evaluation data from patients. Evaluation data can be collected by program staff, volunteers, or evaluators. It is important that anyone involved in data collection completes a comprehensive training program that includes instruction on the following topics: overview of program evaluation, an explanation of the survey development process, an introduction to the survey, discussion of the data collection protocol, informed consent procedures, and survey administration. This material can be covered through large and small group discussions as well as role plays to practice administering the evaluation. Training helps assure that everyone involved in the evaluation follows the procedures systematically (eg, asking questions in the same manner).

Steps 5 and 6: Data Analysis and Using Findings for Program Improvement

Quantitative data analysis can be done with readily available programs such as Excel (see Campbell et al[19] for a detailed evaluation manual for sexual assault service program). Qualitative data can be analyzed using software (eg, NVIVO 7) or by hand. The goal of qualitative analysis is to identify themes in the narrative data. After data are analyzed, it is important that the findings are shared with key stakeholders in the community, as well as the broader community of SANE-SART practitioners and researchers. It can be useful to begin by developing a written report for the SANE-SART program that describes steps 1 through 5. The report should be user-friendly with most information summarized in bullet points and reference tables. There are several ways that the evaluation findings can be utilized. First, the findings can be used for program improvement and implementing an action plan. Second, findings can be shared with program funders and community partners to strengthen support for the program. Finally, evaluation findings can contribute to the field through dissemination at professional conferences (eg, International Association of Forensic Nurses) and publications (eg, *Journal of Forensic Nursing*). See **Table 20-2** for additional resources.

Table 20-2. Additional Resources

Title	Description	Access
National Training Standards for Sexual Assault Medical Forensic Examiners	This is a companion to the *National Protocol for Sexual Assault Medical Forensic Examinations* and includes recommendations for training objectives and topics that will enable an examiner to carry out the recommendations.	US Department of Justice, Office on Violence Against Women. *National Training Standards for Sexual Assault Medical Forensic Examiners.* Rockville, MD: US Dept of Justice, Office on Violence Against Women; 2006.
Evaluation and Management of the Sexually Assaulted or Sexually Abused Patient	This document is a consensus-based set of recommendations for the evaluation and management of the sexually assaulted or abused patient.	American College of Emergency Physicians. *Evaluation and Management of the Sexually Assaulted or Sexually Abused Patient.* www.acep.org/workarea/download asset.aspx?id=8984. Published in June 2009. Accessed March 1, 2011.
The Effectiveness of Sexual Assault Nurse Examiner (SANE) Programs	This document is a brief summation of the currently existing SANE programs here in the United States. The article also discusses current research on the effectiveness of these programs.	Campbell R. *The Effectiveness of Sexual Assault Nurse Examiner (SANE) Programs.* National Online Resource Center on Violence Against Women. http://new.vawnet.org/category/Main_Doc.php?docid=417. Published in November 2004. Accessed March 1, 2011.
Sexual Assault Nurse Examiner (SANE) Development & Operations Guide	The purpose of the guide is to provide those who are starting SANE programs with the knowledge and ability of those who have started programs before them.	Ledray L. *Sexual Assault Nurse Examiner (SANE) Development & Operations Guide.* Washington, DC: Office for Victims of Crime, US Dept of Justice; 1999.
Color Atlas of Sexual Assault	This atlas provides a visual aid in the examination of sexual assault patients.	Girardin B, Faugno D, Seneski P, Slaughter L, Whelan M. *Color Atlas of Sexual Assault.* St. Louis, MO: Mosby; 1997.

(continued)

Table 20-2. *(continued)*

TITLE	DESCRIPTION	ACCESS
Sexual Assault: Victimization Across the Lifespan. A Clinical Guide and a Color Atlas	This 2-volume set is one of the first to bring together the best information available concerning sexual victimization across the entire life span. The atlas provides a wide range of findings and variations that illustrate the observations and histories in sexual assault examinations.	Giardino A, Datner E, Asher J, Girardin B, Faugno D, Spencer M. *Sexual Assault: Victimization Across the Lifespan. A Clinical Guide and a Color Atlas.* St. Louis, MO: G.W. Medical Publishing, Inc; 2003.
Achieving Cultural Competence: A Guidebook for Providers of Services to Older Americans and Their Families	This guidebook is intended for use by providers of services to racially and ethnically diverse older populations. Understanding culture helps service providers avoid stereotypes and biases that can undermine their efforts.	US Department of Health and Human Services, Administration on Aging. *Achieving Cultural Competence: A Guidebook for Providers of Services to Older Americans and Their Families.* http://www.homesteadschools.com/LCSW/courses/Cultural Competence/Chapter08.html Published in January 2001. Accessed March 1, 2011.
Updated US public health service guidelines for the management of occupational exposures to HIV and recommendations for post-exposure prophylaxis	This report updates US Public Health Service recommendations for the management of health care personnel who have occupational exposure to blood and other body fluids that might contain HIV.	Centers for Disease Control and Prevention. Updated US public health service guidelines for the management of occupational exposures to HIV and recommendations for postexposure prophylaxis. *MMWR.* 2005;54(RR09); 1-17.
Sexually transmitted diseases treatment guidelines	These guidelines present updated recommendations for the evaluation and management of sexually transmitted infections resulting from sexual assault or sexual abuse in adults, adolescents, and children.	Centers for Disease Control and Prevention. Sexually transmitted diseases treatment guidelines. *MMWR.* 2006;55 (RR-11):1-94.

(continued)

Table 20-2. Additional Resources *(continued)*

TITLE	DESCRIPTION	ACCESS
Forensic Evidence Collection and the Care of the Sexual Assault Survivor: The SANE-SART Response	This article discusses the components of the SART model and describes its efficacy. It also describes SANE program operation.	Ledray L. *Forensic Evidence Collection and the Care of the Sexual Assault Survivor: The SANE-SART Response.* Violence Against Women Online. http://new.vawnet.org/category/documents.php?docid=817. Published in August 2001. Accessed March 1, 2011.
The Prosecution of Rohypnol and GHB Related Sexual Assaults	This manual and video program provides information to be able to successfully investigate and prosecute drug-facilitated sexual assaults.	American Prosecutors Research Institute. *The Prosecution of Rohypnol and GHB Related Sexual Assaults.* Alexandria, VA: American Prosecutors Research Institute; 1999.
The Provision of Culturally Competent Health Care	This article discusses the significant role health beliefs have in patient treatment outcomes. It also has specific cultural information related to popular folk health care beliefs from South Carolina.	Blue A. *The Provision of Culturally Competent Health Care.* MUSC College of Medicine. http://www.musc.edu/fm_ruralclerkship/culture.html. Accessed March 1, 2011.
Sexual Assault Quick Reference	This pocket-size reference manual provides easy-to-access information on topics related to sexual assault.	Giardino A, Datner E, Asher J, Girardin B, Faugno D, Spencer M. *Sexual Assault Quick Reference.* St. Louis, MO: G.W. Medical Publishing; 2003.
Drug-Facilitated Sexual Assault	This book looks at the history of these crimes over the years and includes an in-depth discussion of the drugs and drug classes in use today. The authors show how to properly collect and analyze evidence and overcome some of the unique difficulties encountered in these types of investigations.	LeBeau M, Mozayani A. *Drug-Facilitated Sexual Assault.* San Diego, CA: Academic Press; 2001.

(continued)

Table 20-2. *(continued)*

TITLE	DESCRIPTION	ACCESS
Abuses Endured by a Woman During Her Life Cycle	This resource describes the violence that may happen throughout the lives of Asian and Pacific Islander women during the life stages of infancy, childhood, adolescence, young adulthood, adulthood, and later life.	Asian & Pacific Islander Institute on Domestic Violence. *Abuses Endured by a Woman During Her Life Cycle.* VAWnet. http://new.vawnet.org/category/Documents.php?docid=765&category_id=586. Published in 2000. Accessed March 1, 2011.
Working with Victims of Crime with Disabilities	This bulletin is a product of the Symposium on Working with Crime Victims with Disabilities, funded by the Office for Victims of Crime and coordinated by the National Organization for Victim Assistance, on January 23-24, 1998, in Arlington, Virginia.	Tyiska CG. *Working with Victims of Crime with Disabilities.* National Organization for Victim Assistance. Available from: http://www.mincava.umn.edu/documents/ovcdisable/ovcdisable.pdf. Published in 2002. Accessed March 1, 2011.

CONCLUSION

The current literature on SANE-SART programs consists primarily of case study reports, with few empirical studies that have tested the effectiveness of SANE-SARTs in multiple domains. Yet, from the information that is available, it appears that SANE-SARTs promote the psychological recovery of rape survivors, provide comprehensive medical care, obtain forensic evidence correctly and accurately, and facilitate the prosecution of rape cases. Through this work, SANE-SARTs can be instrumental in creating interagency collaborative relationships that improve the overall community response to rape. However, such conclusions are tentative because most published studies have not included adequate methodological controls or comparisons to rigorously test the effectiveness of SANE programs. Nevertheless, these preliminary findings can be helpful to SANE-SART practitioners and policy makers because they indicate that this approach to treating sexual assault survivors has merit and should continue for further evaluation and analysis.

To support the continued evaluation of SANE-SARTs, the 6-step process for participatory evaluation was outlined comprehensively. Other programs may find this framework helpful for working with evaluators in a participatory, collaborative way. However, it is important to note that participatory program evaluation requires staff time and commitment, so SANE-SART personnel need to be willing to invest in their evaluators and help them understand their work, and, at the same time, evaluators need to be respectful of practitioners' time. SANE-SART programs should work with their evaluators to determine a level of involvement and engagement that is mutually informative. It may not be necessary for all 6 steps to be carried out jointly, but, overall, this model can help build the evaluation capacity of SANE-SART programs by guiding the process of planning and conducting an internal evaluation.

References

1. Department of Justice. *A National Protocol for Sexual Assault Medical Forensic Examinations: Adults/Adolescents*. Washington, DC: Author; 2004.
2. Ledray L. *Sexual Assault Nurse Examiner (SANE) Development & Operations Guide*. Washington, DC: Office for Victims of Crime, US Dept of Justice; 1999.
3. Barkhurst P, Fowler H, Siadal I, Vokes S. *Attorney General's Sexual Assault Task Force: Sexual Assault Response Team (SART) Handbook* (Version I). http://www.oregonsatf.org/documents/PDFVersionofSARTHandbook.pdf. Published in November 2002. Accessed January 21, 2006.
4. Hutson LA. Development of sexual assault nurse examiner programs. *Emerg Nurs*. 2003;37:79-88.
5. Littel K. Sexual assault nurse examiner programs: improving the community response to sexual assault victims. *Office Victims Crime Bull*. 2001;4:1-19.
6. Young W, Bracken A, Goddard M, Matheson S. Sexual assault: review of a national model protocol for forensic and medical evaluation. *Obstet Gynecol*. 1992;80:878-883.
7. Campbell R, Patterson D, Lichty LF. The effectiveness of sexual assault nurse examiner (SANE) program: a review of psychological, medical, legal, and community outcomes. *Trauma Violence Abuse*. 2005;6:313-329.
8. DiNitto D, Martin PY, Norton DB, Maxwell MS. After rape: who should examine rape survivors? *Am J Nurs*. 1986;86(5):538-540.
9. Cornell D. Helping victims of rape: a program called SANE. *N J Med*. 1998;2:45-46.
10. Ledray L, Simmelink K. Efficacy of SANE evidence collection: a Minnesota study. *J Emerg Nurs*. 1997;23:75-77.
11. Sievers V, Murphy S, Miller J. Sexual assault evidence collection more accurate when completed by sexual assault nurse examiners: Colorado's experience. *J Emerg Nurs*. 2003;29:511-514.
12. Seneski P. Multi-disciplinary program helps sexual assault victims. *The American College of Physician Executives*. 1992;417-418.
13. Aiken MM, Speck PM. Sexual assault and multiple trauma: a sexual assault nurse examiner (SANE) challenge. *J Emerg Nurs*. 1995;2:466-468.
14. Ledray L. The sexual assault nurse clinician: a fifteen-year experience in Minneapolis. *J Emerg Nurs*. 1992;18:217-222.
15. O'Brien C. Sexual assault nurse examiner program coordinator. *Emerg Nurses Assoc*. 1996;22:532-533.
16. Canaff RA. Pediatric sexual assault nurse examination: challenges and opportunities for MDTs in child sexual abuse cases. *NCPCA Update Newsletter*. 2004;16(9):1-3.
17. Crandall C, Helitzer D. *Impact Evaluation of a Sexual Assault Nurse Examiner (SANE) Program*. Washington, DC: National Institute of Justice; 2003.

18. Wilson D, Klein A. *An Evaluation of the Rhode Island Sexual Assault Response Team (SART)*. Washington, DC: National Institute of Justice; 2005.

19. Campbell R, Ahrens CE. Innovative community services for rape victims: an application of multiple case study methodology. *Am J Community Psychol.* 1998;26:537-571.

20. Nugent-Borakove ME, Fanfilk P, Troutman D, Johnson N, Burgess A, O'Connor AL. *Testing the Efficacy of SANE/SART Programs: So They Make a Difference in Sexual Assault Arrest and Prosecution Outcomes?* Washington, DC: National Institute of Justice; 2006.

21. American Nurses Association. *Scope and Standards of Forensic Nursing Practice.* Waldorf, MD: American Nurses Publishing; 1997.

22. Emergency Nurses Association. *Care of Sexual Assault and Rape Victims in the Emergency Department.* http://www.ena.org/SiteCollectionDocuments/Position%20Statements/Sexual_Assault_and_Rape_Victims_-_ENA_PS.pdf. Updated January 2007. Accessed October 26, 2009.

23. Ledray LE, Faugno D, Speck P. SANE: Advocate, forensic technician, nurse? *J Emerg Nurs.* 2001;27:91-93.

24. Lynch VA. *Forensic Nursing.* St. Louis, MO: Elsevier Mosby; 2006.

25. Campbell R, Wasco SM, Ahrens CE, Sefl T, Barnes HE. Preventing the "second rape": rape survivors' experiences with community service providers. *J Interpersonal Violence.* 2001;16:1239-1259.

26. Resnick HS, Holmes MM, Kilpatrick DG, Clum G, Acierno R, Best CL. Predictors of post-rape medical care in a national sample of women. *Am J Prev Med.* 2000;19:214-219.

27. Solola A, Scott C, Severs H, Howell J. Rape: management in a non-institutional setting. *Obstet Gynecol.* 1983;61:373-378.

28. Malloy M. *Relationship of Nurse Identified Therapeutic Techniques to Client Satisfaction Reports in a Crisis Program* [unpublished thesis]. Minneapolis, MN: University of Minnesota; 1991.

29. Campbell R, Patterson D, Adams AE, Diegel R, Coats S. A participatory evaluation project to measure SANE nursing practice and adult sexual assault patients' psychological well-being. *J Forensic Nurs.* 2008;4(1):19-28.

30. Ericksen J, Dudley C, McIntosh G, Ritch L, Shumay S, Simpson M. Clients' experiences with a specialized sexual assault service. *J Emerg Nurs.* 2002;28:86-90.

31. Ciancone A, Wilson C, Collette R, Gerson LW. Sexual assault nurse examiner programs in the United States. *Ann Emerg Med.* 2000;35:353-357.

32. Campbell R. Rape survivors' experiences with the legal and medical systems: do rape victim advocates make a difference? *Violence Against Women.* 2006;12:1-16.

33. Patterson D, Campbell R, Townsend SM. Sexual assault nurse examiner programs' goals and patient care practices. *J Nurs Scholarship.* 2006;38:180-186.

34. Amey AL, Bishai D. Measuring the quality of medical care for women who experience sexual assault with data from the National Hospital Ambulatory Medical Care Survey. *Ann Emerg Med.* 2002;39:631-638.

35. Rovi S, Shimoni N. Prophylaxis provided to sexual assault victims seen at US emergency departments. *J Am Med Women's Assoc.* 2002;57:204-207.

36. Ahrens CE, Campbell R, Wasco SM, Aponte G, Grubstein L, Davidson WS. Sexual assault nurse examiner (SANE) programs: an alternative approach to medical service delivery for rape victims. *J Interpersonal Violence.* 2000;15:921-943.

37. Hatmaker D, Pinholster L, Saye J. A community-based approach to sexual assault. *Public Health Nurs.* 2002;19:124-127.

38. Selig C. Sexual assault nurse examiner and sexual assault response team (SANE/SART) program. *Nurs Clin North Am.* 2000;35:311-319.

39. Smith K, Homseth J, Macgregor M, Letourneau M. Sexual assault response team: overcoming obstacles to program development. *J Emerg Nurs.* 1998;24:365-367.

40. Cousins JB, Earl LM, eds. *Participatory Evaluation in Education: Studies in Evaluation Use and Organizational Learning.* London: Falmer; 1995.

41. Cousins JB, Earl LM. The case for participatory evaluation. *Educ Eval Policy Analysis.* 1992;14:397-418.

42. Cousins JB, Whitmore E. Framing participatory evaluation. *New Dir Eval.* 1998;80:5-23.

43. Rossi PH, Lipsey MW, Freeman HE. *Evaluation: A Systematic Approach.* 7th ed. Thousand Oaks, CA: Sage; 2003.

44. Scriven M. Hard-won lessons in program evaluation. *New Dir Program Eval.* 1993;58:5-92.

45. Scriven M. Truth and objectivity in evaluation. In: Chelimsky E, Shadish WR, eds. *Evaluation for the 21st Century.* Thousand Oaks, CA: Sage; 1997:477-500.

46. Mark MM. Evaluation's future: furor, futile or fertile? *Am J Eval.* 2001;22:457-479.

47. Torres RT, Preskill H. Evaluation and organizational learning: past, present, and future. *Am J Eval.* 2001;22:387-395.

48. Patton MQ. *Utilization-focus Evaluation.* 3rd ed. Thousand Oaks, CA: Sage; 1997.

49. McLaughlin JA, Jordan GB. Using logic models. In: Wholey JS, Hatry HP, Newcomer KE, eds. *Handbook of Practical Program Evaluation.* 2nd ed. San Francisco, CA: Jossey Bass; 2004:7-32.

50. United Way of America Task Force on Impact. *Measuring Program Outcomes: A Practical Approach.* Alexandria, VA: United Way of America; 1996.

51. WK Kellogg Foundation. *Logic Model Development Guide.* Battle Creek, MI: Author; 2004.

52. Dillman DA. *Mail and Telephone Surveys: The Total Design Method.* New York, NY: Wiley; 1978.

53. Dillman DA. *Mail and Internet Surveys: The Tailored Design Method.* 2nd ed. New York, NY: Wiley; 2000.

INDEX

C

E

I

J

K

L

M

N

O

P

Q

R

S

T